The Hippocampal and Parietal Foundations of Spatial Cognition

The Hippocampal and Parietal Foundations of Spatial Cognition

Edited by

N. BURGESS, K. J. JEFFERY and J. O'KEEFE
Department of Anatomy, University College London

Originating from a Discussion
Meeting of the Royal Society of London

DAMAGED

Oxford · New York · Tokyo
OXFORD UNIVERSITY PRESS
1999

Oxford University Press, Great Clarendon Street, Oxford OX2 6DP
Oxford New York
Athens Auckland Bangkok Bogota Buenos Aires Calcutta
Cape Town Chennai Dar es Salaam Delhi Florence Hong Kong Istanbul
Karachi Kuala Lumpur Madrid Melbourne Mexico City Mumbai
Nairobi Paris São Paolo Singapore Taipei Tokyo Toronto Warsaw
and associated companies in
Berlin Ibadan

Oxford is a trade mark of Oxford University Press

Published in the United States
by Oxford University Press, Inc., New York

A catalogue record for this book is available from the British Library

Library of Congress Cataloging in Publication Data
(Data available)

ISBN 0 19 852453 6 (Hbk)
ISBN 0 19 852452 8 (Pbk)

Typeset by Newgen Imaging Systems (P) Ltd, Chennai, India.

Printed and bound in Great Britain by
Biddles Ltd, Guildford and King's Lynn

Preface

Our abilities to find our way through complex environments and to perceive, act upon and remember the objects located around us far outstrip those of man-made devices. Striking recent progress has been made towards an understanding of the neural basis of spatial cognition, centred on two areas of the brain: the hippocampal formation and the parietal cortex. In March 1997 an international selection of the leading groups in these areas presented their work at a Royal Society discussion meeting in London. This book has grown out of the proceedings of the meeting, and includes recent research into how these two areas work, either alone or in cooperation with each other, to support spatial cognition. The research presented is interdisciplinary, ranging across the effects of brain damage in humans, functional imaging of the human brain, electrophysiological recording of single neurones, and computer simulation of the action of the networks of neurons in these brain areas.

The first chapter of the book provides an overall introduction to the field and to the substance of each of the remaining chapters. In this introductory chapter we present a framework in which to consider the diverse spatial and mnemonic functions of the hippocampal formation and parietal cortex. The main body of the book is organized into three sections: the first concentrates on the parietal cortex, the second on the hippocampal formation and the last addresses various aspects of the relationship between the two brain areas. This book should provide a useful starting point and reference for researchers and students of neuroscience, psychology or cognitive science who have an interest in spatial cognition.

N. B.
K. J.
J. O'K.

London
1998

Contents

Contributors   ix

Introduction

1. Integrating hippocampal and parietal functions: a spatial
   point of view   3
   Neil Burgess, Kathryn J. Jeffery, John O'Keefe

Parietal cortex

2. Spatial frames of reference and somatosensory processing:
   a neuropsychological perspective   33
   Giuseppe Vallar
3. Spatial orientation and the representation of space with
   parietal lobe lesions   50
   Hans-Otto Karnath
4. Egocentric and object-based visual neglect   67
   Jon Driver
5. Multimodal integration for the representation of space
   in the posterior parietal cortex   90
   Richard A. Andersen
6. Parietal cortex constructs action-oriented spatial representations   104
   Carol L. Colby
7. A new view of hemineglect based on the response properties
   of parietal neurones   127
   Alexandre Pouget and Terrence J. Sejnowski

The hippocampal formation

8. Robotic and neuronal simulation of the hippocampus and
   rat navigation   149
   *Neil Burgess, James G. Donnett, Kathryn J. Jeffery and
   John O'Keefe*
9. Dissociation of exteroceptive and idiothetic orientation cues:
   effect on hippocampal place cells and place navigation   167
   *Jan Bures, Andre A. Fenton, Yulii Kaminsky, Jerome Rossier,
   Benedetto Sacchetti and Larissa Zinyuk*
10. Variable place-cell coupling to a continuously viewed stimulus:
    evidence that the hippocampus acts as a perceptual system   186
    Alexander Rotenberg and Robert U. Muller

11. Separating hippocampal maps 203
    A. David Redish and David S. Touretzky
12. Hippocampal synaptic plasticity: role in spatial learning or
    the automatic recording of attended experience? 220
    Richard G. M. Morris and Uwe Frey
13. Right medial temporal-lobe contribution to object-location
    memory 247
    Brenda Milner, Ingrid Johnsrude and Joelle Crane
14. The hippocampus and spatial memory in humans 259
    Robin G. Morris, Julia A. Nunn, Sharon Abrahams,
    Janet D. Feigenbaum and Michael Recce
15. Hierarchical organisation of cognitive memory 290
    Mortimer Mishkin, Wendy A. Suzuki, David G. Gadian
    and Faraneh Vargha-Khadem

Interactions between parietal and hippocampal systems in space and memory

16. Memory reprocessing in corticocortical and hippocampocortical
    neuronal ensembles 305
    Yu-Lin Qin, Bruce L. McNaughton, William E. Skaggs and
    Carol A. Barnes
17. The representation of space in the primate hippocampus, and
    its role in memory 320
    Edmund T. Rolls
18. Amnesia and neglect: beyond the Delay–Brion system and
    the Hebb synapse 345
    David Gaffan and Julia Hornak
19. Representation of allocentric space in the monkey frontal lobe 359
    Carl R. Olson, Sonya N. Gettner and Leon Tremblay
20. Hippocampal and parietal contribution to topokinetic and
    topographic memory 381
    Alain Berthoz
21. Hippocampal and parietal involvement in human topographical
    memory: evidence from functional neuroimaging 404
    Eleanor A. Maguire
22. Parietal cortex and hippocampus: from visual affordances to
    the world graph 416
    Michael A. Arbib
23. Visuospatial processing in a pure case of visual-form agnosia 443
    A. David Milner, H. Chris Dijkerman and David P. Carey

Author index 467

Subject index 481

Contributors

Sharon Abrahams Department of Clinical Psychology, Institute of Psychiatry, London, UK

Richard A. Andersen Division of Biology, California Institute of Technology, Pasadena, USA

Michael Arbib USC Brain Project, University of Southern California, Los Angeles, CA 90089-2520, USA

Carol A. Barnes ARL Division of Neural Systems, Memory and Aging, University of Arizona, Tucson, AZ 85724, USA

Alain Berthoz Laboratory of the Physiology of Perception, College of France, CNRS, 121 rue St Jacques, 75231 Paris, France

Jan Bures Institute of Physiology, Academy of Sciences, Videnska 1083, 142 20 Prague 4, Czech Republic

Neil Burgess Dept. of Anatomy and Developmental Biology and Inst. of Cognitive Neuroscience, University College London, London, WC1E 6BT, UK

David P. Carey Department of Psychology, University of Aberdeen, King's College, Aberdeen AB24 2UB, UK

Carol L. Colby Center for the Neural Basis of Cognition and Department of Neuroscience, University of Pittsburgh, Pittsburgh, PA 15260, USA

Joelle Crane Montreal Neurological Institute and the Department of Neurology and Neurosurgery, McGill University, Montreal, Quebec, Canada

H. Chris Dijkerman School of Psychology, University of St Andrews, St Andrews, Fife KY16 9JU, UK

James G. Donnet Department of Anatomy, Institute of Neuroscience, University College London, London, WC1E 6BT, UK

Jon Driver Institute of Cognitive Neuroscience, University College London, London, WC1E 6BT, UK

Janet D. Feigenbaum Department of Clinical Psychology, Institute of Psychiatry, London, UK

Andre A. Fenton Institute of Physiology, Academy of Sciences, Videnska 1083, 142 20 Prague 4, Czech Republic

Uwe Frey Federal Institute of Neurobiology, Brenneckestr. 6, PO Box 1860, D 39006, Magdeburg, Germany

David G. Gadian   Radiology and Physics Unit, Institute of Child Health, University College London Medical School, 30 Guildford Street, London, UK

David Gaffan   Department of Experimental Psychology, University of Oxford, Oxford OX1 3UD, UK

Sonya N. Gettner   Center for the Neural Basis of Cognition, Carnegie Mellon University, 4400 Fifth Avenue, Pittsburgh, PA 15213-2683, USA

Julia Hornak   Department of Experimental Psychology, University of Oxford, Oxford OX1 3UD, UK

Kathryn J. Jeffery   Dept. of Anatomy and Developmental Biology, and Inst. of Cognitive Neuroscience, University College London, London, WC1E 6BT, UK

Ingrid Johnsrude   Montreal Neurological Institute and the Department of Neurology and Neurosurgery, McGill University, Montreal, Quebec, Canada

Yulii Kaminsky   Institute of Physiology, Academy of Sciences, Videnska 1083, 142 20 Prague 4, Czech Republic

Hans-Otto Karnath   Department of Neurology, University of Tübingen, Hoppe-Seyler-Str. 3, D-72076 Tübingen, Germany

Eleanor A. Maguire   Wellcome Department of Cognitive Neurology, Institute of Neurology, Queen Square, London WC1N 3BG, UK

Bruce L. McNaughton   ARL Division of Neural Systems, Memory and Aging, University of Arizona, Tucson, AZ 85724, USA

A. David Milner   School of Psychology, University of St Andrews, St Andrews, Fife KY16 9JU, UK

Brenda Milner   Montreal Neurological Institute and the Department of Neurology and Neurosurgery, McGill University, Montreal, Quebec, Canada

Mortimer Mishkin   Laboratory of Neuropsychology, National Institute of Mental Health, Bethesda, MD 20892, USA

Robin G. Morris   Neuropsychology Unit, Department of Psychology, Institute of Psychiatry, London SE5 8AF, UK

Richard G. M. Morris   Centre for Neuroscience and Department of Pharmacology, University of Edinburgh, Crichton Street, Edinburgh EH8 9LE, UK

Robert U. Muller   Department of Physiology, State University of New York Health Science Center, 450 Clarkson Avenue, Brooklyn, New York 11203, USA

Julia A. Nunn   Department of Psychology, The City University, London, UK

John O'Keefe   Dept. of Anatomy and Developmental Biology and Inst. of Cognitive Neuroscience, University College London, London, WC1E 6BT, UK

Carl R. Olson   Center for the Neural Basis of Cognition, Carnegie Mellon University, 4400 Fifth Avenue, Pittsburgh, PA 15213-2683, USA

Alexandre Pouget   Institute for Cognitive and Computational Science, Georgetown University, Washington, DC 20007-2197, USA

Yu-Lin Qin   ARL Division of Neural Systems, Memory and Aging, University of Arizona, Tucson, AZ 85724, USA

Michael Recce   Department of Computer and Information Science, New Jersey Institute of Technol, Newark, New Jersey, USA

A. David Redish   Computer Science Department, Center for the Neural Basis of Cognition, Carnegie Mellon University, Pittsburgh, PA 15213-3891, USA; and ARL Division of Neural Systems, Memory and Aging, University of Arizona, Tucson, AZ 85724, USA

Edmund T. Rolls   Department of Experimental Psychology, University of Oxford, Oxford OX1 3UD, UK

J. Rossier   Institute of Physiology, University of Lausanne, Rue du Bugnon 7, CH 1005, Switzerland

Alexander Rotenberg   Dept. of Physiology, State University of New York Health Science Center, 450 Clarkson Avenue, Brooklyn, New York 11203, USA

Benedetto Sacchetti   Department of Physiological Sciences, University of Florence, Viale Morgagni 63, 50134 Florence, Italy

William E. Skaggs   ARL Division of Neural Systems, Memory and Aging, University of Arizona, Tucson, AZ 85724, USA

Terrence J. Sejnowski   Howard Hughes Medical Institute, The Salk Institute for Biological Studies, La Jolla, CA 92037, USA

Wendy Suzuki   Laboratory of Neuropsychology, National Institute of Mental Health, Bethesda, MD 20892, USA

David S. Touretzky   Computer Science Dept. and Center for the Neural Basis of Cognition, Carnegie Mellon University, Pittsburgh, PA 15213-3891, USA

Leon Tremblay   Center for the Neural Basis of Cognition, Carnegie Mellon University, 4400 Fifth Avenue, Pittsburgh, PA 15213-2683, USA

Giuseppe Vallar   Department of Psychology, University of Rome, Via dei Marsi 78, 00185, Rome, Italy, and IRCCS S. Lucia, Rome, Italy

Faraneh Vargha-Khadem   Cognitive Neuroscience Unit, Institute of Child Health, University College London Medical School, 30 Guildford Street, London, UK

Larissa Zinyuk   Institute of Physiology, Academy of Sciences, Videnska 1083, 142 20 Prague 4, Czech Republic

Introduction

1

Integrating hippocampal and parietal functions: a spatial point of view

Neil Burgess, Kathryn J. Jeffery and John O'Keefe

1.1 Introduction

As an animal moves through its environment and interacts with it, many of the most important problems it faces involve the processing of spatial information. The animal needs to be able to perceive the locations and orientations of the objects around it relative to itself, to configure and move its receptors and effectors to sense and act upon these objects, and to move bodily through space so as to position itself in favourable locations or to avoid dangerous ones. The difficulty of solving these problems has been regularly demonstrated by the failure of artificial systems to perform such tasks efficiently. By contrast, animals routinely overcome these problems in their everyday life. This book examines some of the neural substrates and mechanisms supporting these remarkable abilities in humans and other mammals.

Several areas of the brain have been implicated in spatial perception, cognition and action, including prefrontal cortex (in particular, the *sulcus principalis*), parietal cortex and the hippocampus. In this book we concentrate upon the respective roles of the latter two areas in spatial cognition. The function of the prefrontal cortex is not our main focus here (but see Chapter 19, and also Roberts *et al.* 1996 for a more general discussion), nor is the question of what contributions the parietal and hippocampal regions might make in non-spatial tasks, although several chapters consider the more general issue of memory beyond that for spatial information. The parietal cortex has long been identified as the neural substrate of an important component of spatial behaviour in humans and lower primates. Compelling evidence ranging from the effects of brain damage in humans to the firing of single neurons in monkeys has implicated various regions within the parietal lobes in both perception and action within 'egocentric' spatial frameworks determined by the position of the eye, head, hand or body. A spatial role for the hippocampus has been also postulated, most particularly following study of the firing of single neurons and the effects of brain damage in rats and, more recently, with regard to results in humans. These findings have implicated the hippocampus in navigation through large-scale space and the representation of spatial relationships within an 'allocentric' framework that is independent of the position of the subject.

Research into the spatial functions of each of these two brain regions has been the subject of rapidly growing interest, and has recently been aided by advances in the non-invasive imaging of human brain function, and the increasing sophistication of artificial models of large networks of neurons. However, research within each field has tended to progress independently of the other, despite the likelihood that both regions contribute to the performance of everyday spatial tasks. For example, returning to a remembered location might be expected to involve the use of allocentric representations of the current and target locations, as well as egocentric representation of the body turns necessary to move in the correct direction and to avoid any obstacles perceived to be in the way. The collection of papers presented here reviews the current state of research into the neural basis of spatial cognition, the respective roles played by the parietal cortex and hippocampal formation, and whether and how they might interact.

In the first two sections of the book we consider the evidence that each area is involved in spatial cognition, and examine the neural mechanisms underlying the generation of the implicated spatial behaviours. In the third section we consider the relative roles of the parietal and hippocampal areas and how each interacts with the other. Here we touch upon some of the broader issues common to both regions. These include problems relating to memory and imagery, such as how an appropriate representation of spatial information might be maintained or produced in the absence of the relevant stimuli, how such representations might be adjusted to take account of actual or intended movement, and how these representations might be used in aiding the storage and recall of other types of information. Indeed, we note that, in humans and primates, the hippocampus has traditionally been thought to play a more general role in memory, beyond the specific contribution to spatial memory so regularly observed in rats.

In the rest of this introductory chapter we set out and briefly discuss the topics covered by the other chapters in this book. As an introduction, we consider the anatomical organization of the hippocampal formation and parietal cortex.

1.2 Anatomy of the parietal cortex and the hippocampal formation

To provide the proper orientation for our discussion of the functional organization of these regions it is useful first to consider their anatomical organization within the brain. In this section we outline the anatomical organization of the various subregions of the parietal cortex and hippocampal formation, and their connections with each other.

Both parietal cortex and the hippocampus are the recipients of highly processed sensory information, much of it visual (particularly in primates). Parietal cortex, in addition, receives inputs from motor and premotor cortex. Ungerleider and Mishkin (1982) have suggested that the visuo-temporal and visuo-parietal pathways carry different information, the former pathway (the ventral or temporal stream) being specialized for the recognition of objects and the latter (the dorsal or parietal stream) being specialized for processing their location. On the basis of more recent neuropsychological data, this hypothesis has been modified to conceive of the dorsal stream as a system for processing visual information for the purpose of guiding and controlling actions such as reaching and grasping (see Fig. 1.3; Goodale 1993; Ch. 23). Furthermore, it appears there are at least three components of the dorsal parietal primary visual cortex stream from (V1): one passing via V2, one via V3 and V3A, and one via V5 (Goodale 1993). In addition to its inputs from primary visual cortex, the dorsal stream also receives visual inputs from the superior colliculus, via the pulvinar (Rodman et al. 1990). There also appears to be a third stream, passing into the superior temporal sulcus (Boussaoud et al. 1990).

Below, we consider the anatomy of the temporal and parietal lobes, before discussing the ways in which they may interact.

Parietal cortex

The parietal cortex in primates is situated caudal to the postcentral gyrus and superior to the Sylvian fissure, and is composed of an anterior part, the postcentral gyrus and the caudal bank of the central sulcus, and a posterior part, which is divided into an upper (superior) and lower (inferior) lobule by the intraparietal sulcus. The anterior parietal cortex includes Brodmann's areas 1, 2, 3 and 43 (the parietal operculum) and contains the primary somatosensory areas. Posterior parietal cortex receives inputs from both sensory and motor cortices (Fig. 1.1), and may be thought of as a higher order polymodal sensorimotor association area. One focus of the present collection of papers is on this region, which appears to subserve complex aspects of spatial behaviour and perception.

Posterior parietal cortex is composed of multiple subdivisions (Fig. 1.1) which differ on cytoarchitectonic and connectivity grounds. It includes Brodmann's areas 5 and 7, area 39 (the angular gyrus) and area 40 (the supramarginal gyrus). Areas 5 and 7 seem to be involved with visuo-motor control. Lesions in humans that produce a corresponding pattern of deficits (optic ataxia) usually involve the intraparietal sulcus and adjacent superior parietal lobule, whereas right inferior parietal lesions are associated with hemineglect (see, for example, Critchley 1953; Kolb and Whishaw 1996; Milner 1996; and below). Posterior parietal cortex is usually further subdivided into the following areas: anterior, lateral, medial and ventral intraparietal areas (AIP, LIP, MIP and VIP, respectively) and 7a and 7b (Fig. 1.2).

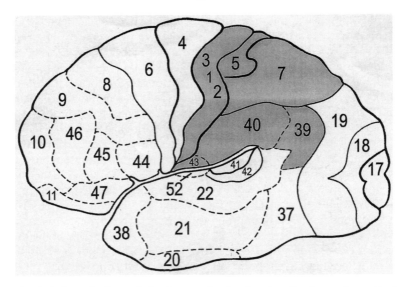

Fig. 1.1 Left lateral view of the human brain showing Brodmann's cortical areas (adapted from Kolb and Whishaw 1990). The parietal areas are shaded.

In the monkey, the intrinsic posterior parietal connections proceed rostro-caudally in two pathways from regions in the postcentral gyrus (Pandya and Seltzer 1982). The upper pathway proceeds from the dorsal half of the post-central gyrus to the posterior part of the superior parietal lobule, and the lower pathway proceeds caudally from the ventral half of the postcentral gyrus to the inferior parietal lobule. Both the superior and rostral inferior parietal lobules also send projections to the parietal operculum and the intraparietal sulcus. The entire postcentral gyrus and portions of the superior and inferior parietal lobules also send projections to the parietal operculum. Many of the posterior parietal zones are reciprocally connected.

The extrinsic cortical connections are mainly with frontal and temporal cortex. Area 5 receives inputs from primary somatosensory cortex and its outputs are to primary motor cortex and to the supplementary motor and premotor areas and to area 7b. Area 7b also receives inputs from primary somatosensory cortex (areas 1, 2 and 3) and from motor and premotor cortex, and projects to the supplementary motor and premotor areas. It also, along with the visual intraparietal areas, receives multimodal sensory information, much of it via the dorsal visual stream of Ungerleider and Mishkin. There are also connections between posterior parietal and prefrontal cortex (Selemon and Goldman-Rakic 1988). The connections between parietal and temporal cortex are shown in Fig. 1.3.

The thalamic inputs to posterior parietal cortex are partially segregated (Schmahmann and Pandya 1990), the superior parietal lobule receiving

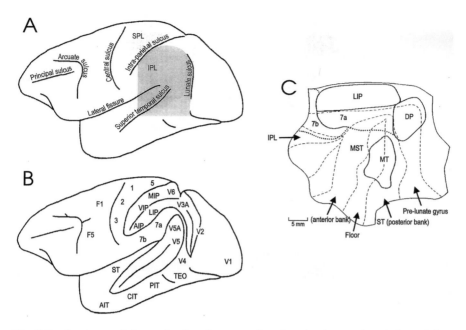

Fig. 1.2 Anatomy of the parietal and temporal regions in the monkey (adapted from Andersen 1995 and Sakata *et al*. 1997). (A) The external surface of the brain, viewed from the left, showing the major sulci: SPL, superior parietal lobule; IPL, inferior parietal lobule. (B) Major cortical regions: F1, primary motor area; F5, hand region of ventral premotor area; 1, 2 and 3, primary somatosensory areas; 5, area 5 of posterior parietal cortex; V1–6, visual areas; AIP, LIP, MIP and VIP, anterior, lateral, medial and ventral intraparietal areas; ST, superior temporal cortex; PIT, CIT, AIT, posterior, central and anterior temporal cortex; 7a and 7b, regions of inferior parietal lobule (Brodmann's area 7). (C) When the shaded region in (A) is unfolded, the parietal areas in the depths and banks of the sulci become visible: MT, middle temporal cortex; MST, medial superior temporal cortex; DP, dorsoparietal cortex.

projections from the more lateral regions of the thalamus (lateral posterior nucleus and pulvinar), while the inferior parietal lobule receives projections from more medial regions. Both lobules also receive inputs from the medio-dorsal, ventroposterior, ventrolateral, intralaminar and limbic nuclei. There is also a projection from the lateral dorsal, lateral posterior and posterior nuclei (Reep *et al*. 1994). Cerebellar information is conveyed via the ventroanterior-ventrolateral thalamic complex (Kakei *et al*. 1997).

Hippocampal formation

In primates, the hippocampus is buried deep within the temporal lobes (Fig. 1.4), while in rats, there is relatively less neocortex and so the hippocampus occupies much of the cerebral hemispheres (Fig. 1.5). It receives two major

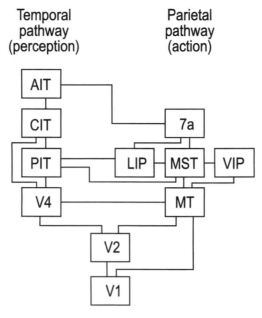

Fig. 1.3 Functional connections of the primary visual and visual intraparietal areas (adapted from Goodale 1993).

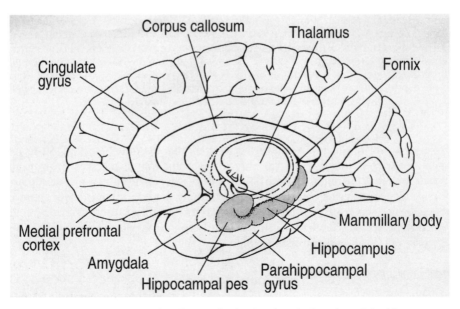

Fig. 1.4 Medial view of the right human brain showing the location of the hippocampus (shaded area) and associated structures.

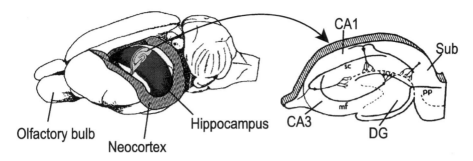

Fig. 1.5 *Left*, the rat brain with the neocortex removed from the left side, showing the underlying hippocampus. *Right*, a cross-section of the hippocampus, showing the major cell layers: DG, dentate gyrus; CA3 and CAl, subfields of the hippocampus proper; Sub, subiculum (Adapted from Amaral and Witter 1989).

sources of information: subcortical inputs, which come from the medial septum via the fornix fiber bundle, and neocortical inputs, which converge on the entorhinal cortex and reach the hippocampus predominantly via the perforant path fibre bundle. These inputs carry highly processed sensory information. Entorhinal cortex in turn receives most of its inputs via the perirhinal and parahippocampal cortices. The main output of the hippocampus is via the subiculum. A diagram of the cortical interconnections with the hippocampus is shown in Fig. 1.6.

In the rat, the left and right hippocampi encircle the thalamus and are joined at the midline anteriorly by the hippocampal commissure but widely separated more posteriorly. The anterior ends lie near the septal nuclei and the ventral (temporal) ends lie near the amygdala and entorhinal cortex. In the primate, the hippocampus has shifted down to lie entirely within the temporal lobe (see Fig. 1.4). The hippocampus consists of two interlocking layers which are composed of morphologically different cell types, and comprises the dentate gyrus (DG), mainly consisting of granule cells, and the hippocampus proper or cornu ammonis (usually abbreviated to CA), which mainly consists of pyramidal cells. The dentate gyrus lies immediately below the hippocampal fissure and curves around so that its two arms encompass the pyramidal cells of the lower arm of the hippocampus proper. The region between the two arms is called the hilus. The subregions of the cornu ammonis are numbered from 1 to 4, starting from its most superficial region and moving around to the dentate hilus. Of these subregions, CA1 and CA3 are the most separable, on histological and physiological grounds. CA4 is usually regarded as a subset of CA3.

The other components of the hippocampal formation are the entorhinal cortex and the subicular complex, which form its major input and target, respectively. The entorhinal cortex is composed of medial and lateral subdivisions. It receives highly processed multimodal sensory information from sensory cortex and projects to the dentate gyrus via a fibre bundle known as

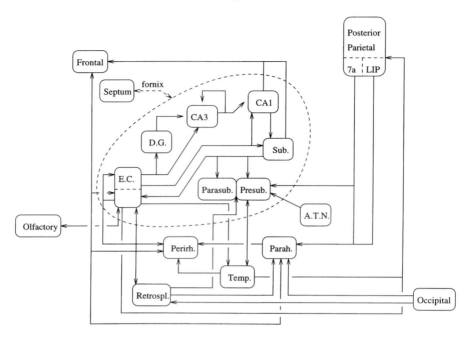

Fig. 1.6 Some of the intrinsic and extrinsic functional connections of the hippocampal formation. The hippocampal formation (inside *dashed line*) includes the hippocampus proper—the dentate gyrus (D.G.) and areas CAl and CA3—as well as the entorhinal cortex (E.C. shown roughly divided into superficial layers I–III above, and deep layers IV–VI below) and the subicular complex (the subiculum, presubiculum and parasubiculum). Connections from the medial septum innervate the hippocampal formation, which in turn projects back to the septum (most notably to the lateral septum), via the fornix. The fornix carries connections to and from other subcortical structures such as the thalamus and mamillary bodies (not shown). The deep layers of the E.C. receive a dense projection from the olfactory system, and the presubiculum receives connections from the anterior thalamic nucleus (A.T.N.). Also shown are extrinsic connections with cortical areas including the perirhinal (Perirh.), parahippocampal (Parah.), temporal (Temp.), retrosplenial (Retrospl.), occipital (i.e. visual), frontal and posterior parietal (shown with area 7a and the lateral intra-parietal area, LIP).

the perforant path. In the rat, input to the lateral entorhinal cortex comes predominantly from the olfactory system. The entorhinal cortex projects to widespread parts of the limbic, paralimbic and olfactory regions of the cortex, and to the septum (mainly the lateral septum) and striatum. The subicular complex receives input from the CAl output of the hippocampus, as well as projecting to and receiving projections from the entorhinal cortex. Its three major subdivisions are the subiculum, presubiculum and parasubiculum. The subiculum projects to parts of the medial prefrontal cortex and provides a prominent projection to the septal complex, the nucleus accumbens, the mammillary nuclei, the amygdala and bed nucleus of the stria terminalis. The only subcortical outputs of the hippocampus proper are a bilateral and unilateral projection to the lateral septum from CA3 and CA1, respectively (Swanson and Cowan 1977; Jarrard 1983).

As well as a large input from the perforant path, the hippocampus receives a sparse but important input from subcortical structures such as the thalamus and hypothalamus, brainstem, septum and amygdala. These inputs presumably carry information about arousal, emotions and autonomic functions.

Connections between parietal cortex and hippocampus

The main area of interaction between parietal cortex and hippocampus occurs in the perirhinal and parahippocampal regions. There is some disagreement about the exact locations of these areas and the correspondence between primates and rodents, but broadly speaking, the term perirhinal cortex is used to mean areas 35 and 36 in the monkey and the rostral parts of these areas in the rat, while parahippocampal cortex is areas TF and TH of the monkey temporal lobe (Burwell *et al.* 1995). No precise parahippocampal equivalent has been delineated in the rat, though Burwell *et al.* have suggested that it may be homologous to the postrhinal cortex, an area consisting of the caudal parts of areas 35 and 36.

The perirhinal and parahippocampal cortices receive polymodal sensory information from the visual, auditory and somatosensory association areas (Suzuki and Amaral 1994) and they also receive extensive projections directly from the posterior parietal region, and indirectly from the hippocampus. The parietal projections proceed indirectly from the caudal third of the inferior parietal lobule via the inferior longitudinal fasciculus to the parahippocampal gyrus, and via a separate pathway to the presubiculum (Seltzer and Pandya 1984). As well as the parietal projections, parahippocampal cortex is reciprocally connected with prefrontal cortex (Goldman-Rakic *et al.* 1984).

These perirhinal and parahippocampal cortices in turn project to entorhinal cortex, and from there to the hippocampus. There are no direct projections from the hippocampus to the parietal cortex, but there is an indirect projection which proceeds via the entorhinal cortex, a highly restricted area of which projects to parietal cortex (Insausti *et al.* 1997).

1.3 Spatial functions of the parietal cortex

The most compelling evidence for the role of the parietal cortex in spatial perception and cognition has come from the human lesion data and from single unit recording in monkeys. We consider the lesion data first, and use the observation of parietal hemineglect to explore which aspects of behaviour depend upon normal functioning of the parietal lobes. We then consider what the data from single unit recording tells us about the neural mechanisms responsible for generating these behaviours. We give particular attention here to the various spatial reference frames in which information appears to be represented in different subregions of the parietal cortex, the way these representations are modulated by actions or by the intention to act, and the ways in which they are combined or used together.

When discussing the spatial functions of the brain, it is natural to ask which type of spatial framework is being used and what is the origin of that framework. Frameworks can be centred on different receptor surfaces, such as the retina, or they can be aligned with a body part, such as the midline of the head or the trunk, or with an effector, such as the arm or the hand. All of these frameworks since they move with the body as it moves through the environment, are collectively labelled 'egocentric'. In contrast, frameworks that are fixed to the environment itself or to individual objects in the environment are called allocentric. The locations of objects within these allocentric frameworks do not change as the subject moves in the environment.

Lesions: parietal hemineglect

Damage to superior posterior parietal regions in humans commonly causes optic ataxia (impaired visually guided reaching), whereas damage to inferior regions, in particular on the right, is often described as resulting in a neglect of the contralateral (i.e. left) half of space. The occurrence of optic ataxia following parietal damage is useful to bear in mind in terms of interpreting the single-unit recordings in monkeys considered below. However, this section focuses on the hemineglect following unilateral parietal damage in humans. This neglect syndrome can affect all modalities and is, therefore, considered to be a spatial deficit rather than a sensory one. The fact that the neglected region of space varies with the movements of the observer has suggested to many that the spatial framework is an egocentric one with its origin fixed to a receptor or body axis (see above). On this view, the lesion results in the loss of the left side of the framework. Attempts to identify the framework with particular receptor or body parts, such as the head or trunk, have met with mixed success. For example, when head and trunk axes were dissociated by requiring the patient to turn the head to the right (e.g. Bisiach *et al.* 1985; Karnath *et al.* 1993) neglect for stimuli occurred on the left side in both frameworks in an additive fashion.

Kinsbourne (1987, 1993) has challenged this view and stressed that the deficits in the neglect syndrome cannot adequately be described as the loss of the left half of a framework or surface in any absolute sense. He cites evidence that the deficit is usually a relative, rather than an absolute, one affecting the left-most of two stimuli anywhere in the entire visual field. Furthermore, the neglect of the left-most stimuli is often associated with increased attention to the right-most stimuli. This suggests to him that the deficit is due to an imbalance in influence between left and right hemispheres with each hemisphere responsible for a gradient of attention towards the contralateral side.

Another alternative view is that parietal neglect reflects damage not to the framework itself but to the mechanism for locating the origin of the spatial axis relative to the body. If this is the case, it might be described better not as a spatial scotoma or loss of a gradient of spatial attention, but rather as a geometric transform of a perceptual or motoric framework relative to the eye, head or trunk. Both Vallar and Karnath (Chapters 2 and 3) present evidence in support of this view, although they disagree as to the exact nature of the transform. Vallar considers neglect in terms of a translation of frameworks, whereas Karnath considers it in terms of a rotation.

An interesting symptom of right-sided parietal damage is 'object centred neglect', in which the left-half of objects or stimuli are neglected despite being presented to the right of the patient's midline. This has been interpreted as evidence for object-centred representations in parietal cortex. Driver (Chapter 4) interprets these findings differently, drawing a parallel with the symptom of extinction, in which a patient can detect single stimuli presented on either side of the midline, but fails to detect the one contralateral to the lesion when both are presented simultaneously. Driver argues that the patient's 'object-centred' deficits can be accounted for in terms of the same defective processing of information within an egocentric frame of reference that causes extinction. In his view, significant visual preprocessing, in which distinct entities have been segmented out and, for example, assigned a major axis, occurs before the passage of information into the compromized spatial system in the damaged parietal cortex. It is the information further to the left of this representation that is neglected. Further evidence indicates that mental rotations may also be performed upon segmented visual stimuli before processing in parietal cortex (see, for example, Buxbaum et al. 1996). Recent experiments on the frontal cortex of the monkey by Olsen et al. (Chapter 19) indicate how an apparently object-based coding might be represented at the level of single cells.

Amelioration of the parietal neglect syndrome by sensory stimulation

One of the most intriguing findings in the parietal neglect literature is that neglect can be ameliorated by sensory stimulation. Caloric stimulation via cold water in the contralateral ear or warm water in the ipsilateral ear, vibratory stimulation of the neck or optokinetic stimuli can all markedly improve the ability of the patient to detect stimuli and to act in the contralesional field. There are several possible interpretations of the cause of these effects. One interpretation is that the stimulation causes a general non-specific increase in arousal or, in a modified interpretation, an increase in neural activity restricted to the side of the damage. According to this view, proper functioning of a cortical region depends on a minimal level of neural activity and one conse-quence of the lesion is to cause the total activation level to drop below this critical minimal level. The effect of the sensory stimulation is to increase the level of activation of the undamaged cortical tissue lying close to the lesion.

An alternative interpretation is that the spatial framework is not, itself, located in the parietal cortex, nor is it permanently fixed to any receptor surface

or aligned with any body part. Instead, the alignment of the egocentric framework is maintained by the overall balance of all the inputs from many different
exteroceptive and proprioceptive inputs. On this view, the parietal cortex contributes information to other brain areas which use it to maintain the axes of the
egocentric coordinate systems in alignment with the eye, head and trunk. Loss of
this information leads to an imbalance in the overall sensory input controlling
axis location, an imbalance which can be compensated for by increased inputs
from non-damaged somatic, vestibular and other sensory inputs.

A particular effect of caloric stimulation, that cold water in the ipsilateral
ear or warm water in the contralateral ear is not effective in reversing the
syndrome and may make it worse (Rubens 1985; Vallar *et al.* 1997), rules out
an explanation in terms of general arousal or amount of activation *per se*. This
effect could be related to the generation of leftward or rightward eye-movements, or vestibular signals indicating head rotation, according to the side and
temperature of the water, although the subjective experience of normal controls
under caloric stimulation is not of such a simple smooth rotation.

Neural representation in egocentric frames of reference

Since the early studies of Hyvarinen and Poranen (1974) and Mountcastle *et al.*
(1975), it has seemed likely that individual neurons in the posterior parietal
cortex of monkeys contribute to the perception of the location of objects or
stimuli around the animal and to its ability to respond to them in various ways
(e.g. pointing at them, looking at them, or grasping them). An interesting
aspect of observed neuronal firing is that neurons in different parietal areas
tend to represent stimuli in terms of their locations within different frames of
reference, often in terms of the sensory modality from which they came, and
in terms of the nature of the action to be performed.

Neurons throughout the region around the intraparietal sulcus have been
found that respond to the location of stimuli from various modalities (see
Chapters 5 and 6 for further details). However neurons in different areas
appear to represent this information in different reference frames(ranging from
those at one end of the spectrum, which are aligned with the sensory receptors
being stimulated, to those at the other end, which are aligned with a part of
the body that might be used to respond to a stimulus but which played no part
in detecting it) For example, neurons in the medial intraparietal area (MIP)
respond to the locations of visual or somatosensory stimuli (often on the hand)
or both, in arm-centred coordinates, with strong responses during reaching to
a visual stimulus that are specific to its location and to which arm is used;
neurons in the nearby ventral intraparietal area (VIP) show visual and
somatosensory receptive fields in head-centred coordinates (i.e. the retinal
location of visual receptive fields shift so as to maintain a fixed location relative
to the head), with strong responses specific to visual stimuli on trajectories
approaching the mouth and independent of eye position (see Chapter 6) the
anterior intraparietal area (AIP) has been related to visually guided grasping

with the hand (see Sakata *et al*. 1995), containing sensory neurons responding to specific object shapes and orientations, and motor neurons responding during specific hand movements.

As one approaches the lateral intraparietal area (LIP) and area 7a, information appears to be encoded in a way more related to the position of the head and body. It is interesting to note that area 7a connects to the hippocampal formation, with its allocentric representations of location and orientation. We consider the functions of LIP and area 7a at greater length below in the context of their role in translating between frames of reference.

Translating information between different frames of reference

It is natural for sensory information received via a particular receptor initially to be encoded in a frame of reference aligned with respect to that receptor. Similarly, the target location for an intended movement needs to be encoded in a frame of reference suitable for guiding actions. Thus, even in a simple task, such as reaching towards a visual stimulus, accurate sensorimotor integration requires the translation of locations from one frame of reference to another. The finding of optic ataxia following superior parietal lesions indicates a role for the parietal cortices in this type of sensorimotor integration. In this section we consider the evidence available at the level of single cells that the parietal lobes, as well as representing information in various egocentric frames of reference, also enable translation between these frames of reference.

A neural correlate of the interaction between eye-centred and head-centred frameworks has been reported by Andersen and colleagues (1985) in areas LIP and 7a of the posterior parietal cortex. The sensory cells in these areas have visual receptive fields coded in retinal coordinates. However, for many of these cells, the gain of the firing rate is modulated by the orientation of the eyes relative to the head (creating an eye-position 'gain field' multiplying the retinal response). The neural response to stimulation of the same retinal field increased or decreased as the eyes were moved to point at different locations in head-centred space. These responses thus contain information regarding the location of the target in a head-centred reference framework, and could be useful for the translation of retinal locations into head-centred coordinates. In about half of these cells in LIP and area 7a, the response is also modulated by the orientation of the head (Brotchie *et al*. 1995). This information would obviously be useful for the translation of head-centred locations into body-centred coordinates. The paper by Pouget and Sejnowski (Chapter 7) presents a computational model of the parietal cortex which shows how the translations between reference frames might be accomplished using units which have inputs from both retina and head position, taking advantage of a gain-field type of encoding. They then show how their model could be applied to explain the neuropsychological data regarding parietal hemineglect, producing a Kinsbourne-like gradient in the responses to stimuli on the left and right by assuming differential loss of cells coding for locations on the left in eye, head and body reference frames.

Information regarding head orientation probably reaches LIP in signals coding for neck proprioception, whereas area 7a receives vestibular inputs coding for absolute accelerations of the head (see Chapter 5). The presence of these vestibular inputs, and the connections of area 7a with the presubiculum and parahippocampal gyrus, might indicate that this area mediates between head-centred and the allocentric or world-centred representations in the hippocampus. The role of vestibular inputs to both parietal and hippocampal systems in humans is explored further by Berthoz (Chapter 20).

Visual constancy, memory and intention

The problem of visual constancy has intrigued researchers for many years, and is worth considering in the light of the functions of the parietal cortex. This problem refers to the perception of a stable visual world despite being seen through constantly moving eyes in a moving head on a moving body. This might be achieved through a series of translations of the incoming visual information from retinal coordinates to head-centred coordinates to body-centred coordinates and finally to some stable world-centred coordinate frame, using the available proprioceptive, vestibular and optic flow information (see Chapter 5). However, the intention to make a movement appears to effect the firing of neurons in LIP and MIP, independently of any sensory feedback resulting from the actual movement. We note that little of a scene is consciously seen at any one time, so that it may not be necessary to translate the entire retinal image. Indeed the parietal lobe may only represent the behaviourally relevant elements of a scene (see Gottlieb *et al.* 1998).

Colby (Chapter 6) explores the argument of Helmholtz that when a command is sent to move the eyes, a copy of the command (termed 'corollary discharge' or 'efference copy') is used to shift our internal image of the world so as to stay in alignment with the visual information to arrive following the movement. She shows how the response of neurons in LIP to a stimulus that is brought into the appropriate retinal receptive field by a saccadic eye movement is maintained even when the stimulus is extinguished before the eye reaches its final location. Indeed, the intention to perform the action appears to be sufficient to effect a remapping of the sensory image: some of the neurons recorded in this task start to fire in advance of the initiation of the eye movement that will bring the stimulus into its receptive field.

1.4 Hippocampus

Representation of spatial location within an allocentric frame of reference

Evidence for a spatial role for the hippocampal formation comes mainly from single-unit recording in freely-moving rats, and from lesion studies which show an impairment of the performance of hippocampally damaged rats on spatial tasks such as the Morris water maze. Neurons in the rat's hippocampus respond to the animal's location within its environment, such that each neuron responds whenever the rat is in a particular place (these neurons are referred to as place cells; O'Keefe and Dostrovsky 1971; O'Keefe 1976). The place cells and neurons in the neighbouring dorsal presubiculum (and other areas, such as the anterior thalamic nucleus) that respond to the direction in which the rat is facing, independent of its location (referred to as head direction cells; Taube *et al.* 1990) together form an allocentric representation of the animal's location and orientation within its environment (a 'cognitive map'; O'Keefe and Nadel 1978). The properties of place cells are briefly reviewed by Burgess and colleagues (Chapter 8), and a model of how the hippocampus could support a spatial memory for the location of a hidden goal is presented. The robustness of the assumptions behind this model, and its behavioural predictions are examined by using it to direct the navigation of a mobile robot.

When comparing the functions of parietal and hippocampal areas, an important point to consider is that sensory information reaches the brain via the surface of the body and therefore arrives in the various egocentric frames of reference of the receptors. It is relatively easy to imagine how this information might be translated into the various egocentric parietal reference frames, via layers of topographically organized cells in sensory cortex. Hippocampal neurons have to go one stage further, however, and translate these inputs into an allocentric framework so that a given place cell can fire whenever the rat is in a particular location (the cell's place field), independent of its orientation or actions. It seems likely that place cells use some types of environmental information in preference to others (such as the distances to environmental walls in given allocentric directions; see O'Keefe and Burgess 1996), and that virtually any external or internal sources of information might be used to support place cell firing if necessary (e.g. Hill and Best 1981).

The internal and environmentally derived sensory inputs that support place cell firing are further investigated in the chapters by Bures and colleagues (Chapter 9) and Rotenberg and Muller (Chapter 10). Bures's group recorded place cells in a featureless arena that could be rotated with respect to the outside room to investigate the contributions of internal signals (e.g. vestibular or proprioceptive) and external signals (e.g. visual). They found that the rat could use either type of input to maintain place cell firing, but that the spatial firing pattern broke down when the two sources of information were placed in conflict. Rotenberg and Muller pursued the contributions of internal and external influences on place cells further by showing that, while a prominent visual cue at the edge of the environment can control the overall orientation of the place fields if slowly rotated, it fails to control them if rotated by a large amount. Following a large rotation, the cue will again control the place field locations during further small rotations despite now having a different overall orientation with respect to the place fields. In addition to locating the animal in a familiar environment, the map may contain information about such things as the location of rewards and landmarks (see O'Keefe 1976). This is consistent with recent evidence that the location of the animal alone does not account for all of the variance of a place cell's firing rate (Chapter 10). Redish and Touretzky (Chapter 11) present a systems level model of the interaction of frames of reference derived from different internal and external signals applied to the production of spatial maps in the rat hippocampus, and the effects of aging on this process (Barnes *et al.* 1997).

A recent finding by Rolls (Chapter 17) may help to bridge the gap between hippocampal representations in rats and primates. He found that a proportion of cells in primate hippocampus had large receptive fields determined by where the animal is looking, but independent of the animal's location or orientation. Some of these cells could also be shown to continue firing when a curtain was placed in front of the wall or objects in the cell's receptive field. Thus these cells could form an allocentric representation of space different from the object-centred representations in frontal areas (see Chapter 19) and from the rat's representation of its current bodily location. The receptive fields of cells reported to date have been located around the walls of the testing room and it will be interesting to see if neurons with fields located more centrally in the testing room are found. The results could, in principle, indicate an evolutionary progression afforded by binocular vision from the rat's hippocampal representation of its location within a room, to a more general representation of locations accessible by moving the eyes. Rolls relates this finding to the needs of an event memory to represent events occurring in the world surrounding the animal's own location. Representing the location of the event would obviously be an important part of such a system, as discussed below.

Episodic memory

Ever since the finding that patient HM had a dense amnesia following bilateral temporal lobectomy (Scoville and Milner 1957), the human hippocampus has been associated with a role in memory. The finding that the orientation of the pattern of hippocampal place fields within an environment can be controlled by a small number of salient cues also relates to this issue, since this pattern of place cell firing can be maintained after the removal of some or all of these cues. A role in memory also fits with the argument presented in Chapter 23 that allocentric rather than egocentric representations are the natural form for long-term storage, as they are not confounded by the animal's temporary position during encoding or recall.

One suggestion made in the original cognitive map theory (O'Keefe and Nadel 1978) was that, in addition to storing information about locations, the hippocampus might also store the times of visits to those locations. Although this was deemed an unnecessary postulate to explain the physiology of the rat hippocampus, it was felt necessary to account for the full range of episodic (or 'event') memory disorders seen following damage to the human medial temporal lobe. Both Morris and Frey (Chapter 12) and Gaffan and Hornak (Chapter 18) suggest that animals as well as humans may have something akin to episodic memory and that the hippocampus is necessary to store these memories. Morris and Frey found that the NMDA receptor, previously implicated in spatial memory formation, is not necessary for the learning of a new spatial task if the animal has previously learned a related spatial task elsewhere. This has led them to suggest that these receptors might be used to incorporate a temporal tag into the spatial maps even in the rat. Gaffan and Hornak show that lesions which damage the fornix, one of the major hippo-campal fibre bundles, has a major effect on the abilities of monkeys to remember which stimuli occurred against which backgrounds. They favour O'Keefe and Nadel's suggestion that the spatio-temporal context in which an event occurs might act as a powerful retrieval cue even when the material to be recalled is not, itself, primarily spatial.

Semantic and recognition memory

A complementary approach to human neuropsychology has been the develop-ment of a primate model of amnesia, in which the effects of lesions were tested on tasks such as delayed match or non-match to sample. In these tasks a monkey has to judge whether or not an object matches that presented a short time before. Hippocampal damage has been claimed to impair performance on these tasks (e.g. Squire 1992), although the nearby perirhinal cortex now appears to be the critical structure (Gaffan and Murray 1992; Meunier et al. 1993; Suzuki et al. 1993).

   Mishkin and colleagues (Chapter 15) report recent evidence that casts doubts on the validity of visual recognition memory as a good task for assessing hippocampal function in primates. They have found that neurotoxic lesions of the amygdala and hippocampus that spare the nearby perirhinal and parahip-pocampal cortices do not produce a measurable deficit in this task even with delays as long as 40 min. Preliminary evidence also suggests that there is no deficit if the information to be remembered is the location of a small number of objects rather than the visual identity of the objects. They also report studies of the memory capacity of three young patients who had suffered bilateral damage to both hippocampi at an early age. Although severely amnesic for events, they showed little deficit in forced choice recognition of words or faces, even after considerable delays. This is consistent with the results of single-unit recordings showing cells in primate perirhinal cortex, but not hippocampus, that respond to the novelty of visual stimuli (see Brown et al. 1987; Fahy et al. 1993) and with the primate lesion studies showing perirhinal cortex to be the crit-ical location in impairments of recognition memory (see above and Chapter 18).

   Interestingly, the children referred to by Mishkin and colleagues also showed a remarkable semantic vocabulary suggesting that their semantic memory sys-tems were compromised to a much smaller extent than their episodic memory systems. Taken together, these pieces of evidence speak against the declarative memory theory of hippocampal function (Squire 1992), which includes both episodic and semantic memories in the hippocampus. They also appear to be inconsistent with the view that the long-term storage of abstracted semantic information in the neocortex is dependent on the short-term storage of similar information in a fast learning hippocampal system (see Chapter 16; McClelland *et al.* 1995).

Spatial memory in humans

Lesion data in humans has implicated the hippocampal formation in memory for the spatial arrangement of objects (the right hippocampal formation in particular, see Chapter 13), and in topographic memory for the layout of buildings and landmarks in the real world (see Chapter 21; Habib and Sirigu 1987). Following a similar line of research, Robin Morris and colleagues (Chapter 14) review a series of experiments on the spatial abilities of patients who have had left and right temporal lobectomies, including removal of the hippocampus. This group found the right temporal lobe patients to be impaired in a variety of tasks designed to be most naturally solved by an allocentric representations of arrays of objects.

These results also mesh nicely with positron emission tomography (PET) imaging work reported by Brenda Milner and colleagues (Chapter 13). They find that memory tasks which required the subject to remember the location of an item on a panel activated the parahippocampal gyrus but not the hippocampus itself. What does activate the hippocampus? The papers from Berthoz and Maguire (Chapters 20 and 21) provide part of the answer: encoding or retrieval of information about large-scale environments activates the human hippocampus. In an encoding experiment, Maguire scanned subjects while they tried to remember what they saw as they watched film clips taken by a camera moving through a small town. Both groups imaged subjects in recall tasks related to navigation through large-scale environments. Berthoz asked subjects to imagine that they were retracing a path they had previously walked along, while Maguire asked London taxi-drivers to construct a route between several locations in London from their long-term knowledge of its geography. Both groups found activation of hippocampal areas during these tasks.

1.5 What is the relationship between the parietal cortex and the hippocampus?

There are currently two main classes of hypothesis about how parietal and hippocampal spatial representations might interact. First, the two structures might form complementary parts of a memory system acting in series on incoming sensory information to form representations suitable for different time scales or levels of abstraction. Second, they might act in parallel to provide two different kinds of spatial representation of the information, to be used for different purposes. Interestingly, these alternative possibilities are not necessarily mutually exclusive (see, for example, Chapter 23). Each alternative is discussed below, followed by an attempt to reconcile them both within a more general picture.

Mnemonic processing on two time scales

The first hypothesis about the interaction of hippocampus and parietal cortex is that both brain areas store the same type of spatial information but that they have different time constants, resulting in different memory properties. According to this hypothesis, the hippocampus stores all information fed into it but does so over a relatively short time scale, while the neocortex abstracts information from the input over several presentations but stores this abstracted information for a long period of time. The most efficient interaction between the two systems might involve the hippocampal system capturing spatio-temporal events on-line and then slowly feeding them to the parietal cortex over time to allow it to abstract, consolidate and store the information for the long term (see Marr 1971; McClelland *et al*. 1995). In search of support for this hypothesis Qin and colleagues (Chapter 16) have simultaneously recorded large numbers of neurons, in both the hippocampus and parietal cortex, as the rat travels along a path, and found evidence that during subsequent sleep episodes there is a rehearsal of the same sequence of spatial cell activations in each area, but less evidence for an increased interaction between the two areas. Rolls (Chapter 17), while finding spatial view cells in the primate hippocampus, has also argued that the hippocampus functions primarily as a system for memory, rapidly storing associations between stimuli of different modalities and enabling it to act in concert with neocortical retrieval of this information, again in a way similar to that proposed by Marr (1971).

Spatial processing in different frames of reference

The second hypothesis derives from the view advanced by Ungerleider and Mishkin (1982): that visual information is processed along parallel ventral and dorsal streams concerned, respectively, with 'what' objects are present and 'where' they are (see Section 1.2). In this view the parietal cortex, as part of the dorsal stream, codes for the spatial location of objects in an egocentric framework which is appropriate for orienting the eyes or hands or body with respect to the appropriate object or objects. In contrast, and extending Ungerleider and Mishkin's hypothesis, the hippocampal formation and its associated parahippocampal cortex, at the meeting point of both streams, might be concerned with the representation of object locations within an allocentric framework. Such a representation would be appropriate for encoding the relative positions of objects, or for finding the distance or allocentric bearing between locations. Thus parietal and hippocampal areas would cooperate in the solution of spatial tasks such as finding ones way through complex environments and interacting with the objects within it, each area addressing the relevant egocentric and allocentric components of the task. This point of view is supported by the influence of head and body movements, as well as eye-movements, on neural firing in parietal area 7a, and the connections of this region to the hippocampal formation (see Chapter 5). Such a system would not be complete, even in terms of the purely spatial component of many tasks. For example, this system would have to interact with object-centred information, such as that found in the supplementary eye field of the frontal lobe (see Chapter 19).

A cooperation between hippocampal and parietal systems in solving allocentric and egocentric components of spatial tasks is consistent with the activations seen in some recent functional imaging studies in humans. Berthoz (Chapter 20) examines the role of the vestibular inputs to both parietal and hippocampal regions, and demonstrates parietal activation in performing a memorized sequence of saccadic eye movements, and hippocampal activation in recall of movement along a previously walked route through Paris. Maguire (Chapter 21) shows parietal and hippocampal activation in the verbal generation of routes through London by taxi-drivers. In a more recent study, Maguire and collaborators (1998) imaged subjects as they found their way between locations within a virtual reality town, and found that activation of the right hippocampus and right inferior parietal cortex correlated with the accuracy of navigation, with right inferior and bilateral medial parietal areas activated by movement through the town in general.

Neural network models of how monkey parietal cortex provides visual affordances for looking and grasping are described by Arbib (Chapter 22) and form the background for a model of the role of the parieto-hippocampal system in navigation in the rat. This model combines the 'taxon-affordances' model, involving the parietal cortex, and the 'world-graph' model relating to hippocampal function. The taxon-affordance model performs the obstacle avoidance and goal approach components of navigation, while the world-graph model both recognizes and links together places as they are traversed, with the links reflecting not only physical proximity but also expectation of future reward. The combined model successfully simulates the behaviour of rats with and without fornix legions in a T-maze alteration task.

A complementary spatial and mnemonic role for the parieto-hippocampal system

A reconciliation of the hypotheses relating to spatial and mnemonic processing is possible when considering the functional requirements of memory systems. Short-term storage of spatial information for the control of current ongoing actions is most efficiently served by egocentric representations related to the body part to be moved. However, long-term storage of spatial information would not be efficiently served by egocentric representations, because their use would depend upon the body being in the same spatial configuration as it was during encoding. On the other hand, allocentric representations are not optimal for guiding immediate responses as they require translation from the egocentric reference frame in which sensory information arrives, and translation back to an egocentric reference frame suitable for controlling action. However, allocentric representations, whether they are the object-centred representation of frontal cortex or the world-centred representation of the hippocampal formation, are the natural way to store long-term information, as they are independent of the current configuration of the body. As an aside we note that some forms of egocentrically encoded information will be stored over the long term, such as when developing motor skills (e.g. how to swing a tennis racket so as to hit a ball on a particular trajectory relative to the body). However, this type of procedural learning appears to be unrelated to the type of memory dealt with in this volume, and does not depend on the hippocampal formation (see Squire 1992).

David Milner and colleagues (Chapter 23) provide evidence for this position in their investigation of what aspects of spatial cognition are spared in a patient with damage to the ventral pathway. She has an impaired ability to recognize objects, although her ability to reach and grasp accurately is relatively unimpaired when there is little or no delay between presentation of the stimulus and responding to it (in contrast to patients showing optic ataxia following superior parietal damage). However, her reaching and grasping is impaired after a delay of two seconds or more, and she is also impaired in immediate grasping of a specially designed stimulus that requires knowledge of the relative locations of holes within it. They have concluded that the ventral stream and the allocentric representations it contains are responsible for immediate conscious perception of objects and for the long-term storage of allocentric spatial information, whereas the dorsal stream uses egocentric encoding of information for the generation of immediate motor responses.

Gaffan and Hornak (Chapter 18), also argue against a simple partition of brain systems into perceptual and memory systems. They believe that amnesic patients may have some as-yet-undefined perceptual problems with scene analysis, finding that amnesic patients were better at recognizing hemi-scenes presented in the hemi-field ipsilateral to the temporal lobe removed than those which were presented in the contralateral hemi-field (Hornak *et al.* 1997). Conversely, they note that parietal neglect patients have 'memory' problems as well as perceptual problems, ignoring the left side of remembered layouts as well as perceived ones. Using this evidence, they argue that long-term memory for scenes is encoded and stored in egocentric coordinates.

In our view, the evidence for recall of long-term spatial memories by patients with parietal neglect seems more consistent with the use of allocentric than egocentric representations in long-term memory. When asked to recall the layout of a familiar location, such as the famous square in Milan (Bisiach and Luzzatti 1978) or the street on which they lived (Meador *et al.* 1987) from a particular perspective, such patients neglect the buildings and features on the left side. However, when asked to view the same location from the opposite end of the square or following a turn of 180° they can recall many of the previously neglected features. This would seem to indicate the existence of an allocentric representation of the entire layout together with the need to transfer this information into a perspective-laden egocentric representation in order to picture and describe the scene (see Kosslyn 1981), although separate storage of a huge number of egocentric representations is hard to rule out. A natural interpretation of this idea would place long-term storage of allocentric information in the hippocampal system, with parietal areas responsible for generating short-term representations reflecting particular viewpoints. Meador *et al.* (1987) also found that recall performance in a neglect patient was modulated by the physical orientation of the eyes/head during recall (recall improving when oriented towards the left), supporting the idea that the parietal cortex is involved in reading out information from a long-term store for visualization from a particular viewpoint. This interpretation relates closely to the analogy of Baddeley and Leiberman (1980) of the visuo-spatial scratch pad as a screen on which long-term spatial information is represented, with neglect patients having a defect in the screen itself or in the process for scanning the screen or in the mechanism which relates the origin of the screen axes to the eye, head, or body.

Finally we note that the neglect patients do not simply recall features from the right-hand side of the visual scene from a given viewpoint, but also recall features that would not be visible from that viewpoint, indicating retrieval from a global allocentric representation, rather than retrieval of a specific retinal visual scene. Interestingly, recent evidence points to a dissociation between neglect in perception and in imagery, with some patients showing only one or the other form (see Anderson 1993; Guariglia *et al.* 1993; Beschin *et al.* 1997; Coslett 1997). Thus different parietal, and possibly frontal (Guariglia *et al.* 1993), areas may be involved in the spatial processing of perceived stimuli and the recall of internal spatial information.

It is interesting to give brief consideration to the possible phylogenetic development of hippocampal and parietal function in moving from rats to monkeys and humans. O'Keefe and Nadel (1978) (see also O'Keefe 1996) have suggested that the ability to represent allocentric spatial locations shown in the rat hippocampus might be combined with the human's more highly developed sense of time to create a memory for episodes in the right hippocampus. They also suggest that the human left hippocampus might have come to process linguistic inputs to provide a long-term structure for language, consistent with impairments in memory for verbal material after left but not right temporal lobectomy (see Chapter 13). In a related analysis of the parietal lobes David Milner and colleagues (Chapter 23) suggest that the dorsal stream might store the locations of stimuli in egocentric coordinates suitable for control of the actions over the short term (around 2 s). In humans, as with the left temporal lobe, the left parietal lobe appears to have taken on some linguistic functions. Interestingly these functions appear to include a critical role in the provision of verbal short-term memory (for stimuli with a total duration of around 2 s), as shown by the classic short-term memory patients such as JB and PV (see Shallice 1988; Baddeley 1986).

1.6 Conclusion

The papers presented here represent part of the considerable recent progress in several complementary areas of research towards elucidating the neural substrates of spatial cognition. An increasingly detailed understanding is emerging of the neuronal representation of the location of stimuli and actions relative to the eye, head and trunk found in the parietal cortex, and of the representation of location within an environment found in the hippocampus. Data from lesion, neuropsychological and functional imaging studies are also beginning to enable a systems level understanding of the functions of sub-regions within the parietal and hippocampal cortices. The resurgence of computational modelling of brain function provides a framework in which to examine and integrate these new data in terms of the mechanisms underlying behaviour at the neuronal and system levels. One restriction on progress has been that, until recently, behaviour in large-scale space has been less well studied than that in smaller scale (table-top and 2-dimensional) tasks, for obvious reasons of convenience and control. However, this imbalance is beginning to be addressed by various approaches used in conjunction with functional imaging, including the recall or imagination of large-scale spatial behaviour and the use of virtual reality. Taken together these advances leave us in a position to begin to put together a coherent picture of the neural processes underlying the extraordinary capacity for spatial cognition demonstrated in our everyday lives. We hope that this volume will provide a suitable starting point for this enterprise.

Acknowledgments

We thank Jon Driver for several useful comments on this manuscript. N.B. is supported by a Royal Society University Research Fellowship, J.O'K and K.J. by an MRC programme grant.

References

Amaral, D. G. and Witter, M. P. (1989) The three-dimensional organization of the hippocampal formation: a review of the anatomical data. *Neuroscience*, **31**, 571–91.

Andersen, R. A. (1995) Coordinate transformations and motor planning in posterior parietal cortex. In: Gazzaniga, M. S. (ed.), *The Cognitive Neurosciences*. London: The MIT Press.

Andersen, R. A., Essick, G. K. and Siegel, R. M. (1985) The encoding of spatial location by posterior parietal neurons. *Science*, **230**, 456–58.

Anderson, B. (1993) Spared awareness for the left side of internal visual images in patients with left-sided extrapersonal neglect. *Neurology*, **43**, 213–16.

Baddeley, A. D. (1986) *Working Memory*. Oxford: Clarendon Press.

Baddeley, A. D. and Leiberman, K. (1980) Spatial working memory. In: Nickerson, R. S. (ed.), *Attention and Performance VIII.* Hillsdale New Jersey: Lawrence Erlbaum Associates.

Barnes, C. A., Suster, M. S., Shen, J. and McNaughton, B. L. (1997) Multistability of cognitive maps in the hippocampus of old rats. *Nature*, **388**, 272–5.

Beschin, N., Cocchini, G., Della-Sala, S. and Logie, R. H. (1997) What the eyes perceive, the brain ignores: a case of pure unilateral representational neglect. *Cortex*, **33**, 3–26.

Bisiach, E. and Luzzatti, C. (1978) Unilateral neglect of representational space. *Cortex*, **14**, 129–33.

Bisiach, E., Capitani, E. and Porta, E. (1985) Two basic properties of space representation. *J. Neurol. Neurosurg. Psychiatry*, **19**, 543–51.

Boussaoud, D., Ungerleider, L. G. and Desimone, R. (1990) Pathways for motion analysis: cortical connections of the medial superior temporal and fundus of the superior temporal visual areas in the macaque. *J. Comp. Neurol.*, **296**, 462–95.

Brotchie, P. R., Anderson, R. A., Snyder, L. H. and Goodman, S. J. (1995) Head position signals used by parietal neurons to encode locations of visual stimuli. *Nature*, **375**, 232–5.

Brown, M. W., Wilson, F. A. and Riches, I. P. (1987) Neuronal evidence that inferomedial temporal cortex is more important than hippocampus in certain processes underlying recognition memory. *Brain Res.*, **409**, 158–62.

Burwell, R. D, Witter, M. P. and Amaral, D. G. (1995) Perirhinal and postrhinal cortices of the rat: a review of the neuroanatomical literature and comparison with findings from the monkey brain. *Hippocampus*, **5**, 390–408.

Buxbaum, L. J., Coslett, H. B., Montgomery, M. W. and Farah, M. J. (1996) Mental rotation may underlie apparent object-based neglect. *Neuropsychologia*, **34**, 113–26.

Coslett, H. B. (1997) Neglect in vision and visual imagery: a double dissociation. *Brain*, **120**, 1163–71.

Critchley, M. (1953) *The Parietal Lobes.* London: Arnold.

Fahy, F. H., Riches, J. P. and Brown, M. W. (1993) Neuronal activity related to visual recognition memory—long-term memory and the encoding of recency and familiarity information in the primate anterior and medial inferior temporal and rhinal cortex. *Exp. Brain Res.*, **96**, 457–72.

Gaffan, D. and Murray, E. A. (1992) Monkeys (*Macaca fascicularis*) with rhinal cortex ablations succeed in object discrimination learning despite 24-hr inter-trial intervals and fail at matching to sample despite double sample presentations. *Behav. Neurosci.*, **106**, 30–8.

Goldman-Rakic, P. S., Selemon, L. D. and Schwartz, M. L. (1984) Dual pathways connecting the dorsolateral prefrontal cortex with the hippocampal formation and parahippocampal cortex in the rhesus monkey. *Neuroscience*, **12**, 719–43.

Goodale, M. A. (1993) Visual pathways supporting perception and action in the primate cerebral cortex. *Current Opinion in Neurobiology*, **3**, 578–85.

Gottlieb, J. P., Kusunoki, M. and Goldberg, M. E. (1998) The representation of visual salience in monkey parietal cortex. *Nature*, **391**, 481–4.

Guariglia, C., Padovani, A., Pantano, P. and Pizzamiglio, L. (1993) Unilateral neglect restricted to visual imagery. *Nature*, **364**, 235–7.

Habib, M. and Sirigu, A. (1987) Pure topographical disorientation: a definition and anatomical basis. *Cortex*, **23**, 73–85.

Hill, A. J. and Best, P. J. (1981) Effects of deafness and blindness on the spatial correlates of hippocampal unit-activity in the rat. *Exp. Neurology*, **74**, 204–17.

Hornak, J., Oxbury, S., Oxbury, J., Iversen, S. D. and Gaffan, D. (1997) Hemifield-specific visual recognition memory impairments in patients with unilateral temporal lobe removals. *Neuropsychologia*, **35**, 1311–5.

Hyvarinen, J. and Poranen, A. (1974) Function of the parietal area 7a as revealed from cellular discharges in alert monkeys. *Brain*, **97**, 673–92.

Insausti, R., Herrero, M. T. and Witter, M. P. (1997) Entorhinal cortex of the rat: cytoarchitectonic subdivisions and the origin and distribution of cortical efferents. *Hippocampus*, **7**, 146–83.

Jarrard, L. E. (1983) Selective hippocampal lesions and behavior: effects of kainic acid lesions on performance of place and cue tasks. *Behav. Neurosci.*, **97**, 873–89.

Kakei, S., Wannier, T. and Shinoda, Y. (1997) Input from the cerebellum and motor cortical areas to the parietal association cortex. In: Thier, P. and Karnath, H.-O. (ed.), *Parietal Lobe Contributions to Orientation in 3D Space. Experimental Brain Research Series 25*. Heidelberg: Springer.

Karnath, H.-O., Christ, K. and Hartje, W. (1993) Decrease of contralateral neglect by neck muscle vibration and spatial orientation of trunk midline. *Brain*, **116**, 383–96.

Kinsbourne, M. (1987) Mechanisms of unilateral neglect. In: Jeannerod, M. (ed.), *Neurophysiological and Neuropsychological Aspects of Spatial Neglect. Advances in Psychology*, **45**. Amsterdam: Elsevier.

Kinsbourne, M. (1993) Orientation bias model of unilateral neglect: evidence from attentional gradients within hemispace. In: Robertson, I. H. and Marshall, J. C. (ed.), *Unilateral Neglect: Clinical and Experimental Studies. Brain Damage, Behaviour & Cognition series*. UK: Lawrence Erlbaum.

Kolb, B. and Whishaw, I. Q. (ed.) (1996) *Fundamentals of Human Neuropsychology*, 4th edn. New York: Freeman and Co.

Kosslyn, S. M. (1981) The medium and the message in mental imagery: a theory. *Psych. Rev.*, **88**, 46–66.

McClelland, J. L., McNaughton, B. L. and O'Reilly, R. C. (1995) Why are there complementary learning systems in the hippocampus and neocortex—insights from the successes and failures of connectionist models of learning and memory. *Psych. Rev.*, **102**, 419–57.

Maguire, E. A., Burgess, N., Donnett, J. G., Frith, C. D., Frackowiak, R. S. J. and O'Keefe, J. (1998) knowing where and getting there: a human navigation network. *Science*, **280**, 921–4.

Marr, D. (1971) Simple memory: a theory for archicortex. *Phil. Trans. Roy. Soc.*, **B 262**, 23–81.

Meador, K. J., Loring, D. W., Bowers, D. and Heilman, K. M. (1987) Remote memory and neglect syndrome. *Neurology*, **37**, 522–6.

Meunier, M., Bachevalier, J., Mishkin, M. and Murray, E. A. (1993) Effects on visual recognition of combined and separate ablations of the entorhinal and perirhinal cortex in rhesus monkeys. *J. Neurosci.*, **13**, 5418–32.

Milner, A. D. (1996) Neglect, extinction and the cortical streams of visual processing. In: Thier, P. and Karnath, H.-O. (ed.), *Parietal Lobe Contributions to Orientation in 3D Space. Experimental Brain Research Series 25*. Heidelberg: Springer.

Mountcastle, V. B., Lynch, J. C., Georgopoulos, A., Sakata, H. and Acuna, C. (1975) Posterior parietal association cortex of the monkey: command functions for operation within extrapersonal space. *J. Neurophysiol.*, **38**, 871–908.

O'Keefe, J. (1976) Place units in the hippocampus of the freely-moving rat. *Exp. Neurol.*, **51**, 78–109.

O'Keefe, J. (1996) The spatial prepositions in English, vector grammar, and the cognitive map theory. In: Bloom, P., Peterson, M. A., Nadel, L. and Garrett, M. F. (eds.), *Language and Space*. Cambridge MA: The MIT Press.

O'Keefe, J. and Burgess, N. (1996) Geometric determinants of the place fields of hippocampal neurons. *Nature*, **381**, 425–8.

O'Keefe, J. and Dostrovsky, J. (1971) The hippocampus as a spatial map: preliminary evidence from unit activity in the freely moving rat. *Brain Res.*, **34**, 171–5.

O'Keefe, J. and Nadel, L. (1978) *The Hippocampus as a Cognitive Map*. UK: Oxford University Press.

Pandya, D. N. and Seltzer, B. (1982) Intrinsic connections and architectonics of posterior parietal cortex in the rhesus monkey. *J. Comp. Neurol.*, **204**, 196–210.

Reep, R. L., Chandler, H. C., King, V. and Corwin, J. V. (1994) Rat posterior parietal cortex: topography of corticocortical and thalamic connections. *Exp. Brain Res.*, **100**, 67–84.

Roberts, A. C., Robbins, T. W. and Weiskrantz, L. (ed.) (1996) Cognitive and executive functions of the prefrontal cortex. *Phil. Trans. Roy. Soc.*, **B 351**, 1387–527. (Discussion meeting issue.)

Rodman, H. R., Gross, C. G. and Albright, T.D. (1990) Afferent basis of visual response properties in area MT of the macaque. II. Effects of superior colliculus removal. *J. Neurosci.*, **10**, 1154–64.

Rubens, A. B. (1985) Caloric stimulation and unilateral visual neglect. *Neurology*, **35**, 1019–24.

Sakata, H., Taira, M., Murata, A. and Mine, S. (1995) Neural mechanisms of visual guidance of hand action in the parietal cortex of the monkey. *Cereb. Cortex*, **5**, 429–38.

Sakata, H., Taira, M., Kusunoki, M., Murata, A. and Tanaka, Y. (1997) The TINS Lecture. The parietal association cortex in depth perception and visual control of hand action. *Trends Neurosci.*, **20**, 350–7.

Schmahmann, J. D. and Pandya, D. N. (1990) Anatomical investigation of projections from thalamus to posterior parietal cortex in the rhesus monkey. *J. Comp. Neurol.*, **295**, 299–326.

Scoville, W. B. and Milner, B. (1957) Loss of recent memory after bilateral hippocampal lesions. *J. Neurol. Neurosurg. Psychiatr.*, **20**, 11–21.

Selemon, L. D. and Goldman-Rakic, P. S. (1988) Common cortical and subcortical targets of the dorsolateral prefrontal and posterior parietal cortices in the rhesus monkey: evidence for a distributed neural network subserving spatially guided behaviour. *J. Neurosci.*, **8**, 4049–68.

Seltzer, B. and Pandya, D. N. (1984) Further observations on parieto-temporal connections in the rhesus monkey. *Exp. Brain Res.*, **55**, 301–12.

Shallice, T. (1988) *From Neuropsychology to Mental Structure*. UK: Cambridge University Press.

Squire, L. R. (1992) Declarative and nondeclarative memory: multiple brain systems supporting learning and memory. *J. Cog. Neurosci.*, **4**, 232–43.

Steward, O. (1976) Topographic organization of the projections from the entorhinal area to the hippocampal formation of the rat. *J. Comp. Neurol.*, **167**, 285–314.

Suzuki, W. A. and Amaral, D. G. (1994) Perirhinal and parahippocampal cortices of the macaque monkey: cortical afferents. *J. Comp. Neurol.*, **350**, 497–533.

Suzuki, W. A., Zola-Morgan, S., Squire, L. R. and Amaral, D. G. (1993) Lesions of the perirhinal and parahippocampal cortices in the monkey produce long-lasting memory impairment in the visual and tactile modalities. *J. Neurosci.*, **13**, 2430–51.

Swanson, L. W. and Cowan, W. M. (1977) An autoradiographic study of the organization of the efferent connections of the hippocampal formation in the rat. *J. Comp. Neurol.*, **172**, 49–84.

Taube, J. S., Muller, R. U. and Ranck, J. B. (1990) Head-direction cells recorded from the postsubiculum in freely moving rats. I. Description and quantitative analysis. *J. Neurosci.*, **10**, 420–35.

Ungerleider, L. G. and Mishkin, M. (1982) Two cortical visual systems. In: Ingle, D. J., Goodale, M. A. and Mansfield, R. J. W. (ed.) *Analysis of Visual Behavior*. Cambridge MA: The MIT Press.

Vallar, G., Guariglia, C. and Rusconi, M. L. (1997) Modulation of the neglect syndrome by sensory stimulation. In: Thier, P. and Karnath, H.-O. (ed.) *Parietal Lobe Contributions to Orientation in 3D Space*. Heidelberg: Springer.

Parietal cortex

This section considers papers on the effects of damage to the parietal lobes, and the neuronal mechanisms of the parietal representation of space. Vallar and Karnath consider the neuropsychology of parietal hemineglect in terms of an impairment to the egocentric frames of reference in which spatial information is processed. The nature of the impairment is considered, respectively, in terms of a translation or a rotation by the two authors. Other aspects of parietal function in humans are considered by Berthoz and David Milner and colleagues in the final section. The phenomena of 'object-centred' neglect is considered by Driver, who concludes that it could be caused by the basic parietal impairment in egocentric processing acting on visual information that has already been extensively processed in the occipital lobe. Single cell data regarding object-centred representations in frontal areas are considered by Olsen and colleagues in the final section. Details of the neural mechanisms of the egocentric representation of the locations of stimuli are presented by Andersen and Colby, who go on to demonstrate how information is translated between egocentric representations and how actions and the intention to act modulates neuronal responses. A neural network model of the posterior parietal representation of space in multiple egocentric frames of reference at once is presented by Pouget and Sejnowski, and used to model the symptoms of parietal hemineglect.

2

Spatial frames of reference and somatosensory processing: a neuropsychological perspective

Giuseppe Vallar

2.1 A hemispheric difference

One basic difference between elementary sensory and motor processes and higher-order mental functions concerns the hemispheric lateralization of their neural basis. The cerebral correlates of language and visuospatial processing are largely asymmetric, with the well-known specialization of the left hemisphere for many linguistic processes, and of the right hemisphere for a variety of spatial processes. By contrast, the neurological organization of sensory–motor systems has a 'contralateral' architecture, so that each hemisphere is primarily concerned with the opposite side of personal (i.e. the body) and extrapersonal space (for example, visual or auditory objects). This state of affairs has implications in the domain of clinical neurology. It is a current view that damage to the specifically committed regions of each cerebral hemisphere brings about somatosensory (hemianaesthesia), visual (hemianopia), and motor (hemiplegia) deficits, contralateral to the side of the lesion (contralesional) with no relevant left–right asymmetries (Rowland 1995; Adams *et al*. 1997).

There is also, however, some evidence of such asymmetries for sensory and motor deficits associated with unilateral lesions. A community-based epidemiological survey has shown that somatosensory, visual half-field, and motor deficits are more frequent after lesions in the right hemisphere, compared with left brain damage (Sterzi *et al*. 1993). In a continuous series of 154 left and 144 right brain-damaged stroke patients the incidence of contralateral somatosensory deficits (position sense) was 37 per cent after damage to the right hemisphere, and 25 per cent after damage to the left hemisphere. The incidence of deficits of sense of pain was 57 per cent in right and 45 per cent in left brain-damaged patients. Similarly, the incidence of contralesional visual half-field deficits was 18 per cent in right brain-damaged patients and 7 per cent in left brain-damaged patients. Finally, 95 per cent of right brain-damaged patients exhibited motor deficits, which were found in only 85 per cent of left brain-damaged patients.

If an analogy is drawn with disorders of linguistic and spatial cognition, this asymmetry may be explained by the existence of a higher-order pathological factor, related to right brain damage, which increases the incidence, and possibly the severity, of left-sided sensory and motor deficits. A plausible candidate is the syndrome of *spatial hemineglect*, which refers to the defective ability of patients with unilateral cerebral lesions to explore the contralesional side and to report stimuli presented in that side. The common trait of the different manifestations of hemineglect is *spatial*: in any given domain (extra-personal and personal space, internally generated images, etc.) the deficit concerns the contralesional part, with reference to a given coordinate system (Vallar 1994). Hemineglect, being more frequent and more severe after lesions in the right hemisphere (reviews in Bisiach & Vallar 1988; Vallar 1993, 1998), shows a hemispheric asymmetry in the same direction as that found in sensory and motor disorders. Furthermore, clinical descriptions of the syndrome include component deficits such as *négligence motrice* or *motor neglect* (the patients' inability to move spontaneously the contralesional arm in the absence of major primary motor deficits: see Garcin *et al.* (1938), Critchley (1953), Castaigne *et al.* (1970) and Mark *et al.* (1996) for a discussion of the terminology), and *sensory inattention* (a deficit in awareness of contralesional stimuli: see Heilman *et al.* (1993)), which may mimic primary motor, somatosensory and visual half-field deficits.

2.2 Preserved sensory processes in neglect-related sensory hemi-syndromes

These hemispheric asymmetries imply that left-sided sensory disorders may be produced by two, possibly additive, pathological factors: (1) a primary sensory component, as maintained by classic neurological views; and (2) a higher-order deficit, such as spatial hemineglect. Their relative contribution may vary across patients but in at least some cases the latter may be the main, if not the only, factor underlying the patients' sensory disorder.

In line with this two-component view, there is evidence that in right brain-damaged patients with visuospatial hemineglect primary sensory processes may be largely preserved, even though awareness of contralesional stimuli is defective. One brain-damaged patient with left hemianaesthesia showed skin conductance responses to stimuli, delivered to the left hand, that he was unable to perceive, as witnessed by a defective verbal report (Vallar *et al.* 1991*a*). Three right brain-damaged patients showed preserved early somatosensory evoked potentials to undetected stimuli (Vallar *et al.* 1991*b*). A similar dissociation between defective phenomenal experience and physiological evidence of preserved perceptual processing has been found in the visual domain. Two right brain-damaged patients with left homonymous hemianopia (Vallar *et al.* 1991*b*) showed largely preserved early visual evoked potentials, in terms of both latency and amplitude, to stimulation of the left visual half-field, that they failed to report and denied perceiving (see also Angelelli *et al*. (1996) for related evidence). These observations suggest that, in at least some patients, the higher-order pathological factor accounts entirely for the somatosensory or visual impairment. These findings also provide a neurophysiological basis to the behavioural evidence, now confirmed many times, of *processing without awareness* in patients with left hemineglect, who have proved to be able to analyse material presented in the left side of space, up to the semantic level (see, for example, Marshall & Halligan 1988; Berti & Rizzolatti 1992; Làdavas *et al*. 1993; McGlinchey-Berroth *et al*. 1993; Vallar *et al*. 1994, 1996*a*). The core finding of these studies is that patients with hemineglect may show relatively preserved *perception* of sensory inputs, but *sensation* (i.e. the phenomenal, conscious, experience of what is perceived) is defective (see the philosophical discussion of the distinction between perception and sensation in Chalmers (1996), p. 18).

The localization of lesions in patients with left visuospatial hemineglect provides a neural substrate to these preserved levels of analysis. Figure 2.1 shows the more frequent anatomical correlate of visuospatial hemineglect in humans: damage to the supramarginal gyrus (Brodmann's area 40) of the inferior parietal lobule, at the temporoparietal junction (Vallar & Perani 1986). Neglect is much less frequent after frontal damage, but a number of reports suggest that damage to both the dorsolateral premotor and the medial (anterior cingulate region, supplementary motor area) frontal regions may be associated with hemineglect (Heilman & Valenstein 1972; Damasio *et al*. 1980). Recently, the suggestion has been made that damage to the dorsal aspect of the right inferior frontal gyrus (Brodmann's area 44, premotor cortex) may be specifically associated with hemineglect (Husain & Kennard 1996). The lesions may

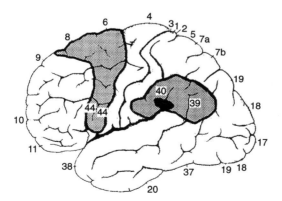

Fig. 2.1 The syndrome of spatial hemineglect: anatomical correlates (grey areas). In the majority of patients the lesion involves the supramarginal gyrus in the inferior parietal lobule, at the temporoparietal junction (black area) (Vallar & Perani 1986). Neglect after frontal damage is much less frequent and is usually associated with dorsolateral lesions of the premotor cortex.

also be confined to subcortical structures such as the basal ganglia, the thalamus and (but much less frequently) the white matter. By contrast, the primary motor, somatosensory and visual cortices are usually spared. In addition, patients with lesions confined to the latter regions usually do not show evidence of spatial hemineglect (see Vallar (1993) and Heilman *et al.* (1994) for reviews of the anatomical correlates of the neglect syndrome).

The lesions of individual patients with left visuospatial hemineglect, as assessed by visuomotor exploratory tasks, and left visual half-field deficits associated with neurophysiological evidence of relatively preserved basic sensory processing largely spare the primary visual cortex (Vallar *et al.* (1991*b*), two patients). By contrast, in patients with contralesional hemianopia not associated with hemineglect the lesions, as expected on the basis of classic neurological notions (Rowland 1995; Adams *et al.* 1997), involved the primary visual cortex and early visual evoked potentials were grossly abnormal or absent (Vallar *et al.* 1991*b*; Angelelli *et al.* 1996). In the somatosensory domain, the empirical evidence is less clear-cut. The patient of Vallar *et al.* (1991*a*) who showed skin conductance responses to unreported tactile stimuli had extensive damage to the right frontotemporoparietal–occipital regions, including the primary somatosensory cortex. In two out of the three patients of Vallar *et al.* (1991*b*) the right primary somatosensory cortex was unaffected, wholly or in part. The neurophysiological evidence of processing without awareness in patients with lesions involving the primary somatosensory cortex is consistent, however, with a positron emission tomography (PET) activation study in one patient with left somatosensory deficits produced by a lesion involving a large portion of the right primary somatosensory and motor areas, the supramarginal gyrus, and, possibly, somatosensory area II (Bottini *et al.* 1995). This patient, during the temporary recovery of left hemianaesthesia after vestibular caloric stimulation (irrigation of the left external ear canal with iced water), showed the activation of the right inferior frontal gyrus, the insula and the putamen. In normal subjects, the two latter areas were activated by both tactile stimulation of the left hand, and by vestibular stimulation. These findings suggest that other brain areas in addition to the primary somatosensory cortex may contribute, in relation to their capacities, to the processing of somatosensory stimuli and to perceptual awareness.

2.3 Defective sensation and spatial hemineglect: modulation by peripheral sensory stimulation

The observations discussed above do not provide any *direct* indication as to the mechanisms whereby patients with hemineglect fail to be phenomenally aware of stimuli they are able to process. The preservation of primary sensory processes suggests that the retinotopic (in the visual domain) and the somatotopic (in the tactile domain) levels of representation may be unaffected, and that the patients' defective awareness of contralesional stimuli may be produced by a disorder of higher-order spatial representations. In line with this view, the main anatomical correlates of hemineglect in humans are lesions of the posterior parietal (inferior parietal lobule) and, although much less frequently, of the premotor regions (Vallar 1993). In the monkey, cells that encode visual stimuli in spatial, body part (head-, arm-centred) coordinates have been described in the posterior parietal and in the premotor cortex (Fogassi *et al.* 1992; Galletti *et al.* 1993; Graziano *et al.* 1994; Battaglini *et al.* 1996).

A major source of evidence for the view that the defective perceptual awareness of contralesional stimuli of patients with hemineglect reflects the disorder of higher-order spatial (e.g. egocentric, with reference to the midsagittal plane of the trunk) representations has been the investigation of the effects of direction-specific sensory stimulations. In recent years, many studies from different laboratories have shown that many manifestations of the neglect syndrome are modulated by vestibular (see, for example, Rubens 1985; Cappa *et al.* 1987), visual (optokinetic) (Pizzamiglio *et al.* 1990), and proprioceptive or somatosensory stimulations (Karnath *et al.* 1993; Vallar *et al.* 1995*d*). Vestibular stimulation has been extensively used, but the results obtained by using other stimulations are similar. In right brain-damaged patients, the modulatory effects concern neglect for objects in extrapersonal space (Rubens 1985; Pizzamiglio *et al.* 1990; Karnath *et al.* 1993), neglect for personal space (the left side of the body: Cappa *et al.* 1987), disorders of monitoring processes, such as anosognosia for hemiplegia (Cappa *et al.* 1987; Vallar *et al.* 1990; Rode *et al.* 1992), and delusional beliefs concerning the left side of the body (somatoparaphrenia: Bisiach *et al.* 1991; Rode *et al.* 1992). Vestibular and optokinetic stimulations producing a nystagmus with a slow phase towards the left, contralesional side, and left-sided transcutaneous mechanical vibration and electrical nervous stimulations temporarily improve these disorders. By contrast, vestibular and optokinetic stimulations producing a nystagmus with a slow phase towards the right, ipsilesional side, and right-sided transcutaneous vibration and electrical stimulations worsen the deficits, or are ineffective (see review in Vallar *et al.* 1997*b*).

Within the somatosensory system, similar results have been obtained by using three types of stimulation: vestibular, electrical transcutaneous and optokinetic. The effects of vestibular stimulation on the deficit of tactile perception of patients with unilateral lesions of the left and of the right hemisphere are shown in Fig. 2.2 (Vallar *et al.* 1993*b*). The irrigation of the left external ear canal with iced water, which produces a nystagmus with a slow phase towards the left side, temporarily improved detection of tactile stimuli, delivered to the left contralesional hand by a von Frey's hair, in 15 out of 17 right brain-damaged patients. Fourteen such patients also showed evidence of left visuo-spatial hemineglect, which was absent in three cases. Similarly, in three right brain-damaged patients this vestibular stimulation (douching of the left canal with iced water) temporarily improved left tactile extinction to double symmetrical (left and right-sided) touches (Fig. 2.3). In nine out of 11 left brain-damaged

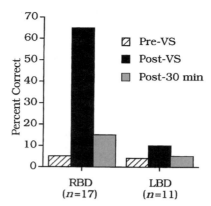

Fig. 2.2 Contralesional somatosensory deficits and vestibular stimulation. Percentage of single tactile stimuli, delivered to the hand contralateral to the hemispheric lesion, detected by right (RBD) and left (LBD) brain-damaged patients, before (Pre) and after (Post) vestibular stimulation (VS), and at a 30 min delay assessment (redrawn from Vallar *et al*. (1993*b*), figure 1, by permission of Oxford University Press).

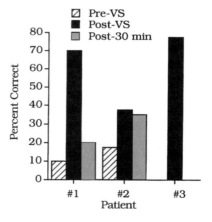

Fig. 2.3 Contralesional tactile extinction to double simultaneous stimulation of the left and of the right hand and vestibular stimulation. Percentage of tactile stimuli delivered to the left hand, detected by three right brain-damaged patients before (Pre) and after (Post) vestibular stimulation (VS) and at a 30 min delay assessment (data from Vallar *et al*. (1993*b*), table 3).

patients, by contrast, vestibular stimulation (irrigation of the right external ear canal with iced water, which produces a nystagmus with a slow phase towards the right side) was ineffective. This vestibular stimulation, however, produced a substantial temporary improvement of the tactile deficit in the right hand in the two left brain-damaged patients, who also showed right visuospatial hemineglect: the patients' performance improved from 2.5 per cent correct responses before stimulation to 37.5 per cent after treatment, with 5 per cent correct responses at the 30 min delay assessment. The effects of vestibular stimulation are related to the direction of the slow phase of the nystagmus and not to the stimulated side (ear). Both irrigation of the left external ear canal with cold water, and of the right canal with warm water, which produce a nystagmus with a slow phase towards the left side, temporarily improve visuospatial hemineglect (Rubens 1985, 17 patients) and left hemianaesthesia (Vallar *et al*. 1990, patient no. 2). By contrast, irrigation of the left external ear canal with warm water, and of the right canal with iced water, which produce a nystagmus with a slow phase towards the right side, temporarily worsened left visuospatial hemineglect in all 17 patients of Rubens' (1985) series.

Transcutaneous electrical nervous stimulation of the left neck improved contralesional left hemianaesthesia in 10 right brain-damaged patients, both with and without visuospatial hemineglect (Fig. 2.4) (Vallar *et al*. 1996*b*). In one right brain-damaged patient with a moderate left somatosensory deficit, the effects of both left-and right-sided transcutaneous electrical stimulation were assessed. Figure 2.5 shows that left-sided stimulation temporarily decreased the somatosensory threshold in the left hand, improving the disorder, whereas right-sided stimulation had negative effects, increasing the threshold. This directional pattern of results is similar to the effects of transcutaneous electrical

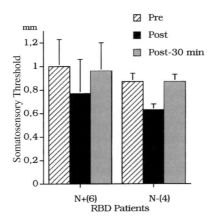

Fig. 2.4 Contralesional somatosensory deficits and transcutaneous electrical nervous stimulation. Average somatosensory thresholds (diameter in millimetres of von Frey's hair) in the contralesional left hand of 10 right brain-damaged (RBD) patients (N + or N −: with or without visuospatial hemineglect) on three successive assessments: before transcutaneous electrical nervous stimulation (Pre); immediately after stimulation of the contralesional left side of the neck (Post); or 30 min after stimulation (Post-30 min) (redrawn from Vallar *et al*. (1996*b*), figure 1, by permission of Cambridge University Press).

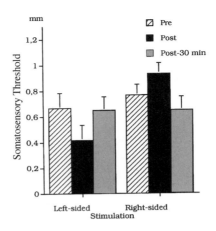

Fig. 2.5 Contralesional somatosensory deficits and transcutaneous electrical nervous stimulation. Average somatosensory thresholds in the contralesional left hand of a right brain-damaged patient with left visuospatial hemineglect, on three successive assessments (see caption to Fig. 2.4). The contralesional (left) and the ipsilesional (right) sides of the neck were stimulated in successive sessions (redrawn from Vallar *et al.* (1996*b*), figure 3, by permission of Cambridge University Press).

stimulation on left visuospatial hemineglect (Vallar *et al.* 1995*d*). Finally, out of the four patients with left hemisphere damage and right-sided somatosensory deficits, stimulation of the right side of the neck reduced the threshold only in the one patient who exhibited also right visuospatial hemineglect.

Finally, two studies investigated the effects of optokinetic stimulation with horizontally moving luminous dots on deficits of position sense in right and left brain-damaged patients in the horizontal (Vallar *et al.* 1993*a*) and the vertical (Vallar *et al.* 1995*a*) plane. A baseline assessment, without optokinetic stimulation, showed, in right and left brain-damaged patients without visuospatial hemineglect, a position sense disorder confined to the contralesional forearm, in line with the traditional neurological views (Rowland 1995; Adams *et al.* 1997). Right brain-damaged patients with visuospatial hemineglect, by contrast, had a much more severe deficit of position sense, which involved not only the contralesional left, but also the ipsilesional right forearm, even though in the latter the disorder was milder. Optokinetic stimulation modulated the severity of the deficit only in right brain-damaged patients with visuospatial hemineglect. Stimulation with a leftward direction of the movement of the luminous dots (contralateral to the side of the lesion) temporarily improved the disorder, in both the left and the right forearms, in both the vertical and the horizontal planes (Fig. 2.6). Stimulation with a rightward direction of the movement (ipsilateral to the side of the lesion) worsened the deficit. No effects of optokinetic stimulation were found, in both right and left brain-damaged patients without visuospatial hemineglect.

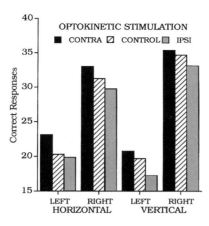

Fig. 2.6 Deficits of position sense of right brain-damaged patients with visuospatial hemineglect and optokinetic stimulation. Mean correct responses in the LEFT and RIGHT forearms, contralateral and ipsilateral to the side of the lesion, by stimulation condition (baseline (CONTROL), optokinetic stimulation with a direction of the movement of the luminous dots contralateral or ipsilateral (CONTRA or IPSI) to the side of the lesion) and by assessed plane (HORIZONTAL or VERTICAL) (redrawn from Vallar *et al*. (1995*a*), figure 2, by permission of Masson).

These studies provide a convergent pattern of results, which may be summarized as two main points.

1. There is a hemispheric asymmetry in the effects of sensory stimulations on the contralesional somatosensory deficits of patients with unilateral lesions. In most patients with right brain damage, the severity of the left-sided impairment was modulated by sensory stimulations in a direction-specific fashion; by contrast, the right-sided deficits of left brain-damaged patients were largely unaffected.

2. There is an association between visuospatial hemineglect and the somatosensory deficits modulated by these stimulations. Most right brain-damaged patients and all of the few left brain-damaged patients who showed temporary recovery of contralesional somatosensory disorders also exhibited visuospatial hemineglect. However, the sensory stimulations also improved detection of left-sided tactile stimuli in a number of right brain-damaged patients without evidence of left visuospatial hemineglect.

This finding, together with the long-known observation that visuospatial hemineglect may occur without associated somatosensory deficits (Bisiach & Vallar 1988; Vallar *et al*. 1993*b*), constitutes a double dissociation. This dissociation suggests that the systems concerned with awareness of somatosensory stimuli, modulated by sensory stimulations, are independent of those subserving the representation of objects in extrapersonal space. All of them, however, share the characteristic of being modulated in a directionally similar fashion by vestibular, optokinetic and proprioceptive or somatosensory stimuli.

These findings provide an explanation, based on experimental studies, of the clinical observation that somatosensory deficits are more frequent after lesions in the right hemisphere than after left brain damage (Sterzi *et al*. 1993). In line with these results, contralesional somatosensory deficits have also been reported to be more severe after lesions (position sense, Vallar *et al*. 1993*a*, 1995*a*) or temporary dysfunction (detection of single and double tactile stimuli, Meador *et al*. 1988) of the right hemisphere (review in Vallar *et al*. 1993*b*). Finally, the observation that also the modulatory effects of direction-specific sensory stimulations occur much more frequently in patients with lesions in the right hemisphere concur to suggest the existence of a specific additional pathological factor associated with right brain damage, over and above the primary somatosensory disorder. The size of the recovery brought about by some treatments, such as vestibular stimulation (see Figs 2.2 and 2.3), suggests that the relative contribution of this factor may be quite substantial.

2.4 Interpretation

This pattern of results supports the view that contralesional somatosensory disorders are produced by two discrete, possibly additive, pathological factors: (1) a primary sensory deficit, which may occur after lesions of either hemisphere, without left–right asymmetries, and (2) a higher-order disorder, closely associated with right brain damage, which is modulated by a number of sensory afferents. The similarity of the effects of sensory stimulations on both left somatosensory deficits and a number of components of the syndrome of left spatial hemineglect suggests that the higher-order pathological factor underlying the greater frequency and severity of left-sided somatosensory deficits may be spatial in nature.

Before accepting this interpretation, however, the possibility that the effects of the modulatory sensory stimulations take place at the level of defective primary sensory processes (in the somatosensory and visual domains, somatotopic and retinotopic levels of representation) should be taken into account. This interpretation is unlikely: there is electrophysiological and, at least in part, anatomical evidence that primary sensory processes may be largely preserved in these patients (Vallar *et al*. 1991*a*, *b*; Angelelli *et al*. 1996). In addition, the existence of a hemispheric asymmetry argues against the view that primary sensory processes are the main target of this sensory modulation. Furthermore, damage confined to the anterior parietal region, including the primary somatosensory cortex, brings about deficits of tactile perception, which do not differ according to the side of the hemispheric lesion (Corkin *et al*. 1970; Pause *et al*. 1989). Finally, as shown in Fig. 2.6 right brain-damaged patients with left hemineglect show a deficit of position sense, modulated by optokinetic stimulation, which also involves the right forearm (Vallar *et al.* 1993*a*, 1995*a*). This ipsilesional deficit, which was not found in right and left brain-damaged patients without visuospatial hemineglect, cannot be ascribed to a primary sensory disorder, but is likely to reflect a higher-order impairment.

The related account of the effects of sensory stimulations in terms of non-specific cerebral or hemispheric activation is also implausible. In addition to the hemispheric asymmetry mentioned above, the effects are direction-specific, related to the direction of the slow phase of nystagmus (vestibular and optokinetic stimulations) or to the side of the transcutaneous (mechanical or electrical) stimulation. These treatments may bring about a temporary recovery, but may also cause a worsening of the disorder, or be ineffective (review in Vallar *et al.* 1997*b*; see also examples in Figs 2.5 and 2.6. The latter effects are not compatible with the hypothesis of a general cerebral activation. Finally, vestibular stimulation temporarily improves a number of components of the neglect syndrome, but not other cognitive disorders, such as aphasia. The observation of these dissociated effects in one left brain-damaged patient with right visuospatial hemineglect and dysphasia makes an interpretation in terms of general hemispheric activation much unlikely (Vallar *et al.* 1995*c*).

The modulatory effects of direction-specific sensory stimulations may then occur at the level of a spatial, non-somatotopic, representation of the body. It has long been known that patients with right hemisphere damage and hemineglect show a pathological displacement of egocentric frames of reference, with the midsagittal plane of the trunk (the subjective 'straight ahead') being lateralized towards the side of the lesion, with a rightward directional error (Heilman *et al.* 1983; Mark & Heilman 1990). This disorder may be conceived in terms of either a rightward pathological translation or, alternatively, a clockwise rotation of egocentric coordinate systems (see a discussion of hemineglect in terms of 'rotation' in Ventre *et al.* (1984); see also Karnath (Ch. 3)). Vallar *et al.* (1995*b*) investigated these hypotheses by requiring patients to report whether sound sources in the front or in the back half of extrapersonal space were perceived to the left or to the right of the subjective midsagittal plane. In right brain-damaged patients with visuospatial hemineglect the subjective midsagittal plane was found to be displaced rightwards in both half-spaces, consistent with an account in terms of a rightward ipsi-lesional translation of egocentric coordinates. Clockwise rotation around the vertical axis, by contrast, would involve an ipsilesional rightward displacement in the front half-space, but a contralesional leftward displacement in the back half-space. The translation hypothesis is also consistent with the results of early studies based on auditory lateralization paradigms, where subjects localized, in the frontal plane passing through the ears, the perceived position of fused sound images generated by dichotic stimuli. Right brain-damaged patients showed a systematic directional error for all stimuli, also when the interaural intensity or time differences (D) were zero, whereas normal subjects localized the fused sound images in the intersection between the midfrontal and the midsagittal planes (the midbody axis) (Teuber 1962; Altman *et al.* 1979;

Bisiach *et al*. 1984). The hypothesis of a rightward rotation of the egocentric coordinate system, by contrast, would predict a normal localization of dichotic stimuli with $D = 0$, because the vertical axis of the body would be unaffected.

Optokinetic and vestibular stimulations modulate this ipsilesional displacement, reducing or increasing the rightward error of patients with left hemineglect, and have similar directional effects in normal subjects (review in Vallar *et al*. 1997*b*). The computation of spatial frames of reference involves the continuous integration of signals from different sensory sources (visual, vestibular, proprioceptive or somatosensory) from the two sides of space and the body (Andersen 1995, and Ch. 5). Unilateral cerebral lesions may bring about an unbalanced activity of the bilateral set of cerebral structures concerned with the building up and operating spatial representations (Ventre *et al*. 1984; Kinsbourne 1993; for a related functional account, see Vallar *et al*. 1993*b*). In patients with lesions in the right hemisphere, one effect of this unbalanced activity is the comparatively minor weight given to left-sided sensory signals. This, in turn, results in impoverished spatial representations, with a left–right gradient, or a rightward distortion (discussion in Vallar *et al*. 1997*b*). The unilateral or direction-specific stimulations discussed above provide a supplementary lateralized signal, which modulates the rightward distortion, restoring, at least in part, or further disrupting the defective spatial representation of the contralesional side.

The view that the contralesional somatosensory deficits of right brain-damaged patients have a spatial component is supported by a number of studies based on an approach complementary to that adopted by the stimulation experiments reviewed above. According to the 'spatial' hypothesis discussed previously, direction-specific stimulations may improve, or worsen, somatosensory deficits of patients with right-sided lesions, reducing, or increasing, the rightward distortion of a spatial representation of the body. Because, however, the ipsilesional right side of such spatial representations is relatively preserved, as suggested by the normal detection of tactile stimuli delivered to the right hand (Vallar *et al*. 1990, 1993*b*) and by the minor deficit of position sense in the right forearm (Vallar *et al*. 1993*a*, 1995*a*), the prediction can be made that left-sided sensory deficits may also be improved by manoeuvres whereby the stimulus is presented in the ipsilesional space, dissociating retinotopic and somatotopic from egocentric (with reference to the midsagittal plane of the trunk) frames of reference. Kooistra & Heilman (1989) found that the left hemianopia of their patient, who had a right thalamic and medial temporo-occipital lesion, improved when her eyes were directed 30° towards the right side. In this condition, where left visual half-field testing fell in the right half-space, the patient's left hemianopia improved significantly. Applying the same logic to left hemianaesthesia, Smania & Aglioti (1995) found that the detection of left-sided tactile stimuli by patients with lesions in the right hemisphere improved when the forearms were crossed, with the left hand being placed in the ipsilesional right half-space. This effect was present during both single and double (two stimuli simultaneously delivered to the left and the right hand) stimulation (see also Moscovitch & Behrmann (1994) for related evidence on tactile extinction).

The results discussed so far provide converging evidence to the effect that spatial egocentric representations contribute to awareness of somatosensory and visual stimuli, and to the perception of the spatial position of body parts (position sense). This perceptual role of spatial frames of reference may be related to their involvement in the conscious organization of movements (for example, of the arm, or of the whole body through locomotion) directed towards specific targets in extrapersonal space, or on the subject's body (review in Andersen 1995). Seen from this perspective, spatial coordinate systems may represent an interface, in which spatial codes are available to both perceptual and premotor representations. If this is the case, the sensory stimulations that modulate spatial frames of reference (review in Vallar *et al.* 1997*b*) and the severity of left somatosensory deficits in right brain-damaged patients may be expected to affect the motor aspects of the syndrome of spatial hemineglect in a similar fashion. In line with this view contralesional hemiplegia, like hemianaesthesia and hemianopia, is more frequent after lesions in the right hemisphere, compared with left brain damage (Sterzi *et al.* 1993). If an analogy is drawn with the hemispheric asymmetry of sensory deficits, this finding suggests that a pathological factor, spatial in nature, may also account for the hemispheric asymmetry of contralesional motor disorders. Were this the case, the direction-specific stimulations that improve left somatosensory deficits would be expected to affect left motor deficits in a similar fashion. The clinical observation in one right brain-damaged patient that vestibular stimulation temporarily improved left hemiplegia supports this hypothesis (Rode *et al.* 1992).

In a recent experimental study (Vallar *et al.* 1997*a*), two right brain-damaged patients with left visuospatial hemineglect were required to flex the fingers of the contralesional paretic hand against a handle, in a baseline condition and during optokinetic stimulation. In line with the results of previous investigations (Pizzamiglio *et al.* 1990; Vallar *et al.* 1993*a*, 1995*a*), optokinetic stimulation with a leftward direction of the movement of the luminous dots improved muscle strength in the left contralesional hand, whereas stimulation with a rightward direction was ineffective. In patient no. 1, magnetic resonance imaging (MRI) showed extensive corticosubcortical damage to the right frontotemporoparietal–occipital cortex. In patient no. 2 the MRI-assessed lesion involved the right inferior parietal lobule, the superior–posterior temporal region, and the occipital cortex. This lesional pattern is frequently associated with hemineglect (see Fig. 2.1). Optokinetic stimulation had no effects on the right-sided motor deficit of two left brain-damaged patients without hemineglect, independent of the direction of the movement. These results suggest that the human ability to organize and produce motor outputs, even as simple as flexing the fingers, requires the availability of an internal representation of the space where movements are to be performed. This spatial medium, the neural bases of which may include the posterior–inferior parietal and premotor frontal regions, may be disrupted by brain damage, and restored, at least in part, by optokinetic stimulation.

Acknowledgements

This work was supported in part by grants from CNR, MURST, and Ministero della Sanità.

References

Adams, R. D., Victor, M. & Ropper, A. H. (eds) 1997 *Principles of neurology*, 6th edn. New York: McGraw-Hill.

Altman, J. A., Balonov, L. J. & Deglin, V. L. 1979 Effects of unilateral disorder of the brain hemisphere function in man on directional hearing. *Neuropsychologia* **17**, 295–301.

Andersen, R. A. 1995 Coordinate transformations and motor planning in posterior parietal cortex. In *The cognitive neurosciences* (ed. M. S. Gazzaniga), pp. 519–548. Cambridge, MA: MIT Press.

Angelelli, P., De Luca, M. & Spinelli, D. 1996 Early visual processing in neglect patients: a study with steady-state VEPs. *Neuropsychologia* **34**, 1151–1157.

Battaglini, P. P., Galletti, C. & Fattori, P. 1996 Cortical mechanisms for visual perception of object motion and position in space. *Behav. Brain Res.* **76**, 143–154.

Berti, A. & Rizzolatti, G. 1992 Visual processing without awareness: evidence from unilateral neglect. *J. Cogn. Neurosci.* **4**, 345–351.

Bisiach, E., Cornacchia, L., Sterzi, R. & Vallar, G. 1984 Disorders of perceived auditory lateralization after lesions of the right hemisphere. *Brain* **107**, 37–52.

Bisiach, E., Rusconi, M. L. & Vallar, G. 1991 Remission of somatoparaphrenic delusion through vestibular stimulation. *Neuropsychologia* **29**, 1029–1031.

Bisiach, E. & Vallar, G. 1988 Hemineglect in humans. In *Handbook of neuropsychology* (ed. F. Boller & J. Grafman), vol. 1, pp. 195–222. Amsterdam: Elsevier.

Bottini, G., Paulesu, E., Sterzi, R., Warburton, E., Wise, R. J. S., Vallar, G., Frackowiak, R. S. J. & Frith, C. D. 1995 Modulation of conscious experience by peripheral stimuli. *Nature* **376**, 778–781.

Cappa, S., Sterzi, R., Vallar, G. & Bisiach, E. 1987 Remission of hemineglect and anosognosia during vestibular stimulation. *Neuropsychologia* **25**, 775–782.

Castaigne, P., Laplane, D. & Degos, J.-D. 1970 Trois cas de négligence motrice par lésion rétro-rolandique. *Rev. Neurol.* **122**, 234–242.

Chalmers, D. J. 1996 *The conscious mind. In search of a fundamental theory*. New York: Oxford University Press.

Corkin, S., Milner, B. & Rasmussen, T. 1970 Somatosensory thresholds. *Archs. Neurol.* **23**, 41–58.

Critchley, M. 1953 *The parietal lobes*. New York: Hafner.

Damasio, A. R., Damasio, H. & Chang Chui, H. 1980 Neglect following damage to frontal lobe or basal ganglia. *Neuropsychologia* **18**, 123–132.

Fogassi, L., Gallese, V., di Pellegrino, G., Fadiga, L., Gentilucci, M., Luppino, G., Matelli, M., Pedotti, A. & Rizzolatti, G. 1992 Space coding by premotor cortex. *Expl Brain Res.* **89**, 686–690.

Galletti, C., Battaglini, P. P. & Fattori, P. 1993 Parietal neurons encoding spatial locations in craniotopic coordinates. *Expl Brain Res.* **96**, 221–229.

Garcin, R., Varay, A. & Hadji-Dimo 1938 Document pour servir a l'étude des troubles du schema corporel. *Rev. Neurol.* **69**, 498–510.

Graziano, M. S. A., Yap, G. S. & Gross, C. G. 1994 Coding of visual space by premotor neurons. *Science* **266**, 1054–1057.

Heilman, K. M., Bowers, D. & Watson, R. T. 1983 Performance on hemispatial pointing task by patients with neglect syndrome. *Neurology* **33**, 661–664.

Heilman, K. M. & Valenstein, E. 1972 Frontal lobe neglect in man. *Neurology* **22**, 660–664.

Heilman, K. M., Watson, R. T. & Valenstein, E. 1993 Neglect and related disorders. In *Clinical neuropsychology* (ed. K. M. Heilman & E. Valenstein), pp. 279–336. New York: Oxford University Press.

Heilman, K. M., Watson, R. T. & Valenstein, E. 1994 Localization of lesions in neglect and related disorders. In *Localization and neuroimaging in neuropsychology* (ed. A. Kertesz), pp. 495–524. San Diego: Academic Press.

Husain, M. & Kennard, C. 1996 Visual neglect associated with frontal lobe infarction. *J. Neurol.* **243**, 652–657.

Karnath, H. O., Christ, K. & Hartje, W. 1993 Decrease of contralateral neglect by neck muscle vibration and spatial orientation of trunk midline. *Brain* **116**, 383–396.

Kinsbourne, M. 1993 Orientational bias model of unilateral neglect: evidence from attentional gradients within hemispace. In *Unilateral neglect: clinical and experimental studies* (ed. I. H. Robertson & J. C. Marshall), pp. 63–86. Hove: Erlbaum.

Kooistra, C. A. & Heilman, K. M. 1989 Hemispatial visual inattention masquerading as hemianopia. *Neurology* **39**, 1125–1127.

Làdavas, E., Paladini, R. & Cubelli, R. 1993 Implicit associative priming in a patient with left visual neglect. *Neuropsychologia* **31**, 1307–1320.

Mark, V. W. & Heilman, K. M. 1990 Bodily neglect and orientational biases in unilateral neglect syndrome and normal subjects. *Neurology* **40**, 640–643.

Mark, V. W., Heilman, K. M. & Watson, R. 1996 Motor neglect: what do we mean? *Neurology* **46**, 1492–1493.

Marshall, J. C. & Halligan, P. 1988 Blindsight and insight in visuo-spatial neglect. *Nature* **336**, 766–767.

McGlinchey-Berroth, R., Milberg, W. P., Verfaellie, M., Alexander, M. & Kilduff, P. 1993 Semantic processing in the neglected visual field: evidence from a lexical decision task. *Cogn. Neuropsychol.* **10**, 79–108.

Meador, K. J., Loring, D. W., Lee, G. P., Brooks, B. S., Thompson, E. E., Thompson, W. O. & Heilman, K. M. 1988 Right cerebral specialization for tactile attention as evidenced by intracarotid sodium amytal. *Neurology* **38**, 1763–1766.

Moscovitch, M. & Behrmann, M. 1994 Coding of spatial information in the somatosensory system: evidence from patients with neglect following parietal lobe damage. *J. Cogn. Neurosci.* **6**, 151–155.

Pause, M., Kunesch, E., Binkofsky, F. & Freund, H. J. 1989 Sensorimotor disturbances in patients with lesions of the parietal cortex. *Brain* **112**, 1599–1625.

Pizzamiglio, L., Frasca, R., Guariglia, C., Incoccia, C. & Antonucci, G. 1990 Effect of optokinetic stimulation in patients with visual neglect. *Cortex* **26**, 535–540.

Rode, G., Charles, N., Perenin, M. T., Vighetto, A., Trillet, M. & Aimard, G. 1992 Partial remission of hemiplegia and somatoparaphrenia through vestibular stimulation in a case of unilateral neglect. *Cortex* **28**, 203–208.

Rowland, L. P. (ed.) 1995 *Merritt's textbook of neurology*, 9th edn. Baltimore: Williams & Wilkins.

Rubens, A. B. 1985 Caloric stimulation and unilateral visual neglect. *Neurology* **35**, 1019–1024.

Smania, N. & Aglioti, S. 1995 Sensory and spatial components of somaesthetic deficits following right brain damage. *Neurology* **45**, 1725–1730.

Sterzi, R., Bottini, G., Celani, M. G., Righetti, E., Lamassa, M., Ricci, S. & Vallar, G. 1993 Hemianopia, hemianaesthesia, and hemiplegia after left and right hemisphere damage: a hemispheric difference. *J. Neurol. Neurosurg. Psychiatr.* **56**, 308–310.

Teuber, H. L. 1962 Effects of brain wounds implicating right or left hemisphere in man: hemisphere differences in vision, audition and somesthesis. In *Interhemispheric relations and cerebral dominance* (ed. V. B. Mountcastle), pp. 131–157. Baltimore: Johns Hopkins Press.

Vallar, G. 1993 The anatomical basis of spatial hemineglect in humans. In *Unilateral neglect: clinical and experimental studies* (ed. I. H. Robertson & J. C. Marshall), pp. 27–59. Hove: Erlbaum.

Vallar, G. 1994 Left spatial hemineglect: an unmanageable explosion of dissociations? *No. Neuropsychol. Rehabil.* **4**, 209–212.

Vallar, G. 1998 Spatial hemineglect in humans. *Trends Cog. Sci.* **2**, 87–97.

Vallar, G., Antonucci, G., Guariglia, C. & Pizzamiglio, L. 1993*a* Deficits of position sense, unilateral neglect, and optokinetic stimulation. *Neuropsychologia* **31**, 1191–1200.

Vallar, G., Bottini, G., Rusconi, M. L. & Sterzi, R. 1993*b* Exploring somatosensory hemineglect by vestibular stimulation. *Brain* **116**, 71–86.

Vallar, G., Bottini, G., Sterzi, R., Passerini, D. & Rusconi, M. L. 1991*a* Hemianesthesia, sensory neglect and defective access to conscious experience. *Neurology* **41**, 650–652.

Vallar, G., Guariglia, C., Magnotti, L. & Pizzamiglio, L. 1995*a* Optokinetic stimulation affects both vertical and horizontal deficits of position sense in unilateral neglect. *Cortex* **31**, 669–683.

Vallar, G., Guariglia, C., Nico, D. & Bisiach, E. 1995*b* Spatial hemineglect in back space. *Brain* **118**, 467–472.

Vallar, G., Guariglia, C., Nico, D. & Pizzamiglio, L. 1997*a* Motor deficits and optokinetic stimulation in patients with left hemineglect. *Neurology* **49**, 1364–1370.

Vallar, G., Guariglia, C., Nico, D. & Tabossi, P. 1996*a* Left neglect dyslexia and the processing of *neglected* information. *J. Clin. Exp. Neuropsychol.* **18**, 733–746.

Vallar, G., Guariglia, C. & Rusconi, M. L. 1997*b* Modulation of the neglect syndrome by sensory stimulation. In *Parietal lobe contributions to orientation in 3D space* (ed. P. Thier & H.-O. Karnath), pp. 555–578. Heidelberg: Springer.

Vallar, G., Papagno, C., Rusconi, M. L. & Bisiach, E. 1995*c* Vestibular stimulation, spatial hemineglect and dysphasia. Selective effects? *Cortex* **31**, 589–593.

Vallar, G. & Perani, D. 1986 The anatomy of unilateral neglect after right hemisphere stroke lesions. A clinical CT/Scan correlation study in man. *Neuropsychologia* **24**, 609–622.

Vallar, G., Rusconi, M. L., Barozzi, S., Bernardini, B., Ovadia, D., Papagno, C. & Cesarani, A. 1995*d* Improvement of left visuo-spatial hemineglect by left-sided transcutaneous electrical stimulation. *Neuropsychologia* **33**, 73–82.

Vallar, G., Rusconi, M. L. & Bernardini, B. 1996*b* Modulation of neglect hemi-anesthesia by transcutaneous electrical stimulation. *J. Int. Neuropsychol. Soc.* **2**, 452–459.

Vallar, G., Rusconi, M. L. & Bisiach, E. 1994 Awareness of contralesional information in unilateral neglect: effects of verbal cueing, tracing and vestibular stimulation.

In *Attention and performance. XV. Conscious and nonconscious information processing* (ed. C. A. Umiltà & M. Moscovitch), pp. 377–391. Cambridge, MA: MIT Press.

Vallar, G., Sandroni, P., Rusconi, M. L. & Barbieri, S. 1991*b* Hemianopia, hemianesthesia and spatial neglect. A study with evoked potentials. *Neurology* **41**, 1918–1922.

Vallar, G., Sterzi, R., Bottini, G., Cappa, S. & Rusconi, M. L. 1990 Temporary remission of left hemianaesthesia after vestibular stimulation. *Cortex* **26**, 123–131.

Ventre, J., Flandrin, J. M. & Jeannerod, M. 1984 In search for the egocentric reference. A neurophysiological hypothesis. *Neuropsychologia* **22**, 797–806.

3

Spatial orientation and the representation of space with parietal lobe lesions

Hans-Otto Karnath

3.1 Introduction

Parietal lobe lesions in humans lead to disturbances of spatial perception and of motor behaviour in space. Due to the usually large extent of lesions affecting the parietal lobe, most clinical cases show a combination of these disturbances. Dissociations arguing for distinct clinical entities combined with small cortical lesions that allow a precise localization of different functions within the parietal lobe are rather rare.

The most established anatomoclinical dissociation within the parietal lobe concerns the disturbances following lesions of the superior and of the inferior lobule. Both lesion locations induce characteristic disturbances of visuospatial behaviour. Patients with inferior (predominantly right) parietal lobe lesions demonstrate a deficient response to stimuli located contralaterally to the lesion and fail to explore the contralesional part of space by eye or limb movements, termed *spatial neglect*. Clinically it becomes apparent, e.g. by omission of objects if located contralesionally, a tendency to spontaneously turn gaze and the body toward the ipsilesional side, or a deviation of drawings or handwriting toward the ipsilesional side on a page. In contrast, superior parietal lobe lesions lead to specific impairments of visually guided pointing and reaching for objects (Perenin 1997), termed *optic ataxia*. Typically, these patients show misreaching with either hand for objects located in the visual half-field contralateral to the lesion.

Different mechanisms of processing spatial information thus have been assumed to be represented in the human inferior and superior parietal lobule. Perenin (1997) has argued that the superior part of parietal cortex is mainly involved in 'direct coding of space for action by means of several effector-specific representations', while the inferior part is responsible for 'more enduring and conscious representations underlying spatial cognition and awareness'. Milner and Goodale (1995) also have argued for distinct functions of superior and inferior parts of parietal lobe. They have suggested that the superior parietal lobe is part of the dorsal stream of visual processing; they have assumed that input transformations carried out via this pathway mediate 'the control of goal-directed actions'. Lesions restricted to the superior part in humans, therefore, lead to disturbances of visuomotor control, such as optic ataxia. Spatial neglect was attributed to lesions of the inferior part of parietal lobe. The authors hypothesized that different from superior parietal lobe function, mechanisms evolved in the human inferior parietal or parietotemporal region deal with abstract spatial processing based on input from the ventral stream. Input transformations via the ventral stream of visual processing were supposed to permit 'the formation of perceptual and cognitive representations which embody the enduring characteristics of objects and their significance'.

The basic pathophysiological principles leading to optic ataxia and to spatial neglect, however, are still an issue of lively debate (e.g. Halligan and Marshall 1994; Milner and Goodale 1995; Perenin 1997). Different mechanisms and possible alterations of neural representations of space have been suggested to explain the behavioural consequences in patients with parietal lobe lesions. The present article tries to contribute to an identification of the functions represented in the parietal lobe by analysing the defective mechanisms of processing spatial information in patients with spatial neglect, i.e. in patients that predominantly suffer from lesions of the inferior part of parietal lobe (Vallar and Perani 1986).

3.2 Does spatial neglect follow a 'lateral gradient of attention' or a 'deviation of egocentric space representation'?—data from *visual search*

One hypothesis on spatial neglect has proposed an altered neural representation of space (Ventre *et al.* 1984; Karnath 1994*a*, 1997). This concept corresponds with recent neurophysiological findings that support the assumption that the brain uses neural representations of space organized in non-retinal, body-centred and/or world-centred coordinates. Parietal cortex seems to provide such a representation of space by transforming the multisensory afferent input into a representation organized in non-retinal coordinates (Andersen 1995; Battaglini *et al.* 1997; Thier and Andersen 1997). The compensatory effects on spatial neglect that had been observed with vestibular (Rubens 1985), optokinetic (Pizzamiglio *et al.* 1990), and neck-proprioceptive stimulation (Karnath *et al.* 1993) are in accordance with the view that spatial neglect might be due to an altered representation of body-centred space. The findings demonstrate that the brain uses the input from these afferent channels to elaborate a unitary representation of egocentric space. In neglect patients, the coordinate transformation seems to work with a systematic error resulting in a deviation of the spatial reference frame to the ipsilesional side (Karnath 1994*a*, 1997).

Kinsbourne (1977, 1987) has proposed an alternative theory. He has assumed an attentional bias with excessive orienting towards the ipsilesional side in patients with spatial neglect due to an imbalance in lateral orienting tendencies. Kinsbourne has argued that attention is directed along the vector resultant from the interaction of paired opponent processors that are controlled by the right and left hemispheres, respectively, each of which directs attention towards the opposite end of a visual display. Activation imbalance in neglect patients biases the vector of attentional orienting and, therefore, elicits ipsilesional shifts of attention and gaze. A crucial prediction of this model is that orienting is not intact within either hemispace in neglect. Rather, a lateral gradient of attention sweeps across both hemispaces, such that attention is always biased into the ipsilesional direction. The gradient is probabilistic and characterizes the probability of, for example, detecting a target. Following the gradient, the probability to detect a target is very low on the extreme contralesional side and increases along the horizontal axis toward the ipsilesional side. According to Kinsbourne (1993), the lateral gradient applies to visual exploration, covert shifting of attention as well as overt gaze deviation.

Within the context of their 'premotor theory', Rizzolatti and co-workers (1985; Rizzolatti and Berti 1990) have also argued for a gradient of severity across the visual field in patients with neglect. They have suggested that neglect results from a lesion of higher order maps or representations of space that are responsible for the organization of motor acts in particular space sectors. The authors have assumed that, in patients with neglect, the whole visual field is affected but with a gradient of severity ranging from a maximum in the extreme contralesional hemifield to a minimum in the extreme ipsilesional field (Rizzolatti et al. 1985). In addition, they have assumed that lesions of those areas leading to neglect liberate competitive actions from the inhibition normally exerted by these areas (Rizzolatti and Berti 1990). The resulting abnormal activation produces additional imbalance in favour of ipsilesional space sectors.

Although based on different concepts, both Kinsbourne's and Rizzolatti's explanations assume that the left as well as the right hemispace are affected in spatial neglect following a gradient ranging from a maximum in the extreme contralesional hemifield to a minimum in the extreme ipsilesional field. The pattern of space exploration that follows such a *gradient* is different from the pattern which should result from a *deviated* representation of egocentric space. Studying the patients' exploratory behaviour in space thus should help to discriminate between the different hypotheses. According to the gradient model, a continuous increase of exploration along the horizontal axis is expected with a minimum on the extreme contralesional side and a maximum on the extreme ipsilesional side (Fig. 3.1). In contrast, the deviation model proposes a displacement of the whole field of exploration toward the ipsilesional side. As in healthy subjects, no lateral gradient should underlie exploration of space (Fig. 3.1).

One way to study space exploration in its natural course is the observation of subjects' spontaneous eye movements. When we explore space, for example, in searching for an object that we expect somewhere in the environment, we usually scan the scene by shifting gaze to various locations in both hemispaces.

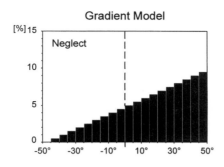

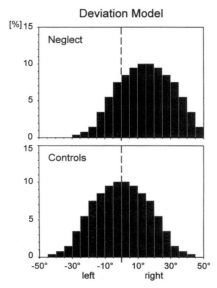

Fig. 3.1 Expected distribution of space exploration (%) along the horizontal axis following two different hypotheses on spatial neglect. According to the gradient model (*top*), a continuous increase of exploration along the horizontal axis is expected with a minimum on the extreme contralesional side and a maximum on the extreme ipsilesional side. In contrast, the deviation model (*middle*) proposes a displacement of the whole field of exploration toward the ipsilesional side. As in controls (*bottom*), no lateral gradient should underlie the patients' exploration of space.

In contrast, eye movement recordings in right brain-damaged patients with neglect show that these patients differ from controls by predominantly fixating on the right side of presented stimuli during visual searching (Chédru *et al.* 1973; Johnston and Diller 1986), looking at different stimuli (Ishiai *et al.* 1987; Rizzo and Hurtig 1992; Jahnke *et al.* 1995; Walker *et al.* 1996), text reading (Karnath and Huber 1992) or scanning while verbally describing simple drawings (Karnath 1994*b*).

All these studies presented visual stimuli while recording exploratory eye movements. The patients' location of gaze was evoked by the visual character-istics of the stimuli. Spatial arrangement and individual significance of stimuli influenced patients' overt orienting of attention, the duration of fixation at different spatial locations, the amplitudes of saccades when shifting gaze from one aspect of the scene or stimulus to another, etc. In other words, subjects directed their gaze to locations that, in part, directly resulted from the experimental set up.

Such *external* ('stimulus-driven') influences on the subject's exploratory behaviour might be disturbing or might even be misleading when the pattern of ocular exploration should serve to identify the *internal* representation of egocentric space in these subjects. Therefore, spontaneous visual search should be investigated under a condition in which no visual stimulus can attract the subject's attention and thus influence the spatial distribution of exploration from outside. A technique which serves for this purpose is the observation of exploratory eye movements while searching for a non-existent target in complete darkness. This can be achieved by transiently presenting a spot of light in a darkened room. After extinguishing the spot, subjects are asked to search for the 'new location' of the spot, which is stated to be located 'somewhere' in the whole room. In fact, the spot is not presented and the subjects thus search in complete darkness with their eye movements being recorded at the same time. It can be assumed that the part of outer space subjects spontaneously explore under this condition is a direct function of the subject's representation of egocentric space. The subject tries to find the (non-existent) target in the 'whole room', i.e. within that part of space which is neurally represented and, of course, is reachable by moving the eyes.

With this technique, Hornak (1992) has recorded eye movements in neglect patients between $\pm 35°$ of azimuth. This area of registration, however, turned out to be too narrow to plot the whole distribution of visual search in patients with neglect from the far left to the far right side. Most of the right part was not recorded and the study did not reveal how the distribution continues further toward the right. The latter, however, is decisive in deciding whether the patients' exploratory eye movements show a deviated but symmetrical distribution or whether they follow a lateral gradient across both hemispaces. According to the gradient model, one would expect a further increase of exploration, while the deviation model predicts a decrease further toward the right (see Fig. 3.1).

The same problem characterizes a recent study by Behrmann *et al.* (1997). In light, the authors recorded eye movements during visual search in an array of randomly presented letters that had a horizontal extent of only $\pm 25°$. Their study could not decide about the distribution of eye movements beyond these narrow boundaries, i.e. in particular beyond $+25°$ further toward the right. Nevertheless, both Hornak's and Behrmann *et al.*'s studies found a distribution with a single peak at about 15–18° on the right side with clearly decreasing frequencies toward the left of this maximum and, at least, a tendency for a decrease (i.e. as far as the area of registration allowed to follow eye movements) also toward the right of this maximum.

Our own studies (Karnath and Fetter 1995; Karnath *et al.* 1996) have recorded exploratory eye movements up to ±50° which have allowed us to observe and plot the whole distribution of visual search along the horizontal axis. Interestingly, visual search of neglect patients showed no skewed distribution of ocular exploration with a maximum on the ipsilesional right side and a minimum on the contralesional left. Exploratory eye movements rather showed a symmetrical, bell-shaped distribution with a maximum around 15° right of the body's midsagittal plane in clear contrast to the prediction of the gradient model but in full accordance with the deviation model.

To strengthen this conclusion, we aimed to record exploratory eye movements in a larger group of neglect patients and over a longer period of time per subject than in our previous studies. In contrast to the short intervals of registration used in these studies, a dense scan pattern should be obtained in each subject to plot a more stable distribution of exploratory eye movements along the horizontal axis. We compared a group of patients with neglect,[1] patients with right brain damage but no neglect (RH-group),[1] and neurological patients without brain damage (NBD-group).[1] Subjects were seated in a spherical cabin with a fixed head/body position and, as described above, were asked to search for the location of a (non-existent) spot which was stated to be located 'somewhere' in the darkened room. Eye movements were recorded within the next 30–40 s. Subsequently, the laser spot was presented at a random location to feign the existence of a real target. The procedure was repeated three times so that the whole duration of registration was between 1.5 and 2 min per subject with a sampling rate of 100 Hz.

The spatial distribution of the subjects' exploratory eye movements is illustrated in Fig. 3.2. Presented is the average percentage of exploration time in discrete five-degree sectors along the horizontal axis. The control groups showed a symmetrical, bell-shaped distribution of exploratory eye movements along the horizontal axis. They explored space with eye movements leading up to ~45° to the left and to the right of their sagittal midplane. Ocular exploration of patients with neglect was also symmetrical and bell-shaped but—compared to both control groups—deviated toward the right. The maximum of exploration lay between +10° and +20° right of their body's sagittal midplane, while it lay around 0° in both control groups.

The results allow us to conclude that neglect patients' exploratory eye movements during visual search in the dark show a bell-shaped distribution with a clear maximum around 15° right of the objective position of the body's midsagittal plane. Ocular exploration decreases symmetrically toward the left *as well as* toward the right side of this maximum. This finding clearly argues against a lateral gradient underlying the bias of space exploration in patients with neglect. The patients did not orient their gaze toward the extreme right

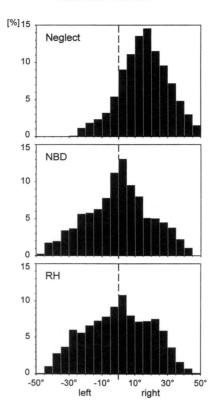

Fig. 3.2 Distribution of ocular space exploration (%) along the horizontal axis in a group of five patients with neglect (*top*), in six non-brain-damaged neurological patients (*NBD*) (*middle*) and in a group of five patients with unilateral right hemispheric lesions but without neglect (*RH*) (*bottom*). 0° = position of subjects' head/body midsagittal plane.

and spent most of the time searching at that location in space. The maximum of exploration rather lay 'only' ~15° right of the peak obtained in controls. Spontaneous visual search clearly decreased toward more eccentric positions on the right.

3.3 Is the ipsilesional deviation due to a 'rotation' or a 'translation' of the egocentric reference frame?

The above findings argue for a deviation of egocentric space representation underlying neglect patients' exploration of space. However, they leave open the actual *gestalt* of the deviated representation. Different hypotheses have been put forward (see Fig. 3.3A). One suggestion has been a *rotation* of the whole

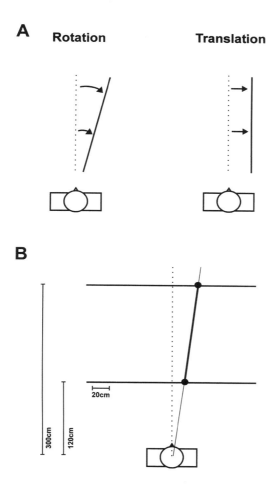

Fig. 3.3 (A) Models of disturbed neural representation of space in spatial neglect leading to a rotation (*left*) of the whole egocentric reference frame around the earth-vertical body axis to the ipsilesional side or to a translation (*right*) of the reference system toward the side of the lesion. The subject's body orientation is illustrated as seen from above; the body is represented by a rectangle, the head by a circle. The *dotted line* represents the body's physical midsagittal plane in the front half-space. The *bold line* illustrates the subjectively perceived orientation of the body's midsagittal plane according to the two different hypotheses. (B) Obtained perception of subjective body orientation in four patients with neglect. The subjects' task was to direct an LED to the position which they felt lay exactly 'straight ahead' of their bodies' midsagittal plane. In order to distinguish between the rotation vs. translation hypotheses, the LED was presented at two different distances by using two parallel guide rails located 120 cm and 300 cm from the subjects at eye level. *Filled circles* indicate average 'straight ahead' judgements measured at the two spatial distances away from the patients' body. The *bold line* connecting the circles illustrates the subjectively perceived orientation of the body's midsagittal plane; its orientation was determined by graphically connecting the two 'straight ahead' positions obtained at the two different spatial distances from the body. The resulting line was then graphically elongated up to the level of the subjects' physical body position.

egocentric reference frame around the earth-vertical body axis toward the ipsilesional side (Ventre *et al.* 1984; Karnath *et al.* 1993), while another has been a *translation* of the whole reference system toward the side of the lesion (Vallar *et al.* 1995).

To distinguish between both hypotheses, we measured neglect patients' perception of subjective body orientation at two different distances away from the subject's body. In complete darkness, a red light emitting diode (LED) was randomly presented either on the left or on the right side of the patients' head/body midsagittal plane. (The area of LED presentation ranged from $-40°$ to $-20°$ on the left or from $+20°$ to $+40°$ on the right side of the head/body midsagittal plane.) The LED could be moved on two parallel, horizontal guide rails located 120 cm and 300 cm from the subjects (see Fig. 3.3B). Subjects sat upright in an armchair, head and body axes were aligned. The subjects' task was to verbally direct the LED to the position which they felt lay exactly 'straight ahead' of their bodies' midsagittal plane. These 'straight ahead' adjustments were conducted at each distance, i.e. 120 cm and 300 cm, from the subjects (see Fig. 3.3B), in an alternating order. Altogether 16 trials of 'straight ahead' adjustments were conducted, eight at each distance. 'Straight ahead' positions were determined for both distances by averaging the respective eight position judgements.

We compared a group of patients with neglect,[2] patients with right brain damage but no neglect (RBD-group),[2] and neurological patients without brain damage (NC-group).[2] Subjective 'straight ahead' judgements of the control groups were close to the objective position of midsagittal plane at both distances from the subjects at eye level. The RBD-group directed the LED to an average position of -2.5 cm (SD 5.0); the NC-group to an average position of $+2.0$ cm (SD 8.3). Significantly different from controls, neglect patients perceived their bodies as being oriented toward the ipsilesional side. Figure 3.3B shows that this egocentric deviation of body representation was clearly due to a *rotation* around the earth-vertical body axis to the ipsilesional side, rather than a translation of the reference system to that side; the ipsilesional displacement of LED position increased linearly with the distance from the subjects.

To explore any possible distortions of perceived space in the vertical dimension, the same procedure for determining 'straight ahead' perception was carried out at two further elevations, i.e. 30 cm above and 30 cm below the individual eye level of the subject. (In fact, the order of measuring 'straight ahead' position at the three spatial levels was randomized between the subjects.) Subjective 'straight ahead' judgements of the controls were again closely scattered around the objective body position. Elevation and distance had no significant effect on their judgements; no relevant differences were observed comparing the judgements at the three different elevations and in the two different distances from the subjects' body. The RBD-group directed the LED to a position of -3.2 cm (SD 7.2) averaged over all six spatial positions; the NC-group to an average position of $+0.4$ cm (SD 7.9) in all six positions.

Figure 3.4 demonstrates the results revealed for the patients with neglect at the three elevations. In contrast to controls, neglect patients showed a marked disparity of subjective and objective body orientation. At all three elevations this egocentric deviation of body representation was due to a rotation around the earth-vertical body axis to the ipsilesional right side rather than a translation of the reference system to that side.

This finding contrasts with the conclusions (not necessarily with the results) drawn from a recent study that used an auditory localization task to determine the subjective midsagittal plane (Vallar *et al.* 1995). The authors found a displacement to the ipsilesional right in the front half-space but also in the back half-space. They interpreted their results in favour of a translation of the whole egocentric coordinate system to the patients' ipsilesional side. Their results,

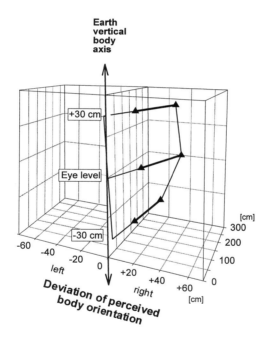

Fig. 3.4 Neglect patients' perception of subjective body orientation in 3-D space. The vertical plane in the centre represents the patients' physical midsagittal plane in the front half-space. *Filled triangles* indicate average 'straight ahead' judgements measured at two spatial distances (120 cm and 300 cm) away from the subject's body. The three *bold lines* connecting the triangles illustrate the subjectively perceived orientation of the body's midsagittal plane in 3-D space as determined at three different elevations (eye level, 30 cm above and 30 cm below eye level). Orientations of the bold lines were determined by graphically connecting the two 'straight ahead' positions obtained at the two different spatial distances from the body. The resulting lines were elongated up to the level of the subjects' physical body position. Illustrated are the average orientations obtained in the patients with neglect.

together with those presently reported, could indicate that the egocentric reference frame is affected differentially in neglect patients, in that it is rotated in the front half-space and translated in the back half-space or, alternatively, that it is rotated to the ipsilesional side in both the front and the back half-space.

However, it is more plausible that the findings of Vallar and co-workers had an origin different from a distortion of space representation. A 'prior entry' advantage for ipsilesional inputs, as has recently been found in patients with parietal lesions and extinction (Rorden *et al.* 1997), could readily explain the observations in that study. Since one of the most important cues for auditory localization is given by interaural time difference, any pathological 'prior entry' for inputs to the ipsilesional ear could produce the auditory mislocation in both front and back half-space.

A further possible explanation of Vallar *et al.*'s results is the normal influence of eye position on auditory lateralization (Lewald and Ehrenstein 1996). When Vallar *et al.*'s subjects had to decide whether the position of the sound source was to the left or to the right of their sagittal midplane, eye position was not restricted. Subjects were free to move their eyes during the experiment. However, various studies (see above) have shown that spontaneous gaze direction in neglect patients is not balanced in both hemispaces but rather demonstrates a characteristic deviation toward the ipsilesional side. This spontaneous bias of eye position could well account for the 'translated' subjective auditory median plane to the ipsilesional side found by Vallar and co-workers in their patients with neglect. As was demonstrated by Lewald and Ehrenstein (1996) in healthy subjects, the subjective auditory median plane shifts with the spatial direction of gaze position. Thus, a spontaneous bias of eye position toward the ipsilesional side in patients with neglect would *physiologically* lead to a shift of their auditory median plane in the same direction (as it is the case in healthy subjects with their gaze directed to that side).

3.4 Does the ipsilesional deviation of egocentric space representation lead to a bias of goal-directed arm movements in the same direction?

To study this question, we have investigated reaching for targets in patients with acute spatial neglect (Karnath *et al.* 1997). We asked whether or not patients who show a severe bias of space exploration toward the ipsilesional side by limb or eye movements, demonstrate a comparable bias in goal-directed arm movements in pointing to targets in peripersonal space. Using an opto-electronic 3-D camera system, the study examined unrestrained, 3-D arm movements during pointing to targets positioned either in the centre or the left and right hemispace. Spatial hand kinematics of five consecutively admitted patients with acute neglect were compared to those of five patients with right hemispheric lesions without neglect and of six non-brain-damaged subjects. Subjects sat in front of a table and performed unrestricted pointing movements with their right hand to three LEDs that lit up in a random order. The LEDs were positioned in front of the subjects at eye level and arranged in a straight line. The central LED was aligned to each subject's sagittal head/trunk midplane, the two other LED's were located in the left and the right hemispace.

All patients were able to point to these targets. In light as well as in darkness, i.e. with or without visual feed-back about actual hand position, terminal accuracy of pointing did not differ between patients with neglect and controls along the horizontal, vertical and anterior–posterior axis. Even more interesting, we found no characteristic differences between the three groups of subjects when actual finger position *during* the pointing movements were compared by plotting them on a straightline hand path between start and target (Fig. 3.5). In particular, the patients with neglect showed no direction-specific deviation of their trajectories toward the ipsilesional, right side. Goal-directed arm movements to single targets in peripersonal space thus seem to be unaffected by the deviated egocentric representation of space that underlies the severe bias of ocular space exploration in these patients.

3.5 Conclusions

The observations reported in this article speak for an altered representation of space associated with the clinical manifestation of 'spatial neglect'. The distribution of the patients' exploratory eye movements during visual search in the dark clearly argues against a lateral gradient (Kinsbourne 1993; Rizzolatti *et al.* 1985) underlying the bias of space exploration in these patients. They rather favour a disturbed input transformation that leads to an ipsilesional deviation of space representation. The ipsilesional deviation causes the patients' contralesional neglect when orienting in space or searching in the surround. Figure 3.6 presents a sketch of the consequences following from this model of altered space representation. It considers that the egocentric deviation is due to a rotation around the earth-vertical body axis to the ipsilesional side rather than a translation to that side.

The kinematic analysis of goal-directed arm movements in patients with acute neglect support the view of dissociated functions in the human superior and inferior parietal lobule. It demonstrates that patients with neglect showing a severe bias of space exploration toward the ipsilesional side, do not exhibit a comparable bias of their hand trajectories when pointing to targets in peripersonal space. The failure to orient toward and to explore the contralesional part of space appear to be distinct from those deficits observed once an object of interest has been located and releases reaching.

The findings argue that (1) *exploratory* and (2) *goal-directed* behaviour do not share the same neural control mechanism. They suggest that neural representation of egocentric space in the inferior parietal lobule serves as a matrix for spatial exploration and for orienting in space but not for visuomotor processes involved in reaching for objects. Disturbances of such processes

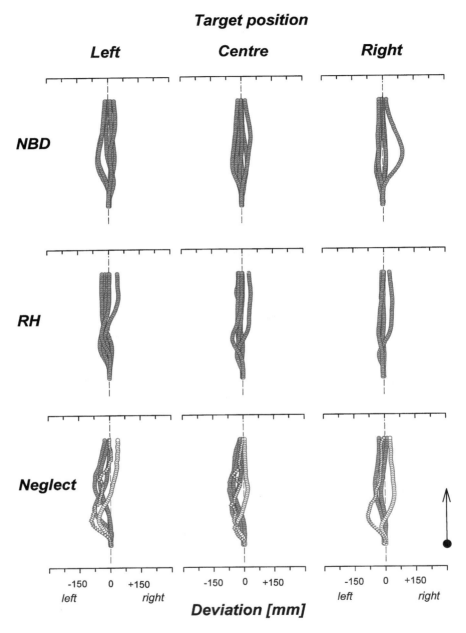

Fig. 3.5 Averaged deviation trajectories along the horizontal axis during pointing in complete darkness. A comparison was made of three groups of subjects: patients with unilateral right hemispheric lesions and neglect, patients with unilateral right hemispheric lesions but no neglect (*RH*) and non-brain-damaged subjects (*NBD*). Subjects

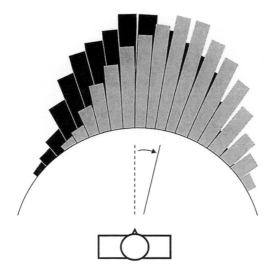

Fig. 3.6 Sketch of the ipsilesional (rightward) deviation of egocentric space representation in patients with spatial neglect. The subject's body orientation is illustrated as seen from above; the body is represented by a rectangle, the head by a circle. The *dashed line* symbolizes the egocentric coordinate system (horizontal dimension) in healthy subjects and the *black histogram* their ocular exploration of space (in %) along the horizontal dimension. The *continuous line* symbolizes the egocentric coordinate system (horizontal dimension) in patients with neglect. It is rotated around the earth-vertical body axis toward the ipsilesional, right side. The *grey histogram* showes the patients' ocular exploration of space along the horizontal dimension. It is suggested that such an ipsilesional deviation of egocentric space representation underlies the bias of space exploration in these patients and their contralesional neglect when orienting in space or searching in the surround.

rather seem to be characteristic for patients with more superior parietal lobe lesions and optic ataxia.

Acknowledgements

This work was supported by grants from the Deutsche Forschungsgemein-schaft and the Bundesministerium für Bildung, Wissenschaft, Forschung und

performed unrestricted pointing movements with their right hand to three LEDs that lit up in a random order. The central LED was aligned to each subject's sagittal head/ trunk midplane (*Centre*), the two other LEDs were located in the left (*Left*) and the right (*Right*) hemispace. A positive value indicates that hand position was right of a straightline path (connecting start and target). A negative value indicates a hand position left of it. Each deviation trajectory represents the average of seven individual trials performed by one subject. *Open symbols* characterize those two neglect patients with the most severe neglect symptoms. (From Karnath *et al*. 1997, p. 441.)

Technologie. I wish to thank Heinke Dick, Susanne Ferber, Michael Fetter, Peter Heidrich and Jürgen Konczak for their collaboration. I am also grateful to Johannes Dichgans, David Milner and Peter Thier for their helpful discussion and comments on the manuscript.

Endnotes

[1] Five patients with neglect were examined (median age = 56 years) in this study of subjects' exploratory eye movements. All five patients suffered from right-sided parietal lobe lesions. Clinical and demographic variables, as well as the neuropsychological examination of three of the five patients, were as previously described (Karnath et al. 1996). The additional two patients with neglect suffered an infarct 8 and 12 days before the examination. CT-scans showed a small hypodense area located in the right parietal cortex in one case and a hypodensity extending from the right temporal cortex to the parieto-occipital junction in the other case.

Five patients with unilateral right brain-damage served as a control group (median age = 59 years). In three of the patients, the lesions were due to infarcts affecting the fronto-temporal region. One patient suffered a basal ganglia hemorrhage and one a temporal lesion due to surgery of a grade IV glioma. None of the five patients showed any signs of neglect. The median time since lesion was 11 days. None of the patients with or without neglect had oculomotor palsies or visual field defects. As an additional control group, five neurological patients without brain damage were examined (median age = 53 years).

[2] Four patients with neglect were examined (median age = 58 years) in this study of subjects' perception of subjective body orientation. All patients suffered from right hemispheric lesions documented by CT and/or MRI scans. In three of the patients, the lesions were due to infarcts affecting the fronto-parietal region in two cases and the temporo-parietal region in one case. The fourth patient suffered a temporo-parietal lesion due to surgery of a grade IV glioma. Time since lesions ranged between 7 and 135 days (median = 12 days). None of the patients had visual field defects as assessed by Goldmann perimetry. Neuropsychological examination included confrontation testing, copying, line bisection, letter cancellation, picture comparison, and the backing tray task. At the time the experiment was conducted, two patients showed severe and two patients moderate left-sided neglect.

The performance of the four patients with neglect was compared with a group of five right brain-damaged patients without any clinical signs of spatial neglect or hemianopia, aged from 26 to 71 years (median = 59). One patient suffered from a grade II oligo-astrocytoma in the right basal ganglia and thalamus. Two patients had a temporal, one other a temporo-parietal lesion due to surgery on a grade IV glioma. One patient sustained an infarct in the right parieto-occipital region. Median time since lesion was 7.5 weeks. As an additional control group, five neurological patients without brain damage aged from 52 to 76 years (median = 60) were examined.

References

Andersen, R. A. (1995). Encoding of intention and spatial location in the posterior parietal cortex. *Cerebral Cortex*, **5**, 457–69.

Battaglini, P.-P., Galletti, C., and Fattori, P. (1997). Neuronal coding of visual space in the posterior parietal cortex. In *Parietal Lobe Contributions to Orientation in 3D Space* (ed. P. Thier and H.-O. Karnath), pp. 539–53. Springer, Heidelberg.

Behrmann, M., Watt, S., Black, S. E., and Barton, J. J. S. (1997). Impaired visual search in patients with unilateral neglect: an oculographic analysis. *Neuropsychologia* **35**, 1445 – 58.

Chédru, F., Leblanc, M., and Lhermitte, F. (1973). Visual searching in normal and brain damaged subjects: contribution to the study of unilateral inattention. *Cortex*, **9**, 94–111.

Halligan, P. W. and Marshall, J. C. (ed.) (1994). *Spatial Neglect: Position Papers on Theory and Practice*. Lawrence Erlbaum, Hillsdale.

Hornak, J. (1992). Ocular exploration in the dark by patients with visual neglect. *Neuropsychologia*, **30**, 547–52.

Ishiai, S., Furukawa, T., and Tsukagoshi, H. (1987). Eye-fixation patterns in homonymous hemianopia and unilateral spatial neglect. *Neuropsychologia*, **25**, 675–9.

Jahnke, M. T., Denzler, P. Liebelt, B., Reichert, H., and Mauritz, K.-H. (1995). Eye movements and fixation characteristics in perception of stationary scenes: normal subjects as compared to patients with visual neglect or hemianopia. *European Journal of Neurology*, **2**, 275–95.

Johnston, C. W. and Diller, L. (1986). Exploratory eye movements and visual hemineglect. *Journal of Clinical and Experimental Neuropsychology*, **8**, 93–101.

Karnath, H.-O. (1994*a*). Disturbed coordinate transformation in the neural representation of space as the crucial mechanism leading to neglect. In *Spatial Neglect: Position Papers on Theory and Practice* (ed. P. W. Halligan and J. C. Marshall), pp. 147–50. Lawrence Erlbaum, Hillsdale.

Karnath, H.-O. (1994*b*). Spatial limitation of eye movements during ocular exploration of simple line drawings in neglect syndrome. *Cortex*, **30**, 319–30.

Karnath, H.-O. (1997). Neural encoding of space in egocentric coordinates? Evidence for and limits of a hypothesis derived from patients with parietal lesions and neglect. In *Parietal Lobe Contributions to Orientation in 3D Space* (ed. P. Thier and H.-O. Karnath), pp. 497–520. Springer, Heidelberg.

Karnath, H.-O. and Huber, W. (1992). Abnormal eye movement behaviour during text reading in neglect syndrome: a case study. *Neuropsychologia*, **30**, 593–8.

Karnath, H.-O. and Fetter, M. (1995). Ocular space exploration in the dark and its relation to subjective and objective body orientation in neglect patients with parietal lesions. *Neuropsychologia*, **33**, 371–7.

Karnath, H.-O., Christ, K., and Hartje, W. (1993). Decrease of contralateral neglect by neck muscle vibration and spatial orientation of trunk midline. *Brain*, **116**, 383–96.

Karnath, H.-O., Fetter, M., and Dichgans, J. (1996). Ocular exploration of space as a function of neck proprioceptive and vestibular input—observations in normal subjects and patients with spatial neglect after parietal lesions. *Experimental Brain Research*, **109**, 333–42.

Karnath, H.-O., Dick, H., and Konczak, J. (1997). Kinematics of goal-directed arm movements in neglect: control of hand in space. *Neuropsychologia*, **35**, 435–44.

Kinsbourne, M. (1977). Hemi-neglect and hemisphere rivalry. *Adv. Neurol.*, **18**, 41–9.

Kinsbourne, M. (1987). Mechanisms of unilateral neglect. In *Neurophysiological and Neuropsychological Aspects of Spatial Neglect* (ed. M. Jeannerod), pp. 69–86. North-Holland, Amsterdam.

Kinsbourne, M. (1993). Orientational bias model of unilateral neglect: evidence from attentional gradients within hemispace. In *Unilateral Neglect: Clinical and Experimental Studies* (ed. I. H. Robertson and J. C. Marshall), pp. 63–86. Lawrence Erlbaum, Hillsdale.

Lewald, J. and Ehrenstein, W. H. (1996). The effect of eye position on auditory lateralization. *Experimental Brain Research*, **108**, 473–85.

Milner, A. D. and Goodale, M. A. (1995). *The Visual Brain in Action*. Oxford University Press, Oxford.

Perenin, M.-T. (1997). Optic ataxia and unilateral neglect: clinical evidence for dissociable spatial functions in posterior parietal cortex. In *Parietal Lobe Contributions to Orientation in 3D Space* (ed. P. Thier and H.-O. Karnath), pp. 289–308. Springer, Heidelberg.

Pizzamiglio, L., Frasca, R., Guariglia, C., Incoccia, C., and Antonucci, G. (1990). Effect of optokinetic stimulation in patients with visual neglect. *Cortex*, **26**, 535–40.

Rizzo, M. and Hurtig, R. (1992). Visual search in hemineglect: what stirs idle eyes? *Clin. Vision Sci.*, **7**, 39–52.

Rizzolatti, G. and Berti, A. (1990). Neglect as a neural representation deficit. *Rev. Neurol. (Paris)*, **146**, 626–34.

Rizzolatti, G., Gentilucci, M., and Matelli, M. (1985). Selective spatial attention: one center, one circuit or many circuits? In *Attention and Performance XI* (ed. M. I. Posner and O. S. M. Marin), pp. 251–265. Lawrence Erlbaum, Hillsdale.

Rorden, C., Mattingley, J. B., Karnath, H.-O., and Driver, J. (1997). Visual extinction and prior entry: impaired perception of temporal order with intact motion perception after unilateral parietal damage. *Neuropsychologia*, **35**, 421–33.

Rubens, A. B. (1985). Caloric stimulation and unilateral visual neglect. *Neurology*, **35**, 1019–24.

Thier, P. and Andersen, R. A. (1997). Multiple parietal 'eyefields': insights from electrical microstimulation. In *Parietal Lobe Contributions to Orientation in 3D Space* (ed. P. Thier and H.-O. Karnath), pp. 95–108. Springer, Heidelberg.

Vallar, G. and Perani, D. (1986). The anatomy of unilateral neglect after right-hemisphere stroke lesions. A clinical/CT-scan correlation study in man. *Neuropsychologia*, **24**, 609–22.

Vallar, G., Guariglia, C., Nico, D., and Bisiach, E. (1995). Spatial hemineglect in back space. *Brain*, **118**, 467–72.

Ventre, J., Flandrin, J. M., and Jeannerod, M. (1984). In search for the egocentric reference. A neurophysiological hypothesis. *Neuropsychologia*, **22**, 797–806.

Walker, R., Findlay, J. M., Young, A. W., and Lincoln, N. B. (1996). Saccadic eye movements in object-based neglect. *Cogn. Neuropsychol.*, **13**, 569–615.

4

Egocentric and object-based visual neglect

Jon Driver

4.1 Introduction

Patients with unilateral neglect characteristically fail to acknowledge or to respond appropriately to information towards their contralesional side, even though initial afferent pathways for such information can be demonstrably intact (see Chapters 2, 3, 7 and 23; Bisiach & Vallar 1988; Driver 1998; Robertson & Marshall 1993). Figure 4.1 provides an example of severe left visual neglect in a copying task. The association of such neglect with lesions centred on the right supramarginal gyrus, in the inferior parietal lobule (see Chapter 2, Fig. 2.1), provides one of the classic links between spatial cognition and the parietal lobe. However, it should be noted that while the area of lesion-overlap across most neglect patients certainly does fall within the right inferior parietal region, each individual case typically has quite extensive damage beyond this area as well, including white-matter. Thus, a rather diffuse network of areas will be impaired in most neglect patients. Correspondingly, recent neuropsychological studies suggest that neglect is a multi-component syndrome, with each neglect patient suffering from a number of problems in accordance with their own particular diffuse brain damage (e.g. Rafal 1994; Thier & Karnath 1997; Mattingley *et al*. 1998).

Nevertheless, there are many similarities across cases, with the common denominator being that information towards the contralesional side (i.e. the left) invariably suffers as a result of the unilateral lesion. A recurrent theme in recent research has been to address the spatial coordinates in which such left neglect might arise; for instance, does the impairment apply to inputs just on the left of the retina, or on the left of the head, of the trunk, of particular limbs, or even towards the left side of individual external objects? (For a review see Bisiach 1997; for some illustrative examples see Driver & Halligan 1991; Karnath *et al*. 1991; Ladavas 1987). Effects due to *all* of these potential frames-of-reference have now been documented for visual neglect, although the results often reflect a mixed influence (e.g. typically both retino-centric *and* trunk-centric position matter, rather than solely one frame of reference). Some authors argue that this conjoint influence of several coordinate frames should be enshrined as a general principle of parietal neglect (see Pouget & Sejnowsji, Chapter 7). Our own view is that while this may be correct, it seems equally

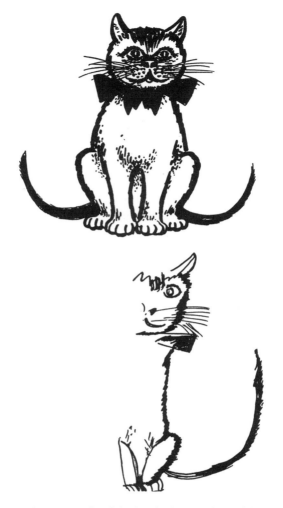

Fig. 4.1 Copying performance of a right-hemisphere patient with severe left neglect—case PP, studied by Marshall & Halligan (1989, and many subsequent studies) and also by Driver & Halligan (1991). (*Top*), the original to be copied; (*bottom*), the patient's free-vision copy.

possible that an influence of multiple coordinate might arise simply because multiple brain systems are usually damaged by the diffuse lesion. If so, more selective lesions might isolate more specific spatial coordinates. Studying the effects of small, reversible unilateral lesions within particular parietal areas of the monkey (Anderson *et al*. 1997) may be particularly revealing on this issue.

The present review focuses on apparent cases of 'object-centred' visual neglect, in patients with the prototypical, large lesion centred on the right-inferior parietal lobule after middle cerebral artery infarction. As we shall see, the term 'object-centred' has been used in the literature with a variety of meanings, and it is important to distinguish these. Perhaps the most famous use of the term was by David Marr (1982), when addressing the problem of how a shape might be recognized as the same across different viewpoints, within his computational theory of vision. A simplified 2-D version of this general shape-recognition problem is shown in Fig. 4.2. The isosceles triangles in this figure have the same shape, but project very different patterns on the retina, due to their different tilts, raising the problem of how their common shape can be coded. Note, however, that relative to their intrinsic axes of symmetry and elongation (dotted lines in Fig. 4.2), the shapes have exactly the same layout. If described relative to this intrinsic axis, rather than in retinal or page-based coordinates, each triangle would thus receive the same description, suggesting that axis-based shape descriptions could help to solve the problem of recognizing shapes across different views. This axis-based idea is fairly old, going back at least to Attneave (1968). Marr's contribution was mainly in appreciating its power, and extending it to 3-D. He also introduced the 'object-centred' terminology for describing such axis-based shape descriptions, on the grounds that intrinsic properties of the external objects (i.e. their elongation and/or symmetry) anchor the coordinate frame. However, as we shall see later, several aspects of such axis-based shape descriptions might still be determined in a purely egocentric manner (in particular, which side of the object's intrinsic axis of elongation or symmetry should be treated as left, and which as right). Moreover, only a few of the putative examples of 'object-centred' neglect in the neuropsychological literature actually refer to the axis-based idea, which motivated Marr's use of the object-centred term. In most cases, research on neglect has used this term in a much looser sense.

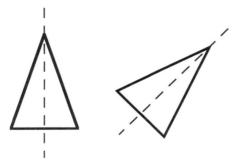

Fig. 4.2 Simplified illustration of the general problem of recognizing shapes as the same across different views. The two isosceles triangles are identical, but project different retinal images. Relative to their intrinsic axes of elongation and symmetry (*dashed lines*) they retain exactly the same layout, despite the different tilts.

4.2 Space-based versus object-based models of *normal* attention

My own entry into the debate about the spatial coordinates of neglect was due to a controversy in the literature on *normal* visual attention, which seemed to bear some potential relation to visual neglect. Attention is the generic term for our various abilities to process incoming sensory information selectively, so that some stimuli get processed more deeply than others even when the initial receptor activity they induce is comparable. Many researchers have argued that neglect can be thought of as a pathological bias in such attentional mechanisms towards the ipsilesional side, so that neglected contralesional stimuli are in effect treated rather like unattended stimuli in normals (e.g. Posner *et al.* 1984; Heilman *et al.* 1985; Kinsbourne 1993; Driver & Mattingley 1995). Length constraints preclude a full assessment of this argument here (see Driver 1994, 1998; Driver *et al.* 1997), though two points can be made. First, the long-running debate over whether neglect should best be considered as a deficit in spatial attention or in spatial representation (see Bisiach 1993) seems likely to concern a false dichotomy, since deficient attention would inevitably have representational consequences, and vice versa. Second, it is perhaps best to judge the fruitfulness of the analogy between neglect and normal attention in terms of the concrete research that it motivates, rather than on philosophical grounds alone.

The last decade has seen a major dispute within the *normal* attention literature over whether visual attention operates in a space-based or an object-based manner. On strictly spatial accounts, attention would operate rather like a 'spotlight' highlighting particular regions of the visual field (e.g. Posner 1980). On object-based accounts, the visual scene would first be segmented by Gestalt principles into those regions that are likely to correspond to separate objects, with attention then being directed to individual candidate objects (see Egly *et al.* 1994; Lavie & Driver 1996; Driver & Baylis 1998, for reviews). The space-based versus object-based distinction may be clarified by the example of eye-movements. These can only operate in a strictly spatial, spotlight-like manner, since the fovea can be moved around at will, but cannot adopt different 'shapes' (since it is anatomically fixed in extent). However, it is possible that internal, covert attention might adopt quite different distributions depending on which object is relevant in the current scene, in a way that mere saccades, or shifting of a spotlight, could not allow. For instance, all the parts of one object, whatever its shape, might be covertly attended to the exclusion of other objects. Moreover, this might be possible even when the different objects are all superimposed, or are spatially intermingled due to partial occlusion. The results of my own studies with colleagues (e.g. Driver & Baylis 1989; McLeod *et al.* 1991; Egly *et al.* 1994; Lavie & Driver 1996; Davis & Driver 1997), plus findings from many other groups (e.g. Duncan 1984; Kramer & Jacobsen 1991) strongly suggest that normal covert visual attention can indeed operate in such an object-based manner, selecting segmented objects for further processing, rather than merely unsegmented regions of space.

In the 1980s, attempts to explain neglect in terms of an impaired ability to shift or 'disengage' a mental spotlight following the lesion were highly influential (e.g. Posner *et al*. 1984). However, if the simple spotlight model was inadequate as a complete account of normal attention, as I believed, then it seemed to me that it should prove equally inadequate as an account of pathological attention in neglect. With this in mind, my colleagues and I set out to determine whether object-based factors could influence neglect, in a similar manner to their influence on normal attention.

4.3 Visual extinction and object-segmentation

One frequent concomitant of right inferior-parietal injury, and thus one common component of the neglect syndrome, is left-sided extinction. The patient can detect sensory events in either visual field when presented in isolation, but typically misses contralesional events when stimulated on both sides simultaneously (see Driver *et al*. 1997, for a recent overview of this phenomenon). Thus, the ipsilesional event is said to 'extinguish' awareness of a contralesional event that would otherwise be detected. This is often attributed to an attentional deficit, since the contralesional event apparently only suffers when it must compete for attention with an ipsilesional event. Certainly, the extinction phenomenon suggests that the lesion produces a competitive disadvantage for contralesional events with respect to ipsilesional events, rather than a total afferent loss on the contralesional side (i.e. the impairment is *relative* in nature).

Extinction seems analogous in some respects to a robust attentional limitation that is found in normal people when brief, masked displays are used to bring performance below ceiling. People are in general quite efficient at monitoring two potential sources of information simultaneously (e.g. both the left and right visual fields) for occasional target events among non-targets. However, performance typically breaks down when two targets occur simultaneously at the two sources, in which case they typically miss one of them (Ostry *et al*. 1976; Duncan 1980; Driver *et al*. 1997). Phenomenologically, it as though attention is drawn to one target at the expense of the other, whereas non-targets do not capture attention in this way. In more objective signal-detection terms, the finding is that normal people can combine a hit and a correct rejection quite efficiently, but have difficulty combining two hits within brief displays. This seems reminiscent of the extinction patient's preserved ability to report a target event on either side when presented in isolation (corresponding to a hit on the stimulated side, plus a correct rejection on the other side), versus their difficulty in detecting two concurrent targets (which requires two hits). Of course, the patient's difficulty can be apparent even with fairly long and salient events that would be trivial for a normal person to detect. Moreover, one can invariably predict which of the two events will be missed by the extinction patient (i.e. the contralesional one). Nevertheless, extinction seems like a spatially-specific, pathological exaggeration of the normal attentional limitation with two concurrent targets (see Driver *et al*. 1997).

Duncan (1984) has reported that the normal limitation only applies when the two concurrent target events involve two separate objects. He found that normals can judge two target attributes concurrently as readily as one, provided both belong to a common object. Subsequent research has supported and extended this general rule (e.g. Baylis & Driver 1993; Duncan 1993*a,b*; Lavie & Driver 1996). If extinction really does relate to the normal two-target cost, as I have proposed, then presumably it too should relate to the number of separate objects that must be judged, rather than the number of attributes. In particular, the patients' difficulty with concurrent left and right events should be reduced if those events are linked into a common object, by analogy with the normal result.

Ward *et al*. (1994) provided the first test of this idea in two right-parietal patients, and confirmed that left-sided extinction was reduced when the two concurrent events were grouped so as to suggest a single object. This general finding has since been replicated and extended in subsequent studies by several independent groups (e.g. Gilchrist *et al*. 1996; Humphreys *et al*. 1996; Mattingley *et al*. 1997). One simple example comes from Driver *et al*. (1997). They briefly presented a circular light in the left visual field, or right visual field, or one in each field concurrently (or, on catch trials, nothing in either field), with the patients' task being to report 'left', 'right', 'both' or 'none' accordingly. As expected, the patients missed the left circle only in the presence of a concurrent right circle. In further blocks of trials, the events were just as described, except that a narrow horizontal line was presented on each trial in addition, such that it connected the two circles when both were present (linking them into one 'dumb-bell' shape). Since this horizontal line was present for every trial-type in such blocks, it never indicated the appropriate response. Nevertheless, extinction was greatly reduced in this situation, with the patients now being able to detect both circles when they were concurrently present. This presumably arose because, when linked, the two circles became allies rather than competitors in the bid to attract attention, as they now belonged to a common object (the dumb-bell).

Having found that extinction is reduced when the two competing events are linked by a connecting line, one can go on to examine whether more subtle object-segmentation factors have a similar effect. For example, in Fig. 4.3A, the two black bars are segmented by normal vision as a single object that is partly occluded by the cube, due to 3-D interpretation of the 2-D image. Would this segmentation still arise in parietal extinction patients, so that less extinction would be found between the two black bars in Fig. 4.3A than for the comparison case in Fig. 4.3B? Mattingley *et al*. (1997) confirmed this to be so.

To summarize, several studies have now shown that parietal extinction can be powerfully modulated by object-segmentation factors. This fits with the

A   B

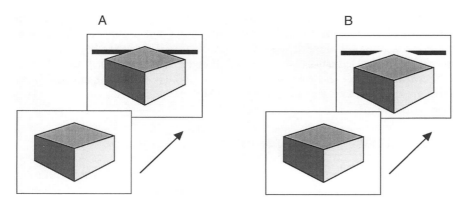

Fig. 4.3 Examples of sequences of display (each shows two successive frames, with the *arrow* indicating time) from a study of extinction by Mattingely *et al*. (1997). Every trial began with a central line-drawing of a cube (*front panels*). The patient's task was to detect the brief onset of black bars; one might appear on the right of the cube, one on the left, or a bar on each side (*back panels*). (A) The two bars appear to form a single partly occluded rod for normal observers, due to image-segmentation processes. (B) The same two black bars now appear quite separate. More extinction was found in displays like (B) than (A), confirming that image-segmentation can determine whether a left event will reach the patient's awareness.

analogy I have drawn between pathological extinction in the patients, and the attentional limit with two concurrent targets in normals, since both limitations apply to segmented objects rather than to fixed retinal positions. The results also imply that various object-segmentation processes can be preserved in the parietal patients, and appear to operate before the level at which their pathological spatial bias arises. This makes considerable sense from an anatomical perspective, given that visual object segmentation is largely thought to arise within occipital extra-striate regions (von der Heydt *et al*. 1984; Mattingley *et al*. 1997), which precede the lesioned parietal areas. (There may also be a role for more ventral areas in object segmentation, but note that these should also be intact in most parietal patients.)

   These influences of object-segmentation upon extinction provide one sense in which parietal patients' deficit might be said to be 'object-based'. Note, however, that this bears no resemblance whatsoever to Marr's use of 'object-centred' terminology involving no axis-based coding. Note also that the underlying spatial bias in extinction (which evidently favours right events over left events) might still be defined in strictly egocentric terms, whether this be retinotopic, or head-centred, etc. The conclusion to be drawn is simply that visual object-segmentation can evidently precede any such egocentric spatial bias. If one were to model neglect in terms of an imbalance or pathological gradient in some representational map(s) of space (as in Pouget & Sejnowski, Chapter 7, plus in every other simulation of neglect to date), then the pathology could be defined egocentrically regarding left versus right, yet still explain the object-based extinction. Note, however, that any such model would have to concede that the pathological gradient or imbalance did not apply to the retinal image *per se*, treated as a pixel map (cf. Pouget & Sejnowski), but instead to some segmented representation of the scene, which treats particular retinal positions quite differently depending on whether they are segmented as parts of separate objects or of a common object.

4.4 Object-based neglect, or relative egocentric position?

I turn now to consider some of the more florid aspects of neglect, and in particular cases where the patient neglects details on the left of individual objects. At first glance, the copy in Fig. 4.1 looks like an example of complete left visual-field loss, suggesting a deficit in strictly retinal coordinates. However, the patient was free to move her eyes when making this copy, so retinal position was not strictly controlled. Moreover, a pure left visual-field loss seems unlikely when one considers that an occipital patient with a strictly retinotopic hemianopia would never produce a copy of this type. Finally, it is fairly simple to demonstrate that neglect for the left side of a shape can arise even *within* the *right* visual field, using brief displays with central fixation. For instance, Fig. 4.4A shows examples of displays from an unpublished study I conducted

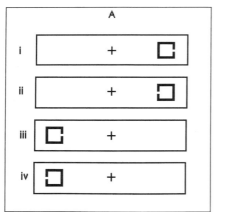 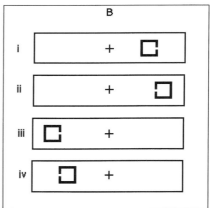

Fig. 4.4 Examples of displays from an unpublished study conducted with right-hemisphere neglect patients. Panel (A) shows four alternative displays. The single fixation cross appeared in the middle of a computer screen throughout. A small square was flashed briefly in either the right visual field (as in (i) and (ii)) or the left visual field (as in (iii) and (iv)). The task was to judge whether this square had a gap in it or not (a gap is shown on the right of the square in (i) and (iii), and on the left of the square in (ii) and (iv)). More gaps were missed in the left visual field, and on the left of a square in either field. Panel (B) shows a follow-up to this study, where any gap always fell at the same eccentricity relative to central fixation (note changes to (i) and (iv)).

with three right-parietal patients. The task was to fixate the cross while judging the presence or absence of a gap in briefly flashed squares (2/3 of the trials did have a gap). All three patients missed significantly more gaps on the left than on the right of each square, regardless of visual field. They were also worse for the left visual field overall.

The neglect for gaps on the left side of a square on the right shows (as do many other results; see Kinsbourne 1993) that neglect can arise within the ipsilesional visual field. It might initially seem tempting to interpret this aspect of the results as evidence for object-based neglect in non-retinotopic coordinates; and, indeed, such a conclusion has frequently been drawn from analogous findings. However, this would be mistaken, since gaps on the left of either square were always further to the left *retinally* than gaps on the right of the same square. Indeed, the entire pattern of results might be explained by retinal position, simply in terms of increasingly poor performance for locations that were further to the left retinally. This would be entirely consistent with the 'graded' egocentric impairment suggested by Kinsbourne (1993) and others, and instantiated in Pouget & Sejnowski's simulation of neglect (Chapter 7). No special mechanism is thus needed to explain cases of apparently 'object-based' neglect, where the comparison between the two sides of an object is confounded with absolute retinal position.

Of course, it seems quite straightforward to control for this particular confound. For instance, Fig. 4.4B shows a modification of the same experiment, which shifted the squares between trials so that gaps on the left versus right of a square always appeared at the same absolute eccentricity. The results were as before, with more misses for gaps on the left of each square (plus worse performance overall in the left visual field). Here one might suppose that since gaps on the left versus right side of the squares fell at the same absolute retinal location in each visual field, the neglect within each field cannot be explained in retinal terms. However, this would overlook the potential importance of *relative* rather than absolute retinal location. Gaps at the right of the squares in Fig. 4.4B have no information to their immediate right on the retina, and thus no competing information that might be advantaged relative to them in egocentric terms. By contrast, gaps on the left of the squares always have the other side of the square further to their right in retinal coordinates (and also in other egocentric frames). This rightwards information might compete with, and dominate, the relatively weaker left information. Thus, the whole pattern of results for Fig. 4.4 might be explained by neglect arising in retinal terms (or in some other egocentric frame), provided that *relative* location rather than absolute location is most critical. Kinsbourne (1993) reviews a substantial body of evidence, which suggests that relative location can indeed be the crucial factor.

In general, I would argue that many cases of apparently object-based neglect can be explained in purely egocentric terms, because the neglected side of the object is typically further to the left in absolute or relative egocentric space. Pouget & Sejnowski (Chapter 7) make effectively the same point in their simulation of Arguin & Bub's (1993) study. This simulation succeeded in producing an apparently 'object-based' pattern of results only because of the role played in the simulation by *relative* retinal location within a display. The other features of their computational model (e.g. the basis–function architecture) are entirely irrelevant to capturing this particular pattern of results. In essence, many examples of putatively 'object-centred' neglect only require that relatively ipsilesional information should be able to compete with, and dominate, relatively contralesional information, where ipsilesional and contralesional are still defined in purely egocentric terms.

In addition, it also seems likely that any such competition must arise at a relatively local scale, in order to produce neglect within an object for just some of its subparts (as in Fig. 4.1 or 4.4). One aspect of the neglect syndrome, which is often overlooked, is that many right-hemisphere patients have a pathological attraction towards fine local details of visual objects, as opposed to the more global overall picture. This local bias is a known consequence of lesions to the right parietal-temporal junction (see Rafal & Robertson 1995), an area that will be damaged in most neglect patients. The combination of an egocentric rightwards bias, plus a general bias for local detail, may thus be responsible for neglect patients' frequent tendency to lock onto just the right side of even quite small objects.

4.5 Further evidence that visual object-segmentation precedes the egocentric bias

Having argued that many examples of patients neglecting the left of individual objects may be explained in strictly egocentric terms, I next want to point out that some of these examples nevertheless force a concession from models such as the Pouget & Sejnowski simulation (Chapter 7). This is an important concession for present purposes, as it is the main conclusion I wish to draw. The conclusion was already sketched in the earlier section on extinction, where I claimed that object-segmentation processes can operate *prior* to the pathological egocentric bias produced by the parietal lesion. In present form, the Pouget and Sejnowski model applies an egocentric bias directly to the raw retinal input. I would argue instead that considerable visual preprocessing precedes the pathological bias, with individual segmented objects then serving as inputs to the biased part of the system, rather than all retinal pixels being input together.

Figure 4.5 illustrates a study by Driver *et al.* (1992), which supports my argument. The right-hemisphere left neglect patient was required to compare the jagged edge in a display like Fig. 4.5A or like Fig. 4.5B, to an isolated central edge appearing shortly afterwards, while fixating centrally throughout. Normal observers see these displays as comprising a white figural shape against a shapeless striped background. Performance by the left neglect patient was better for displays like Fig. 4.5A (critical jagged edge to the left of the patient, but on the right of the white figure) than those like Fig. 4.5B (jagged edge to

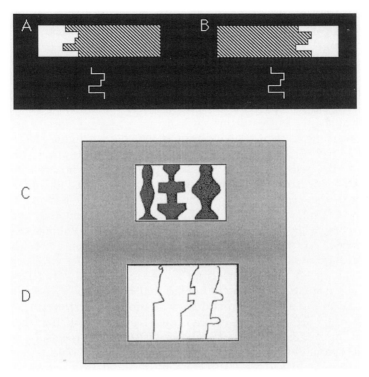

Fig. 4.5 (A) and (B) Each show an example of a display from Driver *et al*. (1992). The task was to fixate the centre of each rectangle, and then compare its jagged edge to the isolated central edge which appeared below shortly afterwards. Normal observers see the rectangles as comprising a small white figural shape against a striped shapeless background. Right-hemisphere neglect patients perform worse for displays like (B), where the critical edge falls to the patients' right, but to the left of the white figure, than for displays like (A), where although the edge falls to the patients' left, it is now on the right of the white figure. (C) Illustration that symmetrical shapes are preferred as figures by normal viewers, a result also found for neglect patients (Driver *et al*. 1992). (D) Copy of (C) produced by a right-hemisphere neglect patient (Marshall & Halligan 1994); note that the patient sketched just the right side of each symmetric shape. See text for further details.

the right of the patient, but now on the left of the white figure). This 'figure-based' neglect has since been replicated in other cases, and observed by other groups (e.g. Marshall & Halligan 1994). Note that it is difficult to account for this pattern of results in terms of an egocentric gradient of impairment applied directly to the retinal image as a whole, because the white figure on the left in Fig. 4.5A has so much competing information to its egocentric right. Instead, the outcome suggests that the white figure was first segmented from its background regardless of where it fell, and that the egocentric bias favouring rightwards information then applied just within the white figure. Thus, individual segmented figures apparently serve as the inputs to the biased part of the system, rather than raw retinal pixels.

This account receives further support from an additional figure-ground phenomenon that we have also studied in neglect patients. Other factors being equal, normal viewers see symmetrical shapes as figures, with adjoining asymmetrical shapes appearing to provide their background (see Fig. 4.5C). Interestingly, neglect patients show this same phenomenon, also choosing symmetrical shapes as figures, which indicates that both sides of each shape must be available to their visual system at the stage of figure-ground assignment (Driver *et al*. 1992; Marshall & Halligan 1994). However, when questioned as to the basis of their choices, such patients make no explicit reference to symmetry. Moreover, if forced to judge whether each individual shape is symmetrical, they cannot do so accurately, presumably because they then neglect the left side of each figure (as in my previous examples), and so have difficulty comparing the two sides explicitly. Figure 4.5D shows the copying performance of one patient (taken from Marshall & Halligan 1994) when asked to copy a figure-ground display that included symmetry. He consistently drew just the right side of each symmetrical shape. As in the study of Driver *et al*. (1992), the sensitivity to symmetry implies that both sides of each shape were available at an initial figure-ground segmentation stage. However, the subsequent loss of the left side for each segmented figure suggests that these figures were then input individually to a subsequent stage of processing, where the egocentric spatial bias arose. This again implies that object-segmentation precedes the pathological bias, with segmented candidate objects serving as the inputs to the spatially biased part of the system, rather than the bias applying to the entire retinal image as in Pouget & Sejnowski's simulation (Chapter 7).

Thus, we are again led to the conclusion that visual neglect can be object-based, in a sense which is non-trivial, yet which bears little relation to Marr's original (1982) use of 'object-centred' terminology. The egocentric spatial bias apparent in parietal neglect can be superimposed upon relatively preserved visual object-segmentation processes. Given current understanding of the anatomy of the visual system, I presume that the latter segmentation processes arise largely within the occipital lobe, which is intact in most neglect patients (the relatively preserved ventral pathway into inferotemporal cortex may also be involved). As a result of the preserved object-segmentation, visual neglect can apply to the left of individual objects, rather than just to fixed positions in space relative to the eye, head or body. Nevertheless, the 'left' in question (i.e. which side of the segmented object will suffer from neglect) still seems to be determined egocentrically.

4.6 Axis-based visual neglect

Our next example of object-based neglect bring us a little closer to the axis-based shape-descriptions associated with Marr's (1982) 'object-centred' terminology. Driver & Halligan (1991) tested whether neglect might operate relative to the intrinsic axis of elongation of unfamiliar shapes. They presented displays like Fig. 4.6A requiring judgements of whether the two shapes in each display were the same or different. Any difference was in a minor detail on one side, as in the illustration. As would be expected, with upright shapes neglect patients miss differences on the left, while detecting equivalent differences on the right. The only noteworthy point so far is that this difference can be highly reliable even with very small shapes, presumably due to the 'local bias' discussed earlier.

The outcome with upright shapes is, of course, consistent with neglect in a variety of possible egocentric coordinates, since differences on the left of the shapes also fell to the left of the patients' eyes, head and body. The critical comparisons were intended to come from displays like Fig. 4.6B, where both shapes were tilted 45°. In the illustrated example, the difference still fell to the left of each shape's principal axis, yet now to the right of the patient's saggital midline. The repeated finding (see Driver 1995) is that such differences are still neglected, which Driver & Halligan (1991) took as evidence for neglect relative to shapes' intrinsic axes of elongation, within Marrian 'object-centred' shape-descriptions.

However, two caveats must be placed on this conclusion. First, one must consider why one side of the proposed axis would be treated as the left of the shape (and thus neglected), while the other would be treated as its right (and thus judged correctly). The shapes in Fig. 4.6 are entirely meaningless and unfamiliar, and thus cannot have any *intrinsic* left versus right. Instead, the assignment of left versus right must still be determined egocentrically, in terms of the layout of the shape *relative to the observer*. Readers who are not immediately convinced of this should consider the following. When looking at Fig. 4.6B, I presume there will be little dispute over which side of the tilted shapes would be assigned as the left and which as the right; people agree that the difference is on the 'left' of the shapes in this example. Now try looking at the same figure from behind the page; the same difference should now appear to be on the *right* of the shapes. This simple demonstration implies that the axis-based shape-descriptions in question cannot be strictly viewpoint-independent (and thus not truly allocentric), because which side of the axis is treated as left and which as right depends on the current viewpoint (e.g. from in front versus behind the page). Indeed, the neglect patients who missed the difference on the left of the tilted shapes in Fig. 4.6B could detect the same difference in the display that is equivalent to viewing Fig. 4.6B from behind the page.

Another way of conveying this point is to suppose that the coordinate system for describing the shapes is Cartesian in nature (I make no assumption that this is true in the brain, but merely adopt the convention here for purposes of exposition). The proposal would be that the intrinsic axis of elongation for each 2-D shape can effectively provide a 'Y-axis' for the coordinates of the shape description, with the 'X-axis' then running orthogonally to this in the picture plane. The assignment of handedness (i.e. the marking of the X-axis with

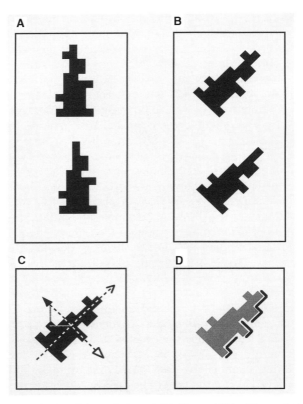

Fig. 4.6 Examples of stimuli from Driver & Halligan (1991). The task for displays like (A) and (B) was to judge whether the two shapes were the same or different. Small differences on the left of each shape were typically neglected, whether the shapes were upright (A) or tilted (B). (C) Shows how a schematic Cartesian coordinate system might be based around the principal axis of elongation (*dashed-line* pointing *top-right*). This could define a Y-axis, with an X-axis then running orthogonally, as shown. Which direction along the latter axis (i.e. in direction of *white solid arrowhead*, or *black solid arrowhead*) gets coded as right versus left may be determined in terms of any egocentric left/right vector component to these directions. For example, the direction indicated by the *black solid arrowhead* (pointing *top-left*) has egocentric-left as one vector component, as shown by the *fine dotted lines*. (D) Illustrates that almost the entire right side of a tilted shape (the regions marked by *thick black lines*) is unique in having nothing to its immediate right. See text for how this alone might explain the neglect results for displays like (B).

respect to left and right, which is the critical question as regards the coordinates of neglect) would then be determined egocentrically. One way for this to proceed would be in terms of whether either direction along the X-axis has some egocentric left or right vector component (see Fig. 4.6C). Note that this specific suggestion predicts that axis-based neglect should disappear for shapes tilted to 90°, as then neither direction along the presumed X-axis would have any remaining egocentric left or right vector component.

Thus, the first caveat to place on Driver & Halligan's (1991) result, for displays like Fig. 4.6B, is that while it may imply neglect that is 'object-centred' in the particular sense of operating relative to shapes' intrinsic axes, the handedness of this neglect must still be determined egocentrically. The second caveat is more serious; on its own, the result might not even require the explicit extraction of axes, once one considers the possible role of *relative* rather than absolute egocentric position that I emphasized earlier. Looking at Fig. 4.6B, the reader can confirm that every point along the left of the outline shape has information to its immediate right in egocentric terms (e.g. retinally), whereas by contrast every point along the right of the shape has no such potentially competing information to its immediate right. Thus, simply applying a retinal (or other egocentric) bias directly to the image could in principle advantage the entire right side of the 45° tilted shape over its left side (see Fig. 4.6D), provided that competition takes place in terms of *relative* rather than absolute retinal position, and moreover does so only locally (i.e. within narrow, retinally horizontal slices; otherwise the entire bottom-half of the object would be neglected, rather than a left side that is equivalent to the axis-based left side). It therefore appears that even tilting a shape through 45° is not sufficient to rule out the potentially powerful influences of purely retinal biases in relative terms.

However, in a further study (Driver *et al.* 1994), we were able to rule out this simple retinal account for axis-based neglect. The task was to detect a gap (present on 2/3 of trials) that could only appear just above fixation, in the upper horizontal edge of a briefly presented equilateral triangle (see Fig. 4.7). We chose to use this particular shape because, unlike the isosceles triangles in Fig. 4.2, or the elongated nonsense shapes in Fig. 4.6, equilateral triangles have no single intrinsic axis of elongation and/or symmetry; instead, they posses several such axes. As first noted by Attneave (1968), shapes with such multiple potential axes are multistable perceptually, and can be seen to 'point' in different directions, depending on which axis predominates at any one time (see Fig. 4.7A and 4.7B). Moreover, it is possible to influence which axis will predominate by embedding such shapes among a biasing configuration, as we did in our experiment (see Fig. 4.7C and 4.7D). We found that more gaps were missed by right-parietal left-neglect patients when the target equilateral triangle was made to 'point' such that the gap in its horizontal edge appeared to fall on its left side (Fig. 4.7D), rather than its right side (Fig. 4.7C). This result is problematic for any account in terms of a rightward egocentric spatial bias applied to the retinal image *per se*. Instead, it supports my proposal that neglect can apply to the left side of an object within an axis-based shape-description, thus bringing us somewhat closer to Marr's (1982) notion of object-centred coding. However, it is critical to realize that the assignment of handedness within the proposed axis-based shape description (i.e. which side of the predominant axis gets treated as left, and which as right) must still be

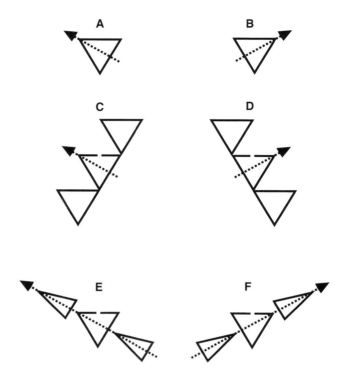

Fig. 4.7 (A) and (B) Illustrate that an equilateral triangle can be seen to point in different directions, depending on which axis (indicated by *dotted lines*) predominates. This can be biased by embedding such a triangle in configurations, as for the middle triangles in (C)–(F). (C) and (D) Use base-alignment with other equilateral triangles, so that the triangles all seem to point away from their aligned bases (as indicated by *arrows*). (E) and (F) Use a symmetry relation with isosceles triangles, so that the triangles all seem to point along the axis of symmetry (indicated by *arrows*). Displays like (C) and (D) were used by Driver *et al.* (1994). The task was to detect any gap in the horizontal edge of the middle triangle, just above central fixation. More left neglect was found for (D) than (C), presumably because the gap then fell to the left of the biased axis. A follow-up found more neglect in the same task for displays like (F) than (E). See text for details.

determined in an egocentric manner, just as I described earlier. Viewing Fig. 4.7 from behind the page reverses which side of the predominant axis counts as left and which as right, exactly as for Fig. 4.6.

Pouget & Sejnowski (Chapter 7) suggest that the effects for Fig. 4.7C and 4.7D might actually be due to the overall tilt of the whole configuration, rather than the influence that this configuration has on the predominant axis within each shape, as I propose. They argue that the slant of the overall configuration may imply a tilted horizon, as if viewed with a tilted head. We doubt their explanation, since there is a large body of normal evidence (e.g. Attneave 1968; Palmer 1980) documenting the influence of such configurations on the predominant axis within each local shape (indeed, that is why we chose to use these stimuli). By contrast, there is no direct evidence for the Pouget & Seknowski proposal that such displays induce an illusion of head-tilt. Further grounds to doubt their interpretation come from a follow-up study, with displays like those in Fig. 4.7E and 4.7F. Here we (Driver & Baylis in prep.) embedded the target equilateral triangle in a context of *isosceles* triangles, aligning these along their axis of symmetry. This is known to bias the predominant axis for the equilateral triangle in the *opposite* direction to any possible head-tilt illusion (Attneave 1968; Palmer 1980). Once again, we found more neglect of the small gap in the target triangle when it fell to the left of the local axis that would be expected to predominate for that shape (i.e. more neglect for Fig. 4.7F than 4.7E).

Such axis-based neglect provides a further restricted sense in which visual neglect may be 'object-based'. In these examples, one component of the shape-description to which neglect applies seems to be determined 'allocentrically'; namely, the principal axis of the shape, which divides it into left and right halves. However, which half is the left, and which the right, would then still be determined egocentrically. Further studies suggests that which direction along the principal axis gets marked as 'up' may be determined by vestibular and visual cues to the gravitational upright in the environment (Ladavas 1987). On all these points, the data from neglect in parietal patients converge nicely with other sources of evidence concerning the coordinate frames used to describe visual shapes during human object recognition (e.g. Rock 1973). They also agree with my general conclusion that considerable visual processing may precede the level of the system at which the egocentric rightward bias arises in parietal patients; this preprocessing can evidently include the extraction of shapes' principal axes.

4.7 Can neglect apply to the intrinsic left of a familiar shape?

Thus far, I have been at pains to emphasize that while visual neglect can be 'object-based' in various senses, these are all consistent with a strictly egocentric spatial bias applying to a preprocessed representation of the visual scene (which has been segmented into candidate objects, with their principal axes extracted). All my studies utilized meaningless nonsense shapes, which had no intrinsic left or right, but at best merely an intrinsic segmentation into figure versus ground, plus intrinsic axes of symmetry and/or elongation for the resulting figures. Perhaps with more familiar and meaningful shapes, truly allocentric neglect could be found for the intrinsic left of an object, rather than merely for its egocentrically-determined left?

Philosophers have long debated whether it is even possible in principle for an object to possess intrinsic handedness. Since Kant's (1770/1929) analysis of the particular example of left versus right hands (and with the added impetus of recent particle physics), intrinsic handedness is now generally accepted as a theoretical possibility. But can such intrinsic handedness influence neglect? I believe that the answer to this question is currently much less clear than for the examples of 'egocentric' object-based neglect that were given above.

Farah *et al.* (1990) presented neglect patients with pictures of meaningful objects (e.g. a rabbit) that had a conventional upright orientation, and which were accordingly considered by the authors to have an intrinsic left versus right (though it is questionable whether this argument would have been accepted by Kant!). These pictures could be presented in a 90°-rotated format, so that their conventional 'top' now fell to the egocentric left or right of the patient, instead of appearing above. No evidence for intrinsic object-centred neglect (i.e. the same region of an object being neglected regardless of its tilt) was found in a task of naming all the letters scattered across such objects. Behrmann & Moscovitch (1994) repeated this finding in a task where the items to be named (colours) were now parts of the meaningful object, rather than merely being superimposed upon it. Studies of this kind provide no evidence for neglect of any object-intrinsic left, though one might question whether the stimuli that were used really possess intrinsic handedness in the first place.

Behrmann & Moscovitch (1994) did report object-intrinsic left neglect in the naming of component colours for another class of stimuli, when tilted through 90°. They found this result for individual letter stimuli, that were each made up of many colours. Moreover, the result was found only for *asymmetric* letters (e.g. K, P, etc.), not for symmetric letters (e.g. A, X, etc.). As noted by Driver *et al.* (1994), one account for this result might be that the assignment of intrinsic handedness is vital for the identification of some asymmetrical letters (e.g. a 'b' is distinguished from a 'd' only by its handedness). The Behrmann & Moscovitch study thus appears to provide a demonstration of intrinsic-handedness influencing neglect, with the added theoretical interest that this seems to arise only in the (rare) situation where handedness matters for correct identification. Unfortunately, however, more recent research (Drain & Reuter-Lorenz 1997) suggests that this pattern of results with letter stimuli may be entirely artefactual because, on average, asymmetric English letters have more jazzy detail on their intrinsic right than on their intrinsic left (e.g. many such letters have only one edge along their left). The patients may thus simply have been attracted to the jazzy details.

Caramazza & Hillis (1990) have described a particularly well-studied case who appears to show visual neglect for one intrinsic side of familiar objects, in the particular task of reading. Atypically, she is a *left*-hemisphere damaged case of neglect, who shows *right*-sided errors when reading words (e.g. HUMID may be reported as HUMAN). The critical finding is that the same part of the word—its ending—is likely to be misreported by this patient even when the letter-string is presented in a spatially transformed manner; for instance, in a columnar rather than horizontal string, or even when mirror-reversed horizontally (so that the right end of the word now falls leftwards on the retina, and vice versa). This unquestionably seems to suggest neglect for one intrinsic side of a familiar object, and so is invaluable as an existence proof. However, the generality of the result can be questioned as regards our current concerns. First, to my knowledge, this pattern has only ever been documented in one case with left-hemisphere damage. The basic manipulation of presenting letter-strings in different spatial formats has been tried in numerous other cases, and egocentric neglect has invariably been found instead (e.g. Riddoch 1991). Second, and more importantly, the particular result for Caramazza & Hillis' (1990) own patient, of neglect that consistently applies to the end of a word, is found even if the letters are presented to her aurally, in spoken sequence, rather than visually. Thus, her deficit presumably arises at some stage of contacting long-term memory representations for words, rather that in dealing with the visual information perceptually, which is my present concern. Indeed, she can always identify all of the individual letters in a visual string, prior to making her mistakes in whole-word reading for just the end letters.

In sum, there seems little evidence for visual neglect that is 'object-centred' in the strong, allocentric sense of applying to one *intrinsic* side of a familiar object, regardless of its current absolute or relative egocentric position. Such evidence is notably sparse in comparison with the more egocentric forms of object-based neglect that were reviewed earlier. The most convincing example of neglect with intrinsic handedness comes from Caramazza & Hillis' (1990) single left-hemisphere case, but it is not clear that her reading errors are based on a strictly visual deficit. It has been suggested (Farah & Buxbaum 1997) that the neglect in this case might arise when she *imagines* what the complete letter-string would look like, after transforming the unconventional format of the sensory input towards its usual form. If so, then even for this patient, purely egocentric neglect might explain the results if arising at a visualization stage.

4.8 Conclusions

The studies reviewed here suggest a variety of senses in which visual neglect may be 'object-based'. These must be carefully distinguished, since some of the senses are more theoretically constraining than others, as I have emphasized. Nevertheless, I have argued that one commonality applies across all the examples (with the one possible exception being Caramazza & Hillis' (1990) unusual case). This common denominator is that the various forms of object-based neglect can all be reconciled with a purely egocentric spatial bias, provided that this bias is applied to a preprocessed representation of the visual scene, rather than to the raw retinal image. If the egocentric spatial bias is applied to individual segmented objects, whose intrinsic axes of elongation and/or symmetry have been extracted, then object-based neglect will result, rather than merely neglect for fixed regions on the retina, or for some fixed sequence of relative positions across it. The 'objects' to which neglect applies in this way may be broadly characterized as segmented blobs, with extracted intrinsic axes and some initial shape description, rather than fully-articulated descriptions of identified and meaningful things. The further issue of whether or not familiar object-identities can exert a top-down influence on neglect (see Farah & Buxbaum 1997) should be considered separately.

In describing these results, I have tended to generalize across neglect patients as though all cases were the same, even though I noted at the outset of this chapter that individual patients can differ in their detailed neuropsychological profile, just as their exact lesions can vary. However, I believe that my main conclusion, that object-based neglect results from an egocentric bias super-imposed on visual preprocessing, should hold true for the vast majority of parietal neglect patients. Certainly, I have found the object-based effects documented in my studies for every case I have tested (provided performance was not at ceiling or floor). I never had to select patients who showed object-based neglect, as distinct from those who did not. I would suggest that a fairly general pattern is found in the behavioural results of these studies because they in turn rest on a very general anatomical pattern. This anatomical pattern is that visual areas in the occipital lobe (and their projections to inferotemporal cortex) are largely intact in most parietal neglect patients. These preserved visual areas are presumably responsible for the preserved object-segmentation and shape-description that leads to object-based visual neglect in the senses I have described.

Acknowledgements

The author's research was supported by the Wellcome Trust, and the Medical Research Council (UK). Thanks to Neil Burgess for helpful comments.

References

Anderson, R. A., Snyder, L. H., Bradley, D. C., & Xing, J. (1997). Multimodal representation of space in the posterior parietal cortex and its use in planning movements. *American Journal of Psychology*, **81**, 447–53.

Arguin, M. & Bub, D. (1993). Evidence for an independent stimulus-centred reference frame from a case of visual hemineglect. *Cortex*, **29**, 349–57.

Attneave (1968). Triangles as ambiguous figures. *American Journal of Psychology*, **81**, 447–53.

Baylis, G. C. & Driver, J. (1993). Visual attention and objects: evidence for hierarchical coding of location. *Journal of Experimental Psychology: Human Perception and Performance*, **19**, 451–70.

Behrmann, M. & Moscovitch. M. (1994). Object-centered neglect in patients with unilateral neglect; effects of left-right coordinates of objects. *Journal of Cognitive Neuroscience*, **6**, 1–16.

Bisiach, E. (1993). Mental representation in unilateral neglect and related disorders: the twentieth Bartlett Memorial lecture. *Quarterly Journal of Experimental Psychology*, **46A**, 435–62.

Bisiach, E. (1997). The spatial features of unilateral neglect. In (P. Thier, & H.-O. Karnath, ed.) *Parietal Lobe Contributions to Orientation in 3D Space*, pp. 465–95. Berlin: Springer-Verlag.

Bisiach, E. & Vallar, C. (1988). Hemineglect in humans. In (F. Boller & J. Grafman, ed.) *Handbook of Neuropsychology: Vol. 1*. Amsterdam: Elsevier.

Caramazza, A. & Hillis, A. E. (1990). Internal spatial representation of written words: evidence from unilateral neglect. *Nature*, **346**, 267–9.

Davis, G. & Driver, J. (1997). Spreading of visual attention to modally versus amodally completed regions. *Psychological Science*, **8**, 275–81.

Drain, M. & Reuter-Lorenz, P. A. (1997). Object-centred neglect: do informational asymmetries play a role. *Neuropsychologia*, **35**, 445–56.

Driver, J. (1994). Unilateral neglect and normal attention. *Neuropsychological Rehabilitation*, **4**, 123–6.

Driver, J. (1995). Object segmentation and visual neglect. *Behavioural Brain Research*, **71**, 135–46.

Driver, J. (1998). The neuropsychology of spatial attention. In (H. Pashler, ed.) *Attention*. Psychology Press.

Driver, J. & Baylis, G. C. (1989). Movement and visual attention: the spotlight metaphor breaks down. *Journal of Experimental Psychology: Human Perception and Performance*, **15**, 448–56.

Driver, J. & Baylis, G. C. (1998). Visual attention and object segmentation. In (R. Parasuraman, ed.) *The Attentive Brain*. Cambridge, MA: MIT Press.

Driver, J. & Halligan, P. W. (1991). Can visual neglect operate in object-centred coordinates?: an affirmative single-case study. *Cognitive Neuropsychology*, **8**, 475–96.

Driver, J. & Mattingley, J. B. (1995). Normal and pathological selective attention in humans. *Current Opinion in Neurobiology*, **5**, 191–7.

Driver, J., Baylis, G. C., & Rafal, R. D. (1992). Preserved figure-ground segregation and symmetry perception in visual neglect. *Nature*, **360**, 73–4.

Driver, J., Baylis, G. C., Goodrich, S. J., & Rafal, R. D. (1994). Axis-based neglect of visual shapes. *Neuropsychologia*, **32**, 1353–65.

Driver, J., Mattingley, J. B., Rorden, C., & Davis, C. (1997). Extinction as a paradigm measure of attentional bias and restricted capacity following brain injury. In (P. Thier & H.-O. Karnath, ed.) *Parietal Lobe Contributions to Orientation in 3D Space*, 401–29. Berlin: Springer-Verlag.

Duncan, J. (1980). The locus of interference in the perception of simultaneous stimuli. *Psychological Review*, **87**, 272–300.

Duncan, J. (1984). Selective attention and the organization of visual information. *Journal of Experimental Psychology: General*, **113**, 501–17.

Duncan, J. (1993a). Coordination of what and where in visual attention. *Perception*, 1261–70.

Duncan, J. (1993b). Similarity between concurrent visual discriminations: dimensions and objects. *Perception & Psychophysics*, **54**, 425–30.

Egly, R., Driver, J., & Rafal, R. (1994). Shifting visual attention between objects and locations: normality and pathology. *Journal of Experimental Psychology: General*, **123**, 161–77.

Farah, M. J. & Buxbaum, L. J. (1997). Object-based attention in visual neglect: conceptual and empirical distinctions. In (P. Thier & H.-O. Karnath, ed.) *Parietal Lobe Contributions to Orientation in 3D Space*, pp. 385–400. Berlin: Springer-Verlag.

Farah, M. J., Brunn, J. L., Wong, A. B., Wallace, M. A., & Carpenter, P. (1990). Frames of reference for allocating attention to space: evidence from the neglect syndrome. *Neuropsychologia*, **28**, 335–47.

Gilchrist, I. D., Humphreys, G. W., & Riddoch, M. J. (1996). Grouping and extinction: evidence for low-level modulation of visual selection. *Cognitive Neuropsychology*, **13**, 1223–50.

Heilman, K. M., Watson, R. T., & Valenstein, E. (1985). Neglect and related disorders. In (K. M. Heilman & E. Valenstein, ed.) *Clinical Neuropsychology*. Oxford: OUP.

Humphreys, G. W., Olson, A., Romani, C., & Riddoch, M. J. (1996). Competitive mechanisms of selection by space and object: a neuropsychological approach. In (A. Kramer & M. Coles, ed.) *Converging Operations in the Study of Visual Attentioin*, pp. 365–94. Washington: APA Press.

Kant, I. (1770, translated 1929). On the first ground of the distinctions of regions in space. (trans. J. Handyside), *Kant's Inaugural Dissertation and Early Writings on Space*. Chicago: Open Court.

Karnath, H.-O., Schenkel, P., & Fischer, B. (1991). Trunk orientation as the determining factor of the 'contralateral' deficit in the neglect syndrome and the physical anchor of the internal representation of body orientation in space. *Brain*, **114**, 1997–2014.

Kinsbourne, M. (1993). Orientational bias model of unilateral neglect. In (I. H. Robertson & J. C. Marshall, ed.) *Unilateral Neglect: Clinical and Experimental Findings*. Hove: Erlbaum.

Kramer, A. F. & Jacobson, A. (1991). Perceptual organization and focused attention. *Perception & Psychophysics*, **50**, 267–84.

Ladavas, E. (1987). Is the spatial deficit produce by right parietal lobe damage associated with retinal or gravitational coordinates. *Brain*, **110**, 167–80.

Lavie, N. & Driver, J. (1996). On the spatial extent of attention in object-based visual selection. *Perception & Psychophysics*, **58**, 1238–51.

McLeod, P., Driver, J., Dienes, Z., & Crisp, J. (1991). Filtering by movement in visual search. *Journal of Experimental Psychology: Human Perception and Performance*, **17**, 55–64.

Marr, D. (1982). *Vision*. San Francisco: Freeman.

Marshall, J. C. & Halligan, P. W. (1989). When right goes left: an investigation of line bisection in a case of visual neglect. *Cortex*, **25**, 503–15.

Marshall, J. C. & Halligan, P. W. (1994). The yin and yang of visuo-spatial neglect: a case study. *Neuropsychologia*, **32**, 1037.

Mattingley, J. B., Davis, G., & Driver, J. (1997). Preattentive filling-in of visual surfaces in parietal extinction. *Science*, **275**, 671–4.

Mattingley, J. B., Husain, M., Rorden, R., Kennard, C., & Driver, J. (1998). Motor function of human inferior parietal lobe revealed in spatial neglect patients. *Nature*, **392**, 179–182.

Ostry, D., Moray, N., & Marks, C. (1976). Attention, practice, and semantic targets. *Journal of Experimental Psychology: Human Perception and Performance*, **2**, 326–36.

Palmer, S. E. (1980). What makes triangles point: local and global effects in configurations of ambiguous triangles. *Cognitive Psychology*, **12**, 285–305.

Posner, M. I. (1980). Orienting of attention. *Quarterly Journal of Experimental Psychology*, **32**, 3–25.

Posner, M. I., Walker, J. A., Friedrich, F. J., & Rafal, R. D. (1984). Effects of parietal injury on covert orienting of attention. *Journal of Neuroscience*, **4**, 1863–74.

Rafal, R. D. (1994). Neglect. *Current Opinion in Neurobiology*, **4**, 231–6.

Rafal, R. D. & Robertson, L. C. (1995). The neurology of visual attention. In (M. Gazzaniga, ed.) *The Coginitive Neurosciences*. Cambridge, MA: MIT Press.

Riddoch, M. J. (1991). *Neglect and the Peripheral Dyslexias*. Hove: Erlbaum.

Robertson, I. H. & Marshall, J. C. (1993). *Unilateral Neglect: Clinical and Experimental Findings*. Hove: Erlbaum.

Rock, I. (1973). *Orientation and Form*. New York: Academic Press.

Thier, P., & Karnath, H.-O. (1997). *Parietal Lobe Contributions to Orientation in 3D Space*. Berlin: Springer-Verlag.

Von der Heydt, R., Peterhans, E., & Baumgartner, C. (1984). Illusory contours and cortical neuron responses. *Science*, **224**, 1489–99.

Ward, R., Goodrich, S., & Driver, J. (1994). Grouping reduces visual extinction: neuropsychological evidence for weight-linkage in visual selection. *Visual Cognition*, **1**, 101–29.

5

Multimodal integration for the representation of space in the posterior parietal cortex

Richard A. Andersen

5.1 Introduction

The posterior parietal cortex and the hippocampus are areas of the brain considered synonymous with spatial cognition. The classic studies of O'Keefe & Nadel (1978) and their colleagues demonstrated cells in the hippocampus of rats selective for places in the environment. Given the amazing spatial properties of these cells, these authors proposed that the hippocampus contained a cognitive map of space. Likewise, lesions to the posterior parietal cortex of humans and non-human primates produce severe deficits in spatial perception. Thus the posterior parietal cortex has been considered essential for the perception of space. In primates the posterior parietal cortex projects to the presubiculum and parahippocampal gyrus and thus there are strong and rather direct connections between these areas. The loss of spatial memories after lesion of the posterior parietal cortex suggests that these memories are laid down there, with the aid of the hippocampus. In rats the posterior parietal cortex contains cells with properties similar to those of cells found in the hippocampus; this observation again suggests that these two structures play an intimate and associated role in the construction of spatial cognition. In this paper, data on how space is processed in the posterior parietal cortex in the macaque monkey are reviewed. An understanding of the spatial role of the parietal areas, when combined with new data that are emerging from studies of the monkey hippocampus (Uno *et al.* 1993; Rolls & Omara 1995; Satoshi *et al.* 1995), will help in understanding the roles these two structures play in spatial cognition. Likewise, the comparison of primates with rats will determine what spatial functions are similar or dissimilar between the two species.

The posterior parietal cortex lies between the visual, auditory and somatosensory areas of the cortex and has long been envisioned as an area 'associating' these different modalities to form a unified, multimodal impression of space. How this is accomplished has not been appreciated until recently. This paper shows that these different modalities are brought together in a very systematic fashion, using multiplicative gain functions to combine different modalities including vision, audition, somatosensation (neck proprioception), eye position, eye movement, and vestibular information. The gain mechanism for combining these signals forms a distributed representation of space across populations of posterior parietal neurones. This distributed representation has the interesting feature that it can be used to construct multiple frames of reference, which can then be used by other parts of the brain.

5.2 Cortical areas

The posterior parietal cortex contains a large number of cortical areas, but this review will concentrate on three: area 7a, the lateral intraparietal area (LIP) and the medial superior temporal area (MST). Although these areas have diverse functions and use a variety of sensory modalities, they have in common the ability to process information about spatial relations. One of the best-understood posterior parietal areas is area LIP, which plays a direct role in the processing of saccadic eye movements. This area has strong anatomical connections to other saccade centres (Asanuma et al. 1985; Lynch et al. 1985; Blatt et al. 1990), the neurones have presaccadic responses (Andersen & Gnadt 1989) and electrical stimulation of the area evokes saccadic eye movements (Mountcastle et al. 1975; Shibutani et al. 1984; Andersen et al. 1987; Kurylo & Skavenski 1987; Their & Andersen 1996). Area MST has neurones selective for complex patterns of motion, including 'optical flow' motion produced during self-motion, and many of its cells are also activated by vestibular stimuli and during smooth pursuit eye movements (Sakata et al. 1985; Tanaka et al. 1986; Newsome et al. 1988; Duffy & Wurtz 1991; Their & Ericksen 1992; Graziano et al. 1994; Bradley et al. 1996). This constellation of inputs suggests that it is important for navigation using motion information. This area may also play a more general role in the perception of patterns of motion (Graziano et al. 1994; Geesaman & Andersen 1996) and their stable localization in space during eye and head movements (Bradley et al. 1996). Area 7a is also a largely visual area, but also has connections with areas of the cortex associated with the highest cognitive functions, including structures associated with the hippocampus (Andersen et al. 1990). Although adjacent to area LIP, area 7a does not appear to play a direct role in saccades (Barash et al. 1991a). Unlike LIP, which has relatively smaller and contralateral visual receptive fields (Blatt et al. 1990), area 7a has large, bilateral fields (Motter & Mountcastle 1981). Area 7a, similar to area MST, has cells sensitive to vestibular inputs. All of the areas listed above are strongly interconnected via corticocortical projections. As will be seen in this review, one of the likely consequences of this interconnectivity is that even areas like LIP and MST, which seem on the surface to be unimodal visual areas, can reveal their multimodal nature when probed with the right set of tasks.

5.3 Representation of space

Combining visual and eye-position signals

Areas 7a and LIP receive a convergence of visual and eye-position signals (Andersen & Mountcastle 1981; Andersen *et al*. 1985); this convergence produces cells with retinal receptive fields that are modulated by the orbital position of the eyes. This modulation produces a 'gain field' because the eye position determines the gain of the visual response. To represent the location of a visual target with respect to the head requires a combining of both eye- and head-position information. One might imagine that an area representing space in a head-centred reference frame would have receptive fields that are anchored in space with respect to the head. The cells in LIP and 7a do not appear to use a head-anchored encoding scheme. Although each neurone receives both necessary input signals, its response for head-centred stimulus location is ambiguous at a single-cell level, because its activity can be varied by changing either the eye position or the retinal location of the stimulus. However, the activity across a population of cells with different eye-position and retinal-position sensitivities will have a unique pattern of firing for each head-centred location. Thus the code of head-centred location in the posterior parietal cortex can be carried as a distributed, population code. When neural networks are trained to transform retinal signals into head-centred coordinates by using eye position signals, the middle layer 'cells' that are responsible for the transformation develop gain fields similar to those of the cells found in the parietal cortex (Zipser & Andersen 1988). This model shows that the gain-field mechanism can be used to code head-centred spatial locations, and that this representation occurs naturally for learning coordinate transformations.

Head position

A knowledge of the orientation of the head with respect to the body is required for coding locations of stimuli in body-centred coordinates. It has recently been shown that approximately half of the 7a and LIP cells that have eye-gain fields also have gain fields for the head (Brotchie *et al*. 1995). Monkeys were trained to orient their direction of gaze with either head movements or eye movements. Interestingly, the eye- and head-gain fields were found to be the same for individual cells; this result indicates that the modulation of the visual signals is a function of gaze direction, independent of whether the head or the eyes are used to direct gaze.

Three possible sources for the head position signal are an efference copy of the command to move the head, a vestibular signal generated by the head movement, and a neck proprioceptive signal generated by the change in the orientation of the head on the body. It was found that even when the head was moved passively to different orientations the head-gain fields were still present (Brotchie *et al*. 1995). Thus efference copy is not the only source of the head-position signal. To test the possible involvement of vestibular signals, the animal's entire body was rotated in a vestibular chair. In this experiment the head remained at the same orientation on the body, but the direction of gaze was shifted by rotating the animal. Rotations were performed in the dark, to remove visual landmarks and optic flow cues. Twenty-eight per cent of cells tested in this manner exhibited vestibularly derived head-gain fields (Snyder et al. 1997). In a second experiment, designed to test for proprioceptive (somatosensory) cues, the animal's body was rotated under the head, with the head fixed relative to the world. In this case there is no vestibular cue, only a neck proprioceptive cue. Forty-nine per cent of cells tested in this paradigm showed proprioceptive gain fields (Snyder et al. 1997). A third test was run in which cells were tested for both proprioceptive and vestibular gain fields. Of 17 cells with gain fields, none had gain modulation for both signals; eight were proprioceptive only and the remaining nine were vestibular only. This is an important result: it indicates that two potential coordinate frames are segregated at a single-cell level. Proprioceptive signals provide information about the location of the head relative to the body and thus can code locations in a body-centred coordinate frame. Vestibular signals indicate the location of the head in space and thus can participate in coding locations in world-centred coordinates. It would be difficult to interpret the presence of both neck proprioceptive and vestibular signals for single parietal neurones; the finding that they do not co-occur fits well with the above scenario. Moreover, the cells with neck proprioceptive signals were found in LIP and the cells with vestibular signals were found in 7a, suggesting that these two areas represent space in different coordinate frames. Area LIP is strongly connected to oculomotor and motor areas and thus a body-centred representation makes good sense in terms of motor control. On the other hand, area 7a projects to the presubiculum and parahippocampal gyrus. Recordings in rats and monkeys have suggested that cells in the hippocampal formation carry information related to place in the world; a world-centred coordinate coding in area 7a is consistent with these observations.

   An additional effect was found in the course of these experiments. Some cells showed no gain fields in the vestibular experiment when the monkey was rotated in the dark. However, if the animal was rotated in the light and then tested in the dark, some neurones were found to have gain fields. This finding suggests that memory of the locations of landmarks in the room, or optic flow generated by the movement, was used to produce the gain fields. This result is of course reminiscent of 'place fields' in the hippocampus of the rat: these also use landmarks in the environment to encode the location of the animal.

Combining auditory and visual information

When a bird sings we perceive the source of the song and the image of the bird as spatially coincident. The multimodal perception of space occurs so effortlessly that we do not recognize what a formidable task it is to bring auditory and visual stimuli into the same coordinate frame. Visual information arrives in the cortex in the coordinates of the retina (eye); auditory stimulus locations are computed into a head-centred reference frame by using intraural time, intraural intensity, and spectral cues arriving at the two ears. How auditory signals are combined with visual signals in the posterior parietal cortex, with special emphasis on how the mismatch in coordinate frames of the two modalities is resolved, has been investigated.

Until recently area LIP was believed to be strictly a visual area involved in processing saccadic eye movements to visual targets. It was recently examined whether LIP would also play a role in processing saccades to auditory targets (Mazzoni *et al*. 1996). It was found that when a monkey is required to memorize the location of an auditory target in the dark, and then make a saccade to it after a delay, neurones in area LIP are active during the presentation of the auditory stimulus, and during the delay period. The LIP cells are multimodal in this task, and the auditory and visual response direction preferences are usually the same; these results suggest that the auditory and visual receptive fields and memory fields overlap one another.

In the experiments outlined above, the animal was fixating straight ahead with its head oriented in the same direction; as a result, the eye and head coordinate frames are aligned and cannot be distinguished. To determine the coordinate frame of the auditory signals in LIP, the auditory fields were mapped with the animal fixating in different directions with respect to the head (Stricanne *et al*. 1996). In these conditions the eye and head coordinate frames are moved apart. The animals performed saccades in darkness to the remembered locations of auditory sounds, and the activity was measured in the delay period between the offset of the sound and offset of the fixation light triggering the saccade. Forty-four per cent of the auditory-responding cells in LIP were found to code the auditory location in eye-centred coordinates during the delay period; in other words, these auditory memory fields actually moved with the eyes. Thirty-three per cent of the cells coded in head-centred coordinates and the remaining 23% were intermediate between the two coordinate frames. Cells of all three types also had gain fields for the eye. The occurrence of cells with eye-centric auditory fields and eye-gain fields suggests that at least this group of LIP neurones shares a common, distributed representation for both auditory and visual signals.

The co-occurrence of head, eye and intermediate coordinate frames also suggests that area LIP is at the source of, or participates in, the transformation from head- to eye-centred coordinates. Further bolstering this view is the finding that all three types of cell are also gain-modulated by eye position. Modelling experiments from the author's laboratory have shown that eye-gain fields can also accomplish the transformation of coordinates from head- to eye-centred; that is, in the opposite direction to the previous examples mentioned above (Xing *et al*. 1995).

Dynamic integration of auditory and visual signals

The finding of auditory responses in LIP is quite novel. In early studies Hyvärinen (1982) and Mountcastle *et al.* (1975) tested posterior parietal neurones with auditory stimuli and found no response. Because area LIP had not been described at that time it is possible that the neurones tested were outside LIP. In the early phases of experiments in LIP neurones were also tested with auditory stimuli and no response was found (R. A. Andersen, unpublished observation). On the other hand, several authors (Sakata *et al.* 1973; Seal *et al.* 1983; Koch & Fuster 1989) have reported auditory responses for neurones in the posterior parietal cortex. These responses were found only when the auditory stimuli were cues for movement. These observations prompted a re-examination of the auditory responsiveness of LIP neurones in two conditions; when the auditory stimuli were irrelevant to the animal, and when they were the targets of eye movements.

Recordings were made from LIP neurones during presentation of auditory and visual stimuli in animals trained to fixate a fixation point for their reward and ignore the presentation of these stimuli (Linden *et al.* 1996). LIP neurones were very responsive to the visual stimuli and absolutely unresponsive to the auditory stimuli. This shows that area LIP is a 'default' visual area. The auditory responsiveness seen in the previous experiments with an auditory memory saccade task could result from training the animals; alternatively, auditory signals could be switched into area LIP when the animals are required to use them for planning saccades. These two possibilities are currently being tested. If the latter, switching operation turns out to be the case, this switching may be required to use area LIP to transform auditory signals into eye-movement coordinates. This model would propose that area LIP is 'multimodal' in a dynamic sense, being auditory only when an auditory saccade is required. This switch would be much more absolute than previously reported attentional phenomenon. Attentional modulation typically changes the gain of sensory responses (Desimone & Duncan 1995; Maunsell 1995), but with the responses still present, and is rarely changed by more than half. The proposed switch would be essentially all-or-nothing. In other words, the decision to make a saccade to an auditory target switches auditory signals into LIP.

If such a gating mechanism for auditory signals is found, it poses the interesting question of why LIP would need to keep out auditory signals so absolutely, except under conditions where the animal requires these signals for saccades. In addition, what is the neural mechanism that can account for such an absolute gating? Finally, will non-spatial, cognitive signals also have gated access to LIP for particular eye movements? For instance, if during driving I wonder if there is enough petrol to get home, I will make a saccade to foveate the petrol gauge. Perhaps LIP receives many signals from numerous parts of the brain for particular, learned eye movement behaviours. The simultaneous input of all these signals may overwhelm the LIP machinery, requiring dynamic switching of specific signals based on the particular task at hand.

Moreover, gain mechanisms may be learned for transforming coordinates under a variety of conditions; limiting the 'pathways' into LIP to only a few at a time may allow very specific learning for making the correct coordinate transformations.

Stabilization of motion signals: integration of retinal motion stimuli with eye pursuit and head pursuit

The brain needs to take into account moving as well as static stimuli when forming stable representations of space. This problem is particularly acute when using optical flow signals for navigation. As outlined below, smooth movements of the eyes during locomotion generate motion signals on the retinas that must be subtracted from the motion signals due to translation in space to determine the path of movement. Human subjects perform this task effortlessly. Another important task is to perceive accurately the locations of motions in the world during eye movements; for instance, the world moves on our retinas when the eyes move yet we perceive the world as stationary and not moving. Whether these two perceptual consequences of integration of retinal motion and extraretinal signals use the same or different neural pathways is not known and will be discussed in more detail below. However, it is now clear that cells of area MSTd, which are sensitive to motion stimuli, shift their tuning properties spatially to compensate for eye movements (Bradley *et al.* 1996). This compensation is produced by an extraretinal eye-movement signal, which appears to operate through a gain-field mechanism similar to that of other parietal areas.

Heading computation by area MSTd

Gibson (1950) proposed that the focus of expansion of the retinal image can be used to determine the direction of heading during observer motion. The focus of expansion corresponds to the direction of heading if the eyes and head do not move. If the eyes are moving, as would occur while fixating a feature on the ground, then a roughly laminar motion (which is opposite in direction to the eye movement) is added to the expansion. In scenes with very little depth variation the retinal-expansion focus is shifted in the direction of eye movement.

Two general methods could be used to compensate for eye movements during observer translation; one uses *retinal cues* in the image, such as motion parallax, and the other uses *extraretinal cues*, such as a signal related to pursuit eye movements. Psychophysical experiments have shown that it is largely extraretinal signals that account for compensation during pursuit eye movements (Royden *et al.* 1992).

Area MSTd is a likely candidate for a cortical area involved in heading computation. Cells in this area have been found to respond to rotations, expansions and contractions, and laminar motion (Sakata *et al.* 1985; Tanaka *et al.* 1986; Duffy & Wurtz 1991; Graziano *et al.* 1994; Lagae *et al.* 1994). The receptive fields of the expansion-selective neurones are also tuned to the location of the expansion focus; this observation provides support for the idea that MSTd plays a role in navigation from optic flow (Duffy & Wurtz 1995). Several studies have documented activity in MST related to the direction of smooth pursuit eye movements (Mountcastle *et al*. 1975; Lynch *et al*. 1977; Komatsu & Wurtz 1988*a,b*; Newsome *et al*. 1988). This coincidence of optic-flow selectivity and pursuit selectivity in MSTd suggests that this area plays a role in heading computation. Area MST also receives angular-rotation vestibular signals, which would result as a consequence of head pursuit (Kawano *et al*. 1980, 1984; Thier & Erickson 1992). The vestibular component during head-pursuit has been measured with a VOR cancellation task in which the monkey maintains fixation on a stimulus that is attached to a rotating vestibular chair in which the animal is seated. The preferred direction of activity during a VOR cancellation task was found to be similar, in individual neurones, to the preferred eye-pursuit direction; this result suggests that the cells are coding smooth gaze movements independently of whether eye or head rotations are used for the gaze pursuit. These results hint that area MSTd may also provide heading compensation during head movements.

The simple condition of an observer moving toward a wall with or without eye movements has recently been examined (Bradley *et al*. 1996). Compensation for pursuit in this condition has been shown to occur when subjects are making eye movements, but not under simulated pursuit conditions where the retinal stimulus is the same but the eyes are not moving. If MSTd is involved in heading computation, then it would be expected that the focus-tuning curves of the expansion-sensitive cells would shift during pursuit eye movements to continue to code the correct heading direction with the eyes moving. It would also be expected, from the human psychophysical results, that movement compensation would not be present when the same retinal stimulus was generated as in the pursuit condition, but without eye movements. Both of these predictions were found to be true; this result provided evidence that area MSTd may play a direct role in heading computation. Moreover, many neurones shifted completely to compensate for the eye movement and showed no shift with the simulated condition. However, other cells shifted only partly and some did not shift at all. In addition, many of the non-shifting cells (as well as shifting cells) showed strong gain modulations of their activity caused by the eye-pursuit signal.

By means of cross-correlation techniques it was found that the average shift of the population of cells recorded from was $18° \pm 3°$ when the pursuit and simulated pursuit conditions were compared. This was approximately a 60% compensation for a focus that was shifted $30°$ during pursuit under the experimental conditions. The fact that many MSTd neurones shift their focus tuning by the right amount, whereas others only shift partly or not at all, suggests two possibilities: (1) only a portion of the MSTd neurones (those with complete compensation) are involved in heading computation and the others are involved in some other function (these being the ones that do not compensate); or (2) the distribution of shifts reflects the *transformatian* from retinal to heading coordinates. In the latter case, the cells with different amounts of compensation would be considered to be at different stages of the transformation process and the output would be derived from the completely shifted group. However, it is also possible that the heading judgment is based on the average shift of all cells; this partial compensation is consistent with psychophysical experiments showing that subjects may only partly correct for pursuit eye movements in heading judgment tasks.

Gain-field effects and a model for the pursuit-compensation mechanism

As indicated above, a fraction of cells in MSTd do not have focus-tuning shifts with pursuit. However, most of these cells do show modulation of their amplitude tuning by pursuit, by an average of $25 \pm 3\%$ for the cells in the sample studied. This finding suggests that shifting may be accomplished by gain modulation. A compensation model has been made, which uses two first-stage neurones whose focus tunings are offset and whose activity is summed by a second-stage neurone, which shifts its focus tuning during pursuit (Bradley et al. 1996). The first-stage cells have non-shifting focus-tuning fields whose gains are modulated by a pursuit signal. The receptive fields were modelled as sine functions; the amplitude, frequency and phase of the receptive fields, as well as two gain parameters that are applied during each of the opposed pursuits, were the parameters of the model that were adjusted and compared to the recording data. For the 36 neurones that clearly shift their focus tuning during pursuit, the fits were extremely good for such a simple model $(r^2 = 0.72 \pm 0.03)$ and much better than those found in single-stage models, which use nonlinear pursuit modulations of the focus-tuning curves (sigmoids, exponentials, thresholded linear functions) (Bradley et al. 1996).

The above model shows how MSTd could correct for the motions due to eye pursuit. However, neither this model, nor the experimental results, can determine in what coordinate frame MSTd represents heading: in the experiments (and model) the position of the eyes, head and body were all aligned. Additional experiments will be needed to dissociate these different coordinate frames by performing the experiments with the eyes, head and body in different positions relative to one another. At some point in the nervous system, heading direction will be represented in body and world coordinates in order to be able to walk or drive through the world, but we do not know if MSTd is yet at the stage where heading is taken out of eye-centred coordinates.

Heading compensation for head rotations

The previous section shows that an eye-velocity signal is required to compensate for heading judgments during eye movements, but it is not known whether a head-velocity signal would also compensate for gaze movements that are performed by moving the head. Current research in the author's laboratory is examining whether human subjects can perceive heading direction during pursuit head movements; it has been found that head-pursuit compensation is present. There are at least three potential sources for the head-movement signal: efference copy, the vestibular system, and neck proprioception. Experiments so far have shown that vestibular signals alone do not lead to compensation. This result is interesting in the light of the observation that simulating the retinal image that would occur if the eyes rotated during observer translation produces a stimulus very similar to what is generated during self motion on a curved path. When subjects view these eye rotation or translation simulations they in fact perceive that they are moving on a curved trajectory; they do not perceive that they are moving on a linear path and rotating their eyes. Such a curved path trajectory would produce vestibular stimulation in the absence of proprioceptive or efference copy signals. Therefore, the psychophysical observation that vestibular stimulation alone does not produce compensation is consistent with the curved-path interpretation made by the subjects: compensation would produce a linear path percept.

As mentioned above, vestibular as well as eye-pursuit signals have been recorded in area MSTd. In preliminary experiments in which animals are rotated in a vestibular chair, evidence has been found that many cells show focus-tuning compensation during head movement as well as during eye movement (Shenoy *et al*. 1996). This result brings up two possibilities. The first is that neurones in area MSTd that compensate for vestibular signals alone are not the final stage for perceiving the path of self motion. Rather, sites downstream from these vestibular-compensating neurones, either within MSTd or in other cortical areas, would be this final site. Thus the computation could be made, but not used if the right set of other stimuli and efference copy signals were not present. The alternative possibility is that area MSTd is not involved in heading computation but rather is computing the head- or body-centred location of motion stimuli in the world and that this computation takes place in a separate network. It is also possible that area MSTd is very general in always compensating for gaze shifts, and that this compensation can be used for either heading computation or egocentric motion perception.

Rotation, spiral and contraction patterns
Area MSTd contains neurones selective for rotation, contraction, laminar flow and spiral motions. During self-motion these various motion patterns can be present, depending on the structure of the environment and the movement of the eyes. For example, when fixating a location forwards and to the side on the ground plane while translating forwards, the motion around the fixation point is in the form of a spiral. Thus stimuli other than just expansion could potentially provide information for computing heading. However, like expansion stimuli, the rotation, contraction and spiral stimuli will shift their retinal focus during pursuit movements. However, these shifts are not in the direction of the eye movement as is the case for expansion. A rotation focus will move orthogonally to the direction of pursuit; a contraction focus will move opposite to the direction of pursuit; and spiral foci will move in oblique paths that depend on the rotation and expansion–contraction components producing the spiral.

In the above experiments, only expansion stimuli were discussed. However, the effects of pursuit eye movements on rotation and contraction neurones have also been investigated. These cells also showed focus-tuning curves and compensated the focus tuning in the correct directions (orthogonal to pursuit for rotation and opposite pursuit for contraction). The cross-correlation results on the population data also showed that the degree of compensation was nearly identical for all three patterns of motion (averaging $18 \pm 3\%$ for expansion, $15 \pm 3\%$ for contraction and $17 \pm 4\%$ for rotation) (Bradley *et al.* 1996).

That pursuit compensation also occurs for rotation- and contraction-sensitive neurones has interesting implications for the role of area MSTd in perceptual functions. Fixation straight ahead while moving over a ground plane leads to expansion on the retina. Tracking points on the ground that are eccentric to the direction of heading leads to rotation in the stimulus, with greater rotation the more eccentric the gaze direction. Thus outward spirals are generally seen (expansion + rotation) when translating while fixating locations on the ground plane. The focus of these spirals can in principle tell us the direction of heading, but only if their locations are corrected for eye velocity. The same arguments pertain to contraction and inward spiral stimuli when looking in directions opposite to the direction of motion. Therefore, the correction of the focus tuning of MSTd neurones for motion patterns other than expansions during eye movements is consistent with the hypothesis that they also assist in heading computation.

A second important perceptual function may be served by compensation for multiple patterns of motion stimuli. The shifts in focus tuning for all flow stimuli may indicate a more general phenomenon of perceptual stability in the face of retinal image motions due to pursuit eye movements. For example, when the eyes track across a spinning umbrella, the umbrella does not appear to move up or down. This idea has recently been tested directly in psychophysical experiments; results showed that subjects do adjust the focus of rotation by using an extraretinal pursuit signal (J. A. Crowell, M. Maxwell, D. C. Bradley & R. A. Andersen, unpublished observation). Thus MSTd may play a general role in compensating for smooth pursuit eye movements by means of extraretinal signals. One important outcome of this compensation may be the ability to compute heading direction, but another may be the perceptual stability of motion in the environment.

5.4 Conclusions

The posterior parietal cortex combines signals from many different modalities to create an abstract representation of space. The modalities involved include vision, audition and somatosensation (neck proprioception), as well as signals derived from the vestibular apparatus and signals indicating eye position and eye velocity. All these signals are combined in a systematic fashion by using the gain-field mechanism. This mechanism can represent space in a distributed format, which is quite powerful, allowing inputs from multiple sensory systems with discordant spatial frames and constructing outputs to other parts of the brain in different coordinate frames. It is possible that humans' unitary impression of space, independent of sensory modality, may be embodied in this abstract and distributed representation of space in the posterior parietal cortex.

References

Andersen, R. A. & Gnadt, J. W. 1989 Role of posterior parietal cortex in saccadic eye movements. In *Reviews in oculomotor research*, vol. 3 (ed. R. Wurtz & M. Goldberg), pp. 315–335. Amsterdam: Elsevier.

Andersen, R. A. & Mountcastle, V. B. 1983 The influence of the angle of gaze upon the excitability of the light-sensitive neurons of the posterior parietal cortex. *J. Neurosci.* **3**, 532–548.

Andersen, R. A., Asanuma, C. & Cowan, W. M. 1985*a* Callosal and prefrontal associational projecting cell populations in area 7a of the macaque monkey: a study using retrogradely transported fluorescent dyes. *J. Comp. Neurol.* **232**, 443–455.

Andersen, R. A., Essick, G. K. & Siegel, R. M. 1985*b* The encoding of spatial location by posterior parietal neurones. *Science* **230**, 456–458.

Andersen, R. A., Essick, G. K. & Siegel, R. M. 1987 Neurons of area 7 activated by both visual stimuli and oculomotor behavior. *Expl Brain Res.* **67**, 316–322.

Andersen, R. A., Snowden, R. J., Treue, S. & Graziano, M. 1990 Hierarchical processing of motion in the visual cortex of monkey. In *Proc. Cold Spring Harbor symp. on the brain*, pp. 741–748.

Asanuma, C., Andersen, R. A. & Cowan, W. M. 1985 Form of the divergent thalamocortical projections form the medial pulvinar to the caudal inferior parietal lobule and prefrontal cortex: a double-label retrograde fluorescent tracer study in macaque monkey. *J. Comp. Neurol.* **241**, 357–381.

Barash, S., Andersen, R. A., Bracewell, R. M., Fogassi, L. & Gnadt, J. 1991 Saccade-related activity in the lateral intra-parietal area. I. Temporal properties. *J. Neurophysiol.* **66**, 1095–1108.

Blatt, G., Andersen, R. A. & Stoner, G. 1990 Visual receptive field organization and cortico-cortical connections of area LIP in the macaque. *J. Comp. Neurol.* **299**, 421–445.

Bradley, D. C., Maxwell, M., Andersen, R. A., Banks, M. S. & Shenoy, K. V. 1996 Neural mechanisms of heading perception in primate visual cortex. *Science* **273**, 1544–1547.

Brotchie, P. R., Andersen, R. A., Snyder, L. H. & Goodman, S. J. 1995 Head position signals used by parietal neurones to encode locations of visual stimuli. *Nature* **375**, 232–235.

Desimone, R. & Duncan, J. 1995 Neural mechanisms of selective visual attention. *A. Rev. Neurosci.* **18**, 193–222.

Duffy, C.J. & Wurtz, R. H. 1991*a* Sensitivity of MST neurones to optic flow stimuli. I. A continuum of response selectivity to large-field stimuli. *J. Neurophysiol.* **65**(6), 1329–1345.

Duffy, C. J. & Wurtz, R. H. 1995 Response of monkey MST neurones to optic flow stimuli with shifted centers of motion. *J. Neurosci.* **15**(7), 5192–5208.

Geesaman, B. J. & Andersen, R. A. 1996 The analysis of complex motion patterns by form/cue invariant MSTd neurones. *J. Neurosci.* **16**(15), 4716–4732.

Gibson, J. J. 1950 *The perception of the visual world*. Boston, MA: Houghton Mifflin.

Graziano, M. S. A., Andersen, R. A. & Snowden, R. J. 1994 Tuning of MST neurones to spiral motions. *J. Neurosci.* **14**(1), 54–67.

Hyvärinen, J. 1982 *The parietal cortex of monkey and man*. Berlin: Springer.

Kawano, K., Sasaki, M. & Yamashita, M. 1980 Vestibular input to visual tracking neurones in the posterior parietal association cortex of the monkey. *Neurosci. Lett.* **17**, 55.

Kawano, K., Sasaki, M. & Yamashita, M. 1984 Response properties of neurones in posterior parietal cortex of monkey during visual-vestibular stimulation. I. Visual tracking neurones. *J. Neurophysiol.* **51**, 340–351.

Koch, K. W. & Fuster, J. M. 1989 Unit-activity in monkey parietal cortex related to haptic perception and temporary memory. *Expl Brain Res.* **76**(2), 292–306.

Komatsu, H. & Wurtz, R. H. 1988*a* Relation of cortical areas MT and MST to pursuit eye-movements. I. Localization and visual properties of neurones. *J. Neurophysiol.* **6**, 580.

Komatsu, H. & Wurtz, R. H. 1988*b* Relation of cortical areas MT and MST to pursuit eye-movements. III. Interaction with full-field visual stimulation. *J. Neurophysiol.* **60**, 621.

Kurylo, D. D. & Skavenski, A. A. 1987 Eye movements elicited by electrical stimulation of area PG in the monkey. *J. Neurophysiol.* **65**, 1243–1253.

Lagae, L., Maes, H., Raiguel, S, Xiao, D. K. & Orban, G. A. 1994 Responses of macaque STS neurones to optic flow components—a comparison of areas MT and MST. *J. Neurophysiol.* **71**, 1597.

Linden, J. F, Grunewald, A. & Andersen, R. A. 1996 Auditory sensory responses in area LIP. *Soc. Neurosci. Abstr.* **22**, 1062.

Lynch, J. C., Graybiel, A. M. & Lobeck, L. J. 1985 The differential projection of two cytoarchitectonic subregions of the inferior parietal lobule of macaque upon the deep layers of the superior colliculus. *J. Comp. Neurol.* **235**, 241–254.

Lynch, J. C., Mountcastle, V. B., Talbot, W. H. & Yin, T. C. T. 1977 Parietal lobe mechanisms for directed visual attention. *J. Neurophysiol.* **40**, 362.

Maunsell, J. H. R. 1995 The brain's visual world representation of visual targets in cerebral cortex. *Science* **270**, 764–769.

Mazzoni, P., Bracewell, R. M., Barash, S., and Andersen, R. A. 1996 Spatially tuned auditory responses in Area LIP of macaques performing delayed memory saccades to acoustic targets. *J. Neurophysiol.* **75**, 1233–1241.

Motter, B. & Mountcastle, V. B. 1981 The functional properties of the light-sensitive neurones of the posterior parietal cortex studied in waking monkeys: foveal sparing and opponent vector organization. *J. Neurosci.* **1**, 3–26.

Mountcastle, V. B., Lynch, J. C., Georgopoulos, A., Sakata, H. & Acuna, C. 1975 Posterior parietal cortex of the monkey: command functions for operation within extra-personal space. *J. Neurophysiol.* **38**, 871–908.

Newsome, W. T., Wurtz, R. H. & Komatsu, H. 1988 Relation of cortical areas MT and MST to pursuit eye movements. II. Differentiation of retinal from extraretinal inputs. *J. Neurophysiol.* **60**, 604–620.

O'Keefe, J. & Nadel, L. 1978 *The hipppocampus as a cognitive map*. Oxford University Press.

Rolls, E. T. & Omara, S. M. 1995 View-responsive neurones in the primate hippocampal complex. *Hippocampus* **5**, 409–424.

Royden, C. S., Banks, M. K. S. & Crowell, J. A. 1992 The perception of heading during eye movements. *Nature* **360**, 583–585.

Sakata, H., Shibutani, H., Kawano, K. & Harrington, T. L. 1985 *Vision Res.* **25**, 453–463.

Sakata, H., Takaoaka, Y, Kawarasaki, A. & Shibutani, H. 1973 Somatosensory properties of neurones in the superior parietal cortex (area 5) of the rhesus monkey. *Brain Res.* **64**, 85–102.

Satoshi, E., Nishijo, H., Kitu, T. & Ono, T. 1995 Neuronal activity in the primate hippocampal formation during a conditional association task based on the subject's location. *J. Neurosci.* **15**, 4952–4969.

Seal, J., Gross, C., Doudet, D. & Bioulac, B. 1983 Instruction-related changes of neuroneal-activity in area 5 during a simple forearm movement in the monkey. *J. Neurosci.* **36**(2), 145–150.

Shenoy, K. V., Bradley, D. C. & Andersen, R. A. 1996 Heading computation during head movements in macaque cortical area MSTd. *Soc. Neurosci. Abstr.* **386**, 167.

Shibutani, H., Sakata, H. & Hyväirinen, J. 1984 Saccade and blinking evoked by microstimulation of the posterior parietal association cortex of monkey. *Expl Brain Res.* **55**, 1–8.

Snyder, L. H., Batista, A. P. & Andersen, R. A. 1997 Coding of intention in the posterior parietal cortex. *Nature* **386**, 167–170.

Stricanne, B., Andersen, R. A. & Mazzoni, P. 1996 Eye-centered, head-centered and intermediate coding of remembered sound locations in area LIP. *J. Neurophysiol.* **76**(3), 2071–2076.

Tanaka, K., Hikosaka, K., Saito, H., Yukie, M., Fukada, Y & Iwai, E. 1986 Analysis of local and wide-field movements in the superior temporal visual areas of the macaque monkey. *J. Neurosci.* **6**(1), 134–144.

Thier, P. & Andersen, R. A. 1996 Electrical microstimulation suggests two different forms of representation of head-centered space in the interaparietal sulcus of rhesus monkeys. *Proc. Natn. Acad. Sci. USA* **93**, 4962–4967.

Thier, P. & Erickson, R. G. 1992 Responses of visual tracking neurones from cortical area MSTd to visual, eye, and head motion. *Eur. J. Neurosci.* **4**, 539–553.

Uno, T., Nakamura, K., Nishijo, H. & Eifuku, S. 1993 Monkey hippocampal neurones related to spatial and nonspatial functions. *J. Neurophysiol.* **70**, 1516–1529.

Xing, J., Li, C.-S. & Andersen, R. A. 1996 The temporal-spatial properties of LIP neurones for sequential eye movements simulated in a neural network model. *Soc. Neurosci. Abstr.* **21**, 28.

Zipser, D. & Andersen, R. A. 1988 A back-propagation programmed network that stimulates response properties of a subset of posterior parietal neurones. *Nature* **331**, 679–684.

6

Parietal cortex constructs action-oriented spatial representations

Carol L. Colby

6.1 Introduction

We construct a representation of the world around us in order to act. This representation must transform sensory information from the coordinates of several receptor surfaces (e.g. retina, cochlea or skin surface) into the motor coordinates needed for each effector system (e.g. eye, head, limb, trunk). The nature of this representation has been the subject of much debate (see Stein 1992, for discussion). The traditional view, strongly supported by subjective experience, is that we construct a single spatial map of the world in which objects and actions are represented in a unitary framework. The alternative view holds that the brain constructs multiple, action-oriented spatial representations in which objects and locations are represented relative to the body (egocentric representations) or relative to extrinsic reference frames not tied to the body (allocentric representations).

Neuropsychological studies support the view that the brain makes use of multiple spatial reference frames and indicate that parietal cortex is central to the construction of these representations. Damage to parietal cortex produces dramatic impairments of spatial perception and action. The most striking of these deficits is neglect, the tendency to ignore objects in the half of space opposite to the side of the lesion (Heilman *et al*. 1985; Bisiach and Vallar 1988). A patient with a right parietal lobe lesion may fail to notice or respond to objects on the left, including food on the left side of a plate or words on the left side of a page. Neglect occurs in all sensory modalities and can be expressed relative to any of several spatial reference frames. A patient with right parietal damage is typically unaware of objects on the left but 'left' may be defined with respect to a variety of axes. Patients may neglect objects on the left with respect to the body, or with respect to the line of sight, or with respect to the object to which they are attending (Gazzaniga and Ladavas 1987; Farah *et al*. 1990; Driver and Halligan 1991; Karnath *et al*. 1991; Moscovitch and Behrmann 1994). For example, a neglect patient may shave only one half of his face (head-centred frame), or dress only one side of his body (body-centred frame).

Neglect can also be expressed relative to spatial reference frames that are extrinsic to the body. A particularly striking example of a deficit expressed in an allocentric spatial reference frame has been described by Moscovitch and Behrmann (1994). They showed that patients neglected a somatosensory stimulus on the left side of the wrist (towards the thumb) when the right hand was palm down. When the hand was turned over so that the palm faced up, the neglected region shifted to the other side (towards the little finger). This demonstrates that the impairment is not of a somatosensory map of the skin surface but rather of an abstract representation of somatosensory space. The dynamic nature of the impairment, changing from moment to moment as a function of body posture, indicates that this representation is constantly being updated. Impairments in different kinds of representations can co-exist and individual patients exhibit different impairments under different behavioural demands (Behrmann and Moscovitch 1994). Multiple frames of reference may even be used simultaneously (Behrmann and Tipper 1994; Tipper and Behrmann 1996). In sum, neuropsychological and behavioural studies support the view that multiple spatial representations are called into play according to the specific demands of the task (Soechting and Flanders 1992; Tipper *et al.* 1992; Sirigu *et al.* 1996).

The deficits in spatial perception described above are matched by corresponding deficits in the generation of spatially directed actions. For example, neglect can be specific for stimuli presented at particular distances. Some patients tend to ignore stimuli presented near the body, in peripersonal space, while responding normally to distant stimuli, or vice versa (Bisiach *et al.* 1986; Halligan and Marshall 1991; Cowey *et al.* 1994). Interestingly, this form of neglect is apparent only when the subject must produce a motor response to the stimulus, and not when spatial perception alone is tested (Pizzamiglio *et al.* 1989). This dependence on action indicates that spatial representations in parietal cortex incorporate both sensory information about distance and information about intended actions. Milner and Goodale (1995) have emphasized the role of parietal cortex in generating spatial representations for the guidance of action.

The variety of deficits observed following parietal lobe damage suggests that parietal cortex must contain more than one kind of spatial representation. In order to understand more precisely how parietal cortex contributes to spatial perception and action, several groups of investigators have carried out recordings from single neurones in alert monkeys, trained to perform spatial tasks. Since the pioneering studies of Hyvarinen, Sakata, Mountcastle, Goldberg and Robinson in the 1970s, physiologists have sought to specify the sensory and motor conditions under which parietal neurones are activated, using tasks which typically require a hand or eye movement toward a visual target. This work in monkeys has provided direct evidence that parietal cortex contains several separate functional areas (Fig. 6.1) and multiple representations of space (Colby *et al.* 1988; Colby and Duhamel 1991, 1996; Stein 1992; Jeannerod *et al.* 1995; Lacquaniti *et al.* 1995; Caminiti *et al.* 1996; Andersen *et al.* 1997;

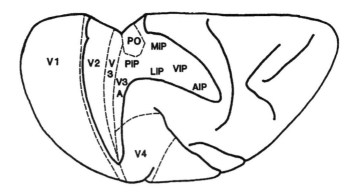

Fig. 6.1   Location of intraparietal areas in the macaque. Dorsal view of macaque right hemisphere with lunate and intraparietal sulci opened to show the location of functionally-defined areas. Adapted from Colby *et al*. (1988).

Rizzolatti *et al*. 1997). Parietal cortical areas are strongly linked with areas of frontal cortex (premotor cortex and the frontal and supplementary eye fields), which themselves encode object locations relative to a variety of reference frames (Rizzolatti *et al*. 1981b, 1994; Gentilucci *et al*. 1983; Goldberg and Bruce, 1990; Graziano *et al*. 1994, 1997; Gross and Graziano 1995). These spatial reference frames have been described either in terms of the body parts to which they are anchored (eye, head, limb) or in terms of the actions to which they contribute (looking, reaching, grasping). Beyond these egocentric representations, recent work has demonstrated the existence of more abstract, allocentric representations that encode stimulus locations and actions in coordinates that are independent of the observer (Olson and Gettner 1995, 1996). The following sections describe evidence for four distinct spatial reference frames used in parietal cortex and consider how motor action contributes to their construction.

6.2 Grasp-related spatial representation

The evidence for a grasp-related representation comes from two newly identified regions in the intraparietal sulcus (IPS). This representation is different from those described below in that the spatial dimension being represented is the desired shape of the hand rather than its position in egocentric space. Visual neurones in the caudal IPS (Kusunoki *et al*. 1993; Shikata *et al*. 1996) and in the anterior intraparietal area (AIP) (Sakata *et al*. 1995) are sensitive to the shape and orientation of objects, while motor neurones are activated in conjunction with specific hand movements. In a memory guided reaching task, AIP neurones are most strongly activated when the monkey is remembering an object with the neurone's preferred object shape (Murata *et al*. 1996). Reversible inactivation of area AIP interferes with the monkey's ability to shape its hand appropriately for grasping an object but does not produce a deficit in reaching *per se* (Gallese *et al.* 1994). Area AIP has a very specific, action-oriented spatial representation dedicated to the visual guidance of grasping with the hand. This representation is used by premotor cortex to control hand shape and grip (Jeannerod *et al.* 1995; Gallese *et al.* 1997). In contrast to the object recognition functions of neurones in ventral stream visual areas, such as inferotemporal cortex, these AIP neurones are involved in constructing an action-oriented representation that translates visual information into motor action.

6.3 Arm-centred and reaching-related spatial representation

An arm-centred spatial representation is one in which the visual receptive field is anchored to the skin surface of the limb: when the arm is moved, the visual receptive field moves with it. The most direct evidence for such a representation comes from experiments in which visual receptive fields are mapped with the arm in different positions. Neurones in premotor cortex have receptive fields that move with the arm (Graziano *et al.* 1994) and neurones encode targets in arm-centred coordinates (Caminiti *et al.* 1991). The arm region of premotor cortex receives input from the medial bank of the intraparietal sulcus (Johnson *et al.* 1993) and spatial representation in the medial intraparietal area (MIP) is thought to be arm-centred as well (Colby and Duhamel 1991). Neurones are specialized for responding to stimuli in a limited spatial range and for acting on them by reaching. A range of response properties is found in MIP, from purely somatosensory, to bimodal, to purely visual, and these response types are encountered sequentially as an electrode is moved from the lip of the sulcus toward the fundus. Purely somatosensory neurones typically have receptive fields on the contralateral limbs, most often on the hand. Bimodal neurones have visual responses to the onset of a stationary visual stimulus, as well as somatosensory responses to passive touch. These neurones are strongly activated when the monkey reaches for a visual target and are specific for both the location of the target and for the arm used to reach toward it. The neurone illustrated in Fig. 6.2 is most strongly activated when the monkey reaches in the light for a visible target using the contralateral hand. The response is strongly diminished by requiring the monkey to reach with the ipsilateral hand or to reach without visual feedback. Below these bimodal neurones is a purely visual region with an unusual response property: some neurones here give visual responses that become stronger when the target is moved to within reaching distance. These 'near' cells presumably signal the presence of a target that can be acquired by reaching.

This progression in sensory receptive field properties through the depth of MIP is mirrored in the motor response properties observed in a directional reaching task. Selectivity for movement direction was prominent during the movement period for more dorsal neurones, while more ventral neurones

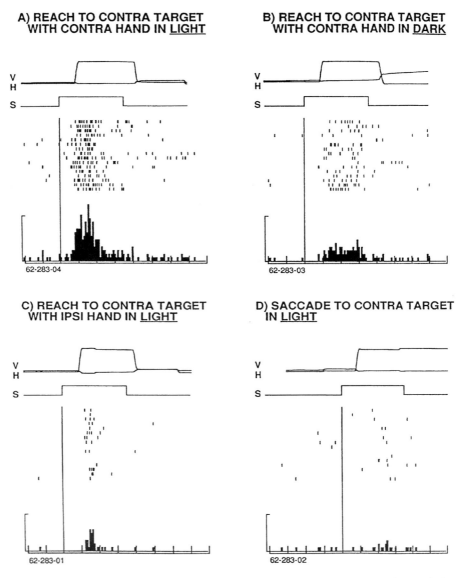

A) REACH TO CONTRA TARGET WITH CONTRA HAND IN LIGHT

B) REACH TO CONTRA TARGET WITH CONTRA HAND IN DARK

C) REACH TO CONTRA TARGET WITH IPSI HAND IN LIGHT

D) SACCADE TO CONTRA TARGET IN LIGHT

Fig. 6.2 Visual and reaching related activation of an MIP neurone. In each panel, the time lines show vertical and horizontal eye position and the onset and offset of a visual target within reaching distance. The rasters and histogram are aligned on time of stimulus onset. (A) Reaching with the contralateral hand under visual guidance produces strong and consistent activation. (B) The same hand and eye movements produce less activation when performed in the dark. (C) Reaching to the same target with the ipsilateral hand produces much less activity. (D) The neurone is not activated by a saccade to the target alone. Adapted from Colby and Duhamel (1991).

showed direction selectivity during the stimulus and delay periods (Johnson *et al.* 1996). Neurones with reaching related activity in MIP have been found to encode both stimulus features, such as location and direction of stimulus motion (Eskander and Assad 1997), and motor parameters (Andersen *et al.* 1997). The existence of visual neurones in MIP that are selective for stimuli within reaching distance suggests that MIP contributes to the construction of a spatial representation designed to control arm movements. Area MIP may be the source of the visual information used by frontal cortex to guide reaching movements.

The spatial reference frame in area MIP is dynamic, reflecting the fact that reaching related representations must be plastic enough to accomodate expansions of reach space. A tennis player experiences the racquet as an extension of his or her arm and some intriguing recent experiments suggest that bimodal neurones in MIP likewise extend their visual receptive fields when the monkey uses a tool. Iriki *et al.* (1996) trained monkeys to use a rake to retrieve distant objects and mapped visual receptive fields before and immediately after tool use. While the somatosensory receptive fields were unchanged, the visual receptive fields expanded when the monkey used the rake as an extension of its hand. The authors interpret this as a change in the body image, or schema: the enlargement of the visual receptive field reflects the neural correlate of a representation of the hand which now incorporates the tool. The visual receptive fields return to their original size within a few minutes after tool use is discontinued, and they do not expand at all if the monkey simply holds the rake without intending to use it. These rapid changes in visual receptive field size indicate that the connections which support the expansion must be in place all along: MIP neurones have access to visual information well beyond the immediately apparent receptive field.

Intended motor actions have an impact on receptive fields and spatial representation in both areas MIP and LIP (see below). These results underscore the importance of looking at the influence of behaviour on sensory representations. In both cases, the changes in spatial representation presumably reflect the impact of feedback projections from frontal motor control centres to parietal cortex (Johnson *et al.* 1996). We usually think of perception as leading to action. Visual signals arriving in cortex are analysed and processed through multiple stages, objects are recognized and locations identified, a decision of some kind is made, and an action is generated. This process is generally conceived of as information moving forward through a system whose output, a motor act, represents the end of the process. Equally important, however, may be the reverse process by which the output is fed back to earlier stages, allowing action to influence perception.

6.4 Head-centred spatial representation

A head-centred representation is one in which visual receptive fields are tied to the position of the head. As long as the head is stationary, the visual receptive

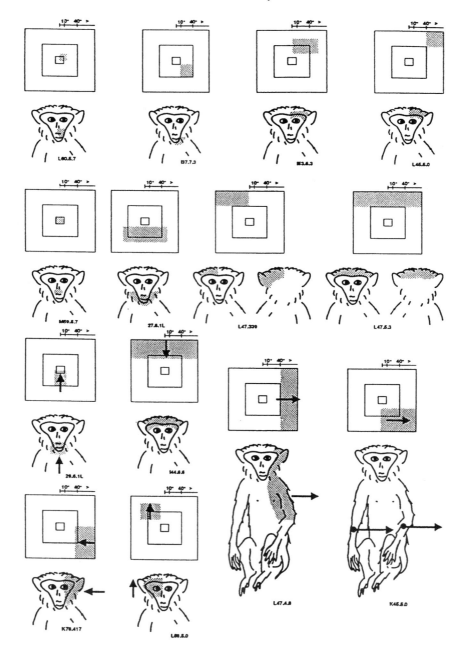

Fig. 6.3 Matching visual and somatosensory receptive fields in area VIP. Shaded regions show the locations of the visual and somatosensory receptive fields for individual VIP neurones. The screen representation is aligned with the skin surface representation. The *arrows* indicate the preferred direction of motion for stimuli in each

field covers the same part of space, regardless of the position of the eyes or the rest of the body. Some neurones in the ventral intraparietal area (VIP) represent locations relative to a head-centred reference frame. Area VIP is a strongly visually responsive area, yet neurones here can be equally well driven by somatosensory stimuli. (Colby and Duhamel 1991; Duhamel *et al*. 1991, 1998). Most VIP neurones have somatosensory receptive fields restricted to the head and face. These tactile receptive fields correspond to the visual receptive fields in three ways (Fig. 6.3). First, they match in location when the monkey looks at a central fixation point: a neurone that responds to a visual stimulus in the upper left visual field also responds when the left side of the brow is touched. The dividing line between somatosensory receptive fields linked to the upper and lower visual fields is not at the level of the eyes, as might be expected for a matching representation, but at the level of the mouth. Neurones with foveal visual receptive fields have somatosensory receptive fields on and around the muzzle, as though the mouth were the fovea of the facial somatosensory system. Second, visual and somatosensory receptive fields match in size. Neurones with small visual receptive fields tend to have restricted somato-sensory receptive fields at a matching location, while those with large, periph-eral visual receptive fields have larger somatosensory receptive fields, which may include the side or top of the head. Third, VIP neurones have matched preferences for the direction in which a stimulus is moved. A neurone that responds to a visual stimulus moving toward the right, but not to one moving left, also responds when a small probe is brushed lightly across the monkey's face in a rightward but not a leftward direction.

The correspondence between visual and tactile receptive field locations immediately raises the question of what happens to the relative locations of these fields in a single cell when either receptor surface moves. If the visual receptive field were purely retinotopic, it would occupy the same portion of the retina regardless of eye position. And if the tactile receptive field were purely somatotopic, it would be unchanged by eye position. There could not be a consistent correspondence in location if both receptive fields were defined solely with respect to their receptor surfaces. The answer is that visual receptive fields move across the retina so as to maintain spatial correspondence with somatosensory receptive fields, that is, visual receptive fields are head-centred. An example is shown in Fig. 6.4. This neurone responds best to a visual stimulus approaching the mouth from any direction (left column, A and C) but does not respond to the same visual stimulus on a trajectory toward the brow (right column, B and D). This pattern of response indicates that the stimulus is not being encoded in a simple retinotopic coordinate frame: stimuli moving through the same portion of visual space evoke quite different responses depending on the projected point of contact. Rather, this neurone is encoding

---

modality. One example is shown of a neurone selective for a visual stimulus moving to the left and joint rotation of the elbow to the left (K45.5.0). Adapted from Duhamel *et al*. (1991).

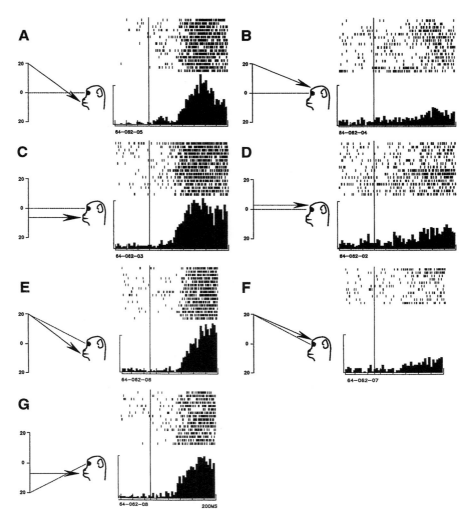

Fig. 6.4 Trajectory selectivity in area VIP. Responses of one VIP visual neurone to stimuli moved toward the mouth (*left column*) or toward the brow (*right column*). The response rate (A)–(D) is more strongly related to the projected point of contact than to either the absolute direction of motion (straight toward vs. down and toward) or the portion of the visual field stimulated (upper vs. lower). Changes in eye position (E)–(G) do not affect trajectory selectivity, indicating that stimuli are coded in a head-centred spatial reference frame. Adapted from Colby *et al*. (1993*b*).

visual information in a head-centred coordinate frame. This was confirmed by having the monkey shift its gaze to different locations (Fig. 6.4, E–G). Regardless of where the monkey looked, the cell continued to respond best to visual stimuli on any trajectory heading toward the mouth and failed to respond to similar trajectories directed toward other points on the face. This neurone has a head-centred receptive field: it responds to a certain portion of the skin surface and to the visual stimulus aligned with it, no matter what part of the retina is activated. Similar trajectory selective neurones have been described by Rizzolatti and co-workers (Fogassi *et al*. 1992, 1996) in regions of premotor cortex that receive input from area VIP. Recent work in VIP shows that head-centred visual receptive fields are not limited to trajectory selective neurones: a quantitative study of VIP neurone responses to fronto-parallel motion indicates that many neurones have head-centred receptive fields (Bremmer *et al*. 1997; Duhamel *et al*. 1997).

The function of the head-centred representation in area VIP is presumably to guide movements of the head, especially reaching with the mouth. This is suggested by the observation of an unusual class of neurones that are responsive only to visual stimuli presented at very close range, within 5 cm of the face (Colby *et al*. 1993*b*). These 'ultranear' neurones are equally well activated by monocular or binocular stimulus presentation, indicating that their distance tuning depends on cues other than disparity. They are similar to the 'near' neurones in MIP that are selective for visual targets within reaching distance of the arm. The ultranear neurones in VIP could signal the presence of a stimulus that can be acquired by reaching with the mouth. This idea fits with the results of anatomical studies showing that area VIP projects to the specific region of premotor cortex involved in the control of head and mouth movements (Matelli *et al*. 1994; Lewis and Van Essen 1996). Neurones in this premotor region, known as area F4, also have bimodal receptive fields, many of which respond best to visual stimuli presented within a few centimeters of the skin surface (Rizzolatti *et al*. 1981*a,b*; Gentilucci *et al*. 1988). Like the trajectory selective neurones in VIP, these premotor neurones also maintain visual responsiveness to stimuli approaching the tactile receptive field, regardless of the direction in which the monkey was looking (Fogassi *et al*. 1992, 1996). In both VIP and F4, locations are represented in terms appropriate for a specific kind of action, namely moving the head.

Multiple spatial representations co-exist in area VIP. The response properties of many neurones in VIP are consistent with a spatial representation in head-centred coordinates: both the ultranear and the trajectory selective neurones encode stimulus location relative to the head, as do many bimodal neurones. Results from electrical stimulation support the idea that some neurones contribute to a head-centred representation. Microstimulation in this region can evoke saccades into a restricted zone in head-centred space, independent of the starting position of the eye (Thier and Andersen 1996). On the other hand, some neurones have purely retinotopic receptive fields and presumably operate in retina-centred coordinates (Duhamel *et al*. 1997). Finally, some VIP neurones are sensitive to vestibular stimuli, which raises the possibility that they encode motion of the head relative to an inertial, or world-based, reference frame (Bremmer *et al*. 1997). Taken together, these findings raise the interesting possibility that neurones in a single cortical area contribute to multiple representations of space, and the guidance of multiple kinds of action.

6.5 Eye-centred spatial representation

At first glance, the map of space in the lateral intraparietal area (LIP) seems to be the simplest of the four described here. LIP neurones have receptive fields at locations defined relative to the retina. These neurones carry visual, memory and saccade-related signals that can be modulated by orbital position (Robinson *et al*. 1978; Bushnell *et al*. 1981; Gnadt and Andersen 1988; Andersen *et al*. 1990; Goldberg *et al*. 1990; Colby *et al*. 1993a). Neural activity in LIP reflects the degree to which spatial attention has been allocated to the location of the receptive field (Colby *et al*. 1995, 1996). The spatial representation in area LIP is not simply retinotopic however. Area LIP combines visual and eye movement information to construct a stable, eye-centred representation of space (Goldberg *et al*. 1990; Duhamel *et al*. 1992a).

This combination is important because neural representations of space are maintained over time and the brain must solve the problem of updating them when a receptor surface is moved. Every time we move our eyes, each object in our surroundings activates a new set of retinal neurones. Despite these changes, we experience the world as stable. More than a century ago, Helmholtz (1866) proposed that the reason the world stays still when we move our eyes is that the 'effort of will' involved in making an eye movement simultaneously adjusts our perception to take that eye movement into account. He suggested that when a motor command is issued to shift the eyes in a given direction, a copy of that command, a corollary discharge, is sent to brain areas responsible for generating our internal image of the world. This image is itself shifted so as to stay in alignment with the new visual information that will arrive following the eye movement. A simple experiment convinces most observers that Helmholtz' account must be essentially true. When the retina is displaced by pressing on the eye, the world does seem to move. In contrast, we are generally oblivious to the changes in the retinal image that occur with each eye movement. This perceptual stability has long been understood to reflect the fact that what we 'see' is not a direct impression of the external world but a construction or internal representation of it. It is this internal representation that is adjusted, or updated, in conjunction with eye movements.

Neurones in area LIP contribute to updating the internal image (Duhamel *et al*. 1992a; Colby *et al*. 1993a). The experiment illustrated in Fig. 6.5 shows that the memory trace of a previous stimulus is updated when the eyes move. The activity of a single LIP neurone is shown in three conditions. In a standard fixation task (left panel), the neurone responds to the onset of a stimulus in the receptive field. In a saccade task (centre), the neurone responds when an eye movement brings the receptive field onto a location containing a visual stimulus. The unexpected result is shown in the right panel. Here the monkey

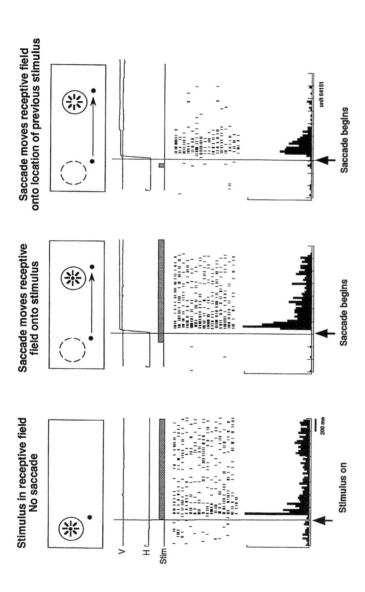

Fig. 6.5 Remapping of memory trace activity in area LIP. Responses of one LIP neurone in three conditions. (*Left*) During fixation, the neurone responds to the onset of a stimulus (starburst) in the receptive field. (Centre) Response following a saccade that moves the receptive field from its original location (*dashed circle*) onto the stimulus location (*solid circle*). (*Right*) Responses following a saccade that moves the receptive field onto a previously stimulated location. The stimulus (hollow starburst) is presented for only 50 ms and is extinguished before the saccade begins. The response is to a memory trace of the stimulus that has been remapped from the coordinates of the initial eye position to those of the final eye position. Adapted from Duhamel *et al.* (1992*a*).

made the same saccade but the stimulus was flashed on for only 50 ms, so that the stimulus was already extinguished before the saccade began. This means that no stimulus was ever physically present in the receptive field. So why did the neurone fire? We infer that an updated memory trace of the stimulus is driving the cell. At the time of stimulus onset, while the monkey is looking at the initial fixation point, the stimulus activates neurones whose receptive fields encompass the stimulated location. Some of these neurones will continue to fire after stimulus offset, encoding a memory trace of the location at which the stimulus occurred (Gnadt and Andersen 1988). At the time of the eye movement, information about the stimulus is passed from these neurones to a new set of neurones whose receptive fields now encompass the stimulated location.

The neural mechanism underlying this information transfer must depend on a corollary discharge of the eye movement command: knowledge about the eye movement causes the memory trace of the stimulus to be updated, or remapped, from the coordinates of the initial fixation point to the coordinates of the new fixation point. Nearly all neurones in area LIP exhibit this kind of remapping of stimulus memory traces. An important implication of this finding is that LIP neurones have access to visual information from the entire visual field and not just from the classically defined receptive field. LIP neurones, like those in area MIP, must already have in place the connections that provide input from distant regions of the visual field.

Remapping updates the internal representation of space in conjunction with eye movements so that it always matches the current eye position. Visual information is thereby maintained in eye-centred coordinates. Such a representation is necessary for the guidance of oculomotor responses directed toward the stimulated location. An eye-centred representation has the advantage, compared to a head-centred or world-centred representation, that it is already in the coordinates of the effector system that will be used to acquire the target. Neurones in area LIP accomplish the sensory to motor coordinate transformation and generate an action-oriented spatial representation for the guidance of eye movements.

Studies of patients indicate that remapping and the construction of an eye-centred representation are impaired as a result of parietal lobe damage. This has been demonstrated using an eye movement task in which two targets are presented sequentially. The subjects' task is simply to look at the targets in order. Because the targets are very brief (on the order of 100 ms), they are no longer present at the time the eye movements are performed. Programming the first saccade is easy. The size and direction of the required saccade exactly match the retinal position of the first target. Programming the second saccade presents a problem. The second target was seen from one location but the saccade toward it will start from a different location. In order to program this second saccade, the system must take into account the difference between the initial eye position and the new eye position. Remapping the memory trace of the second target from the coordinates of the initial eye position to the coordinates of the new eye position accomplishes the necessary transformation. If remapping underlies spatially accurate behaviour, then a lesion in the cortical areas responsible for remapping should manifest itself as a difficulty in compensating for a previous saccade.

This prediction was verified in two studies of patients with unilateral parietal lobe damage (Duhamel *et al.* 1992b; Heide *et al.* 1995). These patients made both saccades accurately when the first saccade was directed into the good (ipsilesional) hemifield. They failed when the first saccade was directed into the contralesional field, exhibiting an inability to update the location of the second target. This is not a memory deficit. Patients occasionally made saccades directly to the second target location, indicating that they both saw and remembered its position. Their problem was that they could not calculate the change in target position relative to eye position. Patients with damage limited to frontal cortex do not show this pattern of results (Heide *et al.* 1995) suggesting that the capacity to use the metrics of a saccade to update the visual representation is a unique property of parietal cortex.

Two conclusions can be drawn from these experiments. First, these patients do not have a simple spatial deficit—they can make visually-guided eye movements to all the targets perfectly well. Instead, they have a deficit that affects updating a spatial representation for use by a particular motor system. Second, updating depends on parietal cortex. The remapping of memory traces, demonstrated in single neurones in area LIP, presumably provides the substrate for the capacity to update an eye-centred spatial representation. Both the physiological and the neuropsychological results indicate that parietal cortex uses information about motor commands to transform visual input from retinal coordinates into an eye-centred representation suitable for the guidance of eye movements. The strong connections between area LIP and the frontal eye fields (Schall *et al.* 1995; Stanton *et al.* 1995) and the discovery of remapped visual responses in the FEF (Goldberg and Bruce 1990; Umeno and Goldberg 1997) suggests that these areas work together to construct an eye-centred representation of oculomotor space. Many questions remain as to how this representation is coordinated with the head, body, or world-centred reference frames that are called into play when the goal of foveating a target requires more than an eye movement (Snyder *et al.* 1993; Brotchie *et al.* 1995; Andersen *et al.* 1997; Krauzlis *et al.* 1997).

6.6 Intention, attention, and spatial representation

The above results show that parietal cortex constructs action-oriented spatial representations: objects and locations are represented in the coordinates appropriate for the effector system to be used. But what exactly is the role of motor action in generating such representations? For example, does the construction of an eye-centred representation depend on the actual perform-ance of an eye movement or is the intention to make a specific saccade enough?

Three experiments show that the intention alone is necessary and sufficient (Goldberg *et al*. 1990; Duhamel *et al*. 1992*a*; Colby 1996).

The intention to make an eye movement can precede the saccade by a long time: in the simplest visually guided saccade task, where the monkey performs the same saccade over and over, the intention to saccade to the target could precede even the appearance of the target and yet the eyes typically do not begin to move until 200 ms after target onset. With such a long lag between intention and action, it might be possible to see the impact of the intention to perform an eye movement in advance of the saccade itself. The eye movement command may be issued quite early in the trial, and a corollary discharge of the command, reflecting the intention to move, could reach parietal cortex well before the eye movement begins.

The LIP neurone illustrated in Fig. 6.6 shows that visual information can be remapped even before the saccade begins. In a standard fixation task (left panel), the neurone responds to the onset of a stimulus in the receptive field with a latency of 70 ms. In the saccade task (centre panel), a stimulus is presented outside the receptive field and the monkey is instructed to saccade to a new fixation point. The stimuli are arranged so that the saccade will move the receptive field onto the stimulus. This LIP neurone starts to respond to the visual stimulus even before the eye movement is initiated. We infer that a corollary discharge of the eye movement command has induced a transient shift in the location of the receptive field so that it encompasses the stimulus location in advance of the eye movement. The intention to make a particular saccade, one that will bring the receptive field onto the stimulus, is sufficient to induce remapping. The corollary discharge alone is enough to transform visual information from retinal to eye-centred coordinates. This process is fast. The visual response latency to the onset of a stimulus that is outside the receptive field (centre histogram) is 83 ms, only 13 ms longer than the response latency in the fixation task. This means that the corollary discharge signal can induce remapping very quickly. About a third of LIP neurones remap visual information in advance. We infer that remapping can be driven by the intention to perform an eye movement.

A second experiment demonstrates that the intention to perform a saccade can induce remapping even when that intention is not fulfilled by the motor system. In this experiment, monkeys did the same sequential saccade task used to test parietal lobe patients. Two lights were flashed briefly and the monkey had to saccade to them in order. The targets were arranged so that, at the end of the first saccade, the neurone's receptive field encompassed the location where the second target had appeared. This arrangement is the same as that used in the single step remapping experiment described above. The only difference in procedure is that the monkey is supposed to make a second saccade to the location of the remapped stimulus memory trace. LIP neurones are strongly activated in this task following the first saccade, just as they are in the single step task, and for the same reason: the stimulus trace of the second target has been remapped to the location of the receptive field. The neurone

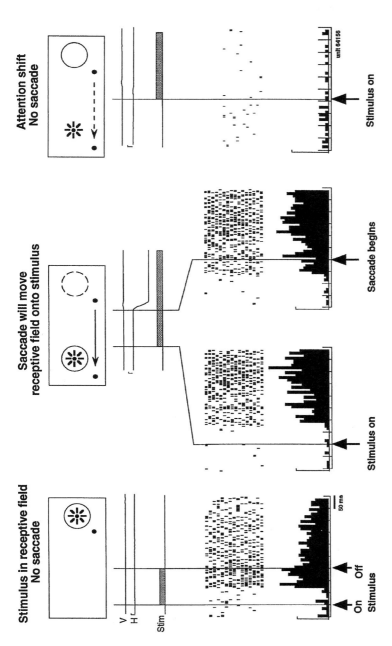

Fig. 6.6 Impact of intention and attention on remapping. (*Left*) In a fixation task, the neurone responds to the onset of a stimulas in the receptive field. (*Centre*) Visual response to a stimulus that is initially outside of the receptive field. The visual stimulus and the new fixation point appear simultaneously. The left raster is aligned on stimulus appearance, right raster on the beginning of the saccade. The neurone responds before the saccade is initiated. (*Right*) In a peripheral attention task, the monkey looks at the fixation point while attending to a peripheral target (*dashed arrow*). The onset of the stimulus produce no response. Adapted from Duhamel *et al.* (1992a) and Colby (1996).

illustrated in Fig. 6.7 is activated following the first saccade (left panel), even though no physical stimulus is currently present in the receptive field. This activity is truncated by the second saccade, which moves the receptive field away from the stimulus memory trace location.

In a long series of trials, the monkey almost always looked at the target locations in the right order but on a few trials made saccades in the wrong order. To our initial surprise, the neurone was still activated in these error trials (centre panel). A saccade directly to the second target location produced a response as though the receptive field had been brought to a stimulated location. The identical saccade produced no response when the monkey simply

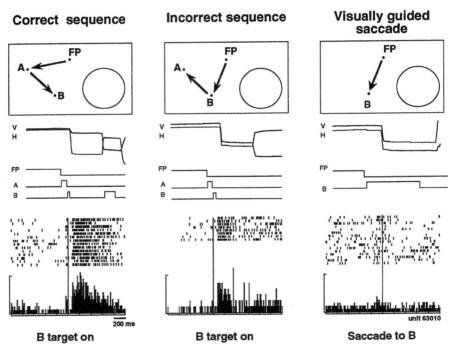

Fig. 6.7 The intention to make a saccade induces remapping regardless of actual performance. Response of one LIP neurone in three conditions. (*Left*) In the sequential saccade task, the neurone fires after the saccade moves the receptive field onto the location of the B stimulus. (*Centre*) The histogram is constructed from error trials (culled from a long series of predominantly correct trials) in which the monkey performed the saccades in reverse order. The neurone still fires after the first saccade, as though the receptive field had been brought to the location of the B stimulus. This indicates that remapping proceeds in accord with the intention to make a correct saccade to target A, even when this intention is not carried out. (*Right*) The neurone does not respond in conjunction with a visually guided saccade direct to the B target.
Adapted from Goldberg *et al*. (1990).

made a visually guided saccade to the B target location (right panel): in this case no other stimulus appeared on the screen and the saccade simply moved the receptive field from one blank location to another. So why does this neurone fire after the same saccade in the error trials? We infer that the monkey intended to perform the sequential saccades in the correct order on every trial, in order to obtain the reward that was withheld on incorrect trials. The initial motor command, and the corollary discharge of that command, stipulated that a saccade to target A would occur. This saccade would move the receptive field to location where the B target appeared. Neurones in area LIP received information about this intention to move the eyes to the A target and proceeded to update the representation of the B target accordingly. The error occured some time after the initial motor command had been issued, downstream from the source of the corollary discharge to parietal. Nonetheless, remapping proceeds as though the saccades were going to be executed in the correct order. As long as the intention to make a specific sequence of saccades is maintained, the transformation from retinal to motor coordinates proceeds, regardless of the actual motor performance. We conclude that remapping depends on a corollary discharge from the neurones that issue the eye movement command, and not on an efference copy signal from the motorneurones that go to the eye muscles.

The above two experiments demonstrate that the intention to perform a saccade is sufficient to induce remapping. Is the intention necessary? A final observation indicates that it is. We asked whether a shift of attention, with no eye movement, can induce remapping of a stimulus representation, i.e. is attention equivalent to the effect of the intention to move the eyes? We used a task that required the monkey to maintain central fixation while attending to a peripheral visual stimulus: the monkey has to release a key when the attentional target changes slightly in luminance without ever breaking fixation. Meanwhile, a new stimulus appears at the screen location that would be in the receptive field if the monkey were permitted to look at the attentional target. If shifting attention to the target were equivalent to intending to move the eyes there, the neurone should respond to the onset of this new stimulus. As shown in Fig. 6.6 (right panel), there was no response. This result contrasts with the result in the centre panel, showing that remapping occurs in accord with the intention to move the eyes. We conclude that a shift in attentional locus alone cannot induce remapping. The intention to move the eyes is both sufficient and necessary.

Intended motor action is essential for constructing a spatial representation in motor coordinates. The failure to update the spatial representation in area LIP in conjunction with an attentional shift suggests that the function of remapping is to maintain the correct alignment between the visual world and its internal representation. With an attentional shift alone, nothing moves on the retina and there is no need to remap the internal representation. Indeed, to do so would be counterproductive because it would introduce a mismatch between the external world and the internal image of it. When a saccade is about to occur, LIP neurones can make use of information about the intended eye movement to anticipate the visual consequences of that saccade and update the stored representation of object locations. The result is the construction of a spatial representation in motor coordinates.

6.7 Conclusions

The primary insight gained from physiological studies of parietal cortex is that our unitary experience of space emerges from a diversity of action-oriented spatial representations. Parietal cortex transforms sensory information from the coordinates of the receptor surfaces into the coordinates of motor effectors: the eye, head, arm or hand. These representations can include information about object shape as well as object location, so as to guide actions in space precisely (area AIP). Moreover, neurones within a single cortical area may participate in multiple spatial representations (area VIP). Spatial representations are dynamically updated in conjunction with self-generated movements, such as saccadic eye movements (area LIP) and tool use (area MIP). The mechanisms that underlie updating of spatial representations may reflect the influence of feedback from frontal cortex to parietal cortex. Finally, updating an action-oriented spatial representation depends on the intention to perform a specific motor act. An attentional shift alone is insufficient because the goal is to construct a spatial representation that tells the organism where the target is in relation to a motor effector that could be used to acquire it. Neuropsychological studies tell us that we use multiple spatial reference frames to act on the world around us. Physiological studies of parietal cortex have begun to show us how these representations could be constructed.

References

Anderson, R. A., Bracewell, R. M., Barash, S., Gnadt, J. W. and Fogassi, L. (1990). Eye position effects on visual, memory, and saccade-related activity in areas LIP and 7a of macaque. *J. Neurosci.* **10**, 1176–96.

Anderson, R. A., Snyder, L. H., Bradley, D. C. and Xing, J. (1997). Multimodal representation of space in the posterior cortex and its use in planning movements *Annu. Rev. Neurosci.* **20**, 303–30.

Behrmann, M. and Moscovitch, M. (1994). Object-centred neglect in patients with unilateral neglect: effects of left-right coordinates of objects. *J. Cog. Neurosci.* **6**, 1–16.

Behrmann, M. and Tipper, S. P. (1994). Object-based attentional mechanisms: evidence from patients with unilateral neglect. In: *Attention and Performance*, (C. Umilta and M. Moscovitch, ed.), vol. 15, pp. 351–75. Cambridge, MA: MIT Press.

Bisiach, E. and Vallar, G. (1988). Hemineglect in humans. In: *Handbook of Neuropsychology*, (F. Boller and J. Grafman, ed.), vol. 1, pp. 195–222. Amsterdam, Elsevier.

Bisiach, E., Perani, D., Vallar, G. and Berti, A. (1986). Unilateral neglect: personal and extra-personal. *Neuropsychologia* **24**, 759–67.

Bremmer, F., Duhamel, J.-R., Ben Hamed, S. and Graf, W. (1997). The representation of movement in near extra-personal space in the macaque ventral intraparietal area (VIP). In: *Parietal Lobe Contributions to Orientation in 3D Space*, (P. Thier and H.-O. Karnath, ed.), pp. 619–31. Heidelberg, Springer-Verlag.

Brotchie, P. R., Anderson, R. A., Snyder, L. H. and Goodman, S. J. (1995). Head position signals used by parietal neurons to encode locations of visual stimuli. *Nature* **375**, 232–5.

Bushnell, M. C., Goldberg, M. E. and Robinson, D. L. (1981). Behavioral enhancement of visual responses in monkey cerebral cortex. I. Modulation in posterior parietal cortex related to sellective visual attention. *J. Neurophysiol.* **46**, 755–72.

Caminiti, R., Johnson, P. B., Galli, C., Ferraina, S. and Burnod, Y. (1991). Making arm movements within different parts of space: the promotor and motor cortical representations of a coordinate system for reaching to visual targets. *J. Neurosci.* **11**, 1182–97.

Caminiti, R., Ferraina, S. and Johnson, P. B. (1996). The sources of visual information to the primate frontal lobe: a novel role for the superior parietal lobule. *Cereb. Cortex* **6**, 319–28.

Colby, C. L. (1996). A neurophysiological distinction between attention and intention. In: *Attention and Performance*, (J. McClelland and T. Inui, ed.), vol. 16, pp. 157–177, Cambridge, MIT Press.

Colby, C. L. and Duhamel, J.-R. (1991). Heterogeneity of extrastriate visual areas and multiple parietal areas in the macaque monkey. *Neuropsychologia* **29**, 517–37.

Colby, C. L. and Duhamel, J.-R. (1996). Spatial representations for action in parietal cortex. *Cog. Brain*, **5**, 105–15.

Colby, C. L., Gattass, R., Olson, C. R. and Gross, C. G. (1988). Topographic organization of cortical afferents to extrastriate visual area PO in the macaque: a dual tracer study. *J. Comp. Neurol.* **269**, 392–413.

Colby, C. L., Duhamel, J.-R. and Goldberg, M. E. (1993a). The analysis of visual space by the lateral intraparietal area of the monkey: the role of extraretinal signals. In: *Progress in Brain Reserach*, (T. P. Hicks, S. Molotchnikoff and T. Ono, ed.), vol. 95, pp. 307–16.

Colby, C. L., Duhamel, J.-R. and Goldberg, M. E. (1993b). Ventral intraparietal area of the macaque: Anatomic location and visual response properties. *J. Neurophysiol.* **69**, 902–14.

Colby, C. L., Duhamel, J.-R. and Goldberg, M. E. (1995). Oculocentric spatial representation in paretial cortex. *Cerebral Cortex* **5**, 470–81.

Colby, C. L., Duhamel, J.-R. and Goldberg. M. E. (1996). Visual, presaccadic and cognitive actvation of single neurones in monkey lateral intraparietal area. *J. Neurophysiol.* **76**, 2841–52.

Cowey, A., Small, M. and Ellis, S. (1994). Left visuo-spatial neglect can be worse in far than near space. *Neuropsychologia* **32**, 1059–66.

Driver, J. and Halligan, P. W. (1991). Can visual neglect operate in object-centred coordinates? An affirmative single case study. *Cog. Neuropsych.* **8**, 475–96.

Duhamel, J.-R., Colby, C. L. and Goldberg, M. E. (1991). Congruent representation of visual and somatosensory space in single neurons of monkey ventral intraparietial cortex area (area VIP). In: *Brain and Space*, (J. Paillard, ed.), pp. 223–36. Oxford, Oxford University Press.

Duhamel, J.-R., Colby, C. L. and Goldberg, M. E. (1992a). The updating of the representation of visual space in parietal cortex by intended eye movements. *Science* **255**, 90–2.

Duhamel, J.-R., Goldberg, M. E., FitzGibbon, E. J., Sirigu, A. and Grafman, J. (1992b) Saccadic dysmetria in a patient with a right frontoparietal lesion: the importance of corollary discharge for accurate spatial behavior. *Brain* **115**, 1387–402.

Duhamel, J.-R., Bremmer, F., BenHamed, S. and Graf, W. (1997). Spatial invariance of visual receptive fields in parietal cortex neurons. *Nature* **389**, 845–8.

Duhamel, J.-R., Colby, C. L. and Goldberg, M. E. (1988). Ventral intraparietal area of the macaque: convergent visual and somatic response properties. *J. Neurophysiol.* **79**, 126–36.

Eskandar, E. N. and Assad, J. A. (1997). Extraretinal activity in posterior parietal cortex (PPC) signals information about inferred stimulus motion distinct from intention to move. *Soc. Neurosci. Abstr.* **23**, 16.

Farah, M. J., Brunn, J. L., Wong, A. B., Wallace, M. A. and Carpenter, P. A. (1990). Frames of reference for allocating attention to space. *Cog. Neuropsych.* **28**, 335–47.

Fogassi, L., Gallese, V., di Pellegrino, G., Fadiga, L., Gentilucci, M., Luppino, G. *et al.* (1992). Space coding by premotor cortex. *Exp. Brain Res.* **89**, 686–90.

Fogassi, L., Gallse, V., Fadiga, L., Luppino, G., Matelli, M. and Rizzolatti, G. (1996). Coding of peripersonal space in inferior premotor cortex (area F4). *J. Neurophysiol.* **76**, 141–57.

Gallse, V., Murata, A., Kaseda, M., Niki, N. and Sakata, H. (1994). Deficit of hand pre-shaping after muscimol injection in monkey parietal cortex. *Neuroreport* **5**, 1525–9.

Gallse, V., Fadiga, L., Fogassi, L., Luppino, G. and Murata, A. (1997). A parietofron-tal circuit for hand grasping movements in the monkey: evidence from reversible inactivation experiments. In: *Parietal Lobe Contributions to Orientation in 3D Space*, (P. Thier and H.-O. Karnath, ed.), pp. 619–31. Heidelberg, Springer-Verlag.

Gazzaniga, M. and Ladavas, E. (1987). Disturbances in spatial attention following lesion or disconnection of the right parietal lobe. In: *Neurophysiological and Neuropsychological Aspects of Spatial Neglect*, (M. Jeannerod, ed.), pp. 203–13. Amsterdam, Elsevier.

Gentilucci, M., Scandolara, C., Pigarev, I. N. and Rizzolatti, G. (1983). Visual responses in the postarcuate cortex (area 6) of the monkey that are independent of eye position. *Exp. Brain. Res.* **50**, 464–8.

Gentilucci, M., Fogassi, L., Luppino, G., Matelli, M., Camarda, R. and Rizzolatti, G. (1988). Functional organization of inferior area 6 in the macaque monkey: I. Soma-totopy and the control of proximal movements. *Exp. Brain Res.* **71**, 475–90.

Gnadt, J. W. and Andersen, R. A. (1988). Memory related motor planning activity in posterior parietal cortex of macaque. *Exp. Brain Res.* **70**, 216–20.

Goldberg, M. E. and Bruce, C. J. (1990). Primate frontal eye fields. III. Maintenance of a spatially accurate saccade signal. *J. Neurophysiol.* **64**, 489–508.

Goldberg, M. E., Colby, C. L. and Duhamel, J.-R. (1990). The representation of visuo-motor space in the parietal lobe of the monkey. *Cold Spring Harbor Symp. Quant. Biol.* **60**, 729–39.

Graziano, M. S. A., Yap, G. S. and Gross, C. G. (1994). Coding of visual space by pre-motor neurons. *Science* **266**, 1054–56.

Graziano, M. S., Hu, X. T. and Gross, C. G. (1997). Visuospatial properties of ventral premotor cortex. *J. Neurophysiol.* **77**, 2268–92.

Gross, C. G. and Graziano, M. S. A. (1995). Multiple representations of space in the brain. *Neuroscientist* **1**, 43–50.

Halligan, P. W. and Marshall, J. C. (1991). Left neglect for near but not far space in man. *Nature*, **350**(6318), 498–500.

Heide, W., Blakenburg, M., Zimmermann, E. and Kompf, D. (1995). Cortical control of double-step saccades: implications for spatial orientation. *Ann. Neurol.* **38**, 739–48.

Heilman, K. M., Watson, R. T. and Valenstein, E. (1985). Neglect and related disorders. In: *Clinical Neuropsychology*, (K. M. Heilman and E. Valenstein, ed.) pp. 131–50. Oxford, Oxford University Press.

Helmholtz, H. (1924/1866). *Treatise on Physiological Optics*. New York, Dover.

Iriki, A., Tanaka, M. and Iwamura, Y. (1996). Coding of modified body schema during tool use by macaque postcentral neurones. *Neuroreport* **7**, 2325–30.

Jeannerod, M., Arbib, M. A., Rizzolatti, G. and Sakata, H. (1995). Grasping objects: the cortical mechanisms of visuomotor transformation. *Trends Neurosci.* **18**, 314–20.

Johnson, P. B., Ferraina, S. and Caminiti, R. (1993). Cortical networks for visual reaching. *Exp. Brain Res.* **97**, 361–5.

Johnson, P. B., Ferraina, S., Bianchi, L. and Caminiti, R. (1996). Cortical networks for visual reaching: physiological and anatomical organization of frontal and parietal lobe arm regions. *Cereb. Cortex* **6**, 102–19.

Karnath, H. O., Schenkel, P. and Fischer, B. (1991). Trunk orientation as the determining factor of the 'contralateral' deficit in the neglect syndrome and as the physical anchor of the internal representation of body orientation in space. *Brain* **114**, 1997–2014.

Krauzlis, R. J., Basso, M. A. and Wurtz, R. H. (1997). Shared motor error for multiple movements. *Science* **276**, 1693–5.

Kusunoki, M., Tanaka, Y., Ohtsuka, H., Ishiyama, K. and Sakata, H. (1993). Selectivity of the parietal visual neurones in the axis orientation of objects in space. *Soc. Neurosci. Abstr.* **19**, 770.

Lacquaniti, F., Guigon, E., Bianchi, L., Ferraina, S. and Caminiti, R. (1995). Representing spatial information for limb movement: role of area 5 in the monkey. *Cereb. Cortex* **5**, 391–409.

Lewis, J. W. and Van Essen, D. C. (1996). Connections of visual area VIP with somatosensory and motor areas of the macaque monkey. *Soc. Neurosci. Abstr.* **22**, 398.

Matelli, M., Luppino, G., Murata, A. and Sakata, H. (1994). Independent anatomical circuits for reaching and grasping linking the inferior parietal sulcus and inferior area 6 in macaque monkey. *Soc. Neurosci.* **20**, 984.

Milner, A. D. and Goodale, M. A. (1995). *The Visual Brain in Action*. Oxford, Oxford University Press.

Moscovitch, M. and Behrmann, M. (1994). Coding of spatial information in the somatosensory system: evidence from patients with neglect following parietal lobe damage. *J. Cog. Neurosci.* **6**, 151–5.

Murata, A., Gallese, V., Kaseda, M. and Sakata, H. (1996). Parietal neurons related to memory-guided hand manipulation. *J. Neurophysiol.* **75**, 2180–6.

Olson, C. R. and Gettner, S. N. (1995). Object-centered direction selectivity in the macaque supplementary eye field. *Science* **269**, 985–8.

Olson, C. R. and Gettner, S. N. (1996). Representation of object-centered space in the primate frontal lobe. *Cog. Brain Res.* **5**, 147–56.

Pizzamiglio, L., Cappa, S., Vallar, G., Zoccolotti, P., Bottini, G., Ciurli, P. *et al.* (1989). Visual neglect for far and near extra-personal space in humans. *Cortex* **25**, 471–477.

Rizzolatti, G., Scandolara, C., Matelli, M. and Gentilucci, M. (1981*a*). Afferent properties of periarcuate neurons in macaque monkeys. I. Somato-sensory responses. *Behav. Brain Res.* **2**, 125–46.

Rizzolatti, G., Scandolara, C., Matelli, M. and Gentilucci, M. (1981*b*). Afferent properties of periarcuate neurons in macaque monkeys. II. Visual responses. *Behav. Brain Res.* **2**, 147–63.

Rizzolatti, G., Riggio, L. and Sheliga, B. M. (1994). Space and selective attention. In: *Attention and Performance*, (C. Umilta and M. Moscovitch, ed.), vol. 15, pp. 231–65. Cambridge, MA: MIT Press.

Rizzolatti, G., Fogassi, L. and Gallse, V. (1997) . Parietal cortex: from sight to action. *Curr. Opin. Neurobio.* **7**, 562–7.

Robinson, D. L., Goldberg, M. E. and Stanton, G. B. (1978). Parietal association cortex in the primate: sensory mechanisms and behavioral modulation *J. Neurophysiol.* **41**, 910–32.

Sakata, H., Taira, M., Murata, A. and Mine, S. (1995). Neural mechanisms of visual guidance of hand action in the parietal cortex of the monkey. *Cereb. Cor.* **5**, 429–38.

Schall, J. D., Morel, A., King, D. J. and Bullier, J. (1995). Topography of visual cortex connections with frontal eye field in macaque: convergence and segregation of processing streams. *J. Neurosci.* **15**, 4464–87.

Shikata, E., Tanaka, Y., Nakamura, H., Taira, M. and Sakata, H. (1996). Selectivity of the parietal visual neurons in 3D orientation of surface of stereoscopic stimuli. *Neuroreport* **7**, 2389–94.

Sirigu, A., Duhamel, J. R., Cohen, L., Pillon, B., Dubois, B. and Agid, Y. (1996). The mental representation of hand movements after parietal cortex damage. *Science* **273**, 1564–8.

Snyder, L. H., Brotchie, P. and Anderson, R. A. (1993). World-centered encoding of location in posterior parietal cortex of monkey. *Soc. Neurosci. Abstr.* **19**, 770.

Soechting, J. F. and Flanders, M. (1992). Moving in three-dimensional space: frames of reference, vectors and coordinate systems. *Annual Rev. Neurosci.* **15**, 167–91.

Stanton, G. B., Bruce, C. J. and Goldberg, M. E. (1995). Topography of projections to posterior cortical areas from the macaqur frontal eye fields. *J. Comp. Neurol.* **353**, 291–305.

Stein, J. F. (1992). The representation of egocentric space in the posterior parietal cortex. *Behav. Brain Sci.* **15**, 691–700.

Thier, P. and Anderson, R. A. (1996). Electrical stimulation suggest two different forms of representation of head-centered space in the intraparietal sulcus of rhesus monkeys. *Proc. Natl. Acad. Sci.* **93**, 4962–5967.

Tipper, S. P., Lortie, C. and Baylis, G. C. (1992). Selective reaching: evidence for action-centered attention. *J. Exp. Psychol. Hum. Percept. Perform.* **18**, 891–905.

Tipper, S. P. and Behrmann, M. (1996). Object-centred not scene-based visual neglect. *J. Exp. Psychol. Hum. Percept. Perform.* **22**, 1261–78.

Umeno, M. M. and Goldberg, M. E. (1997). Spatial processing in the monkey frontal eye field. I. Predictive visual responses. *J. Neurophysiol.* **78**, 1373–83.

7

A new view of hemineglect based on the response properties of parietal neurones

Alexandre Pouget and Terrence J. Sejnowski

7.1 Introduction

The representation of space in the brain is thought to involve the parietal lobes, in part because large lesions of the parietal cortex lead to hemineglect, a syndrome characterized by a lack of response to sensory stimuli that appear in the hemispace contralateral to the lesion (Heilman *et al.* 1985). In what coordinate system are objects represented in the parietal cortex? The answer to this question is not straightforward because neglect appears to affect multiple frames of reference simultaneously, and, to a first approximation, independently of the task. Here, a recent model of the response properties of neurones in the parietal cortex that can account for this observation is presented.

There is evidence that the positions of objects are represented in multiple processing systems throughout the brain, each system specialized for a particular sensorimotor transformation and using its own frame of reference (Stein 1992; Goldberg *et al.* 1990). The lateral intraparietal area (LIP), for example, appears to encode the locations of objects in oculocentric coordinates, presumably for the control of saccadic eye movements (Colby *et al.* 1995). The ventral intraparietal cortex (VIP) (Colby & Duhamel 1993) and the premotor cortex (Fogassi *et al.* 1992; Graziano *et al.* 1994), on the other hand, seem to use head-centred coordinates and might be involved in the control of hand movements towards the face.

This modular theory of spatial representations is not fully consistent with the behaviour of patients with parietal or frontal lesions. According to the modular view, the deficits should be oculocentric for eye movements and head-centred for reaching, and more generally should depend on the task. Instead, clinical studies show a more complex pattern. This point is particularly clear in an experiment by Karnath *et al.* (1993) (Fig. 7.1a). Subjects were asked to identify a stimulus that can appear on either side of the fixation point. In order to test whether the position of the stimuli with respect to the body affects performance, two conditions were tested: a control condition with the head held straight ahead (Cl) and a second condition with the head rotated 15° to the right (where right is defined with respect to the trunk) or, equivalently, with

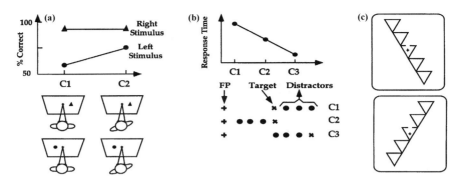

Fig. 7.1 (a) Percentage of correct identification in the experiment of Karnath *et al.* (1993). In condition 1 (C1), subjects were seated with eyes, head, and trunk lined up, whereas in condition 2 (C2) the trunk was rotated by 15° to the left. The overall pattern of performance is not consistent with pure retinal or pure trunk-centred neglect and suggests a deficit affecting a mixture of these two frames of reference. (b) Response times for the experiment by Arguin & Bub (1993) for the three experimental conditions illustrated below the graph (FP, fixation point). The decrease from condition 1 (C1) to condition 2 (C2) is consistent with object-centred neglect, i.e. subjects are faster when the target is on the right of the distractors than when it is on the left, even though the retinal position of the target is the same. The further decrease in reaction time in condition 3 (C3) shows that the deficit is also retinotopic. (c) The two displays used in the experiment of Driver *et al.* (1994). Patients must detect a gap in the upper part of the central triangle. In the top display, the object made out of the triangles is perceived as rotated 60° clockwise; in the bottom display it is perceived as being rotated 60° anticlockwise. Left parietal patients detect the gap more reliably in the bottom display, i.e. when the gap is associated with the right side of the object.

the trunk rotated 15° to the left (where left is defined with respect to the head) (see Fig. 7.1a, C2). In C2, both stimuli occurred further to the right of the trunk than in C1, though at the same location with respect to the head and retina. Moreover, the trunk-centred position of the left stimulus in C2 was the same as the trunk-centred position of the right stimulus in C1.

As expected, subjects with right parietal lesions performed better on the right stimulus in the control condition (C1), a result consistent with both retinotopic and trunk-centred neglect. However, to distinguish between the two frames of reference, performance should be compared across conditions. If the deficit is purely retinocentric, the results should be identical in both conditions because the retinotopic locations of the stimuli do not vary. On the other hand, if the deficit is purely trunk-centred, the performance on the left stimulus should improve when the head is turned right, because the stimulus now appears further towards the right of the trunk-centred hemispace. Furthermore, performance on the right stimulus in the control condition should be the same as performance on the left stimulus in the rotated condition, because they share the same trunk-centred position in both cases.

Neither of these hypotheses is fully consistent with the data. As expected from retinotopic neglect, subjects always performed better on the right stimulus in both conditions. However, performance on the left stimulus improved when the head was turned right (C2), although not sufficiently to match the level of performance on the right stimulus in the control condition (Cl, Fig. 7.1a). Therefore, these results suggest a retinotopically based form of neglect modulated by trunk-centred factors. In addition, Karnath *et al.* (1991) tested patients on a similar experiment in which subjects were asked to generate a saccade towards the target. The analysis over reaction time revealed the same type of results as the one found in the identification task, thereby demonstrating that the spatial deficit is, to a first approximation, independent of the task. Several other experiments have found that neglect affects a mixture of frames of reference in a variety of tasks (Bisiach *et al.* 1985; Calvanio *et al.* 1987; Ladavas 1987; Ladavas *et al.* 1989; Farah *et al.* 1990; Behrmann & Moscovitch 1994).

An experiment by Arguin & Bub (1993) suggests that neglect can be object-centred as well. As shown in Fig. 7.1b, they found that reaction times were faster when a target (the 'x' in Fig. 7.1b) appeared on the right of a set of distractors (C2) instead of on the left side (C1), even though the target was at the same retinotopic location in both conditions. Interestingly, moving the target further to the right led to even faster reaction times (C3), showing that hemineglect is not only object-centred but retinotopic as well in this task. Several other experiments have led to similar conclusions (Bisiach *et al.* 1979; Driver & Halligan 1991; Halligan & Marshall 1994; Husain 1995; Tipper & Behrmann 1996).

Object-centred neglect is also clearly illustrated in an experiment by Driver *et al.* (1994) in which patients were asked to detect a gap in the upper part of a triangle embedded within a larger object (Fig. 7.1c). They reported that patients detected the gap more reliably when it was associated with the right side of the object than when it belonged to the left side, even when this gap appeared at the same retinal location across conditions (Fig. 7.1c).

These results strongly support the existence of spatial representations using multiple frames of reference simultaneously shared by several behaviours. A model of the parietal cortex that has similar properties has recently been developed (Pouget & Sejnowski 1995, 1997). This paper examines whether a simulated lesion of the model leads to a deficit similar to hemineglect. In the model, parietal neurones compute basis functions of sensory signals, such as visual inputs, auditory inputs, and posture signals (e.g. eye or head position). The resulting sensorimotor representation, which is here called a basis-function map, can be used for performing nonlinear transformations of the sensory inputs: the type of transformations required for sensorimotor cordination.

The basis-function hyothesis is briefly summarized in Section 7.2 of this paper. In Section 7.3 the network architecture and the various methods used to assess the network performance in behavioural tests are described. In Section 7.4 the behaviour of a parietal patient is compared with the performance of the network model after a unilateral lesion of the basis-function representation.

7.2 Basis-function representation

The model of the parietal cortex is motivated by the hypothesis that spatial representations correspond to a recoding of the sensory inputs that facilitates the computation of motor commands. This perspective is consistent with the suggestion of Goodale & Milner (1990) that the dorsal pathway of the visual cortex mediates object manipulation (the 'How' pathway) as opposed to simply localizing objects as Mishkin et al. (1983) previously suggested (the 'Where' pathway). In general, the choice of a representation strongly constrains whether a particular computation is easy or difficult to perform. For example, addition of numbers is easy in decimal notation but difficult with Roman numerals. The same is true for spatial representations. With some representations the motor commands for grasping may be simple to perform and stable to small input errors, but in others the computation could be long and sensitive to input errors.

A set of basis functions has the property that any nonlinear function can be approximated by a linear combination of the basis functions (Poggio 1990; Poggio & Girosi 1990). Therefore, basis functions reduce the computation of nonlinear mappings to linear transformations: a simpler computation. Most sensorimotor transformations are nonlinear mappings of the sensory and posture signals into motor coordinates; hence, given a set of basis functions, the motor command can be obtained by a linear combination of these functions. In other words, if parietal neurones compute basis functions of their inputs, they recode the information in a format that simplifies the computation of subsequent motor commands.

As illustrated in Fig. 7.2b, the response of parietal neurones can be described as the product of a Gaussian function of retinal location multiplied by a sigmoid function of eye position. Sets of both Gaussians and sigmoids are basis functions, and the set of all products of these two basis functions also forms basis functions over the joint space (Pouget & Sejnowski 1995, 1997). These data are therefore consistent with the idea that parietal neurones compute basis functions of their inputs and, as such, provide a representation of the sensory inputs from which motor commands can be computed by simple linear combinations (Pouget & Sejnowski 1995, 1997).

It is important to emphasize that not all models of parietal cells have the properties of simplifying the computation of motor commands. For example, Goodman & Andersen (1990) as well as Mazzoni & Andersen (1995) have proposed that parietal cells simply add the retinal and eye-position signals. The output of this linear model does not reduce the computation of motor commands to linear combinations because linear units cannot provide a basis set. In contrast, the hidden units of the Zipser & Anderson model (1988), or the multiplicative units used by Salinas & Abbott (1995, 1996a) have response

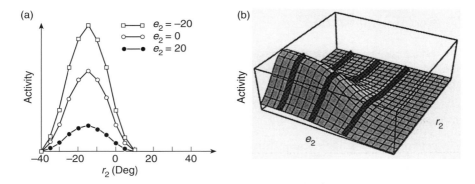

Fig. 7.2 (a) Idealization of a retinotopic visual receptive field of a typical parietal neurone for three different gaze angles (e_x). Note that eye position modulates the amplitude of the resonse but does not affect the retinotopic position of the receptive field (adapted from Andersen *et al.* 1985). (b) Three-dimensional plot showing the response function of an idealized parietal neurone for all possible eye and retinotopic positions, e_x and r_x. The plot in (a) was obtained by mapping the visual receptive field of this idealized parietal neurone for three different eye positions, as indicated by the bold lines.

properties closer to the basis-function units; the basis-function hypothesis can be seen as a formalization of these models (for a detailed discussion, See Pouget & Sejnowski 1997).

One interesting property of basis functions, particularly in the context of hemineglect, is that they represent the positions of objects in multiple frames of reference simultaneously. Thus, one can recover simultaneously the position of an object in retinocentric *and* head-centred coordinates from the response of a group of basis-function units similar to the one shown in Fig. 7.2b (Pouget & Sejnowski 1995, 1997). As shown in the next section, this property allows the same set of units to be used to perform multiple spatial transformations in parallel.

This approach can be extended to other sensory and posture signals and to other parts of the brain where similar gain modulations have been reported (Trotter *et al.* 1992; Boussaoud *et al.* 1993; Bremmer & Hoffmann 1993; Field & Olson 1994; Brotchie *et al.* 1995). When generalized to other posture signals, such as neck-muscle proprioception or vestibular inputs, the resulting representation encodes simultaneously the retinal, head-centred, body-centred, and world-centred coordinates of objects. The problem of the increase in the number of neurones required to integrate further frames of reference is discussed by Pouget & Sejnowski (1997).

Exploration has recently begun of the effects of a unilateral lesion of a basis-function network (Pouget & Sejnowski 1996). The next section describes the structure of this model.

7.3 Model organization

The model contains two distinct parts: a network for performing sensorimotor transformations, and a selection mechanism. The selection mechanism is used when there is more than one object present in the visual field at the same time.

Network architecture

The network has basis-function units in the intermediate layer to perform a transformation from a visual retinotopic map input to two motor maps in head-centred and oculocentric coordinates, respectively (Fig. 7.3)/ The visual inputs correspond to the cells found in the early stages of visual processing and the set of units encoding eye position have properties similar to the neurones found in the intralaminar nucleus of the thalamus)(Schlag-Rey & Schlag 1984). These input units project to a set of intermediate units that contribute to both output transformations. Each intermediate unit computes a Gaussian of the retinal location of the object, r_x, multiplied by a sigmoid of eye position, e_x:

$$o_{ij} = \frac{e^{-(r_x - r_{xi})^2 / 2\sigma^2}}{1 + e^{-\beta(e_x - e_{xj})}}. \tag{7.1}$$

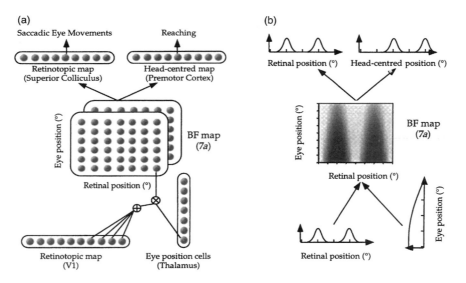

Fig. 7.3 (a) Network architecture. Each unit in the intermediate layers is a basis-function unit with a Gaussian retinal receptive field modulated by a sigmoid function of eye position. This type of modulation is characteristic of the response of parietal neurones. (b) Pattern of activity for two visual stimuli presented at $+10°$ and $-10°$ on the retina with the eye pointing at $+10°$.

Horizontal positions are considered only because the vertical axis is irrelevant for hemineglect. These units are organized in two two-dimensional maps covering all possible combinations of retinal and eye-position selectivities. The only difference between the two maps is the sign of the parameter β, which controls whether the units increase or decrease activity with eye position. The value of β was set to $8°$ for one map and $-8°$ for the other map. The indices (i, j) refer to the position of the units on the maps. Each location is character-ized by a position for the peak of the retinal receptive field, r_{xi}, and the midpoint of the sigmoid of eye position, e_{xj}. These quantities are systematically varied along the two dimensions of the maps in such a way that in the upper right corner r_{xi} and e_{xj} correspond to right retinal and right eye positions, whereas in the lower left they correspond to left retinal and left eye positions.

This type of basis function is consistent with the responses of single parietal neurones found in area 7a. The resulting population of units forms basis-function maps that encode the locations of objects in head-centred and retinotopic coordinates simultaneously.

The activities of the units in the output maps are computed by a simple linear combination of the activities of the basis-function units. Appropriate values of the weights were found by using linear regression to achieve the least mean square error (Pouget & Sejnowski 1997).

This architecture mimics the pattern of projections of the parietal area 7a, which innervate both the superior colliculus and the premotorcortex (via the ventral parietal area (VIP)) (Andersen et al. 1990; Colby & Duhamel 1993), where neurones have retinotopic and head-centred visual receptive fields, respectively (Graziano 1994; Sparks 1991). Figure 7.3b shows a typical pattern of activity in the network when two stimuli are presented simultaneously while the eye is fixated $10°$ toward the right (only the basis-function map with positive $\beta = +8°$ is shown).

Hemispheric biases and lesion model

Although the parietal cortices in both hemispheres contain neurones with all possible combinations of retinal and eye-position selectivities, most cells tend to have their retinal receptive field on the contralateral side (Andersen et al. 1990). Whether a similar contralateral bias exists for the eye position in the parietal cortex remains to be determined, although several authors have reported such a bias for eye-position selectivities in other parts of the brain (Schlag-Rey & Schlag 1984; Galletti & Battaglini 1989; Van Opstal et al. 1995).

In the model, the two basis-function maps are divided into two sets of two maps, one set for each hemisphere (again, the two maps in each hemisphere correspond to two possible values for the parameter, β). Units are distributed across each hemisphere to create neuronal gradients. These neuronal gradients induce contralateral activity gradients, such that there is more activity overall in the left maps than in the right maps when an object appears on the right of the retina and the eyes are turned to the right, with the opposite being true in the right maps.

Several types of neuronal gradients can lead to these activity gradients. The gradients used for the simulations presented here affected only the maps with positive β; that is, maps with units whose activity increases as the eyes turn to the right. In both the right and the left map, the number of units for a given pair of (r_{xi}, e_{xi}) values increased for contralateral values of eye and retinal location, as indicated in Fig. 7.4; this increase is consistent with the experimental observation that hemispheres over-represent contralateral positions.

A right parietal lesion was modelled by removing the right parietal maps and studying the network behaviour produced by the left maps alone. The effect of the lesion is therefore to induce a neuronal gradient such that there is more activity in the network for right retinal and right eye positions.

The exact profile of the neuronal gradient across the basis-function maps did not matter as long as it induced a monotonically increasing activity gradient as objects were moved further to the right of the retina and the eyes fixated further to the right. The results presented in this chapter were obtained with linear neuronal gradients.

Selection model

The selection mechanism in the model was adapted from Burgess (1995), and was inspired by the visual search theory of Treisman & Gelade (1980) and the saliency map mechanism proposed by Koch & Ullman (1985). It was used to model the behaviour of patients when presented with several stimuli

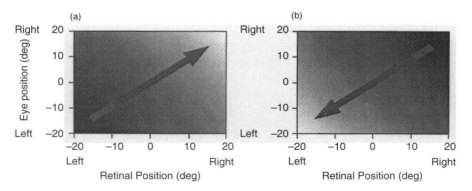

Fig. 7.4 Neuronal gradients in left and right basis-function maps for which the parameter β is positive: the activities of the units increase with eye position. The right map contains more neurones for left retinal and left eye positions, whereas the left map has the opposite gradient.

simultaneously, and it operates on what is here called the *saliency value* associated with each stimulus.

The simultaneous presentation of multiple stimuli induced multiple hills of activity in the network (see, for example, the pattern of activity shown in Fig. 7.1b for two visual stimuli). The stimulus saliency, s_i, is defined as the sum of the activities of all the basis-function units whose receptive field is centred exactly on the retinal position of the stimulus (it is the sum of activities along the dotted line shown on the basis-function map in Fig. 7.3b). The index i varies from 1 to n, where n is the number of stimuli in view at a given time. This method is mathematically equivalent to looking at the profile of activity in the output map of the superior colliculus and defining the saliency of the stimulus as the peak value of activity. Consequently, one need only consider the profiles of activity in the colliculus output map to determine the network's behaviour. Qualitatively similar values could also be obtained by looking at the profile of activation in the head-centred map.

At the first time-step, the stimulus with the highest saliency is selected by a winner-takes-all process, and its corresponding saliency is set to zero to implement inhibition of return. At the next time-step, the second highest stimulus is selected and inhibited, while the previously selected item is allowed to recover slowly. These operations are repeated for the duration of the trial. This procedure ensures that the most salient items are not selected twice in a row, but because of the recovery process, the stimuli with the highest saliencies might be selected again if displayed for long enough.

In this model of selection, the probability of selecting an item is proportional to two factors: the absolute saliency associated with the item, and the saliency relative to that of competing items.

Evaluating network performance

This model was used to simulate several experiments in which patient perform-ance was evaluated according to reaction time or percentage of correct responses.

In reaction-time experiments, it was assumed that processing involves two sequential steps: target selection and target processing. Target-selection time was assumed to be proportional to the number of iterations, n, required by the selection network to select the stimulus by using the mechanism described above. Each iteration was arbitrarily chosen to be 50 ms long. This term matters only when more than one stimulus is present, so that distractors could delay the detection of the target by winning the competition.

The time (RT) for target processing (that is to say, target recognition, target naming, etc.) was assumed to be inversely proportional to stimulus saliency, s_i:

$$RT = 100 + 50n + \frac{500}{1000s_i}. \tag{7.2}$$

The percentage of correct responses to a stimulus was determined by a sigmoid function of the stimulus saliency:

$$p = \frac{0.5}{1+e^{-(s_i - s_0)/t}} + 0.5, \tag{7.3}$$

where s_0 and t are constants.

This model for evaluating performance is based on signal-detection theory, where signal and noise are normally distributed with equal variance (Green & Swets 1966). This is equivalent to assuming that the rate of correct detection (hit rate) is the integral of the probability distribution of the signal from the decision threshold to infinity.

In line-bisection experiments, subjects were asked to judge the midpoint of a line segment. In the network model, the midpoint, m, was estimated by computing the centre of mass of the activity induced by the line in the basis-function, map:

$$m = \frac{\sum_{\text{allunits}} a_i r_{xi}}{\sum_{\text{allunits}} a_i}, \tag{7.4}$$

where r_{xi} is the retinal position of the peak of the visual receptive field of unit i.

7.4 Results

All the results given here were obtained from the lesioned model, in which the right basis-function maps have been removed. For control tasks on the normal network, see Pouget & Sejnowski (1997).

Line cancellation

The network was first tested on the line cancellation test, in which patients were asked to cross out short line segments uniformly spread over a page. To simulate this test, the display shown in Fig. 7.5a was presented and the selection mechanism was run to determine which lines were selected by the network. As illustrated in Fig. 7.5a, the network crossed out only the lines located in the right half of the display, mimicking the behaviour of left-neglect patients in the same task (Heilman et al. 1985). The rightward gradient introduced by the lesion makes the right lines more salient than the left lines. As a result, the rightmost lines always won the competition, preventing the network from selecting the left lines. The probability that the line was crossed out as a function of its position in the display is shown in Fig. 7.5a, where position is defined with respect to the frame of the display. A sharp jump in the probability function was found, such that lines to the right of this break have a probability near to unity of being selected, whereas lines to the left of the break have a probability close to zero (Fig. 7.5b).

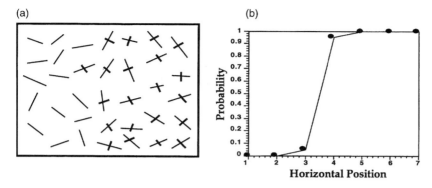

Fig. 7.5 Line cancellation task. (a) The network failed to cross out the line segments on the left side of the page, as in right parietal patients. (b) Probability of crossing a line as a function of its horizontal position in the display. The probability of crossing a bar on the left side of the display is zero, as if the neuronal gradient introduced by the lesion were a step function. The gradient, however, is smooth; the sudden change in behaviour in the centre of the display is the result of the dynamics of the selection mechanism.

The sharp jump in the probability of selection stands in contrast to the smooth and monotonic profile of the neuronal gradient. Whereas the sharp boundary in the pattern of line crossing may suggest that the model 'sees' only one-half of the display, the linear profile of the neuronal gradient shows that this is not the case. The sharp jump is mainly a consequence of the dynamics of the selection process: because right bars are associated with higher saliencies, they consistently win the competition, to the detriment of left bars. Consequently, the network starts by selecting the bar which is furthest to the right and, owing to inhibition of return, moves its way towards the left. Eventually, however, previously inhibited items recover and win the competition again, preventing the network from selecting the leftmost bars. The point at which the network stops selecting bars towards the left depends on the exact recovery rate and the total number of items displayed.

The pattern of line crossing by the network is not due to a deficit in the selection mechanism, but rather is the result of a selection mechanism operating on a lesioned spatial representation. The network had difficulty detecting stimuli on the left side of space not because it was unable to orient toward that side of space—it would orient to the left if only one stimulus were presented in the left hemifield—but because the bias in the representation favoured the rightmost bars in the competition.

Line bisection

In the line-bisection task, the network estimated the midpoint of the line to be slightly to the right of the actual midpoint (Fig. 7.6a) as reported in patients

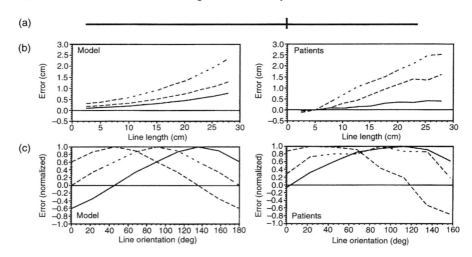

Fig. 7.6 Line bisection task. (a) Network behaviour. The midpoint is estimated too far to the right, owing to the over-representation of the right side of space. (b) Error as a function of line length. As in patients, the error in the model is proportional to the length of the line. (c) Error as a function of line orientation. The curves follow a cosine function for both the model and the patients.

with left neglect (Heilman *et al*. 1985). In contrast, the performance of an intact network was perfect (not shown).

The error does not occur because the lesioned network does not 'see' the left side of the line. On the contrary, the whole line is represented in the lesioned network, but owing to the neuronal gradient, more neurones respond to the right side of the line than to the left side. As a result, the centre-of-mass calculation used to estimate the middle of the line leads to a rightward error.

Increasing the length of the line leads to a proportional increase in the error, a result consistent with what has been observed in patients (Fig. 7.6b). The constant of proportionality between the error and the length of the line varies from patient to patient (Burnett-Stuart *et al*. 1991). A similar variation was found in the present study when the severity of the lesion in the model was varied by changing the slope of the neuronal gradient. Lesions with large slope led to a larger constant of proportionality. Finally, the effect of line orientation was tested: the error followed a cosine function of orientation (Fig. 7.6c). The phase of this cosine function depended on the orientation of the neuronal gradient along the retina. A perfectly horizontal gradient led to a phase of zero (i.e. the maximum error is obtained for a horizontal line) but oblique retinal gradients led to a non-zero phase. A similar cosine relation with variation in the phase across subjects has been reported in patients (Burnett-Stuart *et al*. 1991).

Thus, as assessed by the line cancellation (see above) and line bisection tests, a lesioned network exhibited a behaviour consistent with the neglect syndrome observed in humans after unilateral parietal lesions.

Mixture of frames of reference

The frame of reference of neglect in the model was examined next. Because Karnath *et al*. (1993) manipulated head position, their experiment was simulated in this study by using a basis-function map that integrated visual inputs with head position, rather than with eye position. In Fig. 7.7b, the pattern of activity obtained in the retinotopic output layer of the network is shown in the various experimental conditions. In both conditions, head straight ahead (broken lines) or turned to the side (solid lines), the right stimulus is associated with more activity than is the left stimulus. This is a consequence of the larger number of cells in the basis-function map for rightward position. In addition, the activity for the left stimulus increased when the head was turned to the right. This effect is related to the larger number of cells in the basis-function maps tuned to right head positions.

Because network performance is proportional to activity strength, the overall pattern of performance was found to be similar to that reported in human patients (Fig. 7.1a): the right stimulus was better processed than was the left stimulus, and performance on the left stimulus increased when the head was rotated towards the right, although not sufficiently to match the performance on the right stimulus in condition 1. Therefore, as in humans, neglect in the model was neither retinocentric nor trunk-centred alone, but both at the same time.

Similar principles can be used to account for the behaviour of patients in many other experiments that involve frames of reference (Bisiach *et al*. 1985; Calvanio *et al*. 1987; Ladavas 1987; Ladavas *et al*. 1989; Farah *et al*. 1990; Behrmann & Moscovitch 1994).

Object-centred effect

The network's reaction times in simulations of the experiments of Arguin & Bub (1993) followed the same trends reported in human patients (Fig. 7.1b). Figure 7.7b illustrates the patterns of activity in the retinotopic output layer of the network for the three conditions in those experiments. Although the absolute levels of activity associated with the target (solid lines) in conditions 1 and 2 were the same, the activity of the distractors (broken lines) differed in the two conditions. In condition 1, they had relatively higher activity and thereby strongly delayed the detection of the target by the selection mechanism. In condition 2, the distractors were less active than the target and did not delay target processing as much as they did in condition 1. The reaction time decreased even more in condition 3 because the absolute activity associated with the target was higher. Therefore, the network exhibited retinocentric and

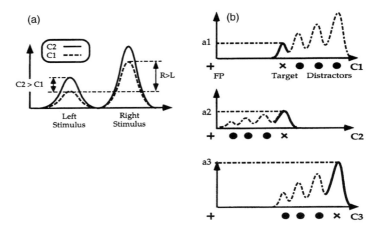

Fig. 7.7 Activity patterns in the retinotopic output layer when simulating the experiments by (a) Karnath *et al*. (1993) and (b) Arguin & Bub (1993). (a) Performance on the left stimulus improved from condition 1 (C1) to condition 2 (C2) because the stimulus saliency increased across conditions. This increase in saliency, however, is not sufficient to match the saliency of the right stimulus in condition 1. (b) Reaction time between conditions 1 and 2 decreased, owing to the change in the relative saliency of the target was the same in these two conditions (a1 = a2). FP, fixation point; C3, condition 3.

object-centred neglect, with the same pattern observed in parietal patients (Arguin & Bub 1993).

The object-centred effect might not have been expected: there was no *explicit* object-centred representation in the model. An explicit object-centred representation would be a picture-like representation of the object, much like the retinotopic map in V1, but normalized for size, translation and rotation. If it exists and if it is mapped onto the cortex in such a way that each side of the object is represented on the contralateral hemisphere, then lesions should automatically induce object-centred neglect.

The results presented here, however, demonstrate that object-based neglect does not necessarily imply that an explicit object-based representation has been lesioned in neglect patients. The form of neglect found in the experiment of Arguin & Bub (1993) could be a consequence of *relative* neglect: the apparent object-based effect could be explained by the relative saliency of the subparts of the object.

Relative saliency, however, cannot explain the results obtained by Driver *et al*. (1994) in the experiment depicted in Fig. 7.1c. In this case, explicit object-centred representations would provide a natural explanation for the behaviour of the patients. There exists, however, an alternative explanation for these results.

The view of an object rotated around an axis perpendicular to the fronto-parallel plane can indicate that either the object *or the viewer* is rotated

(Li & Matin 1995; Matin & Li 1995). In the latter case, the image is used as a cue to infer the orientation of the head in space. For instance, seeing the horizon as tilted is more likely to be the result of the viewer being tilted (flight simulators on computers rely heavily on this illusion). It would therefore make sense for the cortex to integrate general orientation cues in the image with vestibular inputs, the main cue for the determination of the head orientation in space. The right hemisphere in this case would favour vestibular rotation to the *right* and image rotation to the *left*.

Therefore, after a right lesion, a head rotation to the right *or* an object rotation to the left would reduce neglect in the same way that head rotation to the right (this time along an axis perpendicular to the coronal plane) improves subjects' performance in the experiment of Karnath *et al.* (1993) (Fig. 7.1a). There is already evidence that head rotation improves neglect (Ladavas 1987; Farah *et al.* 1990). The experiments by Driver *et al.* (1994) can be interpreted as evidence that rotating an object to the left can have the same effect, assuming that the triangle display illustrated in Fig. 7.1c engages the neural mechanisms responsible for the determination of the head orientation in space. Note that not all visual stimuli may have such cues; this could explain why Farah *et al.* (1990) and Behrmann & Moscovitch (1994) have failed to find object-centred neglect when using images such as a rotated rabbit.

It is therefore possible to reconcile the results of Driver *et al.* (1994) with the basis-function approach without invoking explicit object-centred representations. Further research is needed to determine which interpretation is valid.

Object-centred representation at the single-cell level

Explicit object-centred representations at the neuronal level appear to be supported by the recent work of Olson & Gettner (1995). They trained monkeys to perform saccades to a particular side of an object (right or left, depending on a visual cue) regardless of its position in space, and subsequently recorded the activity of cells if the supplementary eye field to characterize the neural representation involved in the task.

Olson & Gettner found that some cells responded selectively before eye movements directed to a particular side of an object, a response consistent with an explicit object-centred representation. However, *all* the cells recorded by Olson & Gettner can be interpreted as having an oculocentric motor field—they have bell-shaped tuning to the direction of the next saccadic eye movement, where direction is defined with respect to the fixation point—which is gain-modulated by the side of the object (C. R. Olson, personal communication). In a few cases, the modulation could be so strong that a cell fires when the eye movement is directed to one side of the object but not when it is directed to the other side, even if the direction of the saccade is kept constant across these conditions. Nevertheless, the directional tuning is preserved for saccades directed to the side of the object for which the cell responds, a result consistent with the gain-modulation hypothesis. Therefore, object-centred representations may not fundamentally differ from other spatial representations. In all cases, the response of neurones can be interpreted as being a basis function of the input signals. Nonetheless, whether explicit object-centred representations exist remains an empirical issue. There is no incompatibility between the basis-function approach and explicit representations.

7.5 Discussion

The model of the parietal cortex presented here was originally developed by considering the response properties of parietal neurones and the computational constraints inherent in sensorimotor transformations. It was not designed to model neglect, so its ability to account for a wide range of deficits is additional evidence in favour of the basis-function hypothesis.

As has been shown in this paper, the model presented here captures three essential aspects of the neglect syndrome: (1) it reproduces the pattern of line crossing of parietal patients in line cancellation and line bisection experiments; (2) the deficit coexists in multiple frames of reference simultaneously; and (3) the model accounts for some of the object-based effects. These results rely in part on the existence of monotonic gradients along the retinal and eye-position axis of the basis-function map. The retinal gradient is supported by recordings from single neurones in the parietal cortex (Andersen *et al.* 1990), but gradients for the postural signals remain to be demonstrated. The retinal-gradient hypothesis is also at the heart of Kinsbourne's theory of hemineglect (Kinsbourne 1987) and some models of neglect dyslexia and line bisection are based on a similar idea (Mozer & Behrmann 1990; Mozer *et al.* 1996).

The basis-function approach can account for studies beyond the ones considered here by using similar computational principles. It can reproduce, in particular, the behaviour of patients in line-bisection experiments (Halligan & Marshall 1989; Burnett-Stuart *et al.* 1991; Bisiach *et al.* 1994), and a variety of experiments dealing with frames of reference, whether in retinotopic, trunk-centred (Bisiach *et al.* 1985; Moscovitch & Behrmann 1994), environment-centred (i.e. with respect to gravity) (Ladavas 1987; Farah *et al.* 1990), or object-centred coordinates (Driver & Halligan 1991; Halligan & Marshall 1994; Husain 1995). It is also possible to account for the inability of parietal patients to imagine the contralesional side of a visual scene if visual imagery uses a basis-function map as its 'projection screen' (Bisiach & Luzzatti 1978).

In addition, a model with a basis-function map integrating sensory signals with vestibular inputs would also exhibit a temporary recovery after strong vestibular stimulation, as reported in humans after caloric stimulation of the inner ear. The explanation would be identical to that for the performance improvement on left targets observed by Karnath *et al.* (1993) when subjects turn their heads to the right (Figs 7.1a and 7.7a).

The results presented in this paper have been obtained without using explicit representations of the various Cartesian frames of reference (except for the retinotopy of the basis-function map). It is precisely because the lesion affected non-Cartesian representations that the model was able to reproduce these results. The lesion affects the functional space in which the basis functions are defined, which shares common dimensions with Cartesian spaces, but cannot be reduced to them. Hence, a basis-function map integrating retinal location and head position is retinotopic, but not solely retinotopic. Consequently, any attempt to determine the Cartesian space in which hemineglect operates is bound to lead to inconclusive results in which Cartesian frames of reference appear to be mixed.

Finally, recent neurophysiological data and theoretical models are raising the possibility that attention plays a role in spatial perception analogous to that of posture signals. Hence, Connor *et al*. (1996) have found that the position of attention in space can modulate the visual response of V4 neurones just as eye position modulates parietal neurones. Salinas & Abbott (1996*b*), as well as Riesenhubber & Dayan (1997), have pointed out that a population of such neurones provides a basis-function representation in which one of the available frames of reference is centred on attention.

If attentional modulation is distributed in such a way that each hemisphere responds preferentially when attention is oriented toward the contralateral side, one would predict that neglect can be influenced by the position of attention in the same way that it is modulated by postural signals. To our knowledge, this conjecture has not been tested on parietal patients but this would certainly be a subject worth investigating.

Acknowledgements

This research was supported in part by a fellowship from the McDonnell–Pew Center for Cognitive Neuroscience to A. P. and grants from the Office of Naval Research and the Howard Hughes Medical Institute to T. J. S. We thank Daphne Bavelier and Sophie Deneve for their comments and suggestions.

References

Anderson, R., Asanuma, C., Essick, G. & Siegel R. 1990 Corticocortical connections of anatomically and physiologically defined subdivisions within the inferior parietal lobule. *J. Comp. Neurol.* **296**(1), 65–113.

Andersen, R., Essick, G. & Siegel R. 1985 Encoding of spatial location by posterior parietal neurones. *Science* **230**, 456–458.

Arguin, M. & Bub, D. 1993 Evidence for an independent stimulus-centred reference frame from a case of visual hemineglect. *Cortex* **29**, 349–357.

Behrmann, M. & Moscovitch, M. 1994 Object-centred neglect in patients with unilateral neglect: effects of left–right coordinates of objects. *J. Cogn. Neurosci.* **6**(2), 151–155.

Bisiach, E. & Luzzatti, C. 1978 Unilateral neglect of representational space. *Cortex* **14**, 129–133.

Bisiach, E., Luzzatti, C. & Perani, D. 1979 Unilateral neglect, representational schema and consciousness. *Brain* **102**, 609–618.

Bisiach, E., Capitani, E. & Porta, E. 1985 Two basic properties of space representation in the brain: evidence from unilateral neglect. *J. Neurol. Neurosurg. Psychiatr.* **48**, 141–144.

Bisiach, E., Rusconi, M., Peretti, V. & Vallar, G. 1994 Challenging current accounts of unilateral neglect. *Neuropsychologia* **32**(11), 1431–1434.

Boussaoud, D., Barth, T. & Wise, S. 1993 Effects of gaze on apparent visual responses of frontal cortex neurones. *Expl Brain Res.* **93**(3), 423–434.

Bremmer, F. & Hoffmann, K. 1993 Pursuit related activity in macaque visual cortical areas MST and LIP is modulated by eye position. *Soc. Neurosci. Abstr.* no. 1283.

Brotchie, P., Anderson, R., Snyder, L. & Goodman, S. 1995 Head position signals used by parietal neurones to encode locations of visual stimuli. *Nature* **375**, 232–235.

Burgess, N. 1995 A solvable connectionist model of immediate recall of ordered lists. In *Advances in neural information processing systems*, vol. 7 (ed. G. Tesauro, D. Touretzky & T. Leen), pp. 51–58. Cambridge, MA: MIT Press.

Burnett-Stuart, G., Halligan, P. & Marshall, J. 1991 A Newtonian model of perceptual distortion in visuo-spatial neglect. *Neuroreport* **2**, 255–257.

Calvanio, R., Petrone, P. & Levine, D. 1987 Left visual spatial neglect is both environment-centred and body-centred. *Neurology* **37**, 1179–1181.

Colby, C. & Duhamel, J. 1993 Ventral intraparietal area of the macaque: anatomic location and visual response properties. *J. Neurophysiol.* **69**(3), 902–914.

Colby, C., Duhamel, J. & Goldberg, M. 1995 Oculocentric spatial representation in parietal cortex. *Cerebr. Cortex.* **5**(5), 470–481.

Connor, C. E., Gallant, J. L., Preddie, D. C. & Van Essen, D. C. 1996 Responses in area V4 depend on the spatial relationship between stimulus and attention. *J. Neurophysiol.* **75**(3), 1306–1308.

Driver, J. & Halligan, P. 1991 Can visual neglect operate in object-centred co-ordinates? An affirmative single case study. *Cogn. Neuropsychol.* **8**(6), 475–496.

Driver, J., Baylis, G., Goodrich, S. & Rafal, R. 1994 Axis-based neglect of visual shapes. *Neuropsychologia* **32**(11), 1353–1365.

Farah, M., Brunn, J., Wong, A., Wallace, M. & Carpenter, P. 1990 Frames of reference for allocating attention to space: evidence from the neglect syndrome. *Neuropsychologia* **28**(4), 335–347.

Field, P. & Olson, C. 1994 Spatial analysis of somatosensory and visual stimuli by single neurones in macaque area 7B. *Soc. Neurosci. Abstr.* **20**(1), 317.12.

Fogassi, L., Gallese, V., di Pellegrino, G., Fadiga, L., Gentilucci, M., Luppino, G. *et al.* 1992 Space coding by premotor cortex. *Expl. Brain Res.* **89**(3), 686–690.

Galletti, C. & Battaglini, P.1989 Gaze-dependent visual neurones in area V3a of monkey prestriate cortex. *J. Neurosci.* **9**, 1112–1125.

Goldberg, M., Colby, C. & Duhamel, J. 1990 Representation of visuomotor space in the parietal lobe of the monkey. *Cold Spring Harbor Symp. Quant. Biol.* **55**, 729–739.

Goodale, M. & Milner, A. 1990 Separate visual pathways for perception and action. *Trends Neurosci.* **15**, 20–25.

Goodman, S. & Andersen, R. 1990 Algorithm programmed by a neural model for co-ordinate transformation. In *Proc. int. joint cons. on neural networks, San Diego.*

Graziano, M., Yap, G. & Gross, C. 1994 Coding of visual space by premotor neurones. *Science* **266**, 1054–1057.

Green, D. & Swets, J. 1966 *Signal detection theory and psychophysics.* New York: Wiley.

Halligan, P. & Marshall, J. 1989 Line bisection in visuo-spatial neglect: disproof of a conjecture. *Cortex* **25**, 517–521.

Halligan, P. & Marshall, J. 1994 Figural perception and parsing in visuospatial neglect. *Neuroreport* **5**, 537–539.

Heilman, K., Watson, R. & Valenstein, E. 1985 Neglect and related disorders. In *Clinical neuropsychology* (ed. K. Heilman & E. Valenstein), pp. 243–294. New York: Oxford University Press.

Husain, M. 1995 Is visual neglect body-centric? *J. Neurol. Neurosurg. Psychiatr.* **58**(2), 262–263.

Karnath, H., Christ, K. & Hartje, W. 1993 Decrease of contralateral neglect by neck muscle vibration and spatial orientation of trunk midline. *Brain* **116**, 383–396.

Karnath, H., Schenkel, P. & Fischer, B. 1991 Trunk orientation as the determining factor of the 'contralateral' deficit in the neglect syndrome and as the physical anchor of the internal representation of body orientation in space. *Brain* **114**, 1997–2014.

Kinsbourne, M. 1987 Mechanisms of unilateral neglect. In *Neurophysiological and neuropsychological aspects of spatial neglect* (ed. M. Jeannerod), pp. 69–86. Amsterdam: North-Holland.

Koch, C. & Ullman, S. 1985 Shifts in selective visual attention: towards the underlying neural circuitry. *Hum. Neurobiol.* **4**(4), 219–227.

Ladavas, E. 1987 Is the hemispatial deficit produced by right parietal lobe damage associated with retinal or gravitational coordinates? *Brain* **110**, 167–180.

Ladavas, E., Pesce, M. & Provinciali, L. 1989 Unilateral attention deficits and hemispheric asymmetries in the control of visual attention. *Neuropsychologia* **27**(3), 353–366.

Li, W. & Matin, L. 1995 Differences in influence between pitched-from-vertical lines and slanted-from-frontal horizontal lines on egocentric localization. *Percept. Psychophys.* **57**(1), 71–83.

Matin, L. & Li, W. 1995 Multimodal basis for egocentric spatial localization and orientation. *J. Vestib. Res.* **5**(6), 499–518.

Mazzoni, P. & Andersen, R. 1995 Gaze coding in the posterior parietal cortex. In *The handbook of brain theory and neural networks* (ed. M. Arbib), pp. 423–426. Cambridge, MA: MIT Press.

Mishkin, M., Ungerleider, L. & Macko, K. 1983 Object vision and spatial vision: two cortical pathways. *Trends Neurosci* **6**, 414–417.

Moscovitch, M. & Behrmann, M. 1994 Coding of spatial information in the somatosensory system: evidence from patients with neglect following parietal lobe damage. *J. Cogn. Neurosci.* **6**(2), 151–155.

Mozer, M. & Behrmann, M. 1990 On the interaction of selective attention and lexical knowledge: a connectionist account of neglect dyslexia. *J. Cogn. Neurosci.* **2**(2), 96–123.

Mozer, M., Halligan, P. & Marshall, J. 1997 The end of the line for a brain-damaged model of hemispatial neglect. *J. Cogn. Neurosci.* **9**(2), 171–190.

Olson, C. R. & Gettner, S. N. 1995 Object-centered direction selectivity in the macaque supplementary eye. *Science* **269**, 985–988.

Poggio, T. 1990 A theory of how the brain might work. *Cold Spring Harbor Symp. Quant. Biol.* **55**, 899–910.

Poggio, T. & Girosi, F. 1990 Regularization algorithms for learning that are equivalent to multilayer networks. *Science* **247**, 978–982.

Pouget, A. & Sejnowski, T. 1995 Spatial representations in the parietal cortex may use basis functions. In *Advances in neural information processing systems*, vol. 7 (ed. G. Tesauro, D. Touretzky & T. Leen), pp. 157–164. Cambridge, MA: MIT Press.

Pouget, A. & Sejnowski, T. 1996 A model of spatial representations in parietal cortex explains hemineglect. In *Advances in neural information processing systems*, vol. 8

(ed. D. S. Touretzky, M. C. Mozer & M. E. Hasselmo), pp. 10–16 Cambridge, MA: MIT Press.

Pouget, A. & Sejnowski, T. 1997 Spatial transformations in the parietal cortex using basis functions. *J. Cogn. Neurosci.* **9**(2), 222–237.

Riesenhuber, M. & Dayan, P. 1997 Neural models for part-whole hierarchies. In *Advances in neural information processing systems*, vol. 9 (ed. M. C. Mozer, M. I. Jordan & T. Petsche) pp. 17–23 Cambridge, MA: MIT Press.

Salinas, E. & Abbott, L. F. 1995 Transfer of coded information from sensory to motor networks. *J. Neurosci.* **15**(10), 6461–6474.

Salinas, E. & Abbott, L. F. 1996*a* A model of multiplicative neural responses in parietal cortex. *Proc. Natn. Acad. Sci. USA* **93**, 11956–11961.

Salinas, E. & Abbott, L. F. 1996*b* Attentional modulation may underlie shift-invariant visual responses. *Soc. Neurosci. Abstr.* 475.4.

Schlag-Rey, M. & Schlag, J. 1984 Visuomotor functions of central thalamus in monkey. I. Unit activity related to spontaneous eye movements. *J. Neurophysiol.* **51**(6), 1149–1174.

Sparks, D. L. 1991 Sensori-motor integration in the primate superior colliculus. *Sem. Neurosci.* **3**, 39–50.

Stein, J. 1992 The representation of egocentric space in the posterior parietal cortex. *Behav. Brain Sci.* **15**(4), 691–700.

Tipper, S. P. & Behrmann, M. 1996 Object-centred not scene-based visual neglect *J. Exp. Psychol. Hum. Percept. Perform.* **22**(5), 1261–1278.

Treisman, A. & Gelade, G. 1980 A feature integration theory of attention. *Cogn. Psychol.* **12**, 97–136.

Trotter, Y., Celebrini, S., Stricanne, B., Thorpe, S. & Imbert, M. 1992 Modulation of neural stereoscopic processing in primate area V1 by the viewing distance. *Science* **257**, 1279–1281.

Van Opstal, A., Hepp, K., Suzuki, Y. & Henn, V. 1995 Influence of eye position on activity in monkey superior colliculus. *J. Neurophysiol.* **74**(4), 1593-1610.

Zipser, D. & Andersen, R. 1988 A back-propagation programmed network that stimulates response properties of a subset of posterior parietal neurones. *Nature* **331**, 679–684.

The hippocampal formation

This section deals with the allocentric representation of the rat's location in space by place cells in the rat's hippocampus, and the neuropsychology of damage to the hippocampal region in humans. The internal and external signals contributing to place cell firing are reviewed by Burgess and colleagues and incorporated into a neural network model of rat's spatial memory. This model is fully tested by being physically implemented on a mobile robot. Bures and colleagues present a series of experiments looking at the place cell representation of space when the frames of reference indicated by internal and external signals are placed in conflict. Rotenberg and Muller also investigate the properties of hippocampal place cells in the rat, including some intriguing results on the binding between their spatial receptive fields and a polarising visual stimulus at the edge of the environment. A neural network model of the integration of allocentric frames of reference from different sources is presented by Redish and Touretzky, and applied to recent data on the effects of aging on the hippocampal representation of space. Richard Morris and Frey pursue the neural basis of spatial memory at the synaptic level, presenting experiments detailing how synaptic tagging of hippocampal inputs might occur.

Looking at hippocampal function in humans, Brenda Milner and colleagues describe experiments requiring memory for the relative locations of objects in a two dimensional array. Patients with damage to the right medial temporal lobes, including the hippocampus, are impaired on these tasks. Functional imaging of normal subjects in these tasks shows activation of parahippocampal areas, but not of the hippocampus itself. Robin Morris and colleagues attempt to extend these tasks to ensure that an allocentric representation of locations be used by the subject, e.g. using locations on a simulated golf-course or on a table-top that can be walked around. Again, patients with right medial temporal damage are impaired. Mishkin and colleagues report on data from both monkeys and humans that implicate the perirhinal and parahippocampal cortices underlying the hippocampus in some of the non-spatial functions previously assumed to be subserved by the hippocampus. Lesions carefully restricted to the hippocampus in monkeys were found not to impair object recognition memory such as that tested in delayed match or non-match to sample paradigms. They also found that three children with bilateral damage apparently restricted to the hippocampus had reasonably well preserved semantic memory, but impaired memory for personally experienced events.

8

Robotic and neuronal simulation of the hippocampus and rat navigation

*Neil Burgess, James G. Donnett, Kathryn J. Jeffery and
John O'Keefe*

8.1 Introduction

The hippocampus has been implicated as the neural basis of mammalian navigation ever since the discovery of spatially tuned neurons (place cells) in the hippocampus of freely moving rats (O'Keefe & Dostrovsky 1971). The fact that each place cell (PC) tends to fire at a high rate only when the rat is in a particular portion of its environment, independently of local sensory cues such as the odour of the floor covering, prompted the idea that they provide the neural representation of the location of the rat within its environment (O'Keefe & Nadel 1978). It has recently been shown that the firing of PCs does indeed contain sufficient information to localize the rat (Wilson & McNaughton 1993). Lesions of the rat's hippocampus impair its navigational ability, specifically in tasks requiring an internal representation of space such as returning to an unmarked goal location from novel starting positions (see, for example, Morris *et al.* 1982; Jarrard 1993).

More recently, head-direction cells have been found near the hippocampus in the dorsal presubiculum (Taube *et al.* 1990) and elsewhere (Mizumori & Williams 1993; Taube 1995). These cells code for the direction of the rat's head, regardless of its location within the environment. The existence of cells of this type was predicted by O'Keefe & Nadel (1978). Although general amnesia is the primary symptom of lesions of the temporal lobes and hippocampus in humans (Scoville & Milner 1957), evidence is now beginning to emerge relating the human hippocampal region to navigation and topographical memory in neuropsychological (Habib & Sirigu 1987; Maguire *et al.* 1996*a*) and functional imaging (Maguire *et al.* 1996*b*, 1998*a*,*b*) studies.

The behaviour of the spatially tuned neurons in and around the hippocampus of freely moving rats provides an insight into the neuronal basis of mammalian navigation. Understanding the working of these neurons offers the tantalizing prospect of developing control algorithms that directly emulate mammalian navigational abilities. In this paper the spatial properties of place-cell activity are reviewed, and a computational model of the hippocampus as a navigational system implemented on a mobile robot is presented. The use of a robot ensures the realism of the assumed sensory inputs and enables true evaluation of navigational ability. Navigation is driven by place-cell firing in a manner similar to that described by Burgess *et al.* (1994), and is compared to data showing that rats can return to an unmarked goal location from novel starting positions. The behavioural data that show two separate loci for gerbils' search after two cues indicating a single reward site are pulled apart (Collett *et al.* 1986) are also considered. The neurons in the model are compared to single-unit recordings from the corresponding brain regions, where possible.

8.2 What inputs support place-cell firing?

Recent experiments have begun to reveal the nature of the signals underlying the apparently mysterious ability of place cells to restrict their firing to specific portions of an environment. Visual stimuli at or beyond the edge of the rat's reachable environment are sufficient to control the overall orientation of the place (Muller & Kubie 1987; O'Keefe & Speakman 1987) and head-direction (Taube *et al.* 1990) representations. Rotation of these stimuli can be shown to cause rotation of the receptive fields of place and head-direction cells about the centre of a symmetrical environment. However, objects placed within the environment do not show this control (Cressant *et al.* 1997). Interoceptive (possibly vestibular) inputs relating to self-motion also influence the overall orientation of the place (Knierim *et al.* 1995; Sharp *et al.* 1995) and head-direction (Blair & Sharp 1996) representations.

Place cells' receptive fields ('place fields') recorded in a series of uniform, rectangular, walled environments appear to be composed of the thresholded sum of two or more separate Gaussian tuning curves, each peaked at a fixed distance from one wall of the environment (O'Keefe & Burgess 1996) (see Fig. 8.1). Because the walls used in this experiment were indistinguishable, and often interchanged, they can be presumed to be disambiguated on the basis of their allocentric direction from the rat. Recent results (Jeffery *et al.* 1997) have proved consistent with this interpretation: altering the rat's sense of direction by rotating it very slowly (0.15 r.p.m.) in the dark causes the fields to rotate so as to maintain a fixed distance from two walls identified as being in particular directions from the rat relative to its own (rotated) frame of reference. However, if the rat and the box are slowly rotated in the presence of polarizing visual cues in the experimental room, the place fields may rotate with the box, or may stay in fixed orientation with the room, demonstrating the additional effect of extramaze visual cues in determining the rat's sense of direction. Figure 8.2 shows a place field that rotated in the dark, but was not affected by rotation in the presence of the visual room cues: in this case it maintained a fixed distance from two walls identified as being in particular veridical allocentric directions.

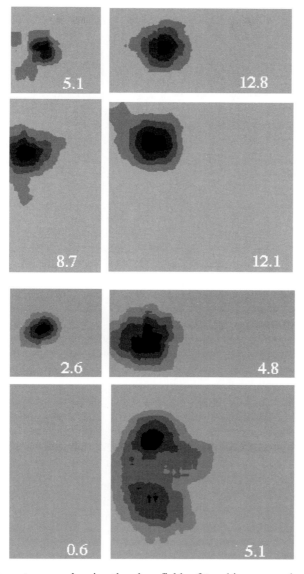

Fig. 8.1   Firing-rate maps showing the place fields of two hippocampal neurons in four rectangular boxes of varying size and shape (the peak firing rate is shown in white on each plot). The place fields maintain fixed distances from two or more walls of the environment. This occasionally leads to bimodal firing-rate maps. See O'Keefe & Burgess (1996).

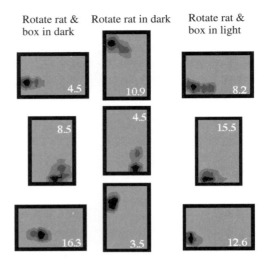

Rotate rat   Rotate rat in dark   Rotate rat &
box in dark   box in light

Fig. 8.2 Effect of internal and external inputs on place-field location. Firing-rate maps as in Fig. 8.1, showing the effect of slowly rotating a rat with and without rotation of the environment and with the polarizing visual room cues either masked (the 'dark' condition) or visibly present (the 'light' condition). *Left column*: rotation of both rat and box in the dark, first 90° anticlockwise and then 90° clockwise, resulted in corresponding rotations of the field. *Middle column*: rotation of the rat alone in the dark by 180° rotated the field by 180° even though the box remained stationary. *Right column*: when the procedure shown in the left column was repeated in the light, the field failed to rotate with the rat and the box, but maintained a constant distance from the south and west walls (as defined in the reference frame of the room).

What types of input are available, and how precise are they?

These remarkable properties of place and head-direction cell firing are apparently derived from relatively unsophisticated sensory inputs. Rats have wide-angle vision (320–360° in the horizontal plane depending on head angle (Hughes 1977)) but do not neccessarily segment stimuli into objects or extract much sensory information beyond the location or motion of the stimulus (see, for example, Dean 1990). The ability of rodents to maintain an estimate of their location and orientation by keeping a cumulative record of their own movements (referred to as 'path integration') is also limited. For example, hamsters err significantly in returning to the start location after an L-shaped route of 1 m per side or after five active rotations or two passive rotations in the dark; see Etienne *et al.* (1996) and Fig. 8.3. Thus, although it is useful for maintaining a sense of direction, path integration is clearly not sufficient to support the firing of place cells over long periods of combined translation and rotation (see Fig. 8.3). However, once established, both the place representation and the locus of searching can be maintained in the dark (O'Keefe 1976; Quirk *et al.*

(a)

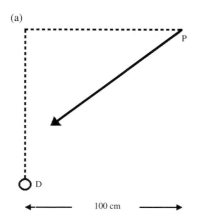

100 cm

(b)

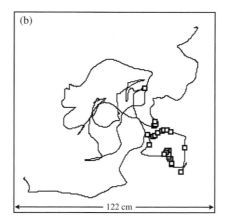

122 cm

Fig. 8.3 Path integration and place-cell firing. (a) The mean return direction (continuous line) of hamsters that had followed an L-shaped path (*broken line*) from a point of departure (D) to the point P in darkness (adapted from Seguinot *et al*. 1993). (b) Typical path of a rat searching for randomly scattered food pellets (37 s shown). The locations at which a place cell fired spikes are shown as black squares. The rat starts in the *top right* corner, initially enters the place field (indicated by a short string of spikes), leaves the place field and performs a long and circuitous trajectory before re-entering the field (indicated by the firing of many spikes) and eventually leaving for the *bottom left* corner. Note that the inaccuracy in path integration (a) implies that it would not be sufficient to support the place-specific firing of place cells (b) on its own.

1990) or in the absence of the environment's polarizing extra-maze stimuli (O'Keefe & Speakman 1987). Uncontrolled auditory, olfactory, and somatosensory cues may contribute to these findings.

Phase coding

Place-cell activity shows interesting temporal as well as spatial properties. Place cells tend to fire in short bursts of between one and four action potentials. The timing of the firing of these bursts has a systematic relation to the concurrently recorded electroencephalogram (EEG). Whenever the rat is involved in head-displacement movements or locomotion, the EEG exhibits a roughly sinusoidal oscillation of 6–11 Hz, called the 'theta' rhythm. As the rat runs through a place field on a linear track, the phase at which spikes are fired is not constant, but shifts in a systematic way (O'Keefe & Recce 1993). When the animal enters the field the firing occurs late in the cycle but shifts to progressively earlier phases as the rat runs through the field.

8.3 The Model

The sensory and motor aspects of the rat are simulated using a robot, see below. Visual estimates of the distances from the robot to the walls of the environment are used to drive the firing of 'sensory cells', entorhinal cells (ECs) and thence place cells (PCs); see Fig. 8.5. The walls are identified by their allocentric direction from the robot. The estimate of the allocentric direction (orientation) of the robot is maintained by odometry and sightings of the north wall, which is visually distinct from the other walls and serves to polarize the environment. When the robot encounters a goal location, a reinforcement signal prompts one-shot Hebbian learning in connections from the place cells to a set of goal cells. The subsequent firing rates of these cells provide a continuous estimate of the direction and proximity of the goal location, enabling navigation (see Burgess *et al.* 1994; Burgess & O'Keefe 1996).

Physical implementation

The model is implemented using a Khepera miniature robot, with on-board video and a ring of short-range infrared proximity detectors to provide artificial visual and haptic information. Two independently driven wheels allow movement around a rectangular environment formed by white walls and a dark floor (see Fig. 8.4a). Visual processing consists solely of filtering for horizontal dark–light edge points formed where a wall meets the floor, and finding the row (y) in the image containing the most dark–light edge points and the column (x) of the centroid of the edge points on that row (see Fig. 8.4b). The distance to the wall is estimated from y; the bearing of the wall to the robot from x. This scheme does not work if the robot accidentally faces directly into a corner; however, the estimated orientation does not drift fast enough for this to happen (see below). One wall (the north wall) is marked by a dark horizontal stripe along the top: its presence is detected by filtering for horizontal light–dark edge points. The infrared proximity detectors detect the presence of a wall within about 4 cm. Their function might be compared to that of a rat's whiskers.

Movement is controlled by setting the speeds of the two independent wheel motors and occasionally monitoring the shaft-encoders on the wheel axles, stopping when the desired amount of turn has been achieved. This control is not precise, so the odometry of the robot is not noticeably superior to that of a rodent (see above). Control of the robot proceeds in steps: the proximity detectors are read and the robot then rotates on the spot to face in the estimated orientations north, south, east and west, capturing an image at each orientation. After each rotation the acquired image is used to estimate the distance to the wall and to correct the robot's estimated orientation to agree with the estimate of its angle to the wall. If no wall was perceived by the proximity detectors the robot moves 3 cm forward in the desired direction.

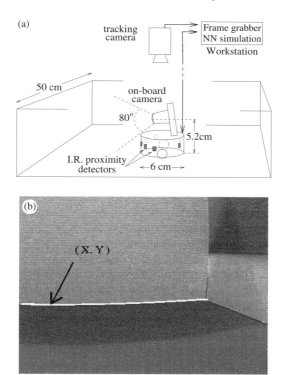

Fig. 8.4 (a) Hardware set-up (see text for further details). (b) Robot's-eye view. Detected horizontal dark–light edge points are shown in white; a black arrow marks the (x, y) position in the image that is returned by the visual processing. The north wall can be identified (on the *right*) by its dark upper half.

If a wall is perceived, the robot moves 3 cm away from the wall, whose direction is estimated from the relative values of the proximity detectors. Each step corresponds to 0.1 s (one theta cycle; see below) implying a speed of 30 cm s^{-1} for the rat, but actually takes around 3 s (processing on a SUN Ultra computer). During exploration, each movement is made in a random direction within 30° of the previous direction (unless a wall is perceived). During navigation, each movement is made in the direction indicated by the goal cells (see below).

The neural network

The visual inputs to the simulated hippocampus are represented by a rectangular array of cells organized such that each row of cells codes for the distance to a particular wall, with each cell tuned to respond maximally at a particular distance (see Fig. 8.5). Note that identifying the walls on the basis

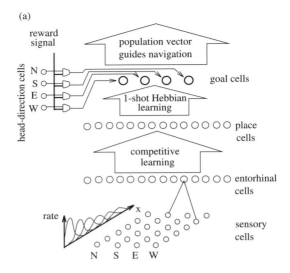

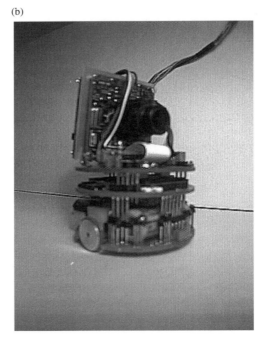

Fig. 8.5 (a) Schematic diagram of the neuronal simulation. There are 60 sensory cells, 900 ECs, 900 PCs and 4 goal cells. Inputs from the sensors on the robot drive the firing of the sensory cells. Activation propagates through the model to form a representation in space in the place-cell layer. Learning in the connections to the goal cells while at the goal location allows them to code for the direction and proximity of the goal location during subsequent movement. (b) The Khepera mobile robot. See text for further details.

of their allocentric direction from the rat solves the 'binding' or 'correspondence' problem of how information regarding a particular wall is channelled to a particular set of cells as the robot moves about. This also suggests a reason for the lack of influence on place-fields of objects within the environment: if the rat moves around an object, its allocentric direction from the rat will vary and information regarding it will not arrive on one constant set of channels.

The tuning of these 'sensory' cells follows the form of the independent place-field components identified by O'Keefe & Burgess (1996); for example, cell i in the row coding for distances from the west wall has firing rate

$$\frac{A\exp[-(x-d_i)^2/2\sigma^2(d_i)]}{\sqrt{2\pi\sigma^2(d_i)}}, \tag{7.1}$$

where x is the distance from the wall (estimated visually), d_i, is the distance at which the cell responds maximally, and the amplitude $A = 500$. The width of the response curve increases with the distance of peak response as $\sigma(x) = \sigma_0(L^2 + x^2)/L^2$. This reflects the decreasing reliability of the estimate of x at large distances. If the rat uses the angle from vertical to the top or bottom of the wall to estimate its distance, then a fixed angular error will produce this form of error as a function of distance (to within a constant). The constants are assigned values $\sigma_0 = 10\,cm$ and $L = 30\,cm$ (half the values given by O'Keefe & Burgess (1996), because the environments used here are about half the size). All connections in the model take a value of 0 or 1 ('on' or 'off'), and each cell fires at a rate proportional to the amount by which its net input exceeds a threshold. Each EC receives hard-wired connections from two sensory cells related to two orthogonal walls (see Fig. 8.5). The connections from the EC layer to the PC layer include an element of learning. Initially, only one connection to each place cell is 'on', and a type of competitive learning turns on connections from a limited number of ECs with nearby receptive fields to the most active PCs at each time-step (0.1 s) as the robot moves about its environment. Learning and activation in the PC layer occurs as follows. At each time-step a threshold is set such that the 50 PCs with the greatest input are active, and connections between maximally active ECs and the four most active PCs are switched on. Each PC has a divisive threshold equal to the number of 'on' connections to it (preventing one PC always being the most active one and always receiving more 'on' connections; see Burgess et al. 1994).

Depending on which connections to a PC have been turned on, its place field will maintain a fixed distance from two orthogonal walls, or reflect more than two inputs, all peaked at a fixed distance from a wall of the environment. Thus, some place fields will change in amplitude and shape when the environment is changed in size or shape. By contrast, the EC-receptive fields will all remain at a fixed distance from two walls and will not change shape or amplitude during changes in the shape and size of the environment.

A simple model of navigation based on place-cell firing could work in the following way. When the rat encounters a 'goal' (i.e. a location in its environment that is associated with reward), a 'goal cell' downstream from the place cells is strongly excited by the attributes of the goal. At the goal, a one-shot Hebbian increment is induced in the synaptic connections to the goal cell from the place cells that are active at the goal location. As the rat moves away from the goal location, the net activity of place cells with strong connections to the goal cell will be a monotonically decreasing fraction of the total place-cell activity. Consequently, the activation of each goal cell will code for the proximity of a goal location, and thus could be used as an evaluation function in a gradient-ascent-type search for the goal, i.e. the rat could return to the goal location simply by moving around so as to increase the firing rate of the appropriate goal cell (see Fig. 8.6a and 8.6b).

In fact, a more complicated model of learning of the goal location is used here, in which one-shot Hebbian association of the PCs active at the goal location to a set of goal cells sets up a 'population vector' (Georgopolous *et al.* 1988) that codes for the direction of the goal during subsequent navigation (see Burgess *et al.* 1994; Burgess & O'Keefe 1996). This has advantages over the simple model, such as enabling rats to take short cuts towards the goal (see, for example, Tolman 1948; Benhamou & Seguinot 1995), and does not require the rat to hunt around to determine the direction in which to move.

The population-vector model depends in part on the information carried by head-direction cells, and in part on the timing of PC firing showing the observed relation to the phase of the theta rhythm of the EEG (O'Keefe & Recce 1993). An implication of this phase relation is that PCs active at a 'late' phase tend to have place fields that are centred ahead of the rat whereas those firing at an 'early' phase tend to have place fields centred behind the rat (Burgess *et al.* 1994). In the simulation, each time-step is divided into two intervals, corresponding to the early and late phases of a 10 Hz theta rhythm. The appropriate phase coding of PCs in the model results from the sensory cells responding to a wall ahead of the rat firing during the late phase, and those responding to a wall behind the rat firing at an early phase.

Briefly, each goal cell receives a projection coding both for the rat's head direction and for the sensory attributes (e.g. food, water, etc.) of a particular goal (see Fig. 8.5). These connections deliver a 'learn now' type of reinforcement signal to a goal cell whenever the rat is at the appropriate goal location and facing in the appropriate direction. If this learning signal arrives at a 'late' phase of the EEG, or if synaptic plasticity is restricted to this phase (see, for example, Pavlides *et al.* (1988) for the relation of long-term potentiation of synapses to the theta rhythm), then the goal cell associated with, for example, the direction north will form active connections from place cells with receptive fields centred to the north of the location of the goal. As the rat looks around in different directions from the goal location, the connection weights to the set of goal cells are incremented such that each is associated with a particular allocentric direction, and will fire maximally at a location displaced from the goal in that direction. Thus the 'population vector', or vector sum of the directions associated with each goal cell weighted by their firing rates, estimates

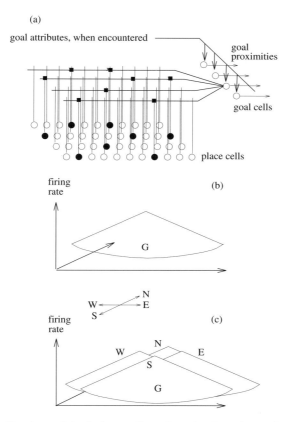

Fig. 8.6 (a) Simple model of place cells and navigation. A 'goal' cell stores a goal's location by taking a snapshot of place cell activity via long-term potentiation (LTP) when a goal cell is excited by the attributes of a particular goal location. *Filled circles*, active place cells; *open circles*, inactive place cells; *filled squares*, potentiated synapses. (b) The firing-rate map of the goal cell in the simple model during subsequent movements of the rat. This shows the cell's firing rate as a function of the location of the rat. It resembles an inverted cone, and codes for the proximity of the goal (G). (c) Population-vector model of place cells and navigation. Each goal location is represented by a group of goal cells. The firing of each cell indicates that the rat is displaced from the goal in a particular direction, such that the population vector of the group of cells represents the direction and proximity of the goal from the rat. The firing-rate maps of four cells corresponding to the directions north, south, east and west are shown. G marks the goal location. Adapted from Burgess & O'Keefe (1995).

the direction of the rat from the goal (for example, whenever the rat is north of the goal, the goal cell associated with north will be firing more strongly than that associated with south; see Fig. 8.6c).

The firing of these goal cells drives navigation of the robot, enabling it to return to a previously visited but unmarked goal location. The goal-cell population vector is an allocentric direction (e.g. north-west) and must be translated into an egocentric direction (e.g. left) before being used. This transformation is simple given that the robot knows its own orientation, and might be expected to occur in the posterior parietal cortex or in the basal ganglia (see Brown & Sharp 1995).

8.4 Performance

The robot was tested in two rectangular environments of size $50\,\text{cm} \times 50\,\text{cm}$ and $50\,\text{cm} \times 75\,\text{cm}$. Its movements were tracked by an overhead camera and tracking system that detected two LEDs on the robot. Figure 8.7 shows the robot's exploration of a square environment. The robot performs well in maintaining estimates of the distance and direction of each wall relative to it. Put another way, relative to its environment, the robot shows good self-localization and maintenance of sense of direction. Figure 8.7 also shows the performance of the robot in returning to an unmarked reward location having visited it once previously. The robot shows generalization in returning to the goal from novel staring locations.

Figure 8.8 shows the effect of expanding the environment after the location of the goal has been learned. When the environment is increased in size along one axis, most simulated place fields remain at a fixed distance from one of the two walls, although some become stretched and bimodal along that axis (see Fig. 8.9). This compares well with observed data, in which the most common pattern was for place fields to maintain fixed positions relative to a wall, although some became stretched or bimodal (O'Keefe & Burgess 1996). By contrast, EC-receptive fields are larger and always remain at a fixed distance from two of the walls, consistent with the reported experimental data (Quirk *et al*. 1992). In terms of the robot's behaviour, expanding the evironment along one axis effectively stretches out the goal-cell representation along that axis, but still results in a unimodal search pattern located between the loci indicated by fixed distances from each of the walls.

The search pattern generated from the hippocampal representation of space depends on the storage and output mechanism that makes use of it. The particular model of this mechanism presented here (i.e. the goal-cell population vector) leads to the above behaviour. The way that phase coding is used in this model in the learning of connection weights to a goal cell leads to the north goal cell effectively being tied most strongly to the north wall, and similarly for the south goal cell and the south wall. Thus, the principal effect of expanding an environment is a separation of the peaks of each goal cell's firing-rate map (the locus of search remaining between them). By contrast, contracting an environment by a large enough factor can cause the locations of peak firing of opposing goal cells to cross over, and produces a more dramatic effect: the robot searches only at the edges of the environment. Whether or not these results predict the actual experimental performance of rats reflects directly on the validity of this

(a)

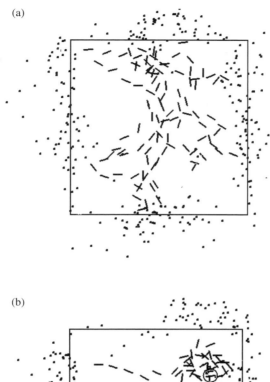

(b)

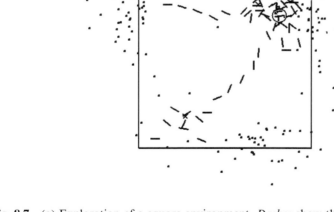

Fig. 8.7 (a) Exploration of a square environment. *Dashes* show the actual path of the robot, each dash representing 0.1 s of simulated time (or about 3 s of real time). *Dots* show the robot's estimate of the locations of the wall at each step. Their proximity to the actual wall locations demonstrates the maintenance of good self-localization. (b) Navigation following exploration. The robot received a (simulated) reward at the location marked O and was then replaced in the environment in two different locations and required to return to the goal location. When searching, the robot follows the direction indicated by the goal cells at each time-step, and is successfully guided back to the goal location.

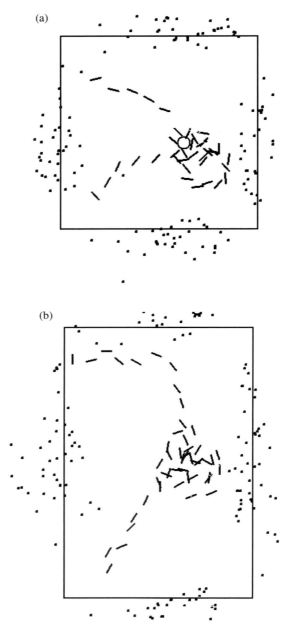

Fig. 8.8 Navigation in a square environment to a goal location (marked by O) before (a) and immediately after (b) expansion of the environment into a long rectangle.

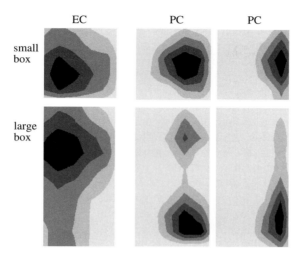

Fig. 8.9 *Top row*: firing rates for an entorhinal cell (EC, *left*) and two place cells (PCs, *middle* and *right*) calculated during exploration in a square environment. *Bottom row*: firing rates for the EC and PCs during exploration immediately after expansion of the square environment into a long rectangular environment. Note that the receptive field of the EC remains at a fixed distance from two of the walls (the *top* and *left* walls), whereas one of the PCs (*middle*) has a bimodal receptive field in the expanded environment.

mechanism. Using a different output mechanism, such as the simple model in Fig. 8.6a and 8.6b, would have different consequences for behaviour.

8.5 Discussion

This model has developed from the work of Burgess *et al.* (1993, 1994) and O'Keefe & Burgess (1996). In terms of the overall aims and structure the work is similar to recent work by Touretzky & Redish (1996). However, their aim is more towards integrating suggested functional roles for many brain regions, whereas our aim is more directed at the details of the neuronal implementation. For example, this model concentrates on the origins of the sensory inputs underlying place-cell firing and on how the firing of place cells could drive navigation (i.e. specifying how a vector-voting hypothesis could be implemented rather than simply postulating its existence).

It is noted that the representation of space in the entorhinal cell layer would be sufficient to enable navigation in a single environment if connected directly to the goal cell layer (presumed to be in the subiculum, immediately downstream of the place cells in region CA1 of the hippocampus). It is supposed that the role of the place cells in regions CA1 and CA3, and in particular of the long-range recurrent collaterals in CA3, is to support navigation in several distinct environments. These recurrent collaterals might enable the model to form an autoassociative memory for those place cells active in a given environment. Different subsets of place cells could then represent different environments, with each subset forming a stable state of the autoassociator (see also McNaughton & Nadel 1990). The different responses of ECs and PCs to changes in environmental shape (Quirk *et al.* 1992) indicate that this response might play a role in environmental recognition. However, modifying the size and aspect ratio of a rectangular environment produced parametric changes in place fields (O'Keefe & Burgess 1996) rather than the discontinuous remapping that might be expected if each environmental shape was represented by place cells as an orthogonal attractor state.

Expansion of an environment after the goal location has been learned stretches the goal-cell representation of goal location. With the current choice of output mechanism (see above) this results in a unimodal locus of search midway between the locations corresponding to maintaining fixed distances from each of the walls that have been pulled apart. These experiments have not yet been performed on rats, but the predicated search behaviour in the expanded environment runs contrary to that implied by simple extension of the result of Collett *et al.* (1986) in which two cylinders indicating the goal location were moved further apart. However, the relative indifference of PCs to objects placed within an environment (Cressant *et al.* 1997) compared with their response to the walls of the environment (O'Keefe & Burgess 1996) may indicate that this task is not mediated by the hippocampus in any case. A second prediction concerns the existence of goal cells, postulated to exist in the subiculum. It remains to be seen whether cells with the appropriate firing behaviour can be found in this part of the brain.

Finally, the likely effect on the model of preventing long-term changes of connection weights is noted. This would lead to an unstable association from ECs to PCs, leading to an unstable mapping of place fields onto place cells. This would be consistent with the finding of Rotenberg *et al.* (1996) in which place fields were recorded in mice genetically engineered not to show long-term potentiation of synapses in region CA1. The second effect of preventing long-term changes of connection weights would be the impermanence of the association from PCs to goal cells, and the loss of the population vector indicating the direction of the goal after the time interval over which any short-term potentiation had occurred. This is consistent with the behaviour of rats in a water maze after pharmacological blockade of long-term potentiation (see Morris & Frey, Chapter 12).

Acknowledgements

A preliminary version of this paper can be found in: the Proceedings of the AISB workshop of *Spatial reasoning in mobile robots and animals*, Manchester, 1997. Technical Report Series, Department of Computer Science, Manchester University, ISSN 1361-6161, report no. UMCS-97-4-1. N.B. is supported by a

Royal Society University Research Fellowship; J. O'K., J. D. and K. J. are supported by a programme grant from the MRC.

References

Blair, H. T. & Sharp, P. E. 1996 Visual and vestibular influences on head-direction cells in the anterior thalamus of the rat. *Behav. Neurosci.* **110**, 643–660.

Benhamou, S. & Seguinot, V. 1995 How to find ones way in the labyrinth of path integration models. *J. Theor. Biol.* **174**, 463–466.

Brown, M. A. & Sharp, P. E. 1995 Simulation of spatial learning in the Morris water maze by a neural network model of the hippocampal formation and nucleus accumbens. *Hippocampus* **5**, 171–188.

Burgess, N. & O'Keefe, J. 1995 Modelling spatial navigation by the rat hippocampus. *Int. J. Neur. Syst.* **7**(suppl.), 87–94.

Burgess, N. & O'Keefe, J. 1996 Neuronal computations underlying the firing of place cells and their role in navigation. *Hippocampus* **6**, 749–762.

Burgess, N., O'Keefe, J. & Recce, M. 1993 Using hippocampal 'place cells' for navigation, exploiting phase coding. In *Advances in neural information processing systems*, vol. 5 (ed. S. J. Hanson, C. L. Giles & J. D. Cowan), pp. 929–936. San Mateo, CA: Morgan Kaufmann.

Burgess, N., Recce, M. & O'Keefe, J. 1994 A model of hippocampal function. *Neur. Networks* **7**, 1065–1081.

Collett, T. S., Cartwright, B. A. & Smith, B. A. 1986 Landmark learning and visuo-spatial memories in gerbils. *J. Comp. Physiol.* **A 158**, 835–851.

Cressant, A., Muller, R. U. & Poucet, B. 1997 Failure of centrally placed objects to control the firing fields of hippocampal place cells. *J. Neurosci.* 2531–2542.

Dean, P. 1990 Sensory cortex: visual perceptual functions. In *The cerebral cortex of the rat* (ed. B. Kolb & R. C. Tees), pp. 75–307. Cambridge, MA: MIT Press.

Etienne, A. S., Maurer, R. & Seguinot, V. 1996 Path integration in mammals and its interaction with visual landmarks. *J. Exp. Biol.* **199**, 201–209.

Georgopoulos, A. P., Kettner, R. E. & Schwartz, A. B. 1988 Primate motor cortex and free arm movements to visual targets in three-dimensional space. II. Coding of the direction of movement by a neuronal population. *J. Neurosci.* **8**, 2928–2937.

Habib, M. & Sirigu, A. 1987 Pure topographical disorientation: a definition and anatomical basis. *Cortex* **23**, 73–85.

Hughes, A. 1977 A schematic eye for the rat. *Visual Res.* **19**, 569–588.

Jarrard, L. E. 1993 On the role of the hippocampus in learning and memory in the rat. *Behav. Neur. Biol.* **60**, 9–26.

Jeffery, K., Donnett, J. G., Burgess, N. & O'Keefe, J. 1997 Directional control of hippocampal place fields. *Exp. Brain Res.* **117**, 131–142.

Knierim, J. J., Kudrimoti, H. S. & McNaughton, B. L. 1995 Hippocampal place fields, the internal compass, and the learning of landmark stability. *J. Neurosci.* **15**, 1648–1659.

Maguire, E. A., Burke, T., Phillips, J. & Staunton, H. 1996a Topographical disorientation following unilateral temporal lobe lesions in humans. *Neuropsychologia* **34**, 993–1001.

Maguire, E. A., Frackowiak, R. S. J. & Frith, C. D. 1996b Learning to find your way: a role for the human hippocampal region. *Proc. R. Soc. Lond.* **B 263** 1745–1750.

Maguire, E. A., Burgess, N., Donnett, J. G., O'Keefe, J. & Frith, C. D. 1998a Knowing where things are: parahippocampal involvement in the encoding of object location in large-scale space. *J. Cogn. Neurosci.* **10**, 61–76.

Maguire, E. A., Burgess, N., Donnett, J. G., Frith, C. D., Frackowiack, R. S. J., & O'Keefe, J. 1998*b* Knowing where and getting there: a human navigation network. *Science* **280**, 921–924.

McNaughton, B. L. & Nadel, L. 1990 Hebb–Marr networks and the neurobiological representation of action in space. In *Neuroscience and connectionist theory* (ed. M. A. Gluck & D. E. Rumelhart), pp. 1–63. Hillsdale, NJ: Lawrence Erlbaum Associates.

Mizumori, S. J. Y. & Williams, J. D. 1993 Directionally sensitive mnemonic properties of neurons in the lateral dorsal nucleus of the thalamus of rats. *J. Neurosci.* **13**, 4015–4028.

Morris, R. G. M., Garrard, P., Rawlins, J. N. P. & O'Keefe, J. 1982 Place navigation impaired in rats with hippocampal lesions. *Nature* **297**, 681–683.

Muller, R. U. & Kubie, J. L. 1987 The effects of changes in the environment on the spatial firing of hippocampal complex-spike cells. *J. Neurosci.* **7**, 1951–1968.

O'Keefe, J. 1976 Place units in the hippocampus of the freely moving rat. *Exp. Neurol.* **51**, 78–109.

O'Keefe, J. & Burgess, N. 1996 Geometric determinants of the place fields of hippo-campal neurones. *Nature* **381**, 425–428.

O'Keefe, J. & Dostrovsky, J. 1971 The hippocampus as a spatial map: preliminary evidence from unit activity in the freely moving rat. *Brain Res.* **34**, 171–175.

O'Keefe, J. & Nadel, L. 1978 *The hippocampus as a cognitive map*. Oxford University Press.

O'Keefe, J. & Recce, M. 1993 Phase relationship between hippocampal place units and the EEG theta rhythm. *Hippocampus* **3**, 317–330.

O'Keefe, J. & Speakman, A. 1987 Single unit activity in the rat hippocampus during a spatial memory task. *Exp. Brain Res.* **68**, 1–27

Pavlides, C., Greenstein, Y. J., Grudman, M. & Winson, J. 1988 Long-term potentiation in the dentate gyrus is induced preferentially on the positive phase of θ-rhythm. *Brain Res.* **439**, 383–387.

Quirk, G. J. Muller, R. U. & Kubie, J. L. 1990 The firing of hippocampal place cells in the dark depends on the rat's experience. *J. Neurosci.* **10**, 2008–2017

Quirk, G. J., Muller, R. U., Kubie, J. L. & Ranck, J. B. 1992 The positional firing properties of medial entorhinal neurons: description and comparison with hippocam-pal place cells. *J. Neurosci.* **12**, 1945–1963.

Rotenberg, A., Mayford, M., Hawkins, R. D., Kandel, E. R. & Muller, R. U. 1996 Mice expressing activated CaMKII lack low frequency LTP and do not form stable place cells in the CA1 region of the hippocampus. *Cell* **87**, 1351–1361.

Scoville, W. B. & Milner, B. 1957 Loss of recent memory after bilateral hippocampal lesions. *J. Neurol. Neurosurg. Psych.* **20**, 11–21.

Sharp, P. E., Blair, H. T., Etkin, D. & Tzanetos, D. B. 1995 Influences of vestibular and visual-motion information on the spatial firing patterns of hippocampal place. *J. Neurosci.* **15**, 173–189.

Taube, J. S. 1995 Head direction cells recorded in the anterior thalamic nuclei of freely moving rats. *J. Neurosci.* **15**, 70–86.

Taube, J. S., Muller, R. U. & Ranck, J. B. 1990 Head-direction cells recorded from the postsubiculum in freely moving rats. I. Description and quantitative analysis. *J. Neurosci.* **10**, 420–435.

Tolman, E. C. 1948 Cognitive maps in rats and men. *Psychol. Rev.* **55**, 189–208.

Touretzky, D. S. & Redish, A. D. 1996 Theory of rodent navigation based on interacting representations of space. *Hippocampus* **6**, 247–270.

Wilson, M. A. & McNaughton, B. L. 1993 Dynamics of the hippocampal ensemble code for space. *Science* **261**, 1055–1058.

9

Dissociation of exteroceptive and idiothetic orientation cues: effect on hippocampal place cells and place navigation

Jan Bures, Andre A. Fenton, Yulii Kaminsky, Jerome Rossier, Benedetto Sacchetti and Larissa Zinyuk

9.1 Introduction

The discovery of hippocampal place cells (PCs) by O'Keefe & Dostrovsky (1971) and the ensuing systematic study of their properties (McNaughton *et al.* 1983; Muller *et al.* 1987; Sharp *et al.* 1990; Bostock *et al.* 1991; O'Keefe & Recce 1993; O'Keefe & Burgess 1996) created an extremely fruitful approach to the study of the cellular substrate of cognition. The idea that a PC firing in a specific region of a familiar environment participates in the neural processes that enable an animal to recognize its position in the charted world has inspired a deluge of ingenious experiments, high-lighted by the papers in this volume.

One consequence of the putative correspondence of PC activity and animal behaviour is that principles used in behavioural studies have been applied to the investigation of single cells. Although PC personification should be avoided, examination of PC activity under certain organism-defined conditions proved to be useful (Markus *et al.* 1995; Gothard *et al.* 1996). This is particularly true for the separation of two sources of information that contribute to spatial representation: exteroceptive inputs derived from environmental features and idiothetic inputs used in path integration (O'Keefe & Nadel 1978; Gallistel 1990).

The same classification presumably applies to PC mapping. Exteroceptive control of PCs has been demonstrated repeatedly (O'Keefe & Conway 1978; Knierim *et al.* 1995; O'Keefe & Burgess 1996). In one experiment a shift of a cue card on the wall of the recording chamber caused a corresponding displacement of firing fields (Muller & Kubie 1987). Idiothetic information must also be able to control PCs: firing fields (FFs) established in light persist in darkness even though in light they are controlled by visual cues (O'Keefe 1976; McNaughton *et al.* 1989*b*; Quirk *et al.* 1990; Markus *et al.* 1994). Thus location-specific PC activity is determined both by exteroceptive and idiothetic information; after elimination of the exteroceptive component, path integration alone can support sustained PC mapping (McNaughton *et al.* 1996). This is in good agreement with behavioural findings that show that place navigation can be directed to new locations by changing the position of extramaze landmarks (Biegler & Morris 1993; Fenton *et al.* 1994) and that sudden darkness does not prevent successful homing (Mittelstaedt & Mittelstaedt 1980; Alyan & Jander 1994).

The equivalence of exteroceptive and idiothetic orientation applies to a stable world where both navigation modes yield the same information and can, therefore, substitute for each other. Thus, exteroceptively based navigation can be supported by path integration in track segments from which no remote landmarks are visible (Liu *et al.* 1994). It is conceivable that equivalence of these two classes of input can be disrupted when the relationship between extramaze landmarks and the animal's locomotion becomes unpredictable. This paper reviews several attempts to assess the changes in PC activity caused by such conditions.

The contribution of PC activity to place navigation is usually implied but only rarely verified by PC recordings in navigation experiments. Because such investigations require distributed exploration of the experimental arena as well as place-directed locomotion, another aim of the research described here was to develop tasks that meet these requirements.

9.2 General methods

Subjects and apparatus

Adult male Long–Evans rats were trained to forage for randomly located food pellets in one of several circular arenas (80–100 cm in diameter). The pellets were dispensed by a computer-controlled feeder either at regular 10 s intervals or after the animal fulfilled some computer-evaluated criteria. The arena was also computer-controlled and could be rotated around its axis at angular velocities ranging from 6 to $30°\,s^{-1}$. The arenas were placed in a room that provided many extra-maze visual cues when the light was switched on, but was completely dark when the light was switched off.

Tracking system

The rat's position was recorded by tracking an infrared light-emitting diode (LED) with an infrared-sensitive television camera connected to a computer-based tracking system. The infrared LED was in the recording head stage (see below) in the electrophysiological experiments and between the rat's shoulders in the purely behavioural studies. The custom-made tracking system operated with a spatial resolution of 0.4–0.5 cm and a temporal resolution of 100 ms. The software permitted interactive control of the experiment. For example, on fulfilment of various behavioural criteria, such as entering and staying in a specified region or moving for a criterion distance or duration, the system could switch the room lights on or off, rotate the arena, apply an electric shock, deliver food pellets, etc..

The position of the rat was plotted in two coordinate systems, either in the x–y coordinate system of the room or in the polar system of the arena where the origin is at its centre. Position in the arena frame was calculated by correcting the room coordinates by the coordinates of a second infrared LED on the arena wall (Bures *et al*. 1997). The arena projection corresponds to a view obtained from a virtual television camera fixed above the centre of the arena and rotating with it. Thus, tracks in the two reference systems are identical when the arena is stationary, but different when the arena is rotating. In the latter case, the track in the room frame records a combination of the animal's active locomotion and the movement of the arena, whereas tracking in the arena frame eliminates the rotation to reflect only the active locomotion.

Unit recording

Under pentobarbital anaesthesia $(40\,\mathrm{mg\,kg}^{-1})$ a driveable bundle of eight Formvar-insulated nichrome electrodes $25\,\mu\mathrm{m}$ in diameter was implanted about 1 mm above the CA1 cell layer of the dorsal hippocampus (3.0 mm caudal from bregma, 2.5 mm lateral from the sagittal suture (Paxinos & Watson 1986)). After several days of recovery the electrodes were slowly advanced until single CA1 units could be isolated. Recording sessions lasted 10 min. Extracellular potentials were first amplified with high-impedance preamplifiers ($10 \times$ gain) in the recording headstage, then amplified another 1000 times and filtered (300–10 000 Hz) before being digitized (32 kHz) and stored in a computer-based system (DataWave, USA).

Analysis of PC activity

Unitary waveforms were discriminated offline with a template-matching algorithm that used a least-square fit to score the match between digitized spike-like events and a waveform template. Those waveforms sufficiently close to only one template were classified as belonging to a single neuron. The discriminated-spike time series for each unit, along with the position time series, were used to construct two-dimensional histograms of the session-averaged firing-rate distribution in $5\,\mathrm{cm} \times 5\,\mathrm{cm}$ pixels. The mean firing rate in a pixel was calculated as the number of spikes recorded in the pixel divided by the total time spent in the pixel. Firing-rate distributions were displayed as grey-scale-coded firing-rate maps. White pixels represented undefined firing rate because the rat was never there. The lightest grey pixels were visited but had a firing rate of zero. The five remaining shades of grey increased in darkness to represent, in increasing order, 31, 25, 19, 14 and 11 per cent of the non-zero firing rates.

Numerical methods were used to describe and compare the averaged firing-rate distributions. A firing field (FF) was defined as an area of at least four pixels ($100 \, cm^2$) where the firing rate was at least two standard deviations above the overall mean firing rate. The pixels included in a field had to share at least one side with another pixel of the same FF. The FF location was defined as the firing-rate-weighted average of the x and y coordinates of the pixels included in the field. The distance between FFs observed in two sessions, i.e. the displacement (D), was used to assess the FF location change. The location was considered changed if the displacement exceeded 5 per cent of the distance from the reference location to the most distant point of the arena. The quality of the location-specific firing was expressed by calculating spatial coherence, concentration and dispersion (Muller & Kubie 1989; Bures *et al.* 1997).

9.3 PC Discharge on a rotating arena

While foraging on a featureless rotating arena, a rat can perceive its position in relation to the immobile surroundings, i.e. to the room cues, or in relation to the surface of the arena, e.g. to the starting point of the movement. Although spatial knowledge is more or less irrelevant for successful pellet chasing, both exteroceptive and idiothetic spatial information is probably recorded automatically because in natural situations this information allows the animals to go straight to a chosen goal or to return to the safe haven of the home. A fundamental difference between exteroceptive-based and idiothetic-based navigation is that the former can generate trajectories to any location of the charted environment, whereas the latter can only generate paths to already visited locations or projected locations along the current track. Whereas the exteroceptive-based navigation requires estimation of the current position and computation of the shortest direction to the goal, the return azimuth to home (or to another point of the current path) is continuously available from the path-integration system and can probably be obtained with shorter latency. This is a vital advantage in case of sudden danger.

Whether either or both classes of information are being utilized can only be verified in behaviourally relevant situations; recording PC activity during pellet chasing can examine how each contributes to PC mapping. A FF characterized on a stationary arena might be activated by one or both classes of information because they are equivalent. In contrast, this equivalence breaks down when the arena rotates. Thus, during slow constant rotation of the arena (one revolution per minute), an FF can:

(1) remain stable in the room frame, i.e. the PC fires when the rat moves into the FF either owing to passive rotation of the arena or by a combination of active and passive movements;

(2) remain stable in the arena frame, i.e. the PC fires when the rat enters a definite region of the arena irrespective of its position in the room; or

(3) disappear or be smeared in both the room and the arena frames.

The first two possibilities indicate that the particular PC responds mainly to exteroceptive or to idiothetic inputs, respectively. The third suggests that such a PC is activated by the coincidence of exteroceptive and idiothetic information. This situation may only occur during the short interval when rotation of the arena brings its surface into the position corresponding to a match between both projections.

Figure 9.1 shows examples of PCs recorded in a cylindrical arena 1 m in diameter with walls 40 cm high. In the first session the arena was stable; in the next, it was rotated (1 rpm) to cause a disagreement between exteroceptive and idiothetic information, and in the third session it was stable again. The rat was not removed from the arena between sessions. In the rotation sessions, the firing-rate distributions were calculated for both the room frame and the arena frame. Figure 9.1a is an example of the most common finding. Although pellet chasing appeared unaffected, an FF characterized on the stationary arena disintegrated in both reference frames during rotation. There was no 'remapping' (Muller & Kubie 1987; Bostock *et al.* 1991; Markus *et al.* 1995) as might be expected for 20 per cent (Thompson & Best 1989) to 50 per cent of PCs (O'Keefe 1979; Wilson & McNaughton 1993).

It was uncommon for FFs to persist during rotation in the light. The few FFs preserved in the room frame (Fig. 9.1b) or in the arena frame (Fig. 9.1c) indicated, however, that exteroceptive or idiothetic information alone may be sufficient to maintain such PCs. In contrast, most PCs retained their FFs when the light was switched off; such FFs were preserved in the arena frame even during rotation in darkness (Fig. 9.2a). It seems that in the rotating arena once darkness diminished exteroceptive information the conflict with idiothetic information was removed and most PCs continued to fire in the arena frame. The above effect of darkness suggests that PCs are disturbed not by rotation alone but rather by the rotation-induced conflict between the two sources of information.

This conflict can be reduced by cues on the rotating cylinder wall. Indeed, the incidence of FFs in the arena frame was markedly increased when a white card was pasted on a 60° segment of the rotating arena wall (Fig. 9.2b). In this situation idiothetic orientation is reinforced by a prominent environmental feature that partly restores the correspondence between idiothetic and exteroceptive information. Although the information from the stable extramaze landmarks in the room continues to disagree with expectations corresponding to idiothetic information, the presence of a visual stimulus confirming these predictions seems to increase the animal's trust in the arena-frame view of the world. Thus, both darkness and visual cues enhance the significance of idiothetic input to the PCs, but the enhancement is achieved by different mechanisms. Darkness eliminated the conflicting salient exteroceptive input, whereas the salient cue card made enough exteroceptive information consonant with the idiothetic input.

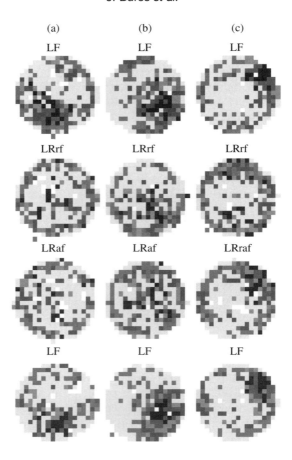

Fig. 9.1 Examples showing three effects of rotating the arena (see text). Firing-rate maps of PCs recorded during 10 min of pellet chasing in light (L) on a fixed arena (F) and on a rotating arena (R). The maps from rotation sessions art presented in either the room reference frame (rf) or in the arena reference frame (af). The grey-scale code increases from the lightest grey (zero rate) to black through five rate-related levels corresponding to 31, 25, 19, 14 and 11 per cent of the non-zero firing rates. (a) An FF characterized in the south on the stable arena disintegrated on the moving arena in both frames and returned to its original form when the rotation stopped. (b) An FF characterized in thc south-east on the stable arena is detectable on the rotating arena in the room frame but not in the arena frame. During rotation the FF was somewhat disorganized but was stronger and in the same room-frame position after the rotation. (c) An FF characterized in the north-east on the stable arena disintegrated during rotation in the room frame but was preserved in the arena frame; the post-rotation FF is closely similar to the initial FF. Black category peak and median firing rates (action potentials per second, AP s^{-1}) from *top* to *bottom*: (a) LF 20.0, 6.0; LRaf 10.0, 3.0; LRaf 10.0, 3.0; LF 20.0, 10.0. (b) LF 8.9, 6.2; LRrf 8.3, 4.3; LRaf 8.3, 4.3; LF 27.8, 13.0. (c) LF 13.0, 7.0; LRrf 20.0, 3.0; LRaf 30.0, 5.0; LF 8.4, 6.0.

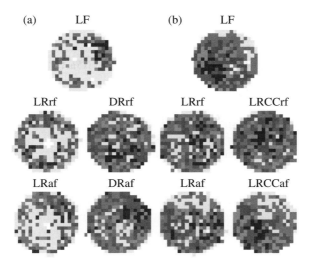

Fig. 9.2 Changes that reduce the conflict between exteroceptive and idiothetic orientation stabilize FFs in the arena frame. (a) An FF in the north-east on the stable arena was abolished by rotation in the light but could be restored in the arena frame during rotation in darkness. (b) An FF in the south-west on the stable arena disintegrated in both frames during rotation in the light but was restored in the arena frame when a cue card (CC) was placed on the wall of the rotating arena. Other conditions as in Fig. 1. Black category peak and median firing rates (AP s^{-1}): (a) LF 10.0, 3.0; LRrf 3.3, 2.3; LRaf 10.0, 2.0; DRrf 11.1, 6.0; DRaf 16.7, 6.0; (b) LF 67.5, 32.0; LRrf 2.0, 8.0; LRaf 15.7, 10.0; LRCCrf 70, 13; LRCCaf 30.0, 15.0.

9.4 Field clamp

The disagreement between idiothetic and exteroceptive orientation had no apparent effect on the rat's performance in the pellet-chasing task; this is probably the reason why prolonged rotation of the arena is tolerated by the PCs. After the rotation stopped, PC mapping returned immediately to the control stationary state. A more serious disturbance of PC mapping can be produced by the field-clamp technique (Zinyuk *et al.* 1996; Bures *et al.* 1997). The pellet-chasing task was used in a ring-shaped arena (25 cm wide, 1 m diameter of the outer wall, 40 cm height of the outer wall). Rotation of the arena in this experiment was used to enhance the disagreement between exteroceptive and idiothetic orientation by confining the animal to a fixed position in the room frame while allowing it to move freely in the arena frame. The field-clamp program controlled the rotation of the arena so that whenever the animal left a specific 30° sector of the ring (e.g. the south-west) the arena moved (30° s^{-1}) to return the rat to the region of the lock. In this way, the animal can travel all over the surface of the ring but nevertheless remain in the same room-frame position. Perhaps this makes the disagreement between the two modes of orientation more conspicuous: idiothetic perception tells the rat it has visited all parts of the arena, but visual perception of the room indicates that it has not moved, or that its attempts to leave the place were frustrated by some strange force. The rats' notorious dislike of restraint might have added emotional distress to the above perceptual disagreement. The slow search that is characteristic for foraging would have required only brief intervals of rotation to bring the animal back to the lock sector, but most rats occasionally ran out of the sector so fast that it sometimes took several seconds to rotate them back into the clamped area.

Changes of PC activity observed in 100 PCs tested in the field-clamp experiments extend the results obtained in the continuously rotating arena. When the field clamp confined the rat to a sector corresponding to the FF previously established in the stationary arena, the FF disappeared in most cases. This suggests that the exteroceptive orientation, asserting that the animal did not leave a definite location in the room, could not resist the more persuasive idiothetic experience telling the animal that it could not be in a place from which it was trying so hard to escape. After termination of the clamp, an FF often appeared in a different location and returned to the original position only after an hour or on the next day. Only 15 PCs had the same FF location during the clamp and afterwards. Seventy PCs showed transient changes of FF location after the clamp; no FF recovery was seen in 15 PCs.

9.5 PC Activity during behavioural testing

Experiments on radial mazes studied how PC activity is controlled by goal locations but did not reveal how PC firing was related to navigation (O'Keefe & Conway 1978; Olton *et al.* 1978; O'Keefe & Speakman 1987; McNaughton *et al.* 1989a). The relation between PC mapping and cognitive behaviour might be examined in experiments that combine standard pellet chasing with place navigation. The well-established characteristics of FFs can then be compared during random foraging and goal-directed locomotion. The effect of conditions that differentially affect the importance of exteroceptive and idiothetic information could be compared as well as the potential influence of appetitive and aversive motivations. The two tasks described on the following pages were developed with the aim of understanding the relationship between PC firing and spatial cognition.

9.6 Place avoidance

One of the most widely used techniques in memory research, the passive avoidance task, is actually a cued spatial avoidance. In the step-down, step-through or two-compartment tasks (see Bures *et al.* (1983) for a review), the rat learns to inhibit visits to a part of the apparatus because it is punished by mild footshock at this location. The region to be avoided is easily discernible and the learned response is to stay in the start compartment. This classic model can be modified into place avoidance when the unmarked region to be avoided is defined by its relation to remote extramaze cues and when the learned response leads to continued foraging on the safe part of the arena and avoidance of the footshock zone (Sacchetti *et al.* 1997).

Method

Under thiopental anaesthesia, a low-impedance silver wire (200 μm diameter, 4 cm long) connected to a miniature socket was implanted under the skin at the back of the neck. The socket was fixed to the skull with anchoring bolts and acrylate. After recovery, the animal was trained to forage for scattered pellets on an elevated circular arena with a metal floor. Through the socket a computer-controlled relay could deliver 0.6 mA of 50 Hz current between the implanted wire and the paws of the animal contacting the grounded metal floor. The infrared LED for tracking was positioned between the rat's shoulders with a latex harness. The rats were first trained for several days in the pellet-chasing task with pellets dispensed at 10 s intervals. A semicircular 'prohibited' area was then designated in one quadrant. Its centre was at the periphery and its radius corresponded to 20 per cent of the arena's diameter. The rat received a mild 0.5 s electric shock whenever it entered the prohibited region for more than 0.5 s. The shock was repeated after 3 s if the animal did not leave the punishment area. Training continued until the animal displayed no apparent fear and continued to forage while avoiding the punishment zone. This initial 'pretraining' was followed by retrieval tests performed under extinction conditions, i.e. in the absence of electric shocks.

Results

The place-avoidance task was used to learn how spatial memories based on distal visual information interact with memories based on path-integration information. Do these two types of information produce independent memories? And if so, how do they interact to mediate spatial behaviour?

Each experimental session began with an 'acquisition' period when footshock punished entries into a rat-specific prohibited area. Acquisition was always in the lit room with the punishment zone defined by room cues. Acquisition training in the light was on either a fixed ($n = 16$) or rotating arena ($n = 22$). Acquisition continued until the animal succeeded in avoiding shock during five consecutive epochs of 2 min duration. Retrieval testing under extinction conditions was then begun by switching off the electric shock, switching off the lights, and setting the rotation condition to either fixed or rotating. Testing continued until the rat regularly entered the prohibited zone. This was measured in each 2 min epoch by calculating the percentage of time

176   J. Bures *et al.*

spent in the prohibited zone compared with the total time spent in the prohibited zone and corresponding areas of the three other quadrants. An analogous calculation was made for the percentage of the total path length in the prohibited zone. The extinction criterion was met when measures of both time and path length were at least 13 per cent in three consecutive 2 min epochs. If this criterion was not reached within 1 h, the rat was given a 60 min to-criterion score. The session continued by switching the lights on and testing for extinction the second time without removing the animal from the arena and without changing the rotation condition.

The results are shown in Fig. 9.3. When both training and testing proceeded on the stable arena, both exteroceptive and idiothetic memories of the place to be avoided were formed during acquisition and the idiothetic memories could support effective place avoidance during extinction testing in darkness

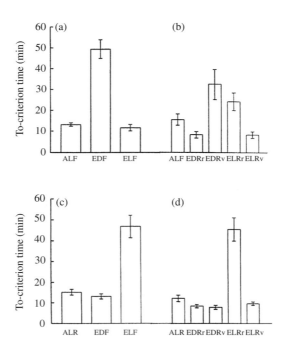

Fig. 9.3 Mean ($\pm$s.e.m.) times to acquisition (A) or extinction (E) criteria of place avoidance. Column labels indicate the experimental conditions: D, darkness; L, light; F, fixed arena; R, rotating arena; r, real camera view (room frame); v, virtual camera view (arena frame). The experiments shown in (a), (c) and (d) were performed on 11 rats each. Five rats were used in the remaining experiment (b). Note that extinction in darkness is slow after acquisition on the fixed arena (a, b) and fast after acquisition on the rotating arena (c, d). Note also that place avoidance acquired on the fixed arena, when tested on the rotating arena, led to avoidance of an arena-frame location in darkness and of a room-frame location in the light (b).

(Fig. 9.3a). In this case, extinction attained in darkness transferred to the subsequent light condition.

The place avoidance acquired on a fixed arena could also be retrieved during testing performed on the rotating arena in darkness. Tracks recorded during a typical experiment (Fig. 9.4b) show that avoidance was seen by the virtual camera in the arena reference frame and not in the room reference frame monitored by the real camera (Fig. 9.3b, EDRv > EDRr, $t_4 = 3.5$, $p < 0.025$). The opposite pattern was seen when the light was switched on in the second testing phase (Fig. 9.3b, ELRv < ELRr, $t_4 = 3.7$, $p < 0.025$). In contrast to extinction in the dark on the stable arena (Fig. 9.3a), extinction in the dark on the rotating arena did not transfer to the light phase. Clear avoidance in the room frame must have been supported by exteroceptive memory traces that were not extinguished in the dark. Although extinction appears accelerated, it was not significantly different from the idiothetic extinction in the previous dark phase (Fig. 9.3b, EDRv > EDRr, $t_4 = 1.2$, n.s.)

Acquisition of place avoidance on the rotating arena resulted in the formation of exteroceptive memories alone. Because any attempts to avoid a region defined in the arena frame may lead to footshock, formation of idiothetic memories for avoidance was probably suppressed. This suppression is manifested by the absence of place avoidance in darkness on either fixed (Fig. 9.3c) or rotating (Fig. 9.3d) arenas. As soon as the light was switched on, avoidance reappeared in the room frame. When both acquisition and retrieval testing proceeded on the rotating arena, avoidance in darkness was seen neither in the room frame (because no room cues were available) nor in the arena frame (because no idiothetic memories were formed during acquisition), but avoidance of the prohibited location defined in the room frame reappeared in the light (Figs. 9.3d and 9.4d).

These results indicate that place-avoidance training has independent exteroceptive and idiothetic components that can be dissociated. During place-avoidance training on the fixed arena the animal learns to avoid a specific location in the room that is identical with a definite sector of the arena. The independence of these two traces makes it possible to solve the task in two different ways: by using just the idiothetic memory in darkness or by using just the exteroceptive memory in light, provided that the idiothetic memory has been eliminated during the preceding extinction in darkness.

The dissociation of exteroceptive and idiothetic place-avoidance memories raises a not immediately apparent prediction. If place avoidance is acquired on a stable arena in the light, its extinction on a rotating arena in the light may lead to an ambiguous solution. This would be manifest as simultaneous avoidance of an exteroceptively defined location (e.g. of the north-west section of the arena) and of an idiothetically defined location (corresponding to the floor region that was in the north-west section of the stable arena during acquisition), which could be seen by the real and virtual cameras, respectively.

The place-avoidance results, compared with the activity changes in PCs induced by rotation, suggest that the PC mapping that is preserved in darkness

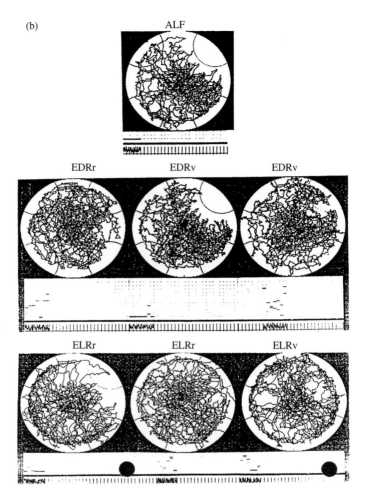

Fig. 9.4 Representative tracks from experiments (b) and (d) and summarised in Fig. 9.3b and 9.3d, respectively. Tracks on the rotating arena are plotted either in the room frame of the real camera view (r) or in the arena frame of the virtual camera view (v). The arcs at the circumference of the arena indicate the prohibited and the three control areas. In each 2-min epoch, two measures of avoidance were calculated: percentage of time and track length in the prohibited area related to the totals for the prohibited and the three control areas. These measures are plotted for each epoch below the tracks. The bottom curve expresses the rat's movement by plotting the rat's distance from an arbitrary point in the reference frame. The rat learned to avoid the north-east region of the rotating arena in (d) and of the fixed arena in (b). Because no idiothetic memories of the shock region were formed in experiment (d), there was no avoidance in darkness

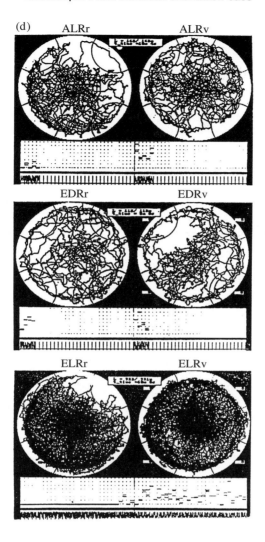

in either reference frame. However, when the light was switched on, the avoidance reappeared in the room frame and lasted for more than 50 min. In experiment (b) avoidance was acquired on the fixed arena and both types of memory were formed. The idiothetic memory was manifested on the rotating arena by avoidance of the prohibited region in the first 12 min and by the gradual development of extinction later. No avoidance was seen in the real camera view. After the light was switched on, the rat avoided the north-east sector of the arena for more than 10 min before extinction set in. This is documented by the real camera view, whereas the virtual camera indicated no avoidance of the part of the arena where the shocks were administered.

on both fixed and rotating arenas can be the basis of continued avoidance of idiothetically defined locations. On the other hand, the disappearance of most location-specific firing during rotation in the light contrasts with the good retrieval of place avoidance on the rotating arena in the light, albeit after previous extinction of the idiothetic memory. It is conceivable that place-avoidance training may increase the percentage of exteroceptively dependent PCs; this increase could support the exteroceptive solution of the task. This is particularly probable in rats that acquire the task on a rotating arena in the light because the importance of exteroceptive input is enhanced by the disutility of idiothetic inputs. The other possibility, that striking exteroceptive place avoidance proceeds in the absence of exteroceptive PC mapping, would require a thorough reappraisal of the role of PCs in place navigation.

9.7 Place-preference task

An obvious disadvantage of the place-avoidance task is that the avoided part of the arena remains unvisited. This drawback is removed in the place-preference task, which permits unlimited exploration of the whole arena (Rossier *et al.* 1997). The task is actually an operant procedure, which requires the animal to visit a specific location on the arena to activate the feeder. After a pellet falls into the arena, the rat leaves the trigger location to search for it. After the pellet is retrieved, the rat runs more or less directly to the trigger area. Thus there is alternation of two modes of spatial behaviour: goal-directed place navigation and random searching.

Method

Five rats were trained to search for pellets in the arena used in the place-avoidance experiments. The pellets were released by the computerized tracking system only when the animal had entered a circular target area (20–36 cm in diameter). Once the pellet was dispensed, the rat had to search for it and stay outside the target area for at least 3 s before the next visit to the target area was rewarded. The rat was placed near the centre of the arena to begin a session that lasted 30 min. The rat's position was recorded every 100 ms. The number of entries into the trigger annulus and the time spent there were compared with control values from analogous annuli in the other three quadrants of the arena. In addition, lengths of the approach and departure trajectories during the 3 s preceding annulus entry were compared in the same way. Analogous values were also compared in the 3 s after departure from an annulus.

Results

After 2 weeks of shaping, the rats were able to release about 100 pellets per session by entering a circular area 36 cm in diameter. A further two weeks of training were necessary to maintain this performance while gradually decreasing the diameter of the trigger annulus to 20 cm, i.e. to 6.25 per cent of the surface of the arena.

Figure 9.5 and Table 9.1 are an example from the place-preference task at the asymptotic performance level. During the 30-min trial, the rat ran 447 m and obtained 94 pellets. The trigger annulus in the north-east quadrant of the arena was visited 104 times. The maps show the tracks generated in the 3 s preceding and 3 s following each visit of the trigger annulus in the north-east quadrant and in the control annuli. Note that the approach paths to the trigger annulus are longer and the departure paths shorter than those leading to the other annuli. This reveals that goal-directed place navigation generates less tortuous and faster locomotion than the random searching that is characteristic of pellet chasing. As soon as the rat hears the pellet fall, locomotion changes from directed to random. This is why the shortest departure paths correspond to the rat's leaving the trigger annulus. Departure paths from the control annuli are often longer because some of them may overlap with approach paths to the trigger annulus that went through a control annulus.

Figure 9.6 summarizes the results after 4 weeks of training. The trigger annulus was visited more frequently (55 per cent) and more time was spent there (58 per cent) than in the other annuli ($F_{3,12} = 82$, $p < 0.001$). The approach paths to the trigger annulus were 56 per cent longer than the departure paths, whereas the departure paths from the control annuli were longer by about 10 per cent than the corresponding approach paths.

PC recordings during this task should help to reveal how PC mapping is related to the rat's behaviour. Because both the random search trajectories and goal-directed trajectories cover the whole arena, it would be possible to compare place-cell activity during these two modes of locomotion that probably reflect different categories of spatial behaviour. It will also be possible to learn how PCs are affected when only exteroceptive (on a rotating arena in the

Table 9.1   The number of entrances, the approach path length and the time spent in these locations in six subsequent 5-min epochs

No.	Entrance					Path length					Time				
	1	2	3	4	%	1	2	3	4	%	1	2	3	4	%
1	13	6	4	11	38	33	35	26	25	16	16	5	6	17	36
2	22	8	10	7	47	44	34	24	33	51	16	11	13	10	31
3	16	9	8	11	36	47	32	22	27	66	12	9	11	14	25
4	16	5	6	10	43	50	45	31	20	66	15	5	6	13	39
5	18	3	8	9	47	48	—	14	25	118	20	2	16	15	37
6	19	6	9	7	46	50	—	24	26	100	24	5	9	9	51

The percentage column indicates the contribution of the trigger area to the total entries or time. In the path-length section, the percentages indicate the excess of the approach path over the departure path. Total food deliveries = 104.

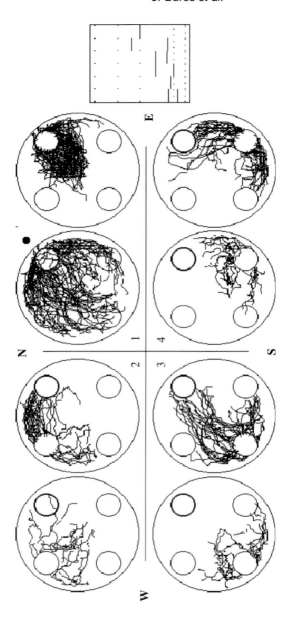

Fig. 9.5 Tracks from an overtrained rat generated during 30 min in the place-preference task. The trigger area was in the north–east quadrant of the arena. Tracks are shown for the 3 s before entering (*left maps*) and after leaving (*right maps*) the trigger zone (1) and the equivalent regions in the other quadrants (2–4). The histogram on the right shows the development of the above values in 5 min bins during the course of the 30 min session.

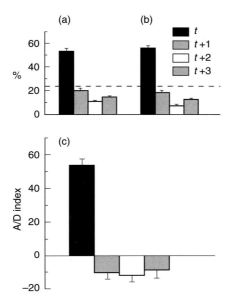

Fig. 9.6 Mean ($\pm$s.e.m.) values of the percentage of entries (a) and of the time (b) spent in each annulus of the arena. t, Target annulus; $t+1$ to $t+3$, remaining annuli in an anticlockwise sequence. (c) Mean ($\pm$s.e.m.) values of the approach/departure (A/D) index calculated according to the equation $(L_1/L_2 - 1) \times 100$, where L_1 and L_2 are the lengths of the 3 s approach and departure tracks for individual visits to the respective annulus.

light) or only idiothetic (in darkness) information is useful for finding the location of the trigger annulus.

9.8 Conclusion

Place navigation in a stable environment is implemented by two cooperating memory mechanisms: one dependent on environmental features (referred to as exteroceptive) and the other dependent on proprioceptive and vestibular cues (referred to as idiothetic). Slow rotation of the experimental arena seems to disrupt the correspondence of the two memories and the animal's position becomes ambiguous: the rat cannot be simultaneously at the two different locations, corresponding to an exteroceptively defined fixed position in the room frame and to an idiothetically defined (or intra-maze cue-dependent) fixed position in the arena frame. This conflict probably accounts for the disorganization of the FFs of most PCs on the rotating arena. The place-avoidance and place-preference tasks make it possible to create situations that increase the behavioural significance of either source of information on a rotating arena. If PC activity is necessary for spatial cognition, then PCs recorded during place-learning tasks should have FFs depending on the behaviourally relevant spatial orientation input. The alternative is either that spatial cognition can be mediated by extra-hippocampal structures or that the location specificity of PCs does not reflect a map-like representation of space in the hippocampus.

Acknowledgements

This research was supported by grant No. 309/97/0555 from the Granting Agency of the Czech Republic.

References

Alyan, S. & Jander, R. 1994 Short range homing in the house mouse, Mus musculus: stages in the learning of directions. *Anim. Behav.* **48**, 285–298.

Biegler, R. & Morris, R. G. M. 1993 Landmark stability is a prerequisite for spatial but not discrimination learning. *Nature* **361**, 631–633.

Bostock, E., Muller, R. U. & Kubie, J. L. 1991 Experience-dependent modifications of hippocampal place cell firing. *Hippocampus* **1**, 193–206.

Bures, J., Buresova, O. & Huston, J. P. 1983 *Techniques and basic experiments in the study of brain and behaviour*. Amsterdam: Elsevier.

Bures, J., Fenton, A. A., Kaminsky, Yu. & Zinyuk, L. 1997 Place cells and place navigation. *Proc. Natn. Acad. Sci. USA* **94**, 243–350.

Fenton, A. A., Arolfo, M. P., Nerad, L. & Bures, J. 1994 Place navigation in the Morris water maze under minimum and redundant extra-maze cue conditions. *Behav. Neurol. Biol.* **62**, 178–189.

Gallistel, C. R. 1990 *The organization of learning*. Cambridge, MA: MIT Press.

Gothard, K. M., Skaggs, W. E., Moore, K. M. & McNaughton, B. L. 1996 Binding of hippocampal CAl neural activity to multiple reference frames in a land-mark based navigation task. *J. Neurosci.* **16**, 823–835.

Knierim, J. J., Kudrimoti, H. S. & McNaughton, B. L. 1995 Place cells, head direction cells, and the learning of landmark stability. *J. Neurosci.* **15**, 1648–1659.

Liu, Z., Francis Turner, L. & Bures, J. 1994 Impairment of place navigation in the Morris water maze by intermittent light is inversely related to the duration of the flash. *Neurosci. Lett.* **180**, 59–62.

Markus, E. J., Barnes, C. A., McNaughton, B. L., Gladden, V. L. & Skaggs, W. E. 1994 Spatial information content and the reliability of hippocampal CA1 neurons: effects of visual input. *Hippocampus* **4**, 410–421.

Markus, E. J., Qin, Y., Leonard, B., Skaggs, W. E., McNaughton, B. L. & Barnes, C. A. 1995 Interactions between location and task affect the spatial and directional firing of hippocampal neurons. *J. Neurosci.* **15**, 7079–7094.

McNaughton, B. L., Barnes, C. A. & O'Keefe, J. 1983 The contributions of position, direction and velocity to single unit activity in the hippocampus of freely-moving rats. *Expl Brain Res.* **52**, 41–49.

McNaughton, B. L., Barnes, C. A., Meltzer, J. & Sutherland, R. J. 1989*a* Hippocampal granule cells are necessary for normal spatial learning but not for spatially-selective pyramidal cell discharge. *Expl Brain Res.* **76**, 485–496.

McNaughton, B. L., Leonard, B. & Chen, L. 1989*b* Cortical–hippocampal interactions and cognitive mapping: a hypothesis based on reintegration of the parietal and inferotemporal pathways for visual processing. *Psychobiology* **17**, 230–235.

McNaughton, B. L., Barnes, C. A., Gerrard, J. L., Gothard, K., Jung, M. W., Knierim, J. J. *et al.* 1996 Deciphering the hippocampal polyglot: the hippocampus as a path integration system. *J. Exp. Biol.* **199**, 173–185.

Mittelstaedt, M. L. & Mittelstaedt, H. 1980 Homing by path integration in the mammal. *Naturwissenschaften* **67**, 566–567.

Muller, R. U. & Kubie, J. L. 1987 The effects of changes in the environment on the spatial firing of hippocampal complex-spike cells. *J. Neurosci.* **7**, 1951–1968.

Muller, R. U. & Kubie, J. L. 1989 The firing of hippocampal place cells predicts the future position of freely moving rats. *J. Neurosci.* **9**, 4101–4110.

Muller, R. U., Kubie, J. L. & Ranck, J. B. Jr. 1987 Spatial firing patterns of hippocampal complex spike cells in a fixed environment. *Neurosci.* **7**, 1935–1950.

O'Keefe, J. 1976 Place units in the hippocampus of the freely moving rat. *Expl Neurol.* **51**, 78–109.

O'Keefe, J. 1979 A review of the hippocampal place cells. *Progr. Neurobiol.* **13**, 419–439.

O'Keefe, J. & Burgess, N. 1996 Geometric determinants of the place fields of hippocampal neurons. *Nature* **381**, 425–428.

O'Keefe, J. & Conway, D. H. 1978 Hippocampal place units in the freely moving rat: why they fire where they fire. *Expl Brain Res.* **31**, 573–590.

O'Keefe, J. & Dostrovsky, J. 1971 The hippocampus as a spatial map. Preliminary evidence from unit activity in the freely-moving rat. *Brain Res.* **34**, 171–175.

O'Keefe, J. & Nadel, L. 1978 *The hippocampus as a cognitive map.* Oxford: Clarendon Press.

O'Keefe, J. & Recce, M. 1993 Phase relationship between hippocampal place units and the EEG theta rhythm: *Hippocampus* **3**, 317–330.

O'Keefe, J. & Speakman, A. 1987 Single unit activity in the rat hippocampus during a spatial memory task. *Expl Brain Res.* **68**, 1–27.

Olton, D. S., Branch, M. & Best, P. J. 1978 Spatial correlates of hippocampal unit activity. *Expl Neurol.* **58**, 387–409.

Paxinos, G. & Watson, M. 1986 *The rat brain in stereotaxic coordinates.* San Diego, CA: Academic Press.

Quirk, G. J., Muller, R. U. & Kubie, J. L. 1990 The hippocampal place cells in the dark reflect the rat's recent experience. *J. Neurosci.* **10**, 2008–2017.

Rossier, J., Kaminsky, Yu., Schenk, F. & Bures, J. 1997 A place preference task allowing dissociation of allocentric and egocentric components of place cell activity in rats. *Physiol. Res.* **46**, 19.

Sacchetti, B., Fenton, A. A. & Bures, J. 1997 Conditioned place avoidance: a tool for dissociating place navigation directed by landmark sighting and by path integration. *Physiol. Res.* **46**, 19.

Sharp, P., Muller, R. U. & Kubie, J. L. 1990 Firing properties of hippocampal neurons in a visually symmetric environment: contributions of multiple sensory cues and mnemonic processes. *J. Neurosci.* **10**, 3093–3105.

Thompson, L. T. & Best, P. J. 1989 Place cells and silent cells in the hippocampus of freely-behaving rats. *J. Neurosci.* **9**, 2382–2390.

Wilson, M. A. & McNaughton, B. L. 1993 Dynamics of the hippocampal ensemble code for space. *Science* **2616**, 1055–1058.

Zinyuk, L., Kaminsky, Yu., Kubik, S. & Bures, J. 1996 Field clamp: a method for dissociating egocentric and allocentric control of hippocampal place cells in rats. *Eur. J. Neurosci.* **S9**, 140.

10

Variable place-cell coupling to a continuously viewed stimulus: evidence that the hippocampus acts as a perceptual system

Alexander Rotenberg and Robert U. Muller

10.1 Introduction

Although place-cell discharge is reliably affected in a variety of ways by the configuration of external ('allothetic') and internal ('idiothetic') cues available to a freely moving rat, a great deal of work has consistently shown that place cells do not behave as if they are sensory units. Place cells do not act as if they are triggered by specific stimulus conditions; they are neither pattern-recognition units nor path integrators. Instead, place cells have been interpreted as components of neural representations of space or 'cognitive maps' since their discovery (O'Keefe & Dostrovsky 1971; O'Keefe 1976; O'Keefe & Nadel 1978; Muller *et al.* 1991), a view that is assumed in this paper.

A complementary way of thinking about place cells is now proposed. This paper attempts to show that place cells are elements of a perceptual system; what is meant by a 'perceptual' system is stated just below. The suggestion that place-cell activity reflects ongoing perceptual processes is not meant to replace the mapping concept. On the contrary, involvement of perception implies that the map has an integrity of its own and that its coupling to the environment is flexible.

This viewpoint is expressed in a quotation from the Introduction of Hebb's *The organization of behaviour* (1949), which is nearing its fiftieth anniversary: 'The central problem with which we must find a way to deal... is the problem of thought: some sort of process that is not fully controlled by environmental stimulation and yet cooperates closely with that stimulation'. This provocative idea can be couched in current notions about the nervous system by using an analogy.

Consider a 'Necker cube' (Fig. 10.1), which is a well known type of 'ambiguous figure' (Gregory 1970). The Necker cube illustrates the distinction to be made here between sensation and perception. At the sensory level, a Necker cube consists of 12 joined line segments in the plane. The six outer segments form a hexagon, and the six inner segments form two Y-shapes.

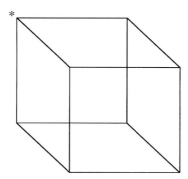

Fig. 10.1 A drawing of a Necker cube. The Necker cube is an example of an ambiguous figure that can be seen to jump between two different states while continuously viewed.

At this level, a Necker cube is a particular retinal image. In contrast, at the perceptual level, the two-dimensional stimulus pattern is interpreted by most people as a cube, even though it is not remotely cubical. The cube interpretation does not depend on binocular processing; it is just as compelling when the stimulus is viewed monocularly.

It is a deep question to ask how two-dimensional images can be reliably interpreted as three-dimensional shapes. The focus of this paper, however, is on the bistability of the Necker cube. At any instant, the viewer sees the cube in one of two configurations. In one, the cube is seen from above, with the accented vertex at the front of the cube; in the other, it is seen from below, and the accented vertex is at the back of the cube. The configuration jumps from one state to the other with time; there is a large literature on the alternation (O'Donnel *et al.* 1988; Peterson & Gibson 1991; Long *et al.* 1992; Gomez *et al.* 1995).

This brings us to a working notion of perception: sensory events shade into the perceptual realm when a single, invariant stimulus is seen in at least two different ways. But how is it possible to know, beyond one's own experience, that a fixed stimulus is indeed able to evoke two or more interpretations? In the context of the connectionist theory of the nervous system, the confirmation must lie in the electrical activity of individual nerve cells; the private experience of seeing the Necker cube jump between configurations must be reflected at the neuronal level.

Consider a thought experiment in which it is possible to non-invasively record from any neuron in a person's nervous system as a Necker cube is viewed. Most likely, retinal neurons would show no correlate of the jumps; variations of cellular activity would not be locked to the instant at which the interpretation shifted. Probably, the same lack of relationship between cell activity and perceptual state would be true of lateral geniculate units, and perhaps of primary visual cortical cells. Nevertheless, on the assumption that perception is causally tied to brain state, it is clear that somewhere in the brain there exists neuronal activity that shifts when the perceived configuration jumps, and that is different depending on which of the cube configurations is current. The signal may be weak, and may be distributed over many cells, but the signal is necessarily there. It is a fundamental assumption of Hebb's resurrection of connectionist theory that 'A particular perception depends on the excitation of particular cells at some point in the central nervous system' (Hebb 1949, p. 17).

The purpose of this paper is to demonstrate that single-cell activity can be coupled to a particular stimulus in a way that strongly resembles expectations from the notions of perception considered above. It is shown that the discharge of individual place cells can be linked in several distinct ways to a single, continuously viewed stimulus. Specifically, the firing field of a place cell can exist stably at more than one angular distance from a white cue card attached to the inside wall of a cylindrical recording chamber. From these findings, the inference is drawn that place cells reflect the operation of a perceptual system. Experimental means of reinforcing the inference are mentioned in Section 10.4.

10.2 Methods

The methods are substantially the same as those used by Muller *et al*. (1987). The experimental task is designed to make the rat visit all parts of the environment so that the positional distribution of place-cell firing can be measured. To this end, rats were trained to retrieve 20 mg food pellets randomly scattered into a grey plywood cylinder (76 cm diameter; 51 cm high). Training lasted about 2 weeks and the rats were thoroughly familiar with the environment and the task before surgery. The floor of the apparatus was a sheet of grey photographic backdrop paper that was replaced each time the rat was removed from the cylinder between sessions. Three nearly identical cylinders in three similar recording rooms were used at different times during the experiment.

Both male and female adult (less than 12 weeks old) Long–Evans hooded rats were used. The animals were initially handled from 30 min to 1 h per day for 1–3 days until they appeared accustomed to the experimenter. During this time, they were fed *ad libitum* standard rat chow mixed with about 5 g of the 20 mg food pellets to motivate the rats to run. After the rats were used to being handled, they were food-deprived to 85% adult body mass and maintained at this level for the duration of the experiment. They received variable amounts of rat chow every evening, depending on the experimenter's estimate of how many 20 mg pellets the animal consumed during the day's experiments.

For training, rats were put into the recording chamber once per day for a session lasting 1–1.5 h. During this session, food pellets were scattered into the cylinder at about six pellets per minute and the rat's behaviour was observed.

If a rat did not search for pellets or ran very little after two or three sessions, it was eliminated from the study. Pre-selection of subjects on the basis of their early performance in training is based on experience that poor runners do not alter their behaviour over long times. Some rats were excluded from the study because signs of respiratory illness were detected. Animals with audible wheezing were not used for fear they would not survive surgery.

Surgical procedures

Surgery was done under sterile conditions and general anaesthesia. After training was complete, rats were anaesthetized with pentobarbital ($40\,mg\,kg^{-1}$ given intraperitoneally) and placed in a stereotaxic instrument. The skin was cut along the midline of the skull and four small holes were drilled in the skull over the right and left olfactory bulbs, left frontal cortex and left parietal cortex. These holes were used for screws to anchor the recording-electrode array. The electrodes themselves were introduced through a 2 mm hole in the lateral portion of the right parietal bone. The exposed dura was cut and reflected back. An electrode array of 10 or 30 microwire, movable electrodes (Kubie 1984) was stereotaxically implanted about 1 mm above the stratum oriens of CA1 of the dorsal hippocampus. The electrodes were positioned so that their tips would pass through 3.3 mm posterior to bregma and 3.1 mm lateral to the midline and therefore through the CA1 layer of the dorsal hippocampus (Paxinos & Watson 1986). Once the electrodes were placed, sterile petroleum jelly was applied to the surface of the brain and around the guide tube of the electrodes. Next, dental acrylic was put over the jelly and around the guide tube to cover the skull hole. Finally, the exposed skull was covered with Grip cement (Ranson and Randolph Ceramics, Maumee, Ohio) and the bottoms of the three drive-screw assemblies were cemented to the skull via the skull screws. The rat was given 3–5 days to recover after surgery before recordings were made. No recordings were made if the rat struggled or vocalized when the recording cable was attached to the connector of the electrode array.

Place-cell recordings

For recordings, the cylinder was placed in the centre of a cylindrical curtain, 2 m in diameter. The inner surface of the cylinder was uniformly grey except for a vertical seam where the single sheet of plywood was joined to complete its circumference. The seam was filled with paint to minimize its contrast with the rest of the interior wall. The seam nevertheless provides a potential orienting cue. It is only one of many 'static background cues' (Sharp *et al.* 1991) that the animal might use to orient itself relative to the laboratory frame.

The only intentionally introduced inhomogeneity in the cylinder was a 60 cm × 51 cm rectangular white cue card. The card extended from the floor to the rim of the cylinder and covered 100° of arc. The reference angular position for the card was with its middle at 0° in the angular coordinate system. When the cylinder is seen from overhead, 0° corresponds to 3:00. Angles are measured in degrees moving anticlockwise, so that 90° corresponds to 12:00.

Recordings were made from CA1 and CA3 complex-spike (pyramidal) cells that showed strong location-specific activity and were therefore classified as place cells. In previous work, no differences had been found between place cells in CA1 and CA3 with regard to control by cue cards; none were seen here. Accordingly, the field of Ammon's horn from which the cell is recorded is ignored. A screening procedure was used to obtain discriminable place cells. The recording cable was attached to the connector on the electrode array and the rat was put into the cylinder. All the wires were then scanned for single-unit activity. If none was seen, the cable was detached and the electrodes were advanced about 40 μm by turning the drive screws. The rat was then returned to its home cage for about an hour to allow any distortion of the brain to relax. The screening procedure was then repeated.

Once at least one recurring waveform of usable amplitude (greater than about 150 μV) was seen, the unit was classified as a complex-spike cell or a theta cell. To be called a complex-spike cell the unit had to meet three criteria.

1. It had to generate complex spikes, which are high-frequency bursts of from two to perhaps six spikes whose amplitudes decrease.
2. It had to commonly show long interspike intervals (>1 s).
3. The duration of the initial phase of the filtered (100 Hz–10 kHz) waveform had to be at least 200 μs.

In contrast, interneurons (theta cells) had to:

1. never generate complex spikes;
2. never fire at rates lower than about 10 spikes s^{-1};
3. have an initial phase of about 100 μs (Ranck 1973; Fox & Ranck 1975; Muller et al. 1987; Kubie et al. 1990).

Waveform discrimination was done in two ways. In the earlier work, three Bak time-and-amplitude window discriminators arranged in series had been used to select waveforms. With this method, the time of each action potential was not saved. Instead, the number of action potentials was accumulated for 1/60 s intervals, the reciprocal of the 60 Hz frequency at which position was measured. Thus, the temporal resolution of spike recording was equal to the temporal resolution of tracking.

In the second discrimination method, waveforms were digitized at 40 kHz per wire with a Datawave workstation. A burst of 32 samples (for a duration of 800 μs) was captured each time the electrode voltage exceeded about 100 μV. Sorting of waveforms into single unit time series was done retrospectively after recording. Often, when the initial negative peak of captured waveforms was plotted against the later positive peak a single elliptic region was seen, as if the positive and negative peaks yielded a two-dimensional Gaussian distribution. A rectangle that encompassed most of the elliptic region was drawn. In this case, all waveforms that fell into the circumscribed rectangle were considered to have been generated by a single unit. If it appeared that two similar waveforms were being classified as a single unit, additional criteria (e.g. spike duration) were used in sorting. It is emphasized, however, that little effort was devoted to extracting any but the largest waveforms, so that in practice this method yielded the same results as the use of the window discriminators.

Tracking

To determine the positional firing distribution for place cells, it is necessary to track the position of the rat's head in parallel with single-cell recordings. To this end, a light-emitting diode (LED) is attached to the electrode carrier and made the brightest source in the view of an overhead television camera. The signal from the camera is sent to a threshold device that detects the LED. At the time of detection, the values in two counters are registered and held until the end of the televisual field. The Y counter holds the number of lines that have been scanned since the beginning of the field; the X counter holds the number of pulses generated by a fast clock that is synchronized with the beginning of each video line. At the end of the field an interrupt causes the X and Y values to be read by a computer. Because the light position is detected once per field, the temporal resolution is 60 Hz. Position was detected in a 64×64 grid of square regions (pixels) 2.4 cm on a side. To calculate firing rate as a function of position, spikes were assigned to the pixel in which the rat's head was detected at the beginning of each 16.7 ms 'sample'. If the LED was not detected for a sample, spikes in the associated 16.7 ms interval were ignored.

Display and analysis

The positional firing distribution for a cell was calculated by dividing the number of spikes fired in each pixel by the total time for which the light was detected in each pixel. Colour-coded firing-rate maps were used to visualize positional firing-rate distributions. Pixel rates were sorted in ascending order and partitioned into six categories encoded in the sequence yellow, orange, red, green, blue, purple. Yellow encodes pixels in which the firing rate was exactly zero, orange the lowest non-zero pixels, and purple the highest non-zero pixels. The boundaries between non-zero firing-rate categories were picked such that the number of pixels in a given category was 0.8 times the number in the next lower rate category. Pixels in the apparatus that were not visited wer coded white, as were inaccessible pixels outside the cylinder. Colour-coded maps were used as the main method of analysis in this paper; visible changes in the positional firing pattern are relied on to demonstrate how experimental manipulations affect place-cell discharge.

Experimental manipulations

The attempt to show that hippocampal place cells are part of a perceptual system is based on investigating the control that the white cue card exerts over place-cell firing. The basic experiment is to change the angular position of the white card on the cylinder wall; such manipulations are called 'card rotations'. The basic question is whether firing fields rotate in register with the card rotations; it is concluded that the cue card has stimulus control if the fields rotate, and that control is absent if the fields stay in the same place. Note that control is defined strictly in terms of what happens to the field and in no way implies that the animal in some sense ignores or is unaware of the stimulus or its altered position. Indeed, the fact that the card can exert strong stimulus control immediately after it had no stimulus control implies that information about the card is continuously available (see below). Because the present experiments involved only cue card rotations of 180° and 45°, the amount of field rotation was easily detected by inspection of the colour-coded firing-rate maps.

Two types of card rotation were done. The first was done with the rat out of the recording chamber. Because these cue-card movements could not be observed by the animal they are referred to as 'hidden'. For hidden rotations the card was put into its standard position and a session was recorded. The rat was taken out of the cylinder and put into its home cage. The card was then rotated (usually by 180°) and a second recording session was run.

The second type of card rotation was done while the animal was inside the recording cylinder. Such rotations could be observed by the animal and are called 'visible'. To make a visible rotation, recording was stopped after a predetermined time had elapsed. The experimenter then stepped through the cylindrical curtain, detached the card from the wall and re-attached it at a new position that was either 45° or 180° away from the previous card position. The experimenter then left the curtained area and the recording room itself and restarted data acquisition. Again, comparisons were made between the amount of card rotation and the amount by which firing fields rotated.

Floor paper was renewed each time the rat was removed from the cylinder. Thus, floor markings made by the rat in the course of a sequence of hidden rotations could not serve as orienting cues in the next session. In contrast, floor markings made during a sequence of visible rotations could serve as orienting cues when the card was in different positions.

10.3 Results

The results were obtained from four different variations of the card-rotation experiment.

Variant 1: hidden card rotations of 180°

In a hidden card rotation, the firing field of a place cell is recorded with the card in its standard position, the rat is put into its home cage, the angular position of the card on the wall is changed, the rat is returned to the cylinder and a second session is done. In previous work, it was shown that hidden card rotations almost always result in equal field rotations, so that the position of the field relative to the card remained constant (see, for example Muller *et al.* 1987; Bostock *et al.* 1991). Additional 180° hidden card rotations were done for this work and the same effect was found, as illustrated for two cells in Fig. 10.2a. The field of cell A1 in Fig. 10.2a was at 7:30 with the card in its standard position (cell A1, Session 1). When a hidden 180° rotation was done, the field also rotated by about 180° to 1:30 (cell A1, Session 2). The effects of the same manipulations on a second cell (cell A2) are also shown in Fig. 10.2a. Hidden 180° rotations caused equal field rotations for six out of seven cells in four rats. Thus, as shown in previous work, the white cue card is salient and its angular position exhibits nearly ideal stimulus control over the angular position of firing fields.

Variant 2: visible 180° card rotations

Does the angular position of the cue card have absolute control over field position? The control demonstrated with hidden rotations could mean that the angular position of the card sets the angular position of firing fields regardless of when or how the card is moved. Alternatively, it could be that the hidden rotations are effective only because they are hidden and that the rat would ignore the card if it could know it had been moved. These possibilities were explored by doing visible card rotations in the rats' presence. It is important that the rats' behaviour indicates that they were aware of the visible card movement. The rat would usually orient toward the card as soon as the experimenter detached it from the wall. The rat would then chase one of the card edges as it was moved along the cylinder wall. When the card rotation was complete, however, the rat always resumed its pellet-chasing activity. Thus, the card-rotation procedure had no long-term effect on behaviour.

It was found that the field stayed at the same angle relative to the laboratory frame in 25 out of 28 cases after visible 180° rotations. (The visible rotations include the first two sessions of the 12 replications of variant 4 described below.) Thus, cue-card control was almost always absent when the card was rotated in the rat's presence. The ineffectiveness of visible 180° rotations is illustrated for two cells in Fig. 10.2b. For one of the remaining three cells, the field rotated after the visible 180° rotation. For the other two cells, the visible 180° rotation caused an apparent 'remapping': the angular position of the field, the radial position of the field and the field shape all changed (Bostock *et al.* 1991). The main conclusion is that moving the cue card by 180° produces very different effects depending on whether the rat can or cannot see the card

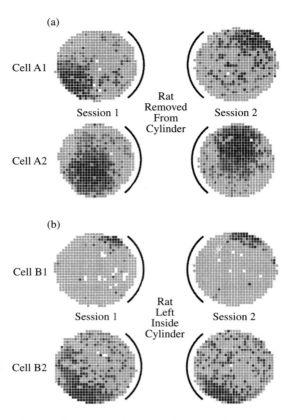

Fig. 10.2 (a) Outcome of experimental variant 1: the effects of hidden 180° cue-card rotations on two independently recorded place cells. The baseline position of the firing field for each cell was established during a standard session (Session 1). For each cell, the rat was removed from the recording room after Session 1 and the cue card was rotated 180°. The rat was then put back in the cylinder for Session 2. Under these conditions, the firing fields rotated by 180°, demonstrating that the cue has strong stimulus control over the positional firing pattern. (b) Outcome of experimental variant 2: the effects of visible 180° cue-card rotations on two independently recorded place cells. The baseline positions of the firing fields were established during Session 1 with the cue card at its standard position. The card was then moved by 180° while the rat was in the cylinder and could view the card. It is evident from the rate maps for Session 2 that the firing field of each example cell stayed at its original angular location in the laboratory frame.

movement. The outcome of the visible 180° rotation makes it clear that cue-card control over the angular position of firing fields is not absolute. In addition, the remappings suggest that in some cases the change in the environment is enough for the hippocampus to produce a new representation rather than 'reattach' the original representation to the card.

Variant 3: visible 45° card rotations

In contrast to visible 180° rotations, visible 45° rotations almost always caused equal firing-field rotations. In addition, firing fields followed sequences of visible 45° rotations so that the field could be caused to rotate by 180° by doing four 45° rotations in a row without removing the rat from the chamber. Thus, there is nothing special about the 180° position itself that precludes fields from following visible rotations. Continuing to do visible 45° rotations after reaching 180° caused fields to continue to rotate, so that after eight such rotations the field was back to its original position.

Two sequences of visible 45° rotations are shown in Fig. 10.3a, where it is clear that each field accurately followed the card position for the four steps that are shown. The same fields continued to follow the card for an additional four sessions so that in the end the fields returned to the original location. A total of five cells in five animals were tested with sequences of eight visible 45° rotations. The fields followed accurately in all cases. It is worth repeating the observation that rats oriented to the card when it was detached and followed one of its edges during the visible 45° rotations, just as was true for the visible 180° rotations. Thus, even though the rat seemed aware that the card was moving, the firing fields were almost ideally controlled by the card.

Variant 4: combinations of visible 180° and 45° card rotations

The discovery that the magnitude of visible card rotations determines whether or not the fields follow the card suggests at least two additional lines of investigation. One experiment would be to vary the magnitude of the visible rotation to look for a threshold: a rotation such that slightly smaller rotations yield cue-card control and slightly larger rotations leave the field fixed in the laboratory frame. The decision was made to ask instead what would happen if visible 45° rotations were done after a visible 180° rotation? That is, would the ordinarily effective visible 45° rotations now fail to cause the field to move, or would they continue to be effective?

A total of 12 sequences were carried out in which a visible 180° rotation was followed by a series of eight 45° rotations all in the same direction. Remarkably, even though the field did not move after the 180° rotation, in five of these experiments in three rats the field rotated with every one of the eight 45° rotations. Two examples of the first six sessions of such sequences are shown in Fig. 10.3b. The key point is that in the sixth session the firing field is 180° away from its angular position in the first, standard session. *Thus, precisely the same configuration of a continuously visible stimulus is associated with two different states of firing of the cell.* In none of these cases was the change in angular relation between the card and the field permanent. On the contrary, in each case when the rat was taken out of the cylinder and replaced, the field resumed its original position relative to the card.

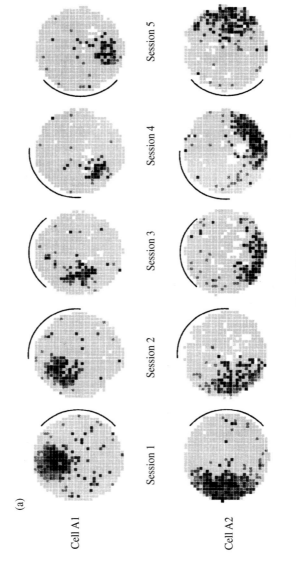

Fig. 10.3(a)

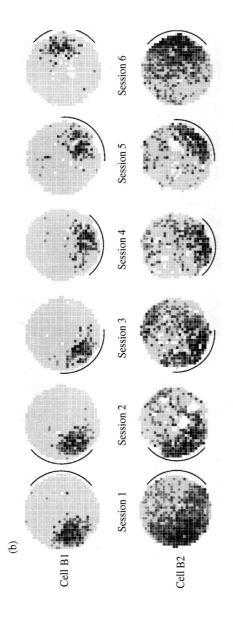

(b)

Cell B1   Session 1   Session 2   Session 3   Session 4   Session 5   Session 6

Cell B2

Fig. 10.3 (a) Outcome of experimental variant 3: the effects of a series of visible 45° cue-card rotations on two independently recorded place cells. The baseline positions of the firing fields were established during Session 1 with the cue card at its standard position. The card was then rotated by 45° between each pair of subsequent sessions while the rat was in the cylinder and could see the card. Each 45° cue-card rotation caused an equal rotation of the firing field. The fields of both cells maintained a constant angular relationship to the cue card for the five consecutive sessions shown and for four additional sessions not included. By Session 5, the cue card was 180° away from its standard position. The firing fields of both place cells also rotated by 180°. Note that the crisper appearance of the firing fields in Session 1 is due to the longer recording time; the baseline sessions lasted 16 min whereas the rotations sessions lasted 4 min (see Muller *et al.* 1987). (b) Outcome of experimental variant 4: the effects of combined visible 180° and 45° cue-card rotations on two independently recorded place cells. The baseline positions of the firing fields were established in Session 1 with the cue card in its standard position. Between Sessions 1 and 2 the cue card was rotated 180° while the animal was in the cylinder and could see the card. Between each pair of sessions after Session 2 the cue card was rotated 45° with the rat in the cylinder. The fields of both cells stayed at their initial position after the 180° rotation. In contrast, the fields followed the subsequent 45° card rotations. Note that by Session 6 the cue card was back to its standard position, but the firing fields were 180° away from the positions seen in Session 1. Thus, place cells can fire in two different ways in response to a single, continuously viewed stimulus. As in Fig. 10.2, the crisper appearance of the fields in Session 1 is because that session lasted 16 min whereas the other sessions lasted only 4 min.

In seven out of 12 cases, the field failed to follow the cue card perfectly for all eight visible 45° rotations. In every case, however, the field was controlled by the visible 45° rotations several times. Moreover, the control generally occurred for several of the rotations in a row. For many of the card rotations that did not produce equal field rotations, the cell was nearly silent. When firing resumed, the field usually began to rotate again, but in a way as if it had 'slipped' relative to the card. That is, for these cells, the field always rotated by less than 360° during the 45° steps. The remaining cell also showed rotations during the sequence of eight 45° rotations. It was anomalous in that its field rotated after the visible 180° rotation.

In summary, all place cells followed at least some visible 45° rotations. Thus, two different field positions were observed for every place cell with the card in its standard location. The effect is most dramatic when the field follows all eight visible 45° rotations, but it is also clear that the angular position of fields is not controlled in an absolute way by either external (allothetic) or internal (idiothetic) cues.

10.4 Discussion

Cue-card control over the angular position of firing fields depends on the magnitude of visible rotations

The work presented bears similarities to several other experiments on place cells and head directional cells in which different sources of sensory information are put into conflict with each other (Sharp *et al.* 1995; Taube & Burton 1995; Blair & Sharp 1995). These studies were designed to test the relative importance of external cues and idiothetic cues. In each case, it was found that visual cues set field position in preference to idiothetic cues, although in each case there were conditions under which idiothetic cues instead controlled firing-field position.

These experiments can be interpreted along similar lines. A single experimental manipulation, namely cue-card rotation in the animal's presence, almost always results in either equal rotation of firing fields or no rotation of firing fields. Specifically, visible rotations of 45° almost always cause 45° rotations of fields, whereas visible 180° rotations almost always leave field position unaffected. Thus, the magnitude of the rotation determines which stimulus class will be prepotent. It could be said that small card rotations cause the place-cell system to 'ignore' static background and idiothetic cues. (Static background cues are potential orienting stimuli that are fixed relative to the labortory frame. Examples are the eccentric position of the overhead commutator, the seam in the cylinder wall or markings of the floor made by the rat. In this case, the idiothetic cue is that the change in card position was not caused by self-motion.) In contrast, it could be said that large card rotations cause the place-cell system to ignore the cue card and to stay in register with static background cues or idiothetic cues or both. It is interesting that the system does not reach a compromise between the two sets of cues but instead seems to go with one or the other. Bistability is not, however, the only possible outcome. In experiments with two cue cards, one black and one white, changing the angular distance between the cards reveals that they exert about equal control over firing fields (Fenton & Muller 1997).

The dependence of the effects of visible rotations on the amount the card is moved has several interesting implications with regard to the place-cell system. First, in agreement with earlier work, the existence of circumstances (visible 180° rotations) in which the card lacks control shows that place cells are not simply triggered by cell-specific cues (Muller & Kubie 1987; Quirk *et al*. 1990; Sharp *et al*. 1990; Markus *et al*. 1994). As we have argued before, findings of this type belie the notion that place cells are properly described as high-order sensory cells or pattern recognition units. In a similar vein, the existence of circumstances (visible 45° rotations) in which the cue card is fully effective in the face of conflict with idiothetic cues that are supported by static background cues suggests that place cells are not dominated by self-motion information. By inference, the place-cell system should therefore probably not be considered to be fundamentally concerned with path integration (see McNaughton *et al*. 1996 for opposite view).

The ineffectiveness of idiothetic and static background cues during small visible rotations has a simple interpretation in terms of a path integration scheme: it can be said that the path integrator is reset so that the 'binding of the cue card to the place cells is maintained. It is, however, unclear why a path integrator should be reset if self-motion cues indicate stability. It is not as if the system *must* reset: field position does not jump when the card rotation is large. We conclude that the results of visible 45° and 180° rotations are as hard to fit into a pattern-integration scheme as they are into a sensory scheme.

The effects of combined visible 180° and 45° rotations suggest that place cells are part of a perceptual system

Is it really proper to conclude that the idiothetic and static background cues are ignored if small cue-card rotations cause equal field rotations? This possibility seems implausible on at least the grounds that the flow of idiothetic information is uninterrupted. It is more satisfactory to imagine that a new binding is made between place cells and idiothetic cues. In path integration terms, one would say that the integrator was reset, but we suggest instead that idiothetic information is just a kind of sensory information that is used when external information is lacking or in great conflict with previous external information.

Similarly, it is tempting, but not necessarily correct, to conclude that the cue card is ignored if large card rotations do not alter field positions. Whether the card is ignored is testable; the results with subsequent small rotations indicate that the card continues to play a role in controlling firing fields. The notion is that the card is rebound in a new position in the angular coordinate of the place-cell system. Moreover, the rebinding is instantaneous within the temporal resolution of our measurements. The process is much faster than the 3–5 min it seems to take to establish a new map (Hill 1978; Bostock *et al*. 1991; Wilson & McNaughton 1993); this difference in speed suggests that different synaptic or cell-level mechanisms are involved in building a map than are required to link the map to external stimuli.

The difference in effectiveness of visible 180° and subsequent visible 45° rotations brings us back to our main theme, that place cells act as if they are part of a perceptual system. This can be seen most clearly when four 45° rotations are made after a single 180° rotation. The surprise is that after the rotation sequence the card is back in its initial state whereas the field is 180° away from its initial position. In those cases in which some of the visible 45° rotations in a sequence failed to cause a 45° field rotation, other card rotations were successful. Therefore, in every repeat of the combined visible 180° and 45° rotations individual cells fired in two different ways relative to an identical cue configuration. This satisfies the criterion that was set out in Section 10.1 to demonstrate that place cells reflect the operation of a perceptual system.

It is of interest whether the preferred directions of head-direction cells would stay in register with the angular locations of firing fields or whether the positional and directional systems would be dissociated in these circumstances. It is our belief that preferred directions in the directional system would show just the same variable coupling to the cue card, so that it would stay in register with the positional system.

We end by suggesting an additional experiment to test the validity of our conclusion. The basic idea for this experiment is similar to the elegant study by Logothetis & Schall (1989) in which monkeys were asked to report the currently perceived direction of motion of a visual pattern under circumstances in which the pattern could be seen to move in either of two ways. When single-cell recordings were made from units in the superior temporal sulcus, most units reflected properties of the retinal light pattern. In contrast, the activity of a fraction of the units shifted in time register with the report of movement direction by the monkey. Logothetis & Schall concluded that the superior temporal sulcus may be involved in the processing of visual movement perception. Note, however, that the changing cellular activity could be coupled to the response itself (if short-term memory of the response is registered) rather than to the subjective perception. In our experiment, it is hard to argue that the altered cell activity is due to altered motor activity, because the behaviour is indistinguishable before and after the visible 180° rotation.

The present work, on the other hand, suffers from the deficit that there is no way for the rat to report that it knows that the environment is different before and after the visible 180° card rotation. It would therefore be interesting to train the rat to go to a certain location on hearing an auditory signal. If the rat went to the original location in the laboratory frame, it would suggest that the place cells and the behaviour were in register. If the rat went to a rotated image of the original location it would indicate that place cells are dissociated from behaviour. It is our prediction, however, that the rat will go first to the original correct position and then to the rotated image; this result would indicate that the rat is aware that two almost equally good interpretations of the environment are available.

Acknowledgement

This work was supported by NIH grant R01-NS20686.

References

Blair, H. T. & Sharp, P. E. 1995 Influences of vestibular and visual motion information on the spatial firing patterns of hippocampal place cells. *J. Neurosci.* **15**, 173–189.

Bostock, E., Muller, R. U. & Kubie, J. L. 1991 Experience-dependent modifications of hippocampal place cell firing. *Hippocampus* **1**, 193–205.

Fenton, A. A. & Muller, R. U. 1997 Place cell discharge is extremely variable during individual passes of the rat through the firing field. *Proc. Natn. Acad. Sci. USA.* **95**, 3182–3187.

Fox, S. E. & Ranck, J. B. Jr 1975 Localization and anatomical identification of theta and complex spike cells in the dorsal hippocampal formation of rats. *Exp. Neurol.* **49**, 299–313.

Gomez, C., Argandona, E. D., Solier, R. G., Angulo, J. C. & Vazquez, M. 1995 Timing and competition in networks representing ambiguous figures. *Brain Cogn.* **29**, 103–114.

Gregory, R. L. 1970 *The intelligent eye*. New York: McGraw-Hill.

Hebb, D. O. 1949 *The organization of behavior*. New York: Wiley.

Hill, A. J. 1978 First occurrence of hippocampal spatial firing in a new environment. *Expl Neurol.* **62**, 282–297.

Kubie, J. L. 1984 A driveable bundle of microwires for collecting single-unit data from freely-moving rats. *Physiol. Behav.* **32**, 115–118.

Kubie, J. L., Muller, R. U. & Bostock, E. M. 1990 Spatial firing properties of hippocampal theta cells. *J. Neurosci.* **10**, 1110–1123.

Logothetis, N. K. & Schall, J. D. 1989 Neural correlates of subjective visual perception. *Science* **245**, 761–763.

Long, G. M., Toppino, T. C. & Mondin, G. W. 1992 Prime time: fatigue and set effects in the perception of reversible figures. *Percept. Psychophys.* **52**, 609–616.

Markus, E. J., Barnes, C. A., McNaughton, B. L., Gladden, V. L. & Skaggs, W. E. 1994 Spatial information content and the reliability of hippocampal CA1 neurons: effects of visual input. *Hippocampus* **4**, 410–421.

McNaughton, B. L. *et al.* 1996 Deciphering the hippocampal polyglot: the hippocampus as a path integration system. *J. Exp. Biol.* **199**, 173–185.

Muller, R. U. & Kubie, J. L. 1987 The effects of changes in the environment on the spatial firing patterns of hippocampal complex-spike cells. *J. Neurosci.* **7**, 1951–1968.

Muller, R. U., Kubie, J. L. & Ranek, J. B. Jr 1987 Spatial firing patterns of hippocampal complex-spike cells in a fixed environment. *J. Neurosci.* **7**, 1935–1950.

Muller, R. U., Kubie, J. L. & Saypoff, R. 1991 The hippocampus as a cognitive graph. Abridged version. *Hippocampus* **1**, 243–246.

O'Donnell, B. F., Hendler, T. & Squires, N. K. 1988 Visual evoked potentials to illusory reversals of the necker cube. *Psychophysiology* **25**, 137–143.

O'Keefe, J. 1976 Place units in the hippocampus of freely moving rat. *Expl Neurol.* **51**, 78–109.

O'Keefe, J. & Dostrovsky, J. 1971 The hippocampus as a spatial map. Preliminary evidence from unit activity in the freely-moving rat. *Brain Res.* **34**, 171–175.

O'Keefe, J. & Nadel, L. 1978 *The hippocampus as a cognitite map.* New York: Oxford University Press.

Peterson, M. A. & Gibson, B. S. 1991 Directing spatial attention within an object: altering the functional equivalence of shape descriptions. *J. Exp. Psychol. Hum. Percept. Perform.* **17**, 170–182.

Quirk, G. J., Muller, R. U. & Kubie, J. L. 1990 The firing of hippocampal place cells in the dark reflects the rat's recent experience. *J. Neurosci.* **10**, 2008–2017.

Ranck, J. B. Jr 1973 Studies on single neurons in doesal hippocampal formation and septum in unrestrained rats. I. Behavioral correlates and firing repertoires. *Expl Neurol.* **41**, 461–555.

Sharp, P. E., Blair, H. T., Etkin, D. & Tzanetos, D. B. 1995 Influences of vestibular and visual motion information on the spatial firing patterns of hippocampal place cells. *J. Neurosci.* **15**, 173–189.

Sharp, P., Muller, R. U. & Kubie, J. L. 1990 Firing properties of hippocampal neurons in a visually symmetrical environment: contributions of multiple sensory cues and mnemonic processes. *J. Neurosci.* **10**, 3093–3105.

Taube, J. S. & Burton, H. L. 1995 Head direction cell activity monitored in a novel environment and during a cue conflict situation. *J. Neurophysiol.* **74**, 1953–1971.

Wilson, M. A. & McNaughton, B. L. 1993 Dynamics of the hippocampal ensemble code for space. *Science* **261**, 1055–1058.

11

Separating hippocampal maps

A. David Redish and David S. Touretzky

11.1 Introduction: reference frames

Hippocampal place cells also show correlations to non-spatial aspects of the world, including environment (Kubie and Ranck 1983; Muller and Kubie 1987; Thompson and Best 1989), task within environment (Markus *et al.* 1995), and even stage within task (Eichenbaum *et al.* 1987; Eichenbaum and Cohen 1988; Cohen and Eichenbaum 1993; Hampson *et al.* 1993; Gothard *et al.* 1996). Some have argued that these experiments imply that place cells should be understood as being general context cells, with space being only one of many parameters to which they are tuned (Eichenbaum *et al.* 1992; Wiener 1993; Eichenbaum 1996).

However, even when a cell shows different firing patterns under two conditions, the cell still show place fields under both conditions. For example, a cell that shows a difference between two tasks performed within the same environment (as reported by Markus *et al.* 1995), still only fires within a constrained place field in each task, if it fires at all. To say that a cell is sensitive to a non-spatial aspect, such as task, means that if the cell has a place field under one condition, it may or may not show a place field under the other, and if two cells both show place fields under both conditions, then the spatial relationships between them may change drastically from one condition to the other. Essentially, a cell's place field under one non-spatial condition (in fact whether it has a place field at all) is independent of its field under other non-spatial conditions.

One way to explain this is the multi-map hypothesis: *multiple maps in the hippocampus* (O'Keefe and Nadel 1978), *active subsets* (Muller and Kubie 1987), *reference frames* (Wan *et al.* 1994a,b; Touretzky and Redish 1996; Redish 1997; Redish and Touretzky 1997a), or *charts* (McNaughton *et al.* 1996; Samsonovich and McNaughton 1997; Samsonovich 1997). All of these authors suggest that the hippocampus includes multiple maps, and that each place cell takes part in one or more of those maps.

There are, however, minor differences among these hypotheses. In this paper, we will concentrate on the two hypotheses that are the most detailed, computationally: *charts* and *reference frames*. The multi-chart hypothesis suggests that the maps are critically a hippocampal property arising from internal dynamics of the hippocampus. In contrast, the reference frame hypothesis suggests that the maps arise from interactions of the hippocampus with extrinsic navigational structures such as a neural path integrator.[1]

Barnes *et al.* (1997) have shown an experiment in which the removal and return of an animal to an environment is sufficient to produce a map transition. In this paper, we present an explanation for this result, with simulations. Our account says that errors in a *path integrator reset* process, which occur on returning to the environment, force a change in reference frame, leading to the appearance of a map transition.

11.2 The reference frame theory

Over the last few years, we have synthesized a theory of rodent navigation, bringing together ideas from the extensive work done on rodent navigation over the last century and showing how the interaction of several subsystems gives rise to a comprehensive, computational theory of navigation (Touretzky and Redish 1996; Redish and Touretzky 1997a, 1998). A complete description of the theory and its correspondence to the experimental literature is given in depth in Redish (1997). Here we will only present a short overview of the theory. Then we will compare its explanation for the Barnes *et al.* (1997) experiment with that of the *multi-chart* model (McNaughton *et al.* 1996; Samsonovich 1997; Samsonovich and McNaughton 1997).

Extending O'Keefe and Nadel (1978), the reference frame theory describes navigation as a consequence of four different functional systems:

(1) taxon navigation (direct approach/avoidance of a landmark);
(2) praxic navigation (a sequence of motor actions, driven from an internal sequencing mechanism);
(3) locale navigation (map-based navigation); and
(4) route navigation (chained stimulus-response mechanisms).

It also describes locale navigation in detail as a consequence of an interaction among five spatial representations:

(1) local view (spatial aspects of external landmarks);
(2) head direction (the orientation of the animal in space);
(3) path integrator (the vector home, represented on a canonical map);
(4) place code (a representation of the animal's location in the current reference frame); and
(5) goal memory (allowing trajectory planning).

The anatomical instantiation suggested for these systems is shown in Fig. 11.1.

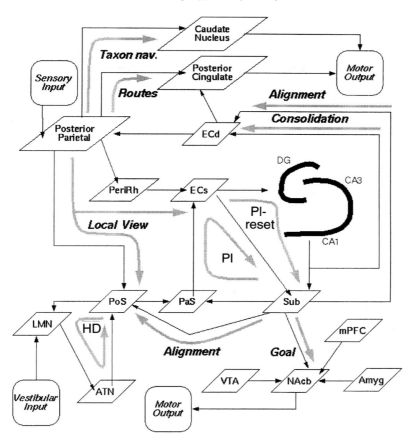

Fig. 11.1 Anatomical realization of a comprehensive model of rodent navigation. From Redish (1997). Amyg: amygdala; ATN: anterior thalamic nuclei; DG: dentate gyrus; CA3, CA1: hippocampus proper; ECs: superficial entorhinal cortex; ECd: deep entorhinal cortex; LMN: lateral mammillary nuclei; mPFC: medial prefrontal cortex. NAcb: nucleus accumbens; PaS: parasubiculum; PeriRh: Perirhinal cortex; PoS: postsubiculum; Sub: subiculum; VTA: ventral tegmental area; HD: Head direction subsystem pathways; PI: Path integration subsystem pathways. Not all anatomical structures or connections are shown. Functional pathways are meant to be indicative only; structures not directly on a labeled pathway may also be involved in that subsystem.

This theory can explain results from a wide range of methodological paradigms, including single- and multi-cell recording, behavioural manipulations, neuropharmacological manipulations, and lesion studies; it is consistent with anatomical data (see Redish 1997). We have simulated most aspects of this theory, demonstrating how it can replicate a variety of results, including:

(1) tracking of head direction by cells in postsubiculum and the anterior thalamic nuclei (Taube *et al*. 1990, 1996; Redish *et al*. 1996; Blair *et al*. 1997; Goodridge *et al*. 1997);

(2) open-field navigation tasks (Collett *et al*. 1986; Saksida *et al*. 1995; Touretzky and Redish 1996);

(3) memory consolidation in the Morris water maze (Morris 1981; Sutherland and Hoesing 1993; Redish and Touretzky 1998);

(4) changes in place fields as a consequence of interactions between a consistent entry point and cue card manipulations (Sharp *et al*. 1990; Redish and Touretzky 1996; Redish 1997); and

(5) consequences of disorientation in rectangular arenas (Cheng 1986; Margules and Gallistel 1988; Gallistel 1990; Wan *et al*. 1994*a*; Touretzky and Redish 1996).

All of the simulations are also detailed in (Redish 1997).

11.3 The experiment of Barnes *et al*. (1997)

Barnes *et al*. (1997) allowed an animal to walk around a figure-eight maze for 25 min. They then removed the animal for 1 h, after which the animal was returned to the maze and allowed to walk around for another 25 min. During each 25-min experience, Barnes *et al*. recorded about three dozen place cells simultaneously.

When young animals were returned to the environment, they used the same set of place cells to encode location. But when old animals were returned to the environment, they sometimes used a completely different set of cells. The ensemble correlation between place fields in the two experiences was always high for young animals (approximately 0.7, indicative of a similar representation between experiences), but was bimodal in old animals (sometimes near 0, indicative of a complete remapping, and at other times near 0.7, indicative of a similar representation). Within a single experience in the environment, place fields were very stable; correlations between the first and second halves of a single run were always high for both old and young animals.

11.4 Two competing explanations

The explanation provided by the multi-chart model

Barnes *et al*. (1997; see also McNaughton *et al*. 1996; Samsonovich 1997; Samsonovich and McNaughton 1997) explain the bimodal distribution in old animals as a problem in *selecting the correct cognitive map*. Their theory includes a set of pre-wired *charts* in the hippocampus, such that the synaptic weight between two cells in the hippocampus is inversely proportional to the minimum of their distances across all of the charts. When combined with global inhibition, this produces a local-excitation-global-inhibition network structure. This type of network has a coherent representation of a single location on a single chart as a stable state (Samsonovich and McNaughton 1997); any other representation, such as noise biased by extra activity at candidate locations suggested by sensory cues, will be unstable and will settle into a stable state.

The major drawback of this theory is that it requires complex pre-wired connections within the hippocampus. Each place cell needs to be more strongly connected to cells with place fields nearby (in some chart) than to cells with place fields that are distant (in all charts). There is evidence that this connection structure exists after exploration (Wilson and McNaughton 1994), but the theory requires that the connection structure be in place *before exploration*.

According to this theory, on entering a novel environment, one location on one *chart* (map) will win the competition among competing representations and become the preferred representation for the entry point. As young animals explore the environment, representations of the local view become bound to places on the currently active chart. Then, on a return visit to the environment entering at the same point as before, the local view representation biases the dynamics in the hippocampus so that the same representation of location on the same chart is reinstantiated. In the case of old animals, deficiencies in LTP (Long Term Potentiation; for a review, see Barnes 1998) prevent the local view from becoming as tightly bound to the currently active chart during initial exploration. Thus, according to the multi-chart model, on returning to the environment, old animals experience a much weaker bias to select the same location on the same chart as before.

The explanation provided by the reference frame model

We propose that the phenomenon seen in older animals is not a consequence of pre-wired chart selection within the CA3 population, but rather an interaction between a non-linearity of the path integrator and the orthogonalization properties of dentate gyrus.

The important points for this experiment, drawn from the theory described in Section 11.2, are:

1. The path integrator is extrinsic to the hippocampus (O'Keefe 1976; Wan *et al.* 1994*b*; Touretzky and Redish 1996; Redish and Touretzky 1997*a*).

2. During normal navigation, place cells require both local view and path integrator input (O'Keefe 1976; Wan *et al.* 1994*b*; Touretzky and Redish, 1996; Redish and Touretzky 1997*a*).

3. The dentate gyrus orthogonalizes the combined local view and path integrator inputs (Marr 1969; McNaughton and Morris 1987; Rolls 1989, 1996; O'Reilly and McClelland 1994) so that if either one changes, a new set of place cells is selected.

4. *Path-integrator reset* occurs on re-entry into an environment (Touretzky and Redish 1996; Redish 1997; Redish and Touretzky 1997a; for similar hypotheses see Rawlins 1985; Rotenberg *et al*. 1996).

Organization of the model

The components required for simulating this experiment are shown in Fig. 11.2. The model includes an extrinsic path integrator (PI), an extrinsic local view (LV), strong random connections from each to the dentate gyrus (DG), and strong random connections from the dentate gyrus to hippocampus (HC). We do not differentiate between CA3 and CA1 in this model, and so HC includes both recurrent connections (as in CA3) and outputs to the path integrator (as in CA1). Both the PI and HC models are composed of excitatory (E) and inhibitory (I) pools.

The path integrator in this model is assumed to consist of a two-dimensional representation of location in which cells show place fields but the fields do not change from environment to environment. Cells in entorhinal cortex and subiculum show these environment-independent place fields (Quirk *et al*. 1992; Sharp 1997). Following these results, we have suggested that the path integrator consists of a loop between three extra-hippocampal structures: subiculum, parasubiculum, and superficial entorhinal cortex (Redish and Touretzky 1997a). The path integrator representation can be updated by offset connections (Zhang 1996; Samsonovich and McNaughton 1997). In addition,

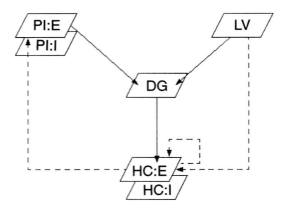

Fig. 11.2 Hippocampal model used to simulate the Barnes *et al*. (1997) experiment. During storage, *solid lines* drive place-cell activity and *dashed lines* show correlational learning; during recall, *dashed lines* show synaptic transmission and drive place-cell activity and path integrator reset. See text for details.

we assume that the path integrator has a local-excitation-global-inhibition network structure. This means that the path integrator reset process can occur by assuming the path integrator is initialized with noise and then biased by input from the place cells (which are in turn biased by the local view). This attractor network structure has been extensively studied both in one dimension (Wilson and Cowan 1973; Amari 1977; Ermentrout and Cowan 1979; Kishimoto and Amari 1979; Kohonen 1982, 1984; Skaggs et al. 1995; Redish et al. 1996; Zhang 1996; Redish 1997) and two (Kohonen 1982, 1984; Droulez and Berthoz 1991; Munoz et al. 1991; Arai et al. 1994; McNaughton et al. 1996; Zhang 1996; Redish and Touretzky 1998; Redish 1997; Samsonovich 1997; Samsonovich and McNaughton 1997).

The reference frame model requires that cells in the path integrator are most strongly connected to other cells with nearby place fields, which is similar to the pre-wired connections required in the hippocampus in the multi-chart model. However, the reference frame model only requires this connection structure to pre-exist for a single map, located outside the hippocampus, which simplifies the model immensely. The model also includes local excitation (within reference frame) connections within the hippocampus, as does the multi-chart model. However, in the reference frame model this complex connection structure is only assumed to exist after exploration. As has been shown by Muller et al. (1991b, 1996; see also Redish 1997; Redish and Touretzky 1998), this connection structure can be learned by random exploration combined with correlational LTP (i.e. Hebbian learning).

Entering a novel environment
When an animal is placed in an environment, we assume that it does not have preconceived path integrator coordinates. The path integrator representation in the model is assumed to initially be random noise. Because the animal has not explored the environment yet, the learnable connections are assumed to have small, uncorrelated random strengths. (The learnable connections, shown by dashed lines in Fig. 11.2, are: LV → HC, HC → PI, and recurrent connections in HC.) Because these connections are very weak, they do not provide any bias to the settling of the path integrator. Therefore, the path integrator settles to a representation of random coordinates (a 'hill' of activation somewhere on the neural sheet) that will serve as the origin or 'reference point' for the new reference frame. We call this settling process the *self-localization* or *PI-reset* process.

In contrast to the learnable connections, the pre-wired connections are assumed to be sparse, and have strong synaptic weights. These connections are indicated by solid lines in Fig. 11.2: LV → DG, PI → DG, and DG → HC.

Activity in the dentate gyrus is a consequence of both the LV and PI representations. In order for a DG cell to fire, it must receive input from both LV *and* PI. Early in the self-localization process, the PI representation is incoherent (i.e. the component neurons show small, random firing rates). This means that early in the self-localization process, DG is effectively silent due to the lack of a coherent representation in PI. This allows the LV → HC → PI pathway to drive the self-localization process.

In contrast, during navigation, the sparse, strong connections passing through DG drive activity in the hippocampus. Because both LV and PI firing fields are spatially localized, a DG cell will show a high firing rate only in a small, compact portion of the environment, the place field of the cell. Because most of the possible LV × PI combinations do not occur in an environment, most DG cells are silent.

Each HC cell receives input from 10 to 20 DG cells. Activity in one DG cell is sufficient to make the HC cell show a high firing rate. HC cells can therefore have varying numbers of place fields, depending on their specific inputs from DG. In practice, we have found that most HC cells simulated with this model show at most one place field within a reference frame, but occasionally, some cells do show two subfields. Cells with multiple subfields have been reported in real animals (e.g. O'Keefe and Nadel 1978; Muller *et al.* 1991a; Wilson and McNaughton 1994; Markus *et al.* 1995).

As the animal explores the environment, LTP occurs along the learnable (dashed) connections. We assume that this LTP is Hebbian and rectified at 0, so that synaptic strength can only increase. We do not model LTD (Long Term Depression).

Returning to a familiar environment

According to the reference frame theory, when young animals return to the environment, LTP has created associations between the LV and HC modules, and between HC and PI. There is a self-localization or PI-reset process each time the animal enters the environment. On a return visit, the learned (dashed) connections that were strengthened by LTP will provide biases to the HC and PI networks. Therefore, upon re-entering the environment, the local view representation instantiates a previous representation in the hippocampus, and this in turn (via the HC → PI) pathway forces the path integrator to reset to the same representation of location as in the young animal's previous experience.

In old animals, however, LTP is deficient (as reviewed by Barnes 1998) and thus there is little or no bias along the LV → HC pathway to reset the hippocampus, and hence via the HC → PI pathway, the path integrator, to the same location. Because each DG cell performs a logical *and* function of its path integrator and local view inputs, if the path integrator representation is not reset correctly, this produces a dramatic change in DG representation, which will be seen in the hippocampus as a low overlap of place codes across different visits to the environment.

Effect of non-linearity

The attractor network structure hypothesized to underlie the path integrator has an important non-linearity dependent on where excitatory bias is input into the network. There are four important cases, depending on the location and magnitude of the extra-population input (Redish 1997; Redish and Touretzky 1997*b*; see also Skaggs *et al.* 1995; Elga *et al.* 1997; Redish *et al.* 1996; Zhang 1996; Samsonovich 1997; Samsonovich and McNaughton 1997 for discussions of specific cases):

1. If an attractor network is in a stable state and receives input (synapsing on excitatory cells) that is peaked at the same position as is currently being represented, then nothing will change. The attractor network will still be in a stable state representing the same position. The overall activity in the attractor network may increase slightly, but the represented position will not change.

2. If the input is offset slightly, then the attractor network will precess until the new representation is centred at the input position.

3. If the input is offset by a large amount but is small in magnitude, it will not be strong enough to affect the current representation, and so the representation will not change.

4. If strong enough input is offset by a large amount, the hill of activiation will jump, i.e. the representation of the current position will disappear and activity will reappear at the offset location.

The effect of this non-linearity is that if the bias supplied by the HC → PI connections is near the position that the path integrator is settling to, it will draw in the representation to match it, whether in strong LTP ('young') or weak LTP ('old') animals. However, if the bias is distant from the position to which the path integrator is settling, the representation will jump only if it is sufficiently strong, i.e. in young animals but not in old animals.

Similarities and differences

The interpretations of this experiment offered by the multi-chart and reference frame models have some similarities and some crucial differences.

Because place cells are active on initial entry into the environment (Hill 1978; Austin *et al.* 1990; Wilson and McNaughton 1994; Tanila *et al.* 1997), there must be some pre-wired connections producing place field activity. In the multi-chart model, the charts are pre-wired in CA3. In the reference frame model, pre-wired connections labelled PI → DG, LV → DG, and DG → HC produce place cells with stable fields on initial entry into the environment. The difference between the pre-wired connections hypothesized by the multi-chart model and those hypothesized by the reference frame model is that the latter are initially random.

Because the place cell instability observed by Barnes *et al.* (1997) is bimodal in older animals, there must be some sort of non-linear process occurring during re-entry. In the chart-model, this non-linearity exists in the competitive dynamics between charts in CA3. In the reference frame model, it is found in the nonlinear settling behaviour of the path integrator.

Because the place cell instability observed by Barnes *et al.* (1997) only occurs on entry into the environment, there must be something special about entry into the environment. We explain this by hypothesizing that the path integrator is only reset on entry into the environment. During normal navigation, the path integrator is not reset; it continues to be driven by internal dynamics more than external. But on returning to an environment, the path integrator is reset and external dynamics can have a strong influence.

11.5 Simulations

Simulations were based on the model shown in Fig. 11.2. All entries to the environment were made at a single location. Each triggered a self-localization process, after which the model was allowed to learn at that location for a short time. The model was then removed from the environment and returned to the same location again, triggering another self-localization. Each self-localization process began with the path integrator reset to random noise. This cycle of removal and return was repeated 10 times for the simulated young animals with normal LTP, and for simulated old animals with weak LTP.

Because the LV → HC and HC → PI connections learned the correct mapping in the simulated young animals, the model always reset the path integrator to the same coordinates (Table 11.1, left). This produced the same PI × LV association, and thus the same DG and CA3 cells became active. All correlations seen were high, as shown in Fig. 11.3a.

Table 11.1 Coordinates represented in the path integrator after each of 10 entries into an environment

Entry	'Young' animals	'Old' animals
1	(120°, 12°)	(120°, 12°)
2	(120°, 12°)	(35°, 131°)
3	(120°, 12°)	(36°, 113°)
4	(120°, 12°)	(91°, 63°)
5	(120°, 12°)	(62°, 109°)
6	(120°, 12°)	(178°, 326°)
7	(120°, 12°)	(128°, 11°)
8	(120°, 12°)	(126°, 12°)
9	(120°, 12°)	(126°, 12°)
10	(120°, 12°)	(125°, 12°)

Since the path integrator was simulated as a torus, the coordinates are expressed as pairs of angles. All entries were to the same location in the same environment. These coordinates can be taken as indicative of the reference point that would be used for any subsequent navigation.

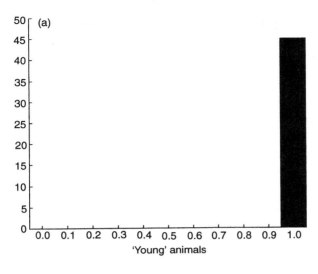

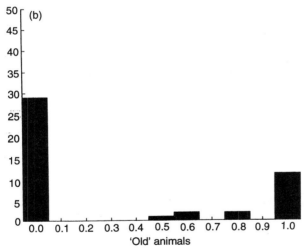

Fig. 11.3 Histograms of correlations between representations of a specific location in the environment after multiple entries into that environment. Simulations were allowed to enter an environment 10 times and the hippocampal representation of a location in the environment was measured. Cross-correlations were made between each pair of experiences in the environment (45 pairs). Plotted are histograms of the correlations found. (a) Simulations with strong LTP (i.e. 'young' animals) always return to the same PI representation, so the correlation is always high. (b) Simulations with weak LTP (i.e. 'old' animals) usually return to different PI representations and so usually have very low correlations, but occasionally return to similar PI representations and thus have rare highly correlated pairs.

However, in the simulated 'old' animals, the path integrator settled to different coordinates on different trials (Table 11.1, right), although the local view had not changed. This changed the PI × LV association, engendering a change in DG and thus the CA3 representations. Typical correlations were around 0. But occasionally the path integrator would reset to a location close to its previous value, producing a rare high correlation (>0.6). See Fig. 11.3b.

As can be seen in the right half of Table 11.1, in the last four trials, the simulated old animals always returned to the same reference point. This occured because LTP built up over time. After enough experience the old animals were able to recognize the environment and reset their path integrator representation correctly. The specific timing of the onset of correct reset is strongly dependent on the parameters chosen for the LTP. In the simulation, old animals had LTP that was 5% that of young animals.

In comparing these results to those reported by Barnes *et al.* (1997), we should note that Barnes *et al.* only examined pairs of experiences and so were unable to examine whether old animals eventually settled on a single location. However, Barnes *et al.* tested all of their animals (young and old) in the hidden-platform water maze (Morris 1981). They report that early in training, histograms of length of path taken by all animals are bimodal: sometimes they find the platform with a short path and sometimes they require a long path. Barnes *et al.* explain the bimodality as a consequence of being on the correct map or not. If the hippocampus represents the correct location on the correct map, the animal should be able to navigate to the goal; but if the hippocampus has an unfamiliar representation, finding the platform will be much more difficult. As young animals gain experience, they transition to the short-path peak in the bimodal histogram. Old animals also show more short-path trials after 4 days of training than they do after 2 days of training, but they continue to be more likely to take a long path than young after 4 days. In agreement with Barnes *et al.*, we take this as an indication that the old animals are learning to return to the correct map, but they learn much more slowly than young animals.

11.6 Discussion

These simulations show that the dramatic non-linearity seen by Barnes *et al.* (1997) does not necessarily imply that there must be pre-wired charts in the hippocampus. A model that includes random pre-wired connections from an external path integrator and an external local view into an orthogonalizing structure (such as dentate gyrus) as well as a single-map pre-wired path integrator is sufficient to produce the observed bimodality in animals with deficient LTP.

This demonstrates why it is important to consider *reference frame* as a property of the entire navigation system and not just the hippocampus. What we are suggesting here is that the old animals are on a different map (different chart, different reference frame) because they are using a different reference point for the path integrator. Because the path integrator representation is changed between experiences, the PI × LV association changes, and this is why the animal constructs a different reference frame.

The work presented in this chapter does not prove that the pre-wired CA3 hypothesis is wrong, only that it is not a necessary conclusion of the bimodality result reported by Barnes *et al.* (1997). The two theories (that DG is orthogonalizing extrinsic path integrator and local view inputs, and that CA3 is pre-wired to form multiple charts) are not incompatible. Further work is being done to examine the interaction between the two hypotheses.

Acknowledgments

This work was supported by National Science Foundation grant IBN-9631336. The results have also been reported in part in (Redish 1997). We thank Carol Barnes, Bruce McNaughton and Jay McClelland for helpful comments and discussions.

Endnotes

[1] Path integration is a process that tracks an animal's position as it moves, allowing it to later return to the starting point using only idiothetic cues (Barlow 1964; Mittelstaedt and Mittelstaedt 1980; Gallistel 1990).

References

S.-I. Amari. Dynamics of pattern formation in lateral-inhibition type neural fields. *Biological Cybernetics*, **27**: 77–87, 1977.

K. Arai, E. L. Keller, and J. A. Edelman. Two-dimensional neural network model of the primate saccadic system. *Neural Networks*, **7**(6/7): 1115–1135, 1994.

K. B. Austin, W. F. Fortin, and M. L. Shapiro. Place fields are altered by NMDA antagonist MK-801 during spatial learning. *Society for Neuroscience Abstracts*, **16**: 263, 1990.

J. S. Barlow. Inertial navigation as a basis for animal navigation. *Journal of Theoretical Biology*, **6**: 76–117, 1964.

C. A. Barnes. Memory changes during normal aging: neurobiological correlates. In (J. L. Martinez, Jr. and R. P. Kesner, ed.), *Learning and Memory: a Biological View*. Academic Press, New York, 1998, pp. 247–273.

C. A. Barnes, M. S. Suster, J. Shen, and B. L. McNaughton. Multistability of cognitive maps in the hippocampus of old rats. *Nature*, **388**(6639): 272–275, 1997.

H. T. Blair, B. W. Lipscomb, and P. E. Sharp. Anticipatory time intervals of head-direction cells in the anterior thalamus of the rat, implications for path integration in the head-direction circuit. *Journal of Neurophysiology*, **1997**, **78**(1), 145–159.

K. Cheng. A purely geometric module in the rat's spatial representation. *Cognition*, **23**: 149–178, 1986.

N. J. Cohen and H. Eichenbaum. *Memory, Amnesia, and the Hippocampal System.* MIT Press, Cambridge, MA, 1993.

T. S. Collett, B. A. Cartwright, and B. A. Smith. Landmark learning and visuo-spatial memories in gerbils. *Journal of Comparative Physiology A*, **158**: 835–851, 1986.

J. Droulez and A. Berthoz. A neural network model of sensoritopic maps with predictive short-term memory properties. *Proceedings of the National Academy of Sciences, USA*, **88**: 9653–9657, 1991.

H. Eichenbaum. Is the rodent hippocampus just for "place?". *Current Opinion in Neurobiology*, **6**: 187–195, 1996.

H. Eichenbaum and N. J. Cohen. Representation in the hippocampus: what do hippocampal neurons code? *Trends in Neurosciences*, **11**(6): 244–248, 1988.

H. Eichenbaum, M. Kuperstein, A. Fagan, and J. Nagode. Cue-sampling and goal-approach correlates of hippocampal unit activity in rats performing an odor-discrimination task. *Journal of Neuroscience*, **7**(3): 716–732, 1987.

H. Eichenbaum, T. Otto, and N. J. Cohen. The hippocampus—what does it do? *Behavioral and Neural Biology*, **57**: 2–36, 1992.

A. N. Elga, A. D. Redish, and D. S. Touretzky. A model of the rodent head direction system. In (J. M. Bower, ed.), *Computational Neuroscience: Trends in Research, 1997*, pp. 623–629. Plenum Press, New York, 1997.

B. Ermentrout and J. Cowan. A mathematical theory of visual hallucination patterns. *Biological Cybernetics*, **34**: 137–150, 1979.

C. R. Gallistel. *The Organization of Learning.* MIT Press, Cambridge, MA, 1990.

J. P. Goodridge, A. D. Redish, D. S. Touretzky, H. T. Blair, and P. E. Sharp. Lateral mamillary input explains distortions in tuning curve shapes of anterior thalamic head direction cells. *Society for Neuroscience Abstracts*, **23**, 1997, p. 503.

K. M. Gothard, W. E. Skaggs, K. M. Moore, and B. L. McNaughton. Binding of hippocampal CAl neural activity to multiple reference frames in a landmark-based navigation task. *Journal of Neuroscience*, **16**(2): 823–835, 1996.

R. E. Hampson, C. J. Heyser, and S. A. Deadwyler. Hippocampal cell firing correlates of delayed-match-to-sample performance in the rat. *Behavioral Neuroscience*, **107**: 715–739, 1993.

A. J. Hill. First occurrence of hippocampal spatial firing in a new environment. *Experimental Neurology*, **62**: 282–297, 1978.

K. Kishimoto and S. Amari. Existence and stability of local excitations in homogenous neural fields. *Journal of Mathematical Biology*, **7**(4): 303–318, 1979.

T. Kohonen. Self-organized formation of topologically correct feature maps. *Biological Cybernetics*, **43**: 59–69, 1982.

T. Kohonen. *Self-Organization and Associative Memory.* Springer-Verlag, New York, 1984.

J. L. Kubie and J. B. Ranck, Jr. Sensory-behavioral correlates in individual hippocampus neurons in three situations: space and context. In (W. Seifert, ed.) *Neurobiology of the Hippocampus*, Chapter 22, pp. 433–447. Academic Press Inc., New York, 1983.

J. Margules and C. R. Gallistel. Heading in the rat: determination by environmental shape. *Animal Learning and Behavior*, **16**(4): 404–410, 1988.

E. J. Markus, Y. Qin, B. Leonard, W. E. Skaggs, B. L. McNaughton, and C. A. Barnes. Interactions between location and task affect the spatial and directional firing of hippocampal neurons. *Journal of Neuroscience*, **15**: 7079–7094, 1995.

D. Marr. A theory of cerebellar cortex. *Journal of Physiology*, **202**: 437–470, 1969. Reprinted in Marr (1991).

D. Marr. *From the Retina to the Neocortex: Selected Papers of David Marr.* Birkhäuser, Boston, 1991. Edited by L. M. Vaina.

B. L. McNaughton and R. G. M. Morris. Hippocampal synaptic enhancement and information storage within a distributed memory system. *Trends in Neurosciences*, **10**(10): 408–415, 1987.

B. L. McNaughton, C. A. Barnes, J. L. Gerrard, K. Gothard, M. W. Jung, J. J. Knierim *et al.* Deciphering the hippocampal polyglot: the hippocampus as a path integration system. *Journal of Experimental Biology*, **199**(1): 173–186, 1996.

M. L. Mittelstaedt and H. Mittelstaedt. Homing by path integration in a mammal. *Naturwissenschaften*, **67**: 566–567, 1980.

R. G. M. Morris. Spatial localization does not require the presence of local cues. *Learning and Motivation*, **12**: 239–260, 1981.

R. U. Muller and J. L. Kubie. The effects of changes in the environment on the spatial firing of hippocampal complex-spike cells. *Journal of Neuroscience*, **7**: 1951–1968, 1987.

R. U. Muller, J. L. Kubie, E. M. Bostock, J. S. Taube, and G. J. Quirk. Spatial firing correlates of neurons in the hippocampal formation of freely moving rats. In (J. Paillard, ed.), *Brain and Space*, Chapter 17, pp. 296–333. Oxford University Press, New York, 1991*a*.

R. U. Muller, J. L. Kubie, and R. Saypoff. The hippocampus as a cognitive graph. *Hippocampus*, **1**(3): 243–246, 1991*b*.

R. U. Muller, M. Stead, and J. Pach. The hippocampus as a cognitive graph. *Journal of General Physiology*, **107**(6): 663–694, 1996.

D. P. Munoz, D. Pélisson, and D. Guitton. Movement of neural activity on the superior colliculus motor map during gaze shifts. *Science*, **251**: 1358–1360, 1991.

J. O'Keefe. Place units in the hippocampus of the freely moving rat. *Experimental Neurology*, **51**: 78–109, 1976.

J. O'Keefe and L. Nadel. *The Hippocampus as a Cognitive Map*. Clarendon Press, Oxford, 1978.

R. C. O'Reilly and J. L. McClelland. Hippocampal conjunctive encoding, storage, and recall: avoiding a trade-off. *Hippocampus*, **4**(6): 661–682, 1994.

G. J. Quirk, R. U. Muller, J. L. Kubie, and J. B. Ranck, Jr. The positional firing properties of medial entorhinal neurons: description and comparison with hippocampal place cells. *Journal of Neuroscience*, **12**(5): 1945–1963, 1992.

J. N. P. Rawlins. Associations across time: the hippocampus as a temporary memory store. *Behavioral and Brain Sciences*, **8**: 479–496, 1985. (See also commentary and response, pp. 497–528.)

A. D. Redish. *Beyond the Cognitive Map: Contributions to a Computational Neuroscience Theory of Rodent Navigation*. PhD thesis, Carnegie Mellon University, Pittsburgh PA, 1997.

A. D. Redish and D. S. Touretzky. Modeling interactions of the rat's place and head direction systems. In (D. S. Touretzky, M. C. Mozer, and M. E. Hasselmo, ed.), *Advances in Neural Information Processing Systems*, **8**, pp. 61–71, 1996.

A. D. Redish and D. S. Touretzky. Cognitive maps beyond the hippocampus. *Hippocampus*, **7**(1): 15–35, 1997*a*.

A. D. Redish and D. S. Touretzky. Implications of attractor networks for cue conflict situations. *Society for Neuroscience Abstracts*, **23**: 1601, 1997*b*.

A. D. Redish and D. S. Touretzky. The role of the hippocampus in solving the Morris water maze. *Neural Computation*, **10**(1): 73–111, 1998.

A. D. Redish, A. N. Elga, and D. S. Touretzky. A coupled attractor model of the rodent head direction system. *Network: Computation in Neural Systems*, **7**(4): 671–685, 1996.

E. T. Rolls. The representation and storage of information in neuronal networks in the primate cerebral cortex and hippocampus. In (R. Durbin, C. Miall, and

G. Mitchison, ed.), *The Computing Neuron*, Chapter 8, pp. 125–159. Addison-Wesley, Reading, MA, 1989.

E. T. Rolls. A theory of hippocampal function in memory. *Hippocampus*, **6**: 601–620, 1996.

A. Rotenberg, M. Mayford, R. D. Hawkins, E. R. Kandel, and R. U. Muller. Mice expressing activated CaMKII lack low frequency LTP and do not form stable place cells in the CA1 region of the hippocampus. *Cell*, **87**: 1351–1361, 1996.

L. M. Saksida, A. D. Redish, C. R. Milberg, S. J. Gaulin, and D. S. Touretzky. Landmark-based navigation in gerbils supports vector voting. *Society for Neuroscience Abstracts*, **21**: p. 1939, 1995.

A. V. Samsonovich. *Attractor Map Theory of the Hippocampal Representation of Space*. PhD thesis, Graduate Interdisciplinary Program in Applied Mathematics, University of Arizona, 1997.

A. Samsonovich and B. L. McNaughton. Path integration and cognitive mapping in a continuous attractor neural network model. *Journal of Neuroscience*, **17**(15): 5900–5920, 1997.

P. E. Sharp. Subicular cells generate similar firing patterns in two geometrically and visually distinctive environments: comparison with hippocampal place cells. *Behavioral Brain Research*, **85**(1): 71–92, 1997.

P. E. Sharp, J. L. Kubie, and R. U. Muller. Firing properties of hippocampal neurons in a visually symmetrical environment: contributions of multiple sensory cues and mnemonic processes. *Journal of Neuroscience*, **10**(9): 3093–3105, 1990.

W. E. Skaggs, J. J. Knierim, H. S. Kudrimoti, and B. L. McNaughton. A model of the neural basis of the rat's sense of direction. In (G. Tesauro, D. S. Touretzky, and T. K. Leen, ed.), *Advances in Neural Information Processing Systems 7*, pp. 173–180. MIT Press, 1995.

R. J. Sutherland and J. M. Hoesing. Posterior cingulate cortex and spatial memory: a microlimnology analysis. In (B. A. Vogt and M. Gabriel, ed.), *Neurobiology of Cingulate Cortex and Limbic Thalamus: a Comprehensive Handbook*, pp. 461–477. Birkhauser, Boston, 1993.

H. Tanila, P. Sipilä, M. Shapiro, and H. Eichenbaum. Brain aging: impaired coding of novel environmental cues. *Journal of Neuroscience*, **17**(13): 5167–5174, 1997.

J. S. Taube, R. I. Muller, and J. B. Ranck, Jr. Head direction cells recorded from the postsubiculum in freely moving rats. I. Description and quantitative analysis. *Journal of Neuroscience*, **10**: 420–435, 1990.

J. S. Taube, J. P. Goodridge, E. J. Golob, P. A. Dudchenko, and R. W. Stack-man. Processing the head direction cell signal: a review and commentary. *Brain Research Bulletin*, **40**(5/6): 477–486, 1996.

L. T. Thompson and P. J. Best. Place cells and silent cells in the hippocampus of freely-behaving rats. *Journal of Neuroscience*, **9**(7): 2382–2390, 1989.

D. S. Touretzky and A. D. Redish. A theory of rodent navigation based on interacting representations of space. *Hippocampus*, **6**(3): 247–270, 1996.

H. S. Wan, D. S. Touretzky, and A. D. Redish. A rodent navigation model that combines place code, head direction, and path integration information. *Society for Neuroscience Abstracts*, **20**: 1205, 1994a.

H. S. Wan, D. S. Touretzky, and A. D. Redish. Towards a computational theory of rat navigation. In (M. Mozer, P. Smolensky, D. Touretzky, J. Elman, and A. Weigend, ed.), *Proceedings of the 1993 Connectionist Models Summer School*, pp. 11–19. Lawrence Earlbaum Associates, Hillsdale NJ, 1994b.

S. I. Wiener. Spatial and behavioral correlates of striatal neurons in rats performing a self-initiated navigation task. *Journal of Neuroscience*, **13**(9): 3802–3817, 1993.

H. R. Wilson and J. D. Cowan. A mathematical theory of the functional dynamics of cortical and thalamic tissue. *Kybernetik*, **13**: 55–80, 1973.

M. A. Wilson and B. L. McNaughton. Reactivation of hippocampal ensemble memories during sleep. *Science*, **265**: 676–679, 1994.

K. Zhang. Representation of spatial orientation by the intrinsic dynamics of the head-direction cell ensemble: a theory. *Journal of Neuroscience*, **16**(6): 2112–2126, 1996.

12

Hippocampal synaptic plasticity: role in spatial learning or the automatic recording of attended experience?

Richard G. M. Morris and Uwe Frey

12.1 Introduction

This paper outlines a new hypothesis about the function of associative synaptic plasticity in the hippocampal formation, namely that it is essential for what is referred to here as the 'automatic recording of attended experience'. This constitutes one component of a larger episodic memory system involving a number of brain regions (Tulving 1983; Tulving & Schacter 1994) and likely to be implemented by several neurophysiological mechanisms of plasticity. The idea is that this part of the episodic memory system of the brain is automatic in the sense that it cannot be switched off in a voluntary manner, although it can be subject to selective disruption by certain kinds of brain damage. Being automatic, it can potentially record everything to which attention is directed, including context, but this recording may only be of markers that an event has happened at a particular place rather than a detailed encoding of sensory or perceptual information. To operate effectively, such a system needs a mechanism of neuronal plasticity that can register event–context associations rapidly in a strictly correlational manner, i.e. without regard to their consistency to an organism's goal-directed actions. N-methyl-D-aspartate (NMDA) receptor-dependent synaptic potentiation in the hippocampus is ideally suited to implementing the rapid online storage of such conjunctive associations. These would be retained temporarily, as changes in synaptic weights, by the early phase of long-term potentiation (LTP) after which they may decay to baseline (i.e. be forgotten). Their temporal persistence may, however, be stabilized by intracellular interactions with the plasticity-related proteins (PPs) that are synthesized by certain patterns of neuronal activation. This variable persistence may be thought of as a type of short-term consolidation of memory. Enhanced persistence of synaptic potentiation in the hippocampus extends the temporal window of opportunity for long-term memory formation by other brain structures that are also part of the episodic memory system, including the diencephalic and frontal lobe areas.

That the hippocampal formation might be part of the episodic memory system of the brain is hardly a new idea: it and structures within the medial temporal and frontal lobes have long been implicated in spatial, episodic and declarative memory (O'Keefe & Nadel 1978; Squire & Zola-Morgan 1991; Tulving & Schacter 1994). What is new, and thus the focus of this paper, is the suggestion that activity-dependent synaptic plasticity in the hippocampus (such as LTP) is functionally relevant to *episodic* memory rather than to the learning of spatial maps or associative conditioning with which it has more often been discussed (see, for example, McNaughton & Morris 1987; Teyler & Discenna 1987; Morris *et al*. 1990; Shors & Matzel 1997). Implicit in this proposal is the notion that episodic memory cannot, therefore, be unique to humans. As hippocampal LTP is present in mammals, 'elements of episodic memory' must exist in these animals also, a claim that is qualified below.

The structure of this paper is as follows. First, evidence implicating NMDA receptor-dependent hippocampal LTP in spatial learning and memory is reviewed. Second, two lines of evidence against this proposal are described: (1) circumstances in which spatial learning occurs in the presence of NMDA antagonists; and (2) data indicating that the learning rule for the acquisition of a spatial map cannot, in practice, be isomorphic with the synaptic learning rule for LTP. Third, based on the notion that episodic memory builds upon a system used for spatial learning in animals (O'Keefe & Nadel 1978; Gaffan 1994), evidence is presented from a delayed-matching-to-place task consistent with this idea and it is shown that the results are exquisitely sensitive to an NMDA antagonist (AP5). Fourth, data pointing to a new property of protein synthesis-dependent LTP (sometimes called 'late-LTP') that would be desirable within an event-memory system are described. Finally, further aspects of the 'automatic recording' hypothesis are spelt out, including ideas about its neural basis, and a number of open issues and speculations that require further experimentation are identified.

12.2 NMDA receptor-dependent hippocampal LTP and its role in spatial learning and memory

It has been known for over a quarter of a century that particular patterns of electrical stimulation in the hippocampal formation can lead to alterations in synaptic efficacy. The classic observations of Bliss & Lomo (1973), who studied the perforant path input to the dentate gyrus of anaesthetized rabbits, now referred to as long-term potentiation (LTP), have been replicated in other mammalian species, *in vitro* as well as *in vivo*, and in several pathways of the hippocampal formation. Contemporary studies have revealed that potentiation of synaptic efficacy in different pathways can have different physiological properties, reflecting distinct underlying mechanisms. The best studied of these has been referred to as 'associative' or 'NMDA receptor-dependent LTP', to distinguish it from other forms of lasting synaptic change such as E–S potentiation (a change in the relationship between EPSP and spike amplitude), mossy-fibre potentiation, long-term depression, neurotrophin-induced potentiation, etc. Although these latter forms of neuronal plasticity are unquestionably important, this paper discusses only the associative NMDA receptor-dependent form, which is referred to, for simplicity, as 'LTP'. A distinction is made only between different temporal phases of its expression. Numerous reviews of LTP have been published (see, for example, Bliss & Collingridge 1993; Bear & Malenka 1994; Fazeli & Collingridge 1996) and the following general understanding of its properties, mechanisms and functional significance has emerged.

With respect to its physiological properties, LTP is defined as a rapidly induced, persistent enhancement in synaptic efficacy lasting at least one hour. Its induction is 'associative', in that weak patterns of stimulation insufficient to induce LTP on their own can none the less result in a persistent synaptic enhancement if they occur in association with depolarization of the target neuron(s) onto which the stimulated pathway is afferent. The resulting LTP is also 'input-specific' in that meeting the conditions for induction results in enhanced synaptic efficacy specific to the synaptic terminals of the activated pathway (or, at least, to closely neighbouring synapses). As noted many times, these properties of persistence, associativity and input-specificity are desirable properties of a physiological mechanism for storing information at synapses. Later (Section 12.6), a further property of hippocampal LTP is described, whereby the persistence of an induced change in synaptic efficacy can be extended by other heterosynaptic patterns of neural activity.

With respect to its underlying neural mechanisms, there is a consensus that activation of a subclass of excitatory postsynaptic glutamatergic receptors, the so-called N-methyl-D-aspartate (NMDA) receptor, is an essential first step in LTP induction. The NMDA receptor, now known to be a complex protein consisting of a number of individual subunits, has the intriguing property of being both ligand- and voltage-gated. When activated by glutamate and at a particular level of postsynaptic depolarization, calcium (Ca^{2+}) enters the dendrite via the NMDA receptor ion-channel, where it activates a chain of intracellular events leading to altered synaptic efficacy. Theories about how the resulting change in synaptic efficacy is achieved include activation of Ca^{2+}-dependent enzymes that phosphorylate receptors and trigger gene expression. Some of these biochemical events are responsible for short-lasting changes (often referred to as early-LTP); others cause the early change to be stabilized, i.e. made persistent (late-LTP), with the latter involving mechanisms activated by other than just glutamatergic inputs (see Section 12.7).

With respect to the functional significance of LTP, studies have been conducted exploring whether there is any correlation between behavioural learning and the occurrence or persistence of LTP (for recent reviews, see Alkon *et al*. 1991: Morris & Davis 1994; Barnes 1995; Cain 1997; Jeffery 1997; Shors & Matzel 1997). Inevitably, as LTP was first discovered in the hippocampus, such studies have tended to focus on types of learning broadly held to be 'hippocampal-dependent' (i.e. thought to engage hippocampal activity and/or be impaired by hippocampal lesions). Correlations have been observed between the persistence of LTP and how long such types of memory are retained, as well as between the occurrence of particular types of learning and the activation of the various Ca^{2+}-dependent enzymes. Studies with the use of drugs that antagonize the NMDA receptor, or targeted mutations of NMDA receptor subunits, have also revealed behaviourally selective learning impairments. The interpretation of many of these studies is very controversial: the techniques used to manipulate LTP generally have multiple effects on brain function.

Early support for the idea of a link between LTP and spatial learning came from several studies. One was the finding of Morris *et al.* (1986) that blockade of NMDA receptors by chronic intraventricular (ICV) infusion of the selective NMDA antagonist AP5 resulted in an impairment of spatial learning, but not of visual-discrimination learning, in the open-field watermaze. This inhibition of spatial learning is dose-related and occurs across a range of estimated extracellular concentrations of D-2-amino-5-phosphopentanoate (D-AP5) in the hippocampus *in vivo* comparable to those that block LTP *in vitro* (Davis *et al.* 1992). Application of AP5 after learning is without effect on performance (Morris 1989). Acute intrahippocampal infusion of nanomolar quantities of AP5, revealed radioautographically to be restricted to the hippocampus, are also sufficient to cause an impairment of spatial learning (Morris *et al.* 1989). Other pharmacological studies have also shown deficits in spatial learning with both competitive and non-competitive NMDA antagonists (Danysz *et al.* 1996; cf. Cain 1997).

A recent replication of the basic observation is shown in Fig. 12.1 (Bannerman *et al.* 1995, experiment 1). Rats were trained to find the hidden escape platform over eight trials, at one trial per day, with transfer tests (platform absent) conducted before the first trial, half-way through training, and at the end. Before training, the animals were implanted with an osmotic minipump containing either artificial cerebrospinal fluid (aCSF) or D-AP5 (30 mM in aCSF). Connected via a catheter to a cannula implanted into the lateral ventricle, this pumped continuously into the brain of the rat at $0.5\,\mu l\,h^{-1}$ (i.e. $15\,nmol\,h^{-1}$). The results were that aCSF animals showed a gradual decline in escape latency across training, reflecting learning of the platform's location, but the D-AP5-treated group did not (Fig. 12.1a). Similarly, in the transfer tests, the aCSF group gradually came to concentrate its search in the correct quadrant as training progressed (transfer tests TT2 and TT3), whereas the D-AP5 group did not (Fig. 12.1b). These behavioural effects occurred at measured intracerebral concentrations of the drug sufficient to block dentate LTP under urethane anaesthesia.

Pharmacological studies such as this have been complemented by work using targeted molecular engineering. Deletion of the R2A subunit of the NMDA receptor causes both a blockade of NMDA receptor-dependent LTP and impairments of spatial learning in mice (Sakimura *et al.* 1995). Elegant experiments by Tonegawa and his colleagues have recently established that site-specific deletion of the NMDA-R1 subunit from CA1 pyramidal cells results in a blockade of LTP at the Schaffer collateral input to CA1, an

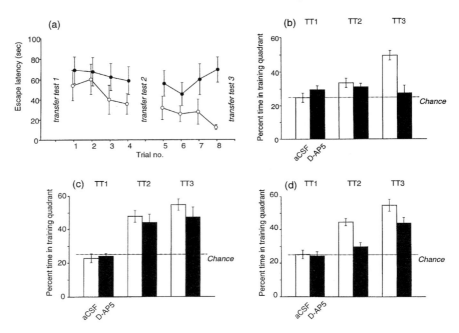

Fig. 12.1 Dissociation between components of spatial learning by using an NMDA receptor antagonist. (a) Experiment 1: escape latency (s ±1 s.e.m.) across training by the experimentally naive aCSF- (*open symbols*) and AP5-treated (*filled symbols*) groups. Note blockade of learning by the AP5-treated group. (b) Experiment 1: percentage time (±1 s.e.m.) spent in the training quadrant during TT1 (before training), TT2 (halfway through) and TT3 (after training). Note absence of searching in the training quadrant by the AP5-treated group. (c) Experiment 2: in animals given spatial pretraining in a watermaze in a separate room, AP5 has no significant effect on the percentage of time spent searching in the training quadrant during the second task. (d) Experiment 4: in animals given random search pretraining in a separate room, AP5 impairs learning of the platform location during the second task. The deficit is not as substantial as in experimentally naive animals (Experiment 1). For other experiments in this series, Bannerman *et al.* (1995).

impairment of spatial learning, and changes in the size and specificity of CA1 place-fields (McHugh *et al.* 1996; Tsien *et al.* 1996a,b). Collectively, these studies would appear to offer strong support for the notion that NMDA receptor-dependent synaptic plasticity is involved in spatial learning.

12.3 Dissociation between NMDA receptor-dependent and NMDA receptor-independent components of spatial learning

Some recent studies have, none the less, called into question the notion that NMDA receptor-dependent mechanisms are always necessary for spatial learning. In the authors' own work, for example, Bannerman *et al*. (1995, experiment 2) found that rats that had previously been trained a spatial task in one watermaze were relatively unaffected by AP5 when trained in a second watermaze in a different room. The thinking behind this study was twofold.

First, although learning in a watermaze is conveniently categorized as a 'spatial', it is misleading to think that spatial learning is the only type of learning that occurs in the apparatus. Multiple types of learning can occur simultaneously, coupled with the formation of distinct memories. Animals that are experimentally naive have to learn to swim away from the side walls to find the platform at all (i.e. overcome thigmotaxis) and to learn that climbing on the platform when they find it is the appropriate thing to do (i.e. incentive learning). These and other behavioural processes engaged by the watermaze task may also be AP5-sensitive. It follows that it cannot be unambiguously concluded that the failure of experimentally naive, AP5-treated animals to learn a spatial task (as in Fig. 12.1a and 12.1b) is necessarily because AP5 interacts directly with spatial learning mechanisms *per se*. Second, although animals may be 'experimentally naive', they will nevertheless have had previous experiences that could influence their subsequent learning. To explore this in a controlled way, the possibility was considered that spatial training of animals probably enables them to learn more than just the particular layout of cues in the training room. They may also learn behavioural or even abstract 'strategies' that could influence their performance in other spatial tasks in the future. For example, they may learn that there is a single place to escape and that, once it is found, one should always approach that place. Such a strategy might generalize from one spatial environment to another. Learning a strategy, as distinct from learning a specific set of spatial cues, may also be sensitive to AP5.

To address both issues, additional experiments were conducted in which rats were first trained in one watermaze before drug treatment and then, under AP5 or aCSF, taken to a second laboratory room housing a different watermaze and trained in the same spatial task as the one described in Fig. 12.1. Bannerman *et al*. (1995, experiment 2) found, surprisingly, that AP5-treated animals then learned the second task remarkably well. Their escape latencies showed a steady decline across training (although they were slightly longer than those of aCSF-treated animals) and their performance in TT2 and TT3 was indistinguishable from that of controls (Fig. 12.1c). Control procedures were instituted to ensure that there was minimal generalization between the two laboratory rooms. At the end of training, the AP5-treated animals revealed a near-complete blockade of dentate LTP *in vivo*, together with whole-tissue drug concentrations indistinguishable from those obtained in the earlier experiment.

In another study (Bannerman *et al*. 1995, experiment 4), the rats were first trained on a random search task. For this, curtains were drawn around the pool to occlude extramaze cues, and the hidden platform was moved to a different location in the pool between trials. There is little other than incentive learning in such a task; the rats search around randomly and learn to use the platform as a refuge when it is found. After the same number of trials as in the spatial pretraining used in experiment 2 above, the rats were given mini-pumps and trained in the second spatial task. A drug-induced deficit was now obtained (see also Morris 1989). Escape latencies during training were longer in AP5-treated rats and their performance during TT2 and TT3 was impaired relative to that of controls (Fig. 12.1d). The AP5-treated animals were, however, not as impaired as the experimentally naive animals of experiment 1.

These findings allow three separate points to be made. First, as non-spatial pretraining affected the sensitivity of subsequent spatial learning to AP5, there must be aspects of watermaze training that are non-spatial and that depend on NMDA receptor activation. These may include learning that the platform is a refuge. Second, as spatial pretraining caused subsequent spatial learning to be insensitive to AP5, spatial learning may be dissociable into components that depend on NMDA receptor activation in the hippocampus and those that do not. Learning the spatial layout of an environment, which it had hitherto been thought would depend critically upon the associativity of LTP (e.g. representing the associative relationships between landmarks) appears to be insensitive to the drug with this training schedule of one trial per day. The animals have, presumably, acquired some kind of spatial strategy during spatial pretraining that can transfer to a new environment, and it is this component of spatial learning that is AP5-sensitive. Third, although these results are similar to Saucier & Cain's (1995) finding of normal spatial learning under AP5 in certain circumstances, they do not support their argument that the effects of NMDA antagonists on performance in spatial tasks can be explained exclusively in terms of whether they induce sensorimotor disturbances. Not only were these minimal in the one-trial-per-day procedure, but such disturbances cannot explain the differential effects of pretraining.

12.4 Blocking in the spatial domain

The notion that allocentric spatial learning is divisible into a number of dissociable components is also suggested by a recent strictly behavioural study of landmark learning. The idea was to explore whether the incorporation of information into a spatial map of the environment obeyed a correlational rule or depended also on an animal's goal-directed expectations; the classic phenomenon of blocking was used to make this distinction.

The rationale was as follows. O'Keefe & Nadel (1978) claimed that two dissociable learning systems can be used for navigation: the 'locale' and the 'taxon' system. The former is the cognitive mapping system in which the locations of landmarks are rapidly encoded as a result of exploration of the environment. Exploration is triggered by novelty, such as mismatches between the animal's memory of the environment and its perception of it. This learning system is thought to be located in the hippocampal formation and critically depends on place cells (Burgess *et al.*, Chapter 8). Importantly, it is not thought to be goal-driven; that is, learning about space is thought to be unaffected by the animal's needs or expectations. If this is correct, the incorporation of information into a spatial map may follow a Hebbian learning rule in being sensitive only to correlations between information about the relative locations of landmarks. This idea raises the intriguing possibility that the 'behavioural' learning rule determining the incorporation of information into an animal's representation of the environment may be isomorphic to the 'synaptic' learning rule underlying hippocampal LTP.

There are, however, at least two reasons to be suspicious of this idea. First, the experiments with AP5 described in Section 12.3 suggest that NMDA receptor-dependent mechanisms are not critical for learning about the spatial layout of an environment even if they do play some unidentified role in spatial 'strategy' learning. Second, most forms of associative learning are sensitive to an animal's expectations about the availability of reward. Learning tends to take place only to the extent that an animal needs to learn. The well-studied phenomenon reflecting this selectivity is called 'blocking'.

Blocking refers to the ability of a previously trained stimulus (A) that predicts reinforcement R to prevent or 'block' conditioning to a second or added stimulus (B) when B is arranged to predict R as well (Kamin 1969). Learning about the B–R association fails to occur despite B being correlated with R and repeatedly presented before it at an appropriate interstimulus interval. This phenomenon has had an important influence on the formulation of modern associative learning theory (Rescorla & Wagner 1972; Dickinson 1980; Mackintosh 1983) according to which learning can be adequately described by the accumulation of associative connections between events, according to goal-driven error-correcting learning rules. It is widely accepted as a parsimonious account of animals' associative learning abilities.

To investigate whether blocking would occur in the spatial domain, Biegler & Morris (1997) trained two groups of rats to find food hidden at a particular location in a large arena (as in Biegler & Morris 1993, 1996). The arena had several centimetres of sawdust on the floor and the food (hidden inside a small computer-activated feeder that could rise to the surface of the sawdust) was placed at a set distance from an array of landmarks. These were distinctive objects (such as white cylinders, a pyramid-shaped object, and a stack of golf balls glued together); they were placed in an array that was systematically changed across training and test phases.

At the start of training (phase 0, days 1–5), the location of the food (F+) was cued by two identical landmarks that, on their own, could not unambiguously specify the location of food (Fig. 12.2a). In the later phase 1 (days 6–28) and phase 2 (days 28–37) of a conventional blocking design, other landmarks were added to provide disambiguating directional information. The experimental group had one additional landmark added at the start of

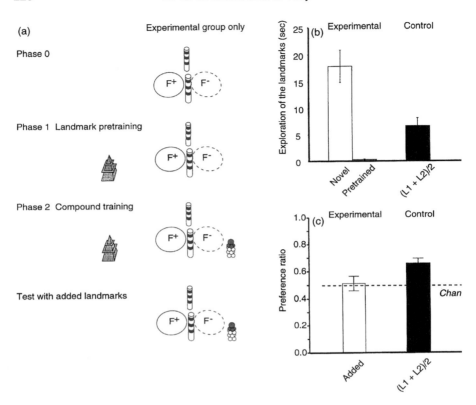

Fig. 12.2 Blocking in the spatial domain. (a) The experimental design consisted of successive phases. For the experimental group (shown), the animals were first trained (phase 0) to find food (F+) in relation to two identical white towers. In phase 1, a landmark (*grey pagoda symbol*) was then added to disambiguate the situation and the animals trained until search was focused at F+ rather than F−; in phase 2, a second landmark was then added (*stack of golf balls*) and additional training given for several days; finally, a test was conducted with this added landmark (and the two identical landmarks). For the control group (not shown), the landmark used in phase 1 was visually distinctive and in a different geometric location. (b) Searching of the added landmarks during trial 1 of phase 2 (time spent (in seconds) in circle of radius 20 cm around each landmark ±1 s.e.m.). The control group explores both added landmarks (L1+L2/2); the experimental group directs search to the novel landmark added on that trial. (c) Searching during the transfer test with the landmark added at the start of phase 2 for the experimental group (preference ratio $-T_{F+}/(T_{F+}+T_{F-})\pm 1$ s.e.m.). The control group shows a bias towards searching at F+ but the experimental group does not. Based on Biegler & Morris (1997).

phase 2 (as shown); the control group was trained with a visually different landmark in a different geometric location during phase 1, but then given the same two landmarks as the experimental group at the start of phase 2 (not shown). Thus, the key difference between the groups in phase 2 was that, for the experimental group, the location of the hidden food was already cued by the landmark trained in phase 1, whereas for the control group, both landmarks added in phase 2 were novel. There were four training trials per day, of which one was non-rewarded and without landmarks. This schedule ensured that the landmarks served as conditional cues, signalling the availability of reward.

The transition from phase 1 to phase 2 was one focus of attention: whether the experimental group would react to and explore the novel added landmark. The second focus of attention was whether this group would incorporate the added landmark into its spatial map of the landmark array. To measure this, a series of post-training probe tests were conducted at the rate of one test per two days, interleaved with additional training at asymptote. The key test among these examined how well the animals could search appropriately for the food with only the single landmark added in phase 2 (as well as the two identical landmarks present throughout training).

Two main findings were obtained. First, during the transition from phase 1, both groups explored the added landmarks. Exploration was measured by recording the amount of time spent searching in a 20-cm radius around each of the landmarks during the first trial of phase 2. For the control group, both landmarks were novel and both were explored. For the experimental group, only one landmark was novel and only it was explored (Fig. 12.2b). In keeping with O'Keefe & Nadel's (1978) theory, exploration is triggered and guided by a mismatch between the animal's stored and perceived representations of space. The animals of the experimental group were not so intent on finding the food that they ignored the added landmark.

However, the second finding was that this exploration (which habituated rapidly over the course of the next 1–2 trials) was insufficient for the location of the added landmark to be incorporated into the experimental group's spatial map. In the post-training test after the end of phase 2, the extent to which both groups searched preferentially in an area of 20-cm radius around the F+ and F−locations on either side of the two identical landmarks was measured (Fig. 12.2c). The control group learned about both landmarks that had been added together in phase 2 and used each of them to disambiguate the locations of F+ and F−. Both were incorporated into the animals' representation of the landmark array and either could be used alone to localize F+. In contrast, the experimental group noticed the added landmark and explored it, but then ignored it. It failed to search preferentially at F+. Thus, blocking occurs in the spatial domain. Spatial learning is influenced by the extent to which the animals need to learn about the location of landmarks to find a desired goal (see also Rodrigo *et al.* 1997).

There are several implications of these results for the study of spatial learning. The key point in the present context is that the incorporation of information into an animal's representation of space cannot be explained fully in terms of a simple Hebbian type of correlational rule. The learning rule must be more complex and probably involves at least two processes: (1) perception of mismatch followed by exploration and the short-term retention of information that could prove of value, followed by (2) some decision-making process governing the incorporation of the temporarily stored information into the animal's long-term representation of the environment. The former process can be thought as a kind of novelty-detection, guided by the animal's existing and activated knowledge base (its spatial map in this case). The latter can be thought of a selective process, and perhaps as an aspect of memory consolidation in which errors are corrected as a function of need. A goal-driven error-correcting learning rule is engaged if the animal is required to alter its representation of the environment to find the goal. This study did not address the issue of whether hippocampal synaptic plasticity is engaged in either of these processes. However, to anticipate the argument, it is surmised that the 'automatic recording' process is likely to be involved in only the first of these two processes.

12.5 The role of NMDA receptors in delayed matching to place: a form of event memory?

Two distinctive features of 'event memory' are that it refers to memory for something that may happen once only (rather than repeatedly) and that singular events happen in specific spatial contexts. A memory system capable of keeping track of events must therefore have the ability to encode information very rapidly. Moreover, because it may be helpful to distinguish between similar events occurring in different spatial contexts, an event-memory system will disambiguate more effectively if it encodes where an event happened in addition to information about its nature. As Gaffan (1994; Chapter 18) has cogently argued, episodic memory may be fundamentally spatial in origin, although not necessarily linked to navigation through space or to the detailed geometric representation of space. Certain phenomena, such as food-cacheing (Sherry *et al.* 1992; Jacobs 1994), illustrate this 'episodic' aspect of spatial memory.

A complication in thinking about event-memory in animals arises from the fact that, in humans, the occurrence of events is normally reported via language. The question therefore arises of whether it is possible to devise tasks for animals that reflect event memory unambiguously. Broadly speaking, there are two views one can take on this question. One view holds that animals do not possess 'episodic memory' in 'quite' the same way as humans (Tulving 1983, p. 1). Thus such tasks cannot be devised. The present authors favour the alternative view that animals are capable of event memory, but that few laboratory tasks developed so far are unambiguous reflections of such a memory process. The watermaze, as it is usually run (i.e. as a reference-memory task), is a case in point. Animals are given repeated training trials to find a fixed hidden platform. The events that happen on each of these trials contribute, usually incrementally, to their eventual 'semantic' knowledge of the task. There is no obligation on the part of the animals to remember 'explicitly' any specific event that has happened during training. When placed into the water on trial N, there is no necessity for them to have a 'recollective experience' of what happened on trial $N-1$. All that is required is that they develop knowledge about the environment, about the location of the hidden platform, and some kind of behavioural strategy to perform the task. The animals may remember their previous experience in the pool, but this is not required. In animal learning theory, this idea is sometimes referred to as the 'independence of path assumption'.

To model episodic memory in animals more effectively, the challenge is therefore to devise new tasks in which having a 'recollective experience' would be helpful (or even required). More formally, such a task should distinguish between *changes in behaviour that occur because an animal remembers some prior event* and *changes in behaviour that occur happen because some prior event has occurred*. This distinction, although subtle, is absolutely fundamental to the claim that animals possess 'elements of episodic memory'. Such a task might also help in investigating comparative aspects of the character of event memory and its neural mechanisms.

Steele & Morris (1998) have recently developed a modification of the water-maze task that goes some way towards this. The procedure is as follows. Rats are trained to find the hidden platform in the pool at a rate of four trials per day. Importantly, the platform moves from one random location to another random location each day so that, on trial 1 of the day, the animals have no way of knowing where the platform is located. Having found the platform on trial 1, the animals may be able to remember the 'event' of having got out of the water at this location during the second and succeeding trials, and so use this trial-unique information to escape faster on trials 2–4. The results show that this is precisely what happens (Fig. 12.3a). Early in training, the escape latency on trial 2 is quite long. After a few days, trial 2 latencies drop substantially and stabilize at a level that improves no further. Trial 1 latencies average about 60 s. By this stage of training, the animals are familiar with the environment and have a stable spatial representation that could provide a framework in which to remember where events happen in the environment.

This delayed matching-to-place (DMP) task cannot, however, be unambiguously described as an event-memory task. It is different from strict 'working-memory' tasks of the kind described by Olton *et al.* (1979) because in these, information is retained and used within a single trial. In the DMP task, information acquired in one trial is used in subsequent trials, but is not necessarily of value for the purpose of creating a lasting long-term memory However, what is unclear is whether the animals remember the recent event of escaping at that place, or merely a recent place; moreover, recently visited places might simply acquire a relative increase in 'familiarity' compared with other places in the room, obviating the need for 'recollective experience'. However, in comparison with the spatial reference-memory task used in the earlier experiments, the capacity to remember selectively what has happened most recently is clearly a useful component of event memory. If so, disruption of the system responsible for encoding recent events would be expected to cause

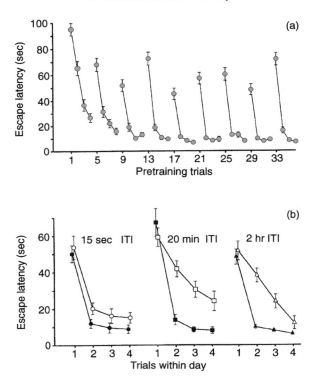

Fig. 12.3 Delayed matching to place. (a) Escape latency (± 1 s.e.m.) over the 9 days of pretraining, four trials per day, with the escape platform moving location each day. Note that latency on trial 1 stabilizes at around 60 s, whereas trial 2 latencies drop over the course of training from 65 s to less than 20 s. The saving between trial 1 and trial 2 reflects memory of platform location on trial 1. Normal animals in Fig. (a) (grey symbols). (b) Performance of the DMP task during the subsequent nine days of testing in the presence of AP5 (*filled symbols*) or aCSF (*open symbols*) when the data are subdivided as a function of the intertrial interval between trials 1 and 2 (the ITI between trials 2, 3 and 4 was always 15 s). Note the delay-dependent effect of AP5; savings are equivalent at the short ITI, but decline in the AP5-treated group as ITI is lengthened. Based on Steele & Morris (1998).

memory deficits, particularly if the interval between trial 1 and the subsequent trials was lengthened. It was therefore asked whether this DMP task was sensitive to the NMDA-receptor blockade in a delay-dependent manner.

To determine this, rats were first trained as normal rats (i.e. before drug administration) over 9 days with four trials per day. The hidden platform was located in a different position each day (nine locations) and the animals were allowed 30 s on the platform after escaping from the water. This gave them an opportunity to encode the location where they escaped. During this pretraining, three different intertrial intervals (ITIs) were used between trials 1 and 2. On 3 days (randomly intermixed), the ITI was 15 s; on 3 days it was 20 min; on the remaining 3 days it was 2 h (these are averaged in Fig. 12.3a). The ITI between trials 2 and 3, and between 3 and 4, was always 15 s. The animals were then divided into two groups given AP5 or aCSF via minipumps as before. Both groups were then retrained on the task over 9 days with nine new platform locations. As in pretraining, the ITI between trials 1 and 2 was varied between the three intervals.

The AP5-treated animals showed a striking delay-dependent pattern (Fig. 12.3b). When the interval between trials 1 and 2 was 15 s, they performed well and indistinguishably from the aCSF-treated animals. Both groups took approximately 1 min to find the platform on trial 1 but only 20 s on trial 2. This 'saving' in escape latency reflects their ability to remember, on trial 2, the location that the platform had occupied on trial 1. However, when the ITI between trials 1 and 2 was lengthened to 20 min and 2 h, the AP5-treated animals were impaired. Whereas the aCSF group continued to be able to remember back to trial 1 without difficulty, the drug-treated group showed much longer escape latencies on trial 2 and thus much less saving. The change in performance showed up in the analysis of both trial 2 latencies and T1–T2 savings scores as a highly significant statistical interaction between groups and delay interval, i.e. there was a true delay-dependent effect.

What are the implications of these findings? In Section 12.3 it was shown that prior spatial training on a reference-memory task resulted in subsequent spatial training in a new environment being insensitive to AP5. From this and other results (Saucier & Cain 1995), it might be supposed that NMDA receptor activation is not critical for spatial learning. However, it was also seen that changing the pretraining from a spatial task to a random search task (with extramaze cues obscured) had the effect of restoring, at least partly, the sensitivity of subsequent spatial learning to AP5. The effects of AP5 on the new DMP task take this a step further, bearing out the notion that spatial learning is divisible into AP5-sensitive and AP5-insensitive components. The DMP task also uses pretraining of normal animals to develop the strategy, but, instead of requiring learning of a new environment under AP5, its performance requires memory of the most recently visited location within a now familiar environment (i.e. a recent event–context association). On trial 2 of each day, the animals are attempting to remember what happened to them the last time they were in the pool. AP5-treated animals can only do this over a short period.

12.6 Synaptic tagging and the variable persistence of hippocampal synaptic plasticity

In describing the physiological properties of LTP (Section 12.3), its persistence for at least 1 h was identified as the defining property of the phenomenon. It is clear that persistence is a necessary condition for a putative synaptic mechanism of information storage underlying any kind of long-term memory.

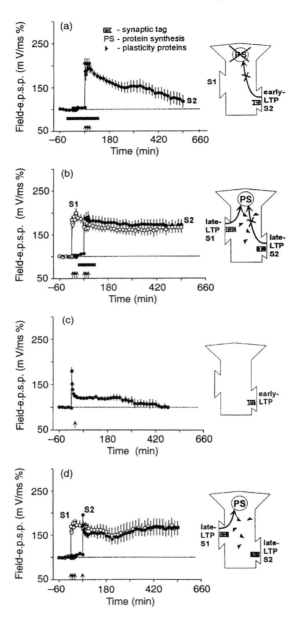

Fig. 12.4 Synaptic tagging and long-term potentiation. (a) Induction of short-lasting long-term potentiation (early LTP) on pathway S2 in response to a strong tetanus (three trains of 100 Hz for 1 s, *arrow symbols*) given in the presence of anisomycin (*black bar*). The cartoon inset shows that a synaptic tag has been set on pathway S2 but protein synthesis is blocked (*cross symbol*). (b) Prior induction of late LTP on pathway S1 now allows late LTP to be induced on pathway S2 even when the strong tetanus is given in

A prominent characteristic of event memory is, however, that some events are remembered for a long time, others only for a short time. In fact, the human capacity to remember the inconsequential events of the day for any length of time is quite limited, although we are generally able to remember such events for a few hours. It follows that, if NMDA receptor-dependent plasticity is an essential prerequisite for event memory, factors contributing to the variable persistence of LTP could be of functional significance with respect to the strength or accessibility of memory 'traces'.

The issue of variable temporal persistence is made more complicated by the possibility that events happening closely in time may be part of a single 'episode', where an episode is defined as a sequence of related events. It would clearly make sense for the encoding system to be organized in such a manner that most or all events associated with an episode are recalled together. Spatial context may be one important feature of this 'binding' process because, if events are remembered with respect to where they happen, this could provide a basis for considering them as part of a single episode. A common spatio-temporal context is, of course, likely to be only one of several determinants of this binding process.

These speculations form part of the intellectual context of a new series of experiments on the persistence of protein-synthesis-dependent late LTP (Frey & Morris 1997). The immediate aim of this study was to address the issue of how the input-specificity of late LTP is realized. The early phase of NMDA receptor-dependent LTP, lasting less than 3 h (early LTP), can be dissociated from LTP lasting longer (late LTP) by using inhibitors of protein synthesis. However, whether synthesized in the cell body (arguably the more important site (Frey *et al.* 1989)) or in dendrites (Feig & Lipton 1993; Steward & Wallace 1995; Torre & Steward 1996), the question arises of how the input-specificity of late LTP is achieved without elaborate protein trafficking. One way might be via the creation of a short-lasting 'synaptic tag' at each activated synapse at the time of LTP induction (Fig. 12.4). This tag would have the potential to sequester plasticity-related proteins to stabilize early LTP at that synapse and so render it long-lasting. In the simplest case, a single strong input to a population of afferent fibres could (1) induce early-LTP, (2) set synaptic tags locally in the postsynaptic compartment of each of the activated synapses, and

---

the presence of anisomycin. The cartoon inset shows synaptic tags set on both S1 and S2, and events at the synapses activated by S1 capable of triggering protein synthesis. Plasticity-related proteins (*triangles*) diffuse through the dendrites, where they are sequestered by the tags set at both pathways. (c) Induction of early LTP on pathway S2 in response to a single short tetanus (one train of 100 Hz for 200 ms). No drugs to limit protein synthesis are necessary. The early LTP induced decays over 3–4 h. (d) Prior induction of late LTP on pathway S1 also allows late LTP to be triggered in response to single-tetanus activation of S2. The tag set at S2 can sequester plasticity proteins synthesized in response to activation of S1. Based on Frey & Morris (1997).

(3) trigger the biochemical cascades that increase the synthesis of plasticity-related proteins (PPs). The diffuse travel of these newly synthesized PPs inside the cell's dendrites would result in tag–protein interactions only at previously activated synapses. This hypothesis makes an intriguing prediction. Provided the creation of these tags is independent of protein synthesis, there is no reason why tags set in the presence of drugs that inhibit protein synthesis should not 'hijack' PPs synthesized earlier and so stabilize any early LTP induced after protein synthesis has been shut down. Paradoxically, the synaptic-tag mechanism for realising input-specificity allows for the possibility that protein-synthesis-dependent LTP can be induced during the inhibition of protein synthesis.

Stimulation and recording were conducted in the stratum radiatum of area CA1 *in vitro* by using extracellular techniques. Figure 12.4a shows that when a strong tetanus was applied to a pathway (S2) in the presence of anisomycin, a decaying early LTP was induced but not late LTP. The cartoon insert shows that protein synthesis cannot be induced during the application of anisomycin. In Fig. 12.4b, S1 is strongly tetanized before anisomycin application. S2 is also strongly tetanized, but only after protein synthesis has been inhibited by the drug. Late LTP none the less develops on S2 because PPs synthesized in response to tetanization of S1 are captured by the tag set on S2. The same phenomenon can be displayed by using weaker patterns of stimulation that cannot, on their own, trigger protein synthesis. Figure 12.4c shows that weak tetanization of S2 only induces early LTP. In Fig. 12.4d, weak tetanization of S2 is preceded by strong tetanization of S1. Late LTP develops on pathway S2 because the tag set by weak stimulation of S2 sequesters proteins synthesized in response to the stimulation of S1. Further experiments of this series indicated that the putative 'synaptic tag' lasts less than 3 h (see Frey & Morris 1997).

There are three immediate implications of these findings. First, they support the synaptic-tag hypothesis. Second, the input-specificity and temporal persistence of LTP must be determined somewhat separately. Whereas input-specificity is determined by the local synaptic activation of NMDA receptors, temporal persistence appears to be determined, at least in part, by the history of activation of the neurone. Third, weak afferent events that usually only give rise to transient changes in synaptic efficacy can be made to cause lasting changes in neurones in which the synthesis of PPs has previously been upregulated. These findings are relevant to the general hypothesis of this paper, as discussed below.

12.7 General discussion

The aim of this paper has been to present a series of experiments that collectively point to a new way of thinking about the functional role of NMDA- dependent hippocampal synaptic plasticity. Specifically, in contrast to the current emphasis upon its serving a role in associative and/or spatial learning, this paper has summarized findings more consistent with its playing a role in one aspect of event memory.

Summary of experimental findings

The evidence here summarized against a Hebbian correlational rule being sufficient to account for spatial learning is at two levels. First, varying the character of pretraining given before animals are later trained on a spatial reference memory task can change this second task from one that is sensitive to an NMDA antagonist (if no pretraining is given) to one that is insensitive (after spatial pretraining in a different environment). This differential sensitivity suggests, at a minimum, that spatial learning in a watermaze is more complex than previously recognized and that NMDA-receptor activation is not critical for learning the spatial relationships between extramaze cues (the usual way of thinking about this type of learning). Second, at a purely behavioural level, the observation that 'blocking' occurs in the spatial domain also indicates that the determinants of spatial learning must be quite complex. The results here presented show that rats are sensitive to differences between their perception and stored representation of a landmark array, and that their reaction to mismatch is expressed in the form of exploratory behaviour. Exploration of a novel landmark is, however, no guarantee that its location will be incorporated into the animal's spatial map. Incorporation only occurs to the extent that information is needed to locate a goal. That exploration of the novel landmark declines over trials indicates that some information about it is rapidly encoded; the possibility that this includes information about its location cannot be excluded. However, if this does happen, it is not in a form that can later be used to guide search behaviour. Our view is that the hippocampally based automatic recording system has access to the animal's currently activated spatial map and that it triggers exploratory behaviour (directed attention) in situations where there is mismatch. If the information it then acquires is needed—for example to find the goal in a new place—the effortful components of the long-term memory system are engaged and the animal's spatial representation of the environment updated. When it is not needed to find the goal, there will be no 'reinforcement signal' of a goal-directed character and, thus, the error-correcting learning rule used for long-term memory need not be engaged.

The positive evidence in favour of hippocampal LTP playing a role in event-memory is also at two levels. First, it was shown that, after animals have been pretrained in the DMP task to a stable level of profiency, chronic infusion of AP5 causes a severe delay-dependent impairment. This finding implies that blocking NMDA receptors does not affect the use of spatial information *per se*, but might impair the capacity to form or recall recent events in relation to a previously learned spatial framework. In this case, and unlike the study by Bannerman *et al.* (1995), the behavioural strategy that the animals acquire during pretraining is one that continues to call upon event memory for its deployment. Second, we have uncovered a novel property of LTP—synaptic tagging—that is suggestive of LTP playing a role in episodic memory. A synaptic tag provides a way of marking that an event has happened and has been recorded as a recent distributed alteration of synaptic strengths. It also extends the opportunity for creating a more lasting long-term memory as a function of other events happening around the same time. The determinants of persistence of synaptic enhancement extend beyond the particular pattern and strength of activation at the time of LTP induction; the history of activation of the neuron is also important.

The automatic recording of attended experience

The theoretical proposal for integrating these findings is that the neural mechanisms underlying hippocampal NMDA-dependent synaptic plasticity underlie temporary information storage within a network responsible for the 'automatic recording of attended experience'. This recording system is part of a larger 'episodic memory' system of the brain (Tulving 1983). In making this proposal, a distinction is drawn between functions of the hippocampus itself and our proposed function of NMDA-dependent hippocampal synaptic plasticity. This is an important distinction: there may be other functions, including information retrieval from cortex, in which the hippocampus participates (and specifically, fast synaptic transmission) but in which changes in synaptic efficacy are unnecessary.

Beyond this, we make the following further comments about the hypothesis. First, the inclusion of 'automaticity' within the definition emphasizes the need to distinguish between automatic and effortful aspects of memory encoding. Many types of memory experiment in humans, such as remembering lists of words accurately, or recalling the details of complex pictures, require careful and deliberate scanning of the stimulus material and an effortful process of encoding. This type of memory requires the integrity of structures in the medial temporal lobe (Squire & Zola-Morgan 1991) and there is evidence from functional imaging studies that it also activates the frontal lobe (Kapur *et al.* 1994; Shallice *et al.* 1994; Tulving *et al.* 1996). Our supposition is that 'episodic memory' might usefully be subdivided into an automatic subsystem involved in 'online' information capture (medial–temporal?) and a second subsystem involved in the deliberate creation of veridical memory traces as a function of task demand (frontal?). If a task requires accurate recall of a large amount of information, it is generally necessary to go over the stimulus information several times before a lasting veridical memory can be formed from the online record. This distinction has points of similarity to Moscovitch's (1995) important idea of a distinction within the domain of episodic memory between the conscious experience of an event (that he believes to be hippocampal) and the task of working with episodic memories during encoding and retrieval (involving the frontal lobes). Second, the reference to it as a recording of 'experience' constitutes a recognition that information cannot be processed automatically in a manner that is divorced from its spatiotemporal context (O'Keefe & Nadel 1978; Gaffan 1994). Events happen at particular places and particular times; human memory for events necessarily includes remembering where (and sometimes when) an event actually happened. Our supposition is that the system is tuned to record events with respect to the scenes or places where they occur, rapidly forming event–context associations. These associations serve the important function of helping to disambiguate similar stimuli occurring in different places. Third, we also consider 'automatic recording' a subsystem of episodic memory in which attended information is processed preferentially. Selective attention acts as a filter controlling the access of information to the system.

There are numerous facets of the hypothesis that need to be developed more formally if it is to be predictive. As we are proposing that hippocampal LTP plays a critical role in this type of temporary information storage, it follows that all mammals displaying LTP (with the properties we have described) should be capable of at least 'elements' of episodic memory. The extent to which this challenges Tulving's claim (1983, p. l) that only humans are capable of this type of memory is largely one of emphasis. After all, his book recognized that certain phenomena studied in animals (such as the studies by Olton *et al.* (1979) of 'working memory' in the radial maze) may be analogous to episodic memory in humans. Our suspicion, guided in part by later writings (Tulving & Markowitsch 1994), is that Tulving has always been sceptical about whether animals are capable of remembering events in 'quite' the same way as humans (his emphasis). Underlying this scepticism may be the supposition that, because animals are unable to report events via the medium of language, they have no need of 'recollective experiences'. We prefer the alternative view that event memory evolved because it is useful to an organism in its own right, with the communication of information about events being a separate matter. The division of episodic memory into (1) a subsystem involved in the online capture of events and (2) a system for integrating information as a function of task demand could be valuable in all mammalian species. The challenge for neuroscientists investigating memory in animals is, therefore, to devise ways of distinguishing between changes in behaviour that occur because of true memory for events and those that occur simply because an event has happened. We do not yet offer any solution to this important problem.

A separate point is that the proposal for subdividing episodic memory is in the tradition of seeing an important link between memory and understanding. This link is rarely discussed by proponents of declarative memory (cf. Squire *et al.* 1993), but has been a key aspect of the 'cognitive mapping' theory of O'Keefe & Nadel (1978). Briefly, we believe that the processing of information within the automatic recording system is strongly influenced by the current activated knowledge of the animal (or human). Animals do not just process attended information; they notice mismatches between what they perceive and what they know. In spatial learning, these mismatches immediately trigger exploration and such behaviour ensures that some record of the newly attended information is processed. In the delayed matching-to-place task, the capacity to respond appropriately to information acquired in a single trial relies upon the animal's having some activated representation of the space in which that event happens. Thus, the capture of new information is guided by what the animal already knows, focusing processing effort onto novel information. The notion that the memorability of information is importantly influenced by existing activated knowledge has long been appreciated in the human literature also (Bransford & Johnston 1972; Longuet-Higgens 1983). However, because we see a distinction between the automatic and effortful components of episodic memory, information captured temporarily may not be stored permanently. Memory consolidation is a selective process, guided in part by task demand and so by goal-directed error-correcting learning rules.

Neural implementation within the hippocampal formation

The neural mechanisms of episodic memory are poorly understood. Pieces and patches are emerging from functional imaging studies, but these have so far been restricted to discoveries about localization within the brain and the sequence of mental processes involved, rather than underlying neural mechanisms. Our proposal is that NMDA receptor-dependent LTP in the hippocampus displays properties ideal for an 'automatic recording' subsystem (rapid associative induction using a correlational rule, input-specificity, variable persistence). The concept of the synaptic tag is relevant to this idea, as it affords a way of extending the persistence of synaptic changes induced by recent events as a function of their temporal proximity to other events. We conclude by focusing on the implications of synaptic tagging for event memory.

In physiological experiments designed to identify the mechanisms by which changes in synaptic efficacy are triggered, high-frequency stimulation of afferents can induce either a short or a prolonged increase in synaptic strength as a function of the prior (and perhaps subsequent) activity state of the neuron. With respect to LTP, it has already been noted that an early phase can be dissociated from a late phase because only the latter requires the synthesis of new macromolecules. Activation of NMDA receptors and the subsequent influx of Ca^{2+} ions, possibly acting via the cytoplasmic tail of the NMDA receptor signalling complex, triggers several intracellular cascades. These are now thought to include the phosphorylation of kinases, of receptors and of target proteins as well the synthesis of plasticity-related proteins (PPs) (Malinow et al. 1988; O'Dell et al. 1991; Deisseroth et al. 1996; Rostas et al. 1996; for reviews see Goelet et al. 1986; Walaas & Greengard 1991; Bliss & Collingridge 1993; Schulman 1995).

The stimulation pattern that ordinarily results in early LTP activates only some of these intracellular processes. We have argued that they must also include, beyond expressing the change in synaptic efficacy itself, the setting of input-specific synaptic tags. The job of these tags is to sequester PPs to stabilize temporary synaptic changes. Identifying the molecule(s) that serve as synaptic tags is clearly a very important goal of future research. A parsimonious speculation, in the spirit of Goelet et al. (1986), is that such molecules are likely to be on the same biochemical pathway that gives rise to the synthesis of PPs.

They are therefore likely to be downstream of the NMDA receptor, and possibly at, or upstream of, the protein kinase A (PKA) signalling pathway that activates transcription factors in the cell nucleus. The type of experiment needed to identify a candidate tag will, therefore, involve the two-pathway S1–S2 paradigm used by Frey & Morris (1997), with strong tetanization of S1 followed by tetanization of S2 during the application of selective enzyme-inhibiting drugs. Pharmacological studies would, of course, have to be complemented by relevant molecular and cell-biological work.

Increasing the strength of the stimulation needed to induce early LTP also activates mechanisms responsible for the synthesis of PPs. Identification of these PPs is also an important priority of current research. A clue to what might be involved is the finding of a transient increase in intracellular levels of cyclic AMP (cAMP) in CA1 after both strong tetanization that results late LTP (Frey *et al.* 1993) and pharmacological activation of the NMDA receptor (Chetkovitch & Sweatt 1993). This increase probably then activates a somatically located cAMP-response element (CRE) that triggers immediate gene expression (Deisseroth *et al.* 1996). Interestingly, an input-*non*-specific late LTP can be induced by application of a membrane-permeable cAMP analogue which activates cAMP-dependent protein kinase A (PKA). This late LTP is prevented by simultaneous application of anisomycin, indicating the necessity for protein synthesis. Electrically induced, input-specific late LTP is also blocked by a PKA inhibitor applied during tetanization (Frey *et al.* 1993). Collectively, these data point to a multifunctionality of the cAMP–PKA pathway: it could be linked both to the synthesis of plasticity-related proteins and to the setting of synaptic tags. An additional point is that Frey *et al.* (1993) found that the increase in cAMP concentrations after strong tetanization was blocked by antagonists of the dopaminergic D1-receptor, a receptor that is positively coupled to adenylate cyclase. Late LTP is blocked by D1-receptor antagonists (Frey *et al.* 1990) and induced by D1 or D5 receptor agonists (Huang & Kandel 1995). Dopamine could have reinforcement properties, controlling the transformation of early LTP into late LTP. Other transmitter systems than just glutamate have to be brought into the picture in relation to the synthesis of PPs (see also Matthies 1989).

Conclusion

Assuming these biochemical mechanisms can be identified, how might the synaptic tagging mechanism help the automatic recording system to achieve selectivity? We end with two speculations: the first concerned with a distinction between short- and long-term consolidation, the second with how episodes could be constructed from a succession of events.

First, variable persistence is important because it allows the duration of synaptic changes triggered by events to be influenced by other temporally adjacent events. We have argued that early LTP implements the on-line recording of information in an 'associative' manner, linking information presented to the hippocampal network about events (such as briefly presented stimuli, or an animal's own actions) to more stable information about the context in which they occur. The synthesis of PPs is likely to be increased if other events happening around the same time also trigger LTP in a common pool of neurons. This synthesis will, synergistically, increase the chance that temporally related events are sustained for longer in the hippocampal network (short-term consolidation). Long-term consolidation (stabilization of intra-cortical connections) also requires time; it is more likely to be successful if the automatic but temporary record is more persistent. Short-term consolidation extends the opportunity for the creation of lasting episodic memories or the incorporation of newly acquired information into an animal's or person's long-term semantic memory, a process that probably involves interaction with other brain areas (e.g. the frontal lobe).

Second, whereas synaptic tagging provides a mechanism for realizing variable persistence, it could also be useful in a number of distinct circumstances for enhancing the memorability of stimuli that might otherwise be poorly remembered. With respect to the circumstances surrounding emotionally significant events, it is not uncommon to remember numerous apparently trivial details. This phenomenon is sometimes referred to as 'flashbulb memory' (Brown & Kulik 1977). If emotionally charged events activate reinforcing inputs to the hippocampal formation (such as the dopaminergic system), incidental stimuli associated with these events could trigger changes in synaptic plasticity in the hippocampus and set synaptic tags against a background of the greater availability of PPs. Memory of these incidental stimuli would then be longer-lasting. A different way in which trivial events might be rendered more memorable would be if the neural representation of two (or more) events in the hippocampus shared a common pool of neurones. This would be most likely if two events occurred in a common spatial location. For example, if events were represented as sparsely coded but orthogonal patterns of activation on glutamatergic input pathways to the hippocampus, the construction and binding together of 'episodes' might occur when these patterns activated a common pool of place cells. Under these circumstances, a weak event might innervate a substantially similar population of cells as a stronger event and so benefit from the latter triggering the synthesis of PPs. Place–event associations may thereby provide a way of constructing coherent episodes. As O'Keefe & Nadel (1978) and Gaffan (1994) before us have argued, spatial memory provides the evolutionary foundation upon which the elaborate scaffold of human episodic memory is built.

Acknowledgements

This work was supported by grants from the UK Medical Research Council, the Wellcome Trust, the Human Frontiers Science Programme and the German Land Sachsen-Anhalt. We are grateful to David Bannerman, Robert

Biegler and Bob Steele for their collaboration on some of the experimental work we describe.

References

Alkon, D. L., Amaral, D. G., Bear, M. F., Black, J., Carew, T. J., Cohen, N. J. *et al.* 1991 Learning and memory. *Brain Res. Rev.* **16**, 193–220.

Bannerman, D. M., Good, M. A., Butcher, S. P., Ramsay, M. & Morris, R. G. M. 1995 Distinct components of spatial learning revealed by prior training and NMDA receptor blockade. *Nature* **378**, 182–186.

Barnes, C. A. 1995 Involvement of LTP in memory: are we 'searching under the street light'? *Neuron* **15**, 751–754.

Bear, M. F. & Malenka, R. C. 1994 Synaptic plasticity: LTP and LTD. *Curr. Opin. Neurobiol.* **4**, 389–399.

Biegler, R. & Morris, R. G. M. 1993 Landmark stability is a prerequisite for spatial but not discrimination learning. *Nature* **361**, 631–633.

Biegler, R. & Morris, R. G. M. 1996 Landmark stability: further studies pointing to a role in spatial learning. *Q. J. Exp. Psychol.* **49B**, 307–345.

Biegler, R. & Morris, R. G. M. 1998 Blocking in the spatial domain with arrays of landmarks. *J. Exp. Psychol. Anim. Behav. Proc.* (In press.)

Bliss, T. V. P. & Collingridge, G. L. 1993 Long term potentiation: a synaptic model of memory. *Nature* **361**, 31–39.

Bliss, T. V. P. & Lomo, T. 1973 Long-lasting potentiation of synaptic transmission in the dentate area of the anaesthetized rabbit following stimulation of the perforant path. *J. Physiol.* **232**, 331–356.

Bransford, J. D. & Johnston, M. K. 1972 Contextual prerequisities for understanding: some investigations of comprehension and recall. *J. Verb. Learn. Verb. Behav.* **11**, 717–726.

Brown, R. & Kulik, S. 1977 Flashbulb memory. *Cognition* **5**, 73–99.

Cain, D. P. 1997 LTP NMDA, genes and learning. *Curr. Opin. Neurobiol.* **7**, 235–242.

Chetkovitch, D. M. & Sweatt, J. D. 1993 NMDA receptor activation increases cyclic AMP in area CA1 of the hippocampus via calcium/calmodulin stimulation of adenyl cyclase. *J. Neurochem.* **61**, 1933–1942.

Danysz, W., Zajaczkowski, W. & Parsons, C. G. 1996 Modulation of learning processes by ionotropic glutamate receptor ligands. *Behav. Pharmacol.* **6**, 455–474.

Davis, S., Butcher, S. P. & Morris, R. G. M. 1992 The *N*-methyl-D-aspartate receptor antagonist 2-amino-5-phos-phonpentanoate (AP5) impairs spatial learning and LTP *in vivo* at comparable intracerebral concentrations to those that block LTP *in vitro*. *J. Neurosci.* **12**, 21–34.

Deisseroth, K., Bito, H. & Tsien, R. W. 1996 Signaling from synapse to nucleus: postsynaptic CREB phosphorylation during multiple forms of hippocampal synaptic plasticity. *Neuron* **16**, 89–101.

Dickinson, A. 1980 *Contemporary animal learning theory.* Cambridge University Press.

Fazeli, M. S. & Collingridge, G. L. 1996 *Cortical plasticity: LTP and LTD.* Oxford: Bios Publishers.

Feig, S. & Lipton, P. 1993 Pairing the cholinergic agonist carbachol with patterned Schaffer collateral stimulation initiates protein synthesis in hippocampal CA1 pyramidal dendrites via a muscarinic, NMDA-dependent mechanism. *J. Neurosci.* **13**, 1010–1021.

Frey, U. & Morris, R. G. M. 1997 Synaptic tagging and long-term potentiation. *Nature* **385**, 533–536.

Frey, U., Krug, M., Brodemann, R., Reymann, K. & Matthies, H.-J. 1989 Long-term potentiation induced in dendrites separated from rat's CA1 pyramidal somata does not establish a late phase. *Neurosci. Lett.* **97**, 135–139.

Frey, U., Schroeder, H. & Matthies, H.-J. 1990 Dopaminergic antagonists prevent long-term maintenance of posttetanic LTP in the CA1 region of rat hippocampal slices. *Brain Res.* **522**, 69–75.

Frey, U., Huang, Y.-Y. & Kandel, E. R. 1993 Effects of cAMP simulate a late stage of LTP in hippocampal CA1 neurons. *Science* **260**, 1661–1664.

Gaffan, D. 1994 Scene-specific memory for objects: a model of episodic memory impairment in monkeys with fornix transection. *J. Cogn. Neurosci.* **6**, 302–320.

Goelet, P., Castellucci, V. F., Schacher, S. & Kandel, E. R. 1986 The long and the short of long-term memory—a molecular framework. *Nature* **322**, 419–422.

Huang, Y.-Y. & Kandel, E. R. 1995 D1/D5 receptor agonists induce a protein synthesis-dependent late potentiation in the CA1 region of the hippocampus. *Proc. Natn. Acad. Sci. USA* **92**, 2446–2450.

Jacobs, L. F. 1994 The ecology of spatial cognition. In *Behavioural brain research in naturalistic and semi-naturalistic settings* (ed. E. Alleva), pp. 301–322. Amsterdam: Kluwer.

Jeffery, K. J. 1997 LTP and spatial learning—where to next? *Hippocampus* **7**, 95–110.

Kamin, L. J. 1969 Predictability, surprise, attention and conditioning. *In Punishment and aversive behavior* (ed. B. A. Campbell & R. M. Church), pp. 276–296. New York: Appleton–Century–Crofts.

Kapur, S., Craik, F. I. M., Tulving, E., Wilson, A. A., Houle, S. & Brown, M. 1994 Neuroanatomical correlates of encoding in episodic memory: levels of processing effect. *Proc. Natn. Acad. Sci. USA*, **91**, 2012–2015.

Longuet-Higgens, P. 1983 *Mental models.* Cambridge University Press.

Mackintosh, N. J. 1983 *Conditioning and associative learning.* Oxford University Press.

Malinow, R., Madison, D. V. & Tsien, R. W. 1988 Persistent protein kinase activity underlying long-term potentiation. *Nature* **335**, 820–824.

Matthies, H. 1989 In search of cellular mechanisms of memory. *Prog. Neurobiol.* **32**, 277–349.

McHugh, T. J., Blum, K. I., Tsien, J., Tonegawa, S. & Wilson, M. 1996 Impaired hippocampal representation of space in CA1-specific NMDAR1 knockout mice. *Cell* **87**, 1339–1349.

McNaughton, B. L. & Morris, R. G. M. 1987 Hippocampal synaptic enhancement and information storage within a distributed memory system. *Trends Neurosci.* **10**, 408–415.

Morris, R. G. M. 1989 Synaptic plasticity and learning: selective impairment of learning in rats and blockade of long-term potentiation *in vivo* by the *N*-methyl-D-aspartate receptor antagonist, AP5. *J. Neurosci.* **9**, 3040–3057.

Morris, R. G. M., Anderson, E., Lynch, G. S. & Baudry, M. 1986 Selective impairment of learning and blockade of long-term potentiation by an *N*-methyl-D-aspartate receptor antagonist, AP5. *Nature* **319**, 774–776.

Morris, R. G. M., Butcher, S. P. & Davis, S. 1990 Hippocampal synaptic plasticity and NMDA receptors: a role in information storage? *Phil. Trans. R. Soc. Lond.* B **329**, 187–204.

Morris, R. G. M. & Davis, M. 1994 The role of NMDA receptors in learning and memory. In *The NMDA receptor*, 2nd edn (ed. G. L. Collingridge & J. C. Watkins), pp. 340–374. Oxford University Press.

Morris, R. G. M., Halliwell, R. F. & Bowery, N. 1989 Synaptic plasticity and learning. II. Do different kinds of plasticity underly different kinds of learning? *Neuro-psychologia* **27**, 41–59.

Moscovitch, M. 1995 Recovered consciousness: a hypothesis concerning modularity and episodic memory. *J. Clin. Exp. Neuropsychol.* **17**, 276–290.

O'Dell, T. J., Kandel, E. R. & Grant, S. G. 1991 Long-term potentiation in the hippocampus is blocked by tyrosine kinase inhibitors. *Nature* **353**, 558–560.

O'Keefe, J. & Nadel, L. 1978 *The hippocampus as a cognitive map.* Oxford University Press.

Olton, D. S., Handelmann, G. E. & Becker, J. T. 1979 Hippocampus, space and memory. *Behav. Brain Sci.* **2**, 313–365.

Rescorla, R. A. & Wagner, A. R. 1972 A theory of Pavlovian conditioning: variations in the effectiveness of reinforcement and non-reinforcement. In *Classical conditioning. II. Current research and theory* (ed. A. H. Black & W. F. Prokasy), pp. 66–99. New York: Appleton–Century–Crofts.

Rodrigo, T., Chamizo, V. D., McLaren, I. P. L. & Mackintosh, N. J. 1998 Blocking in the spatial domain. *J. Exp. Psychol.* (In press.)

Rostas, J. A. P., Brent, V. A., Voss, K., Errington, M. L., Bliss, T. V. P. & Gurd, J. W. 1996 Enhanced tyrosine phosphorylation of the 2B subunit of the *N*-methyl-D-aspartate receptor in long-term potentiation. *Proc. Natn. Acad. Sci. USA* **93**, 10452–10456.

Sakimura, K., Kutsuwada, T., Ito, I., Manabe, T., Takayama, C., Kushiya, E., Yagi, T., Aizawa, S., Inoue, Y., Sugiyama, H. & Mishina, M. 1995 Reduced hippocampal LTP and spatial learning in mice lacking NMDA R2 subunit. *Nature* **373**, 151–155.

Saucier, D. & Cain, D. P. 1995 Spatial learning without NMDA-receptor-dependent long-term potentiation. *Nature* **378**, 186–189.

Schulman, H. 1995 Protein phosphorylation in neuronal plasticity and gene expression. *Curr. Opin. Neurobiol.* **5**, 375–381.

Shallice, T., Fletcher, F., Frith, C. D., Grasby, P., Frackowiak, R. S. J. & Dolan, R. 1995 Brain regions associated with acquisition and retrieval of verbal episodic memory. *Nature* **368**, 633–635.

Sherry, D. F., Jacobs, L. F. & Gaulin, S. J. C. 1992 Spatial memory and adaptive specialization of the hippocampus. *Trends Neurosci.* **15**, 298–303.

Shors, T. J. & Matzel, L. 1997 Long term potentiation: what's learning got to do with it? *Behav. Brain Sci.* **20**, 597–655.

Squire, L. R. & Zola-Morgan, S. 1991 The medial temporal lobe memory system. *Science* **253**, 1380–1386.

Squire, L. R., Knowlton, B. & Musen, G. 1993 The structure and organization of memory. *A. Rev. Psychol.* **44**, 453–495.

Steele, R. J. & Morris, R. G. M. 1997 Delay-dependent impairment of a hippocampal-dependent matching-to-place task with chronic and intrahippocampal infusion of the NMDA antagonist D-AP5. (In preparation.)

Steward, O. & Wallace, C. S. 1995 mRNA distribution within dendrites: relationship to afferent innervation. *J. Neurobiol.* **26**, 447–458.

Teyler, T. J. & DiScenna, P. 1986 The hippocampal memory indexing theory. *Behav. Neurosci.* **100**, 147–154.

Torre, E. R. & Steward, O. 1996 Protein synthesis within dendrites: glycosylation of newly synthesized proteins in dendrites of hippocampal neurons in culture. *J. Neurosci.* **16**, 5967–5978.

Tsien, J. Z., Chen, D. F., Gerber, D., Tom, C., Mercer, E. H., Anderson, D. J., Mayford, M., Kandel, E. R. & Tonegawa, S. 1996a Subregion- and cell type-restricted gene knockout in mouse brain. *Cell* **87**, 1317–1326.

Tsien, J. Z., Huerta, J. & Tonegawa, S. 1996*b* The essential role of hippocampal CA1 NMDA receptor-dependent synaptic plasticity in spatial memory. *Cell* **87**, 1327–1338.

Tulving, E. 1983 *Elements of episodtc memory*. Oxford: Clarendon Press.

Tulving, E. & Markowitsch, H. J. 1994 What do animal models of memory model? *Behav. Brain Sci.* **17**, 498–499.

Tulving, E. & Schacter, D. 1994 *Memory systems*. Cambridge, MA: MIT Press.

Tulving, E., Markowitsch, H. J., Craik, F. I. M., Habib, R. & Houle, S. 1996 Novelty and familiarity activations in PET studies of memory encoding and retrieval. *Cerebr. Cortex* **6**, 71–79.

Walaas, S. I. & Greengard, P. 1991 Protein phosphorylation and neuronal function. *Pharmacol. Rev.* **43**, 299–349.

13

Right medial temporal-lobe contribution to object-location memory

Brenda Milner, Ingrid Johnsrude and Joelle Crane

13.1 Introduction

The study of patients undergoing unilateral brain operation for the relief of epilepsy has revealed impairments after right anterior temporal lobectomy on a variety of spatial learning and spatial memory tasks, but only if the removal encroached extensively upon the hippocampus and/or the parahippocampal gyrus. The tasks sampled ranged from simple delayed recall of the position of a point on a line (Corsi 1972; Rains and Milner 1994) to more complex ones, such as stylus maze learning, both visual (Milner 1965) and tactual (Corkin 1965), and spatial conditional associative learning (Petrides 1985). These results for spatial memory are in marked contrast to the findings for complex visual patterns, such as faces, abstract designs, or the figurative detail in representational drawings, where an impairment in recognition memory is demonstrable after right temporal-lobe removals, even when the hippocampal region is spared (Kimura 1963; Milner 1968; Burke and Nolan 1988; Pigott and Milner 1993). They also contrast with those for verbal material, where memory impairment is typically seen after left temporal lobectomy but not after right.

The domain of spatial memory is broad and heterogeneous. This paper will focus on one conspicuous aspect, namely the ability to remember the location of objects in the environment. In what follows, findings are presented from lesion studies in patients and from positron emission tomography (PET) studies in normal volunteers to examine the contribution of the right hippocampal region to the processes underlying object-location memory.

13.2 Lesion studies: the recall of the location of objects in an array

Smith and Milner (1981, 1984, 1989) have demonstrated a clear impairment after right temporal lobectomy on a task requiring the recall, after an interval of 4 min, of the locations of 16 toy objects within an array, the occurrence of the deficit being contingent upon inclusion of the bulk of the hippocampus and/or parahippocampal gyrus in the removal. No impairment was seen after corresponding removals from the left temporal lobe, nor after large frontal-lobe removals from either hemisphere. Notably, the impairment of the right temporal-lobe group with extensive hippocampal lesions (RTH) was manifested in both a greater than average displacement of each object from its original position (its absolute location) and an impaired recall of each object's position relative to its neighbours (its relative location). The presence of an intra-trial interval was, however, critical in eliciting the deficit: at zero delay all groups performed normally, thus showing that the impaired recall after 4 min was due to rapid forgetting of information that had been accurately perceived.

Crane *et al.* (1995) have since extended Smith and Milner's findings to a learning paradigm, in which subjects were first instructed to name and remember the locations of 12 objects randomly distributed in fixed positions on a board. The array was then removed from view, and the subjects were given an identical set of objects and required to place them in the corresponding positions on an empty board. Placements that fell within a radius of 5 cm of the target position were judged correct, and the subjects were informed as to the total number correct on that trial. This process was repeated over successive trials, with an inter-trial interval of 2–3 min, until all 12 items had been correctly placed on a given trial, or until 10 trials had been completed.

This study broke new ground by including not only patients tested after left or right temporal lobectomy, but also those who had undergone a selective left or right amygdalohippocampectomy (LAH or RAH), sparing the lateral and polar temporal neocortex and thus permitting observations of the effect of the medial temporal-lobe lesion on task performance. Figure 13.1 displays the mean trials to criterion for the various temporal-lobe subgroups and for a normal control group (NC) matched to the patient groups with respect to age and education. Subsequent analysis showed both the RTH and RAH groups to be impaired relative to the NC group but not to differ from one another. In contrast to their impaired learning over multiple trials, the RTH and RAH groups performed normally on the first recall trial. It seems probable therefore, in the light of Smith and Milner's findings, that their impaired learning stems from abnormally rapid forgetting during the 2–3 min inter-trial intervals.

These findings for the human right hippocampal region accord well with the results of lesion studies in the monkey, where both bilateral hippocampectomy (Parkinson *et al.* 1988) and fornix transection (Gaffan and Saunders 1985; Gaffan and Harrison 1989) have been shown to impair the acquisition and retention of object-place associations. The present authors' own findings are also consistent with those models of hippocampal function that emphasize the role of this structure in spatial memory, notably the cognitive map hypothesis of O'Keefe and Nadel (1978) and the personal memory hypothesis of Gaffan and Harrison (1989). Nevertheless, several important questions remain to be

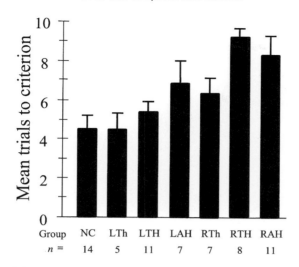

Fig. 13.1 Spatial-array learning. Number of trials required to reach criterion. Each subject was tested on two arrays, and the mean trials-to-criterion value that is given is an average for these two tests. NC: normal control; LTh: left temporal-lobe resection, small hippocampal removal (<1.5 cm); LTH: left temporal-lobe resection, large hippocampal removal; LAH: left selective amygdalohippocampectomy; RTh, RTH, RAH: groups of patients with corresponding resections from the right temporal lobe. Error bars give the standard error of the data. Compared to NC subjects, performance was significantly impaired in the RTH and RAH groups. ($p < .01$ and $p < .05$ respectively).

addressed. First, it is not clear whether the right hippocampal system is critically involved in mediating associations between object and place, or whether the impairment observed on object-location memory tasks after right hippocampal lesions can be reduced to a deficit in memory for location as such. It is also not clear, from a neuroanatomical standpoint, whether damage to the hippocampus itself is responsible for the deficits seen, or whether the parahippocampal gyrus plays an equal or preponderant role in the performance of the selected tasks. We therefore had recourse to blood-flow activation studies in normal subjects using positron emission tomography (PET) and magnetic resonance imaging (MRI), in an attempt to resolve these issues.

13.3 PET studies of object-location memory

In the following two experiments, the relative distribution of cerebral blood flow (CBF) was measured by using the bolus $H_2{}^{15}O$ method with averaged image subtraction (Raichle *et al.* 1983; Fox *et al.* 1985). A high-resolution

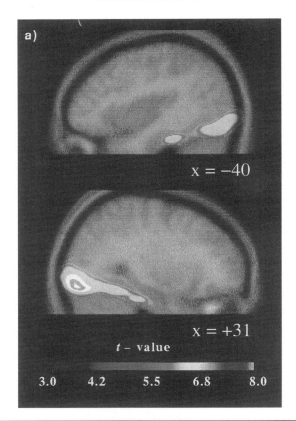

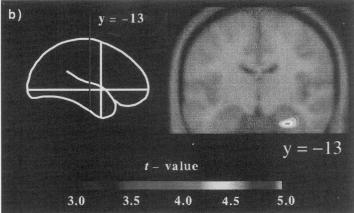

Fig. 13.2 Object-location memory versus memory for simple location. In this and subsequent figures presenting imaging data, the averaged PET subtraction images are shown superimposed on the corresponding averaged MRI scans (*n* = 12), transformed

MR image was obtained for each subject and co-registered with the corresponding PET images; each matched pair of MR and PET data sets was linearly transformed into stereotaxic space (Collins *et al*. 1994; Talairach and Tournoux 1988). The PET data were normalized for global differences in CBF and the mean CBF-change image volumes were obtained. The presence of significant focal changes was tested according to the method of Worsley *et al*. (1992).

Object-location memory versus memory for simple location

In this first PET study (Owen *et al*. 1996), 12 normal volunteers were scanned while performing a computerized version of the object-location memory task, which first required them to monitor and encode the positions of eight representational drawings of common objects, presented successively on a computer touch screen. Retrieval was tested in a separate scanning condition, 8 min later, in which they had to select, from two alternatives, the correct location for each of these objects. In two analogous conditions, designed to look at memory for location alone, the subjects were required to encode, and then to retrieve, eight distinct locations represented by identical white boxes on the computer screen.

It was predicted that, when blood-flow in either of the location conditions was subtracted from that in the corresponding object-location condition, activation would be seen in the ventral visual pathway (Ungerleider and Mishkin 1982), brought about by the introduction of representational drawings as compared with empty boxes. This was borne out by the results, as illustrated for *encoding* in Fig. 13.2a, which shows, in sagittal section, significant activation in the anterior fusiform gyrus and the prestriate cortex bilaterally when bloodflow in the *encoding location* condition was subtracted from that in the *encoding object-location* condition.

The second prediction, and the motive for the study, was that increased blood-flow in the right hippocampal region should also be seen when activation in the *retrieving location* condition was subtracted from that in the *retrieving object-location* condition, if this region were indeed critically involved in

into the standardized stereotaxic space of Talairach and Tournoux (1988). Subtraction of one condition from another yields focal changes in blood flow, which are shown as a *t*-statistic image, whose range is coded by the scale placed underneath each illustration. (a) *Encoding object-location* minus *encoding location*: the sagittal sections illustrate the significant rCBF increases observed in inferior visual associative cortices, extending into the anterior fusiform gyrus, bilaterally. (b) *Retrieving object-location* minus *retrieving location*: the coronal slice illustrates the significant rCBF increase observed in the right anterior parahippocampal gyrus in the region corresponding to the entorhinal cortex (Talairach coordinates: $x = 28$, $y = -13$, $z = -29$; $t = 4.89$). From Owen *et al*. (1996).

memory for object-place associations. This prediction was partly confirmed: although no changes were elicited in the hippocampus itself, an increase in blood-flow was seen in the anterior part of the right parahippocampal gyrus (corresponding to the entorhinal cortex), as shown in coronal section in Fig. 13.2b. The fact that no such change was seen in the *encoding* subtraction is consistent with the finding that patients with right-hippocampal lesions show normal recall of object-location at zero intratrial delay.

The negative findings for the hippocampus itself do not conflict with the notion that this structure is critically involved in spatial memory. In this particular study, as Owen *et al*. (1996) point out, all four scanning conditions involved memory for spatial information, the neural correlates of which may well have been subtracted out, leaving only those changes in blood flow specifically related to memory for the location of objects. A second PET experiment, described below, was designed to overcome this difficulty.

Object-location memory: shifted versus fixed array

In this study, modelled closely upon the one by Owen *et al*. (1996) and illustrated in Fig. 13.3, an attempt was made to enhance activation in the hippocampal formation in two ways. We incorporated a baseline visual discrimination task (shown in Fig. 13.3f), which was without a mnemonic component, and which could be performed on the basis of object-feature cues alone, without reference to spatial cues. Subjects merely had to touch the leaf on each trial and disregard the hammer. Second, the object-location retrieval task was made more difficult by changing the absolute positions of the stimuli, while maintaining constant the spatial relationships among the set of items. Before scanning, 12 subjects performed an encoding task similar to that of Owen *et al*. (1996), except that two featureless square landmarks were present in fixed locations on the screen during the encoding trials (Fig. 13.3a). Retrieval was then tested in four different scanning conditions. In the two *shifted* conditions, the array, composed of the eight object drawings and the landmarks, effectively shifted position from trial to trial, although the individual elements maintained the same spatial relations to each other. In one of these conditions, the landmarks themselves were presented as cues to the configuration of the stimuli (Fig. 13.3c), whereas in the other *shifted* condition, two other objects from the array served as cues (Fig. 13.3e). In the two *fixed* retrieval conditions, the array was static, in the same position as during encoding. Once again, either the two landmarks (Fig. 13.3b) or two other objects (Fig. 13.3d) were also visible on any given trial.

In this brief report, no detailed account of the results of the various subtractions can be given. Instead, this paper focuses on the findings with respect to the hippocampal region. When activity in the *visuomotor* control condition was subtracted from that in each of the *retrieval* scans involving

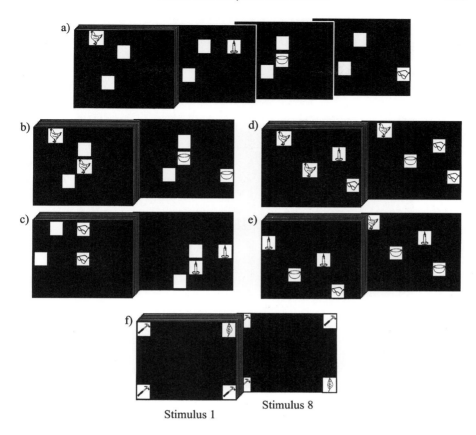

Stimulus 1   Stimulus 8

Fig. 13.3 Object-location memory: shifted array versus fixed array. Schematic drawings showing examples from experimental tasks. (a) *Encoding object-locations* (10 min prior to first scan); (b) *retrieval of fixed-array location using landmark cues*; (c) *retrieval of shifted-array location using landmark cues*, the subject selects correct location for that object relative to the landmarks; (d) *retrieval of fixed-array location using object cues*, subject selects the correct position of the duplicated object relative to the two other objects; (e) *retrieval of shifted-array location using object cues*; (f) *visuomotor control task*, subject touches the screen.

landmark cues, significant activation foci were observed in the right para-hippocampal gyrus bordering on the hippocampus, as shown in coronal section in Fig. 13.4a and 13.4b for *fixed* and *shifted* landmarks, respectively. Thus this region appears to be involved in the retrieval of object-location information, regardless of whether the retrieval task emphasizes the position of objects relative to a fixed external reference frame, as in the *fixed-array* tasks, or the

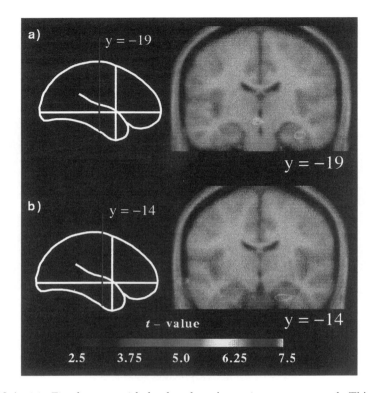

Fig. 13.4 (a) *Fixed array with landmarks* minus *visuomotor control*. This coronal section illustrates the significant rCBF increase observed in the right anterior parahippocampal gyrus (Talairach coordinates: x = 36, y = −19, z = −23; t = 3.31). The other two activation foci observed in this image are artefactual. (b) *Shifted array with landmarks* minus *visuomotor control*. This coronal section illustrates the significant rCBF increase observed in the right hippocampus/parahippocampal gyrus (Talairach coordinates: x = 21, y = −14, z = −27; t = 3.54).

location of objects relative to each other (as in the *shifted-array with landmarks* task).

The introduction of the simple visuomotor baseline task failed to bring out any important contribution from the hippocampus itself to the retrieval of object-location information. Nor did hippocampal CBF increase disproportionately in the *shifted-array* compared with the *fixed-array* conditions. Instead, subtraction of blood-flow during *fixed-array* from that during the *shifted-array* analogues yielded significant activation in the right posterior inferotemporal cortex (Brodmann's area 37), as shown in Fig. 13.5. Thus some lateralization of visual memory function within the neocortex was observed, a finding in accordance with a recent PET study by Moscovitch *et al.* (1995).

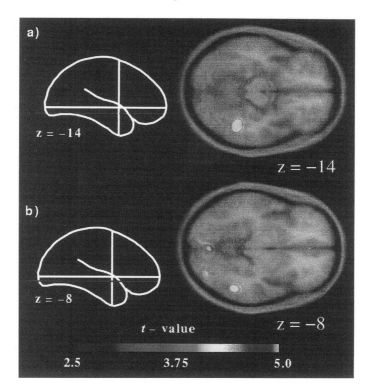

Fig. 13.5   Object-location memory: shifted array versus fixed array. Significant rCBF increases in the two higher-order subtractions. (a) This section illustrates the significant rCBF increase observed in right posterior inferotemporal cortex (BA 37) in the *shifted array with landmarks* minus *fixed array with landmarks* subtraction (Talairach coordinates: x = 44, y = −45, z = −14; *t* = 3.99). (b) This horizontal section illustrates the significant rCBF increase observed in right posterior inferotemporal cortex (BA 37) in the *shifted array with objects* minus *fixed array with objects* subtraction (Talairach coordinates: x = −51, y = −50, z = −8; *t* = 3.53).

13.4 Discussion

These findings as a whole point to a strong hemispheric asymmetry in the processes mediating memory for the location of objects. Surgical excision of the right medial temporal region, but not of the left, impaired the delayed recall of the locations of real objects in an array, in both single- and multi-trial studies, a result consonant with the authors' own earlier findings for other spatial-memory tasks, as well as with a recent study by Abrahams *et al.* (1997). A similar emphasis on the right hemisphere emerged from the two PET experiments in normal volunteer subjects, where activation was observed consistently in the right anterior parahippocampal gyrus, probably corresponding to entorhinal cortex, during retrieval of information about the location of objects on a computer screen, with no corresponding activation in the left hemisphere.

As Owen *et al.* (1996) have emphasized, the entorhinal area occupies a pivotal position within the hippocampal system (Amaral *et al.* 1993; Van Hoesen 1982): it is known that in the monkey selective lesions of entorhinal and adjacent perirhinal cortex impair learning and memory for both objects and locations (Murray and Gaffan 1993; E. A. Murray, personal communication). Furthermore, single-cell recording studies in the monkey have identified entorhinal neurones that respond selectively to objects (Quirk *et al.* 1992; Suzuki *et al.* 1995) and to a combination of both (Rolls *et al.* 1989). On the basis of studies in the rat, Eichenbaum and Bunsey (1995) have proposed that the parahippocampal region (including the entorhinal cortex) has the capacity to hold stimulus representations for extended periods of time, and that in so doing, it could combine simultaneously occurring stimuli into associated representations in memory (Gluck and Myers 1995). It may be that object-place associations are a special instance of this.

Whereas the work reported here provides strong evidence for a contribution from the right parahippocampal-gyrus region to memory for object location, in neither of the PET studies could clear activation in the hippocampus itself be elicited, despite the introduction of an ostensibly non-spatial baseline task in the second study. It seems possible, therefore, that the object-location memory task, at least in its two-dimensional computerized form, was too static to provoke increased blood-flow in the hippocampus itself, whereas tasks with a more navigational component may do so (Ghaem *et al.* 1997; Maguire *et al.* 1996; Morris *et al.* 1982). Against this interpretation, Aguirre *et al.* (1996) present evidence from a functional magnetic resonance imaging study, showing medial temporal-lobe activity confined to the parahippo-campal gyri, and not involving the hippocampus itself, during the learning and recall of topographical information. It is clear that more work needs to be done to delineate the role of the human hippocampus in spatial learning and spatial memory.

Acknowledgements

We thank Adrian Owen for his collaboration in the PET studies, and the staff of the McConnell Brain Imaging Unit (coordinator Alan Evans) for facilitating this research. This work was supported by the McDonnell-Pew Program in Cognitive Neuroscience and by the Medical Research Council of Canada through Special Project Grant SP-30 to A. Evans, and through operating Grant MT 2624 and a Career Investigatorship award to B. Milner. Joelle Crane holds a Medical Research Council studentship. All research protocols were approved by the Research Ethics Committee of the Montreal Neurological Institute and Hospital.

The authors would also like to thank MIT Press, Adrian Owen, Michael Petrides and Alan Evans for their permission to reproduce published material (Fig. 13.2).

References

Abrahams, S., Pickering, A., Polkey, C. E. and Morris, R. G. (1997). Spatial memory deficits in patients with unilateral damage to the right hippocampal formation. *Neuropsychologia*, **35**, 11–24.

Aguirre, G. K., Detre, J. A., Alsop, D. C. and D'Esposito, M. (1996). The parahippo-campus subserves topographical learning in man. *Cerebral Cortex*, **6**, 823–9.

Amaral, D. G., Witter, M. P. and Insausti, R. (1993). The entorhinal cortex of the monkey: a summary of recent anatomical findings. In *Brain Mechanisms of Perception and Memory: from Neuron to Behavior*, (ed., T. Ono, L. R. Squire, M. E. Raichle, D. I. Perret and M. Fukuda), pp. 228–40. Oxford University Press.

Burke, T. and Nolan, J. R. M. (1988). Material specific memory deficits after unilateral temporal neocorticectomy. *Society for Neuroscience Abstracts*, **14**, 1289.

Collins, D. L., Neelin, P., Peters, T. M. and Evans, A. C. (1994). Automatic 3D intersubject registration of MR volumetric data in standardized Talairach space. *Journal of Computer Assisted Tomography*, **18**, 192–205.

Corkin, S. (1965). Tactually-guided maze-learning in man: effects of unilateral cortical excisions and bilateral hippocampal lesions. *Neuropsychologia*, **3**, 339–51.

Corsi, P. M. (1972). Human memory and the medial temporal region of the brain. Unpublished D.Phil. thesis. McGill University.

Crane, J., Milner, B. and Leonard, G. (1995). Spatial-array learning by patients with focal temporal-lobe excisions. *Society for Neuroscience Abstracts*, **21**, 1446.

Eichenbaum, H. and Bunsey, M. (1995). On the binding of associations in memory: clues from studies on the role of the hippocampal region in paired-associate learning. *Current Directions in Psychological Science*, **4**, 19–23.

Fox, P. T., Perlmutter, J. S. and Raichle, M. E. (1985). A stereotactic method of anatomical localization for positron emission tomography. *Journal of Computer Assisted Tomography*, **9**, 141–53.

Gaffan, D. and Harrison, S. (1989). Place memory and scene memory: effects of fornix transection in the monkey. *Experimental Brain Research*, **74**, 202–12.

Gaffan, D. and Saunders, R. C. (1985). Running recognition of configural stimuli by fornix-transected monkeys. *Quarterly Journal of Experimental Psychology*, **37**B, 61–71.

Ghaem, O., Mellet, E., Crivello, F., Tzourio, N., Mazoyer, B., Berthoz, A. *et al.* (1997). Mental navigation along memorized routes activates the hippocampus, precuneus, and insula. *Neuroreport*, **8**, 739–44.

Gluck, M. A. and Meyer, C. A. (1995). Representation and association in memory: a neurocomputational view of hippocampal function. *Current Directions in Psychological Science*, **4**, 23–9.

Kimura, D. (1963). Right temporal-lobe damage. *Archives of Neurology*, **8**, 264–71.

Maguire, E. A., Frackowiak, R. S. J. and Frith, C. D. (1996). Learning to find your way: a role for the human hippocampal formation. *Proceedings of the Royal Society of London, B*, **263**, 1745–50.

Milner, B. (1965). Visually-guided maze-learning in man: effects of bilateral hippo-campal, bilateral frontal and unilateral cerebral lesions. *Neuropsychologia*, **3**, 317–38.

Milner, B. (1968). Visual recognition and recall after right temporal-lobe excision in man. *Neuropsychologia*, **6**, 191–209.

Morris, R. G. M., Garrud, P., Rawlins, J. N. P. and O'Keefe, J. (1982). Place navigation impaired in rats with hippocampal lesions. *Nature*, **297**, 681–3.

Moscovitch, M., Kapur, S., Köhler, S. and Houle, S. (1995). Distinct neural correlates of visual long-term memory for spatial location and object identity: a positron emission tomography study in humans. *Proceedings of the National Academy of Sciences, USA*, **92**, 3721–5.

Murray, E. A. and Gaffan, D. (1993). Effects of lesions of rhinal cortex, hippocampus, or parahippocampus gyrus in rhesus monkeys on object and spatial reversals. *Society for Neuroscience Abstracts*, **19**, 438.

O'Keefe, J. and Nadel, L. (1978). *The Hippocampus as a Cognitive Map*. Clarendon Press, Oxford.

Owen, A. M., Milner, B., Petrides, M. and Evans, A. C. (1996). A specific role for the right parahippocampal gyrus in the retrieval of object-location: a positron emission tomography study. *Journal of Cognitive Neuroscience*, **8**, 588–602.

Parkinson, J. K., Murray, E. A. and Mishkin, M. (1988). A selective mnemonic role for the hippocampus in monkeys: memory for the location of objects. *Journal of Neuroscience*, **8**, 4159–67.

Petrides, M. (1985). Deficits on conditional associative-learning tasks after frontal- and temporal-lobe lesions in man. *Neuropsychologia*, **23**, 601–14.

Pigott, S. and Milner, B. (1993). Memory for different aspects of complex visual scenes after unilateral temporal- or frontal-lobe resection. *Neuropsychologia*, **31**, 1–15.

Quirk, G. J., Muller, R. U., Kubie, J. L. and Ranck, J. B. (1992). The positional firing properties of medial entorhinal neurons: description and comparison with hippocampal place cells. *Journal of Neuroscience*, **12**, 1945–63.

Raichle, J. E., Martin, W. R. W., Herscovitch, P., Mintum, M. A. and Markham, J. (1983). Brain blood flow measured with intravenous $H_2{}^{15}O$. II. implementation and validation. *Journal of Nuclear Medicine*, **24**, 790–8.

Rains, G. D. and Milner, B. (1994). Right-hippocampal contralateral-hand effect in the recall of spatial location in the tactual modality. *Neuropsychologia*, **32**, 1233–42.

Rolls, E. T., Miyashita, Y., Cahusac, P. M. B., Kesner, R. P., Niki, H., Feigenbaum, J. D. and Bach, L. (1989). Hippocampal neurons in the monkey with activity related to the place in which a stimulus is shown. *Journal of Neuroscience*, **9**, 1835–45.

Smith, M. L. and Milner, B. (1981). The role of the right hippocampus in the recall of spatial location *Neuropsychologia*, **19**, 781–93.

Smith, M. L. and Milner, B. (1984). Differential effects of frontal-lobe lesions on cognitive estimation and spatial memory. *Neuropsychologia*, **22**, 697–705.

Smith, M. L. and Milner, B. (1989). Right hippocampal impairment in the recall of spatial location: encoding deficit or rapid forgetting? *Neuropsychologia*, **27**, 71–81.

Suzuki, W. E., Miller, E. K. and Desimone, R. (1995). Object and place memory in the monkey entorhinal cortex. *Society for Neuroscience Abstracts*, **15**, 10.

Talairach, J. and Tournoux, P. (1988). *Co-planar Stereotactic Atlas of the Human Brain: 3-Dimensional Proportional System: an Approach to Cerebral Imaging*, Georg Thieme Verlag, Stuttgart and New York.

Ungerleider, L. G. and Mishkin, M. (1982). Two cortical visual systems. In *Analysis of Visual Behavior*, (ed., D. J. Ingle, M. A. Goodale and R. J. W. Mansfield), pp. 549–86. MIT Press.

Van Hoesen, G. W. (1982). The parahippocampal gyrus: new observations regarding its cortical connections in the monkey. *Trends in Neuroscience*, **5**, 345–50.

Worsley, K. J., Evans, A. C., Marrett, S. and Neelin, P. (1992). Determining the number of statistically significant areas of activation in subtracted activation studies from PET. *Journal of Cerebral Blood Flow and Metabolism*, **12**, 900–18.

14

The hippocampus and spatial memory in humans

Robin G. Morris, Julia A. Nunn, Sharon Abrahams, Janet D. Feigenbaum and Michael Recce

14.1 Introduction

In common with many other species, human subjects determine their spatial orientation in novel environments and are able to do this using a combination of directional cues and establishing a cognitive representation of their spatial domain (Gallistel 1990). It is fair to say that the neuronal structures or mechanisms that support these processes have not been investigated extensively in humans to date; the main developments in this area relate to studies of rodents and non-human primates. The purpose of this chapter is to review a series of recent investigations that we have conducted into spatial memory in humans with focal temporal lobe lesions, all involving the hippocampus. Such studies have had the primary aim of elucidating the pattern of memory function through the development of novel paradigms and relating spatial memory impairment to structural brain lesions.

The hypothesis that the hippocampus is responsible for spatial memory has strong support across different species of animals. For example, in rodents, bilateral lesions of the hippocampus produce pronounced deficits in spatial working memory, investigated using a variety of paradigms (e.g. Morris *et al.* 1982; Olton *et al.* 1978). The additional demonstration of place cells within the hippocampus by O'Keefe (1976) provides very convincing evidence for the physiological basis of spatial mnemonic processing, with the more recent demonstration that these can be recorded in a simultaneous multiple fashion (Wilson and McNaughton 1993). Likewise, in non-human primates, deficits following hippocampectomy on spatial delayed response tasks have been observed, provided long delays are used or the memory load is increased by testing for more than one spatial location simultaneously (Angeli *et al.* 1993; Zola-Morgan and Squire 1985). Furthermore, electrophysiological recordings in primates have shown neurones that respond differentially to spatial stimuli or the place in which stimuli are presented, irrespective of the orientation of the animal, suggesting an allocentric representation of the spatial domain (Feigenbaum and Rolls 1991; Rolls, 1996).

Such findings have led to the notion that there is a physiologically distinct system that integrates the memory of spatial locations into a single representation, the so-called cognitive mapping hypothesis (O'Keefe and Nadel 1978). The mapping system, dependent on the hippocampus, enables a 'viewer independent' or allocentric representation of the environment, coding distances and directions. The subsequent elucidation of the properties of place cells, combined with computational modelling, has led to further developments of this theory (Burgess and O'Keefe 1996; O'Keefe 1991; O'Keefe and Burgess 1996). Others, however, have argued against a specific system suggesting that the hippocampus acts as multimodal store for declarative memory, having a general role in forming associative links utilising neural network neuronal architecture. For example, this includes Marr's (1969, 1971) proposal of the early auto-associative memory model, adapted by Treves and Rolls (1994), by McNaughton and Nadel (1990), and, more recently Harris and Recce (1996).

In humans, there is evidence for a specialized system in so much as visuo-spatial memory impairment is associated with damage to the right hippocampal formation. This is independent of deficits in visuospatial perceptual or manipulation abilities and has been observed across a range of tasks. The main patient group that has been used to establish this finding consists of those who have undergone unilateral temporal lobectomies (TL), an operation used to treat patients with intractable epilepsy, which involves removal of the anterior temporal lobe and amydgala, and varying amounts of the hippocampus (see below). Patients with left temporal lobectomies are impaired on tasks requiring verbal memory and learning (Corsi 1972; Petrides 1985; Smith and Milner 1981), whilst those with right TL are impaired in their memory for items that are difficult to verbalize, including visuospatial material (Corkin 1965; Jones-Gotman 1986; Milner 1967, 1968; reviewed also in Smith 1989). In humans, the challenge has been to dissociate cognitively different aspects of mnemonic function, for example, the visual or pattern recognition aspect from the spatial, and also to take into account the mental various strategies brought to bear in 'solving' a spatial memory task. However, one difficulty is that, whilst studying patients with focal lesions is a powerful method for localization of function, experimental control of the lesion is denied to the research, which relies on the outcome of brain damage or surgical procedure.

14.2 The substrate for neuropsychological study

Many investigations of visuospatial memory in patients with unilateral temporal lobectomies have been conducted on patients at the Montreal Neurological Institute (MNI). In such studies, the patients were subdivided into groups according to the size of hippocampal removal; the size was based on the surgeon's drawings and the report of the operation. The hippocampal lesion is classed as 'small' if the hippocampus is spared entirely, or if removal does not extend beyond the pes (the anterior region). The 'large' operation involves removal beyond the pes into the main body of the hippocampus or the corresponding part of the hippocampal gyrus. Several studies conducted in Montreal have shown that the level of spatial memory impairment in right TL patients is dependent on whether the large operation was performed, including, for example, recall of spatial location, maze learning and recall of designs (Jones-Gotman 1986; Smith and Milner 1981, 1989).

The Maudsley/King's Neuroscience Centre *en bloc* resection, used on the patients included in the studies described below, are closer to the Montreal 'large operation'. This operation, described by Polkey (1987) involves removal of between 5.5 cm and 6.5 cm of temporal lobe tissue from the anterior pole in the posterior direction, with relative sparing of the superior temporal gyrus in the language dominant hemisphere. Additionally, the amygala and approximately the anterior 2 cm of the hippocampus are removed.

The extent of the operation is shown in Figs 14.1 and 14.2, investigated using a post-operative Magnetic Resonance Imaging (MRI) scan. This shows the complete removal of the anterior temporal lobe, with perirhinal and entorhinal cortices non-existent on the operated side. The parahippocampal gyrus is shown to be present, but only towards the posterior hippocampal region, as shown in the series of MRI slices in Fig. 14.1. Recently, Nunn, Morris and colleagues have applied a lesion analysis to a cohort of 19 left and 19 right TL patients (Graydon *et al.* in preparation). The brain was scanned using 1.5 mm contiguous slices, with the analysis conducted on the temporal lobe from the temporal pole to the posterior limit of the hippocampus. The temporal lobe was segmented into four regions using a radial division technique, as shown in Fig. 14.2; namely, Superiorlateral (SL), Inferolateral (IL), Basal (B) and Mesiotemporal (MT). The latter was rated separately for parahippocampal gyrus and hippocampus. These five regions were rated by eye according to the intactness of the regions or structures for each slice with a four-point scale varying from 'total resection/no tissue present' to 'intact/all tissue present'. An aggregate score was then computed for each region to assess the degree of preservation of tissue. This score was then correlated against psychometric measures of verbal and spatial memory functioning. The analysis revealed a significant correlation only between preservation of the hippocampus and visuospatial memory ($r^2 = 0.46$; $p < 0.05$), the latter measured using a delayed recall version of the Rey–Osterrieth complex figure test, in which a complex figure is copied and the drawn from memory after a 40-min delay (Visser 1980; cf Morris *et al.* 1995*a*) (verbal memory functioning, and intellectual measures, were not correlated with the brain scanning data).

In our study, the measurement technique exploited natural variations in the extent of removal within the same type of operation. Since this variation occurs with respect to removal of the posterior hippocampus, this may suggest additionally that the degree of damage to this region is related specifically to visuospatial memory function. Of note, this corresponds topographically to the dorsal hippocampus in rodents; parallels can be drawn between the two areas of research. In rodents, spatial learning impairment relates specifically to the

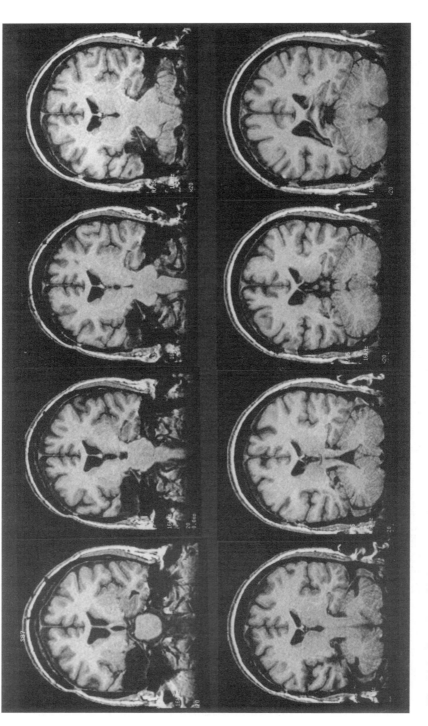

Fig. 14.1 Sequence of 1.5 mm coronal magnetic resonance imaging slices covering the hippocampal region. Every third slice is shown.

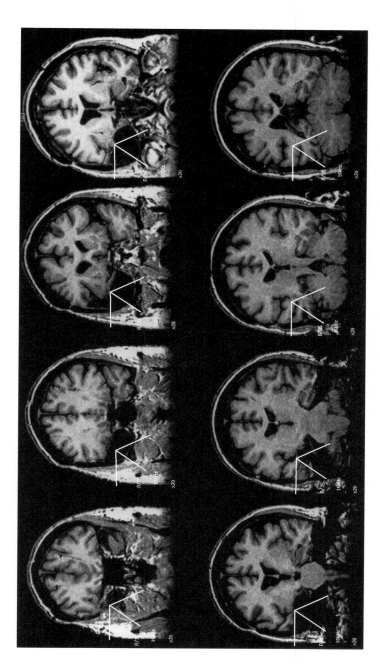

Fig. 14.2 Sequence of 1.5 mm coronal magnetic resonance imaging slices across the temporal lobe using the ANALYZE program to segment the structure into the different regions described in the text. The sequence shows every sixth slice. The radial segmentation is explained fully in the text: within the temporal lobe, and in the anticlockwise direction, there exists (1) the superiorlateral (temporal lobe above the horizontal line); (2) inferolateral; (3) basal and; (4) mesiotemporal segments (temporal lobe above the oblique line). The same radial segmentation was used across the temporal lobe to measure the intactness of structures. The mesiotemporal segment was split into parahippocampal and hippocampal regions by inspection. Note that the 'segmentation' is only applicable for the posterior slices, the areas where intactness was rated.

magnitude of dorsal hippocampal lesions, but is hardly present following ventral lesions (Moser *et al*. 1993). Additionally, ischaemic damage to the hippocampus using short-duration occlusion produces selective damage to the dorsal hippocampus in rodents and an associated substantial spatial impairment (Nunn and Hodges 1994; Nunn *et al*. 1994).

14.3 Investigation of spatial memory

Support for a specific impairment in spatial memory following the right TL has come from a series of studies that have investigated memory for place. For example, in what is now regarded as one of the main studies in this field, Smith and Milner (1981) required right and left TL patients to inspect 16 toy objects laid out on a blank piece of paper. The patients had to price the object and subsequently were tested both for their memory of the objects, using recall and recognition, and their memory of the spatial locations. Whilst both groups showed normal object name recall, only the right TL group were impaired on recall of location. This was observed after a 24-h delay and, moreover, the extent of deficit was contingent on there being a radical excision of the hippocampus (the 'large hippocampal excision'). Additional deficits in object name recall were found at this delay for both the left and right TL groups. Subsequent studies from the same centre have confirmed the spatial location deficit, for example, using filled delays (Smith and Milner 1989) or embedding the objects in scenes (Pigott and Milner 1993).

Spatial memory versus object memory

Such studies suggest that the right hippocampus supports spatial memory function, but may not have an exclusive role, because of the additional non-spatial memory deficits associated with the right TL. This raises the question as to whether purely spatial and other types of long-term memory can be dissociated, given that they have been shown to share the same regional substrate? According to a cognitive framework, the spatial memory might utilize the same neuronal structures, but exist as a separate system; if spatial memory exists neuronally as a broader class of declarative memory (Cohen and Eichenbaum 1993; Squire 1992), then the same physiological mechanisms would be invoked as well. One method of exploring dissociation, applied previously to amnesic patients, is the technique of titration. Either the delay between presentation of material and test or the exposure of the material is manipulated to equate patient and control performance on one type of memory, with simultaneous comparison on the other type of memory. In some studies with amnesic patients a disproportionate spatial memory impairment has been revealed in cases where non-spatial memory has been matched in this fashion (MacAndrew and Jones 1993; Shoqeirat and Mayes 1991).

Nunn *et al*. (1998*a*) have recently used this technique with an adaptation of the Smith and Milner paradigm (1981, 1989), first tried on amnesic patients by Cave and Squire (1991). This technique was further modified and involved presenting the 16 toys in a pseudo-random spatial array and then testing for object recall after the retention interval, followed by object recognition memory and then memory for location of the objects. Pre-testing had determined the delay needed to match each group approximately in terms of object recall or recognition. For the left TL patients this was 1 h, for the right TL 2 h and for the controls 3 h. This method of *temporal titration* revealed a large deficit in spatial memory in the right TL patients only. Because the patients included in this study were the same as those who had undergone the lesion analysis described above, comparisons with the extent of tissue removal could be made. For the right TL group, the extent of hippocampal resection was found to be inversely related to the extent of spatial memory functioning ($r^2 = -0.58$; $P < 0.05$).

This result, at least suggests that the right hippocampus may play a disproportionate role in spatial memory, in comparison to memory for objects. It confirms the exclusive involvement of the right hemisphere in spatial memory. However, the correlation with object name recall also indicates that it may share this function with memory for other types of material, in this case the names of objects.

Spatial versus visual memory

Object recall and recognition can be thought of as 'impure' tests of memory in relation to specific modalities, because of the possibility of 'dual encoding' in which memory traces are formed representing either the name (verbal) or the appearance (visual) of the object (Pavio 1971). If so, there may be separate explanations for the object recall deficits in left and right TL patients. Thus the left TL group might be impaired due to a verbal memory deficit, whilst the right due to a visual memory impairment.

A number of studies have shown that right TL patients are specifically impaired in visuospatial memory tasks that emphasize pattern recall or recognition rather than spatial relationships. This includes memory for faces (Milner 1968; Morris *et al*. 1995*a*; Rains 1981) and for complex designs (Jones-Gotman 1986) and photographs of doors (Morris *et al*. 1995*b*). In some of these, for example, faces or the doors from the Baddeley *et al*. (1994) 'Doors and People' test, the patient has to rely almost exclusively on visual 'pattern' to facilitate memory performance. This raises the possibility that the right hippocampus supports both 'visual' and 'spatial' memory functioning. The question is whether these aspects dissociate in the same way as object recall and spatial memory were observed to do in the study described above. The dissociation between these two types of memories may reflect a more fundamental neuroanatomical dissociation, arising in both human and non-human primates. Specifically, there is substantial evidence for a ventral or *occipito-temporal* pathway that specializes in object perception, contrasting with the *occipito-parietal* pathway that is involved in spatial perception and manipulation (Ungerleider and Mishkin 1982). These two routes have been dissociated behaviourally through lesion and electrophysiological studies in non-human primates (Gross 1973) and is mirrored in humans where temporal lobe deficits can give rise to impairments in object recognition, whilst parietal lobe damage results in difficulties with spatial manipulation (De Renzi 1982; Farah *et al.* 1988; Morris and Morton 1995).

Recently Nunn *et al.* (1998*b*) conducted an experiment addressing this question, based on the Smith and Milner (1981, 1989) memory for location paradigm. Instead of objects, eight abstract designs (taken from Jones-Gotman 1986) were placed in different locations within a 60-cm square piece of white paper (see Fig. 14.3). After a variable delay, the subjects had to draw the designs from memory (visual memory test) and distinguish them from individually matched distracter items (recognition). Left and right TL patients were included in this study, with the delay between presentation and test manipulated to match performance, in this case a 2-h delay for the Left TL patients and controls, and a delay of 1 h for the right TL patients. All groups were then tested on their memory of the spatial locations by requiring each subject to indicate the original position of the design and measuring deviation from the

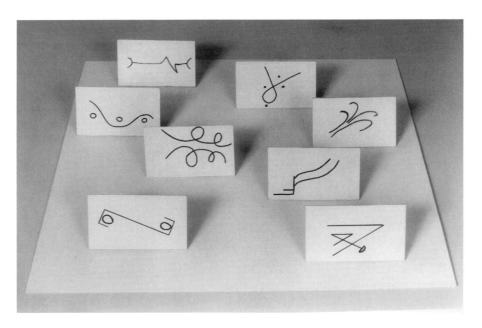

Fig. 14.3 The abstract designs using in the experiment by Nunn *et al.* (1998*b*). The subject has to remember the appearance of the patterns as well as their spatial location on the board.

true position. This revealed a specific impairment in the right TL group only, with a significantly lower level of spatial (but not visual) memory functioning in this group. In other words, by manipulating the retention interval, the spatial memory deficit in the right TL patients was shown to be dissociated from visual memory impairment. For the patients used in this study, MRI structural measurements were available in the manner described above, showing a significant correlation between preservation of hippocampus and spatial recall in only the right TL group. An additional correlation was found with parahippocampal preservation, but this applied also the left TL group as well.

Summary

In summary:

(1) Patients with right TL only have been shown to have spatial and visual memory deficits.

(2) The spatial memory impairment appears to dissociate from that related either to object recall or visual memory.

In both experiments described above, the degree of preservation of posterior hippocampus was significantly related to memory for location, reinforcing the notion of hippocampal involvement in spatial memory, perhaps operating as a separate system.

14.4 Human analogues of animal studies

An issue with animal experiments is the extent to which the results are directly applicable to humans, given the obvious differences in brain structure, but also because of the types of tests used to measure memory function. Many of the animal studies relating hippocampal lesions to spatial memory have used a spatial maze task originally developed by Olton (Olton *et al*. 1978). Here the animal has to traverse a number of runways that radiate out from a central platform, the radial arm maze. A main feature is that each of the arms are baited only once and the animal has to remember not to return to arms previously traversed in order to receive a food reward. Many versions of this test have been developed showing hippocampal lesion-induced impairments in rodents. Although the term 'working' memory has been used to characterize the type of memory function studied, the cognitive operations used to perform the task requires a capability that corresponds most closely to the long-term episodic aspect of declarative memory studied in humans.

The EXECUTIVE-GOLF task

Analogous tasks have been developed for humans, and variations of these form the basis for the remaining series of experiments described below. The first of these tests is illustrated in Fig. 14.4 and is now termed the EXECUTIVE-GOLF task. The subject is presented with the representation of a 'golf putting area' on the visual display unit (VDU) of a computer, fitted with a touch-sensitive screen. The display consists of a 'golfer' in the distance and a number

(a)

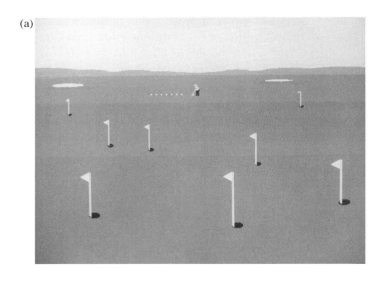

(b)

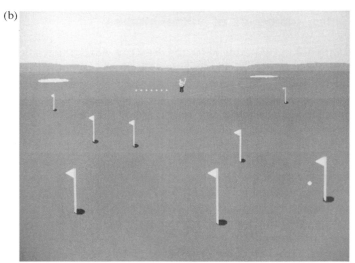

Fig. 14.4 The appearance of the EXECUTIVE-GOLF task on the VDU of the computer. To-be-remembered spatial locations are represented by the golf holes: (a) the arrangement prior to the first touch of the subject; (b) the arrangement when a correct touch has been made, with the ball 'flying' through the air to enter the correct hole.

of golf holes, representing the to-be-remembered spatial locations. The subject is instructed initially to discover which hole the golfer is planning to 'putt' the ball into. They search by touching each hole in turn until the pre-determined one is selected, at which point the golfer putts the ball. The subjects are then told that the golfer will never 'putt' into the same hole twice and they should search around for a further pre-determined location. This then continues until all the holes have been used, analogous to searching on the Olton maze in which the animal eventually visits all the baited arms. This task was administered to 20 left and 20 right TL patients with a further age and IQ matched control group.

The difficulty of the task can be varied by altering the number of holes, in this case using a series of trials with four, six or eight holes. The patient can make two types of errors, a *Within Search Error*, in which the subject returns to the same hole within a search; and a *Between Search Error* in which they return to a hole that was successful on a previous search. For *Within Search Errors* there were no significant differences between any of the groups. This result suggests that within a very short period of time and a limited number of locations to remember there is no reliance on hippocampal function, perhaps akin to a 'visuospatial scratchpad' memory system, in which a subject holds 'on line' small amounts of spatial information, with evidence that this system relies on support from other systems, such as prefrontal or parietal cortices (Miotto *et al.* 1996). The *Between Search Error* measure showed a different pattern, with a significant impairment in the right TL patients, but not the left, the level of impairment increasing with the memory difficulty.

This pattern of results mirrors those found using the spatial delayed response task in non-human primates. Here, short delays (approximately 10 s) do not seem to produce impairments in animals with bilateral hippocampectomies (Correll and Scoville 1967; Diamond *et al.* 1989), whilst long delays or using more than one location do produce an impairment (Angeli *et al.* 1993; Parkinson *et al.* 1988). In both cases, it is not clear whether the length of delay is the critical factor or whether it is the degree of visual distraction. For example, in the current task, the patient is distracted from remembering 'holes' that have been used by the process of subsequent searches; in the non-human primate studies, long delays increase the probability of distraction. One additional factor may be the added complexity of having multiple searches, in producing the *Between Search Errors*. This may be akin to the added complexity caused by requiring more than one spatial location to be remembered on the modified delayed response task developed by Angeli *et al.* (1993), which also showed impairments associated with hippocampectomized monkeys.

One feature of this task is the possibility for subjects to develop specific strategies to help avoid going back to previously used holes. The main strategy was to always start the search with a particular location, switching only when this location was successfull, and can be measured by counting the number of different starting locations used in a series of searches. Neither TL group showed a deficit in strategy formation, suggesting that this factor could not account for the spatial memory deficit in the right TL group. In contrast, other patient groups, for example, those with prefrontal cortical lesions, have shown strategy formation deficits that account for a significant proportion of their deficit on this task (see Fig. 14.5 for an illustration of this deficit) (Miotto *et al*. 1996).

Allocentric spatial memory

One feature of the above task is that a 'three-dimensional space' is created by the computer program; the subject 'sees' the spatial array in three dimensions. Nevertheless, the space is viewed only from a single vantage point and so emphasizes egocentric or viewer-dependent spatial processing and memory. It also increases the likelihood of the patient forming a 'snapshot' memory for

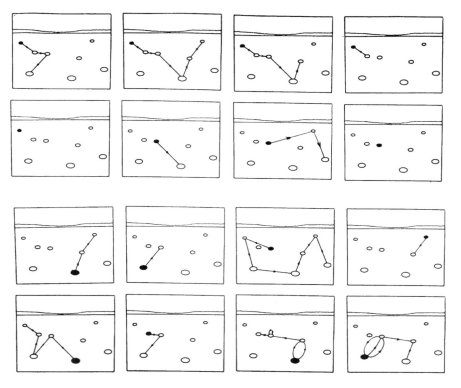

Fig. 14.5 Illustration of the strategy used by patients on the EXECUTIVE-GOLF task. The patient starts the search path using the same location until this becomes the target. They then switch to another starting location. The top set of frames shows an efficient use of this strategy. Patients with unilateral temporal lobectomies were not impaired on strategy formation; this contrasted with patients with right frontal neurosurgical lesions, as illustrated by the poor strategy used by one patient shown in the bottom frames (from Miotto *et al*. 1996).

each relevant configuration. In most animal tasks, the subject is immersed in the spatial domain. For example, in the Olton maze, the animal moves within a spatial environment, whilst the geometric relations between locations is invariant, the view changes continously. A central feature of such a task is that it facilitates the formation of an allocentric memory representation, as envisaged in theories concerning cognitive mapping (O'Keefe and Nadel 1978). In order to incorporate this feature into the task above, a second task was developed, termed the Rotating Spatial Memory task (ROTATE; Feigenbaum *et al.* 1996).

The layout for this task is shown in Fig. 14.6. A large graphically represented 'disc' is shown in the centre of the VDU, with a number of locations on the upper surface of the disc. Just as in the previous task, the subject searches around the locations to find the target one. At this point, the disc 'rotates' with the locations also rotating around a central point. Thus, within the represented three dimensional space, the distance between the locations remain the same, whilst their position and inter-relationships differ on the VDU screen. The subject then searches for a new location, avoiding the one that has been successful before. In this task, the disc either rotates between 90° and 180° or rotates the equivalent distance and back again. In both cases, the number of *Within Search Errors* were minimal in all three groups, but the right TL group only were significantly impaired. Of note, the error rates were approximately equivalent to the EXECUTIVE-GOLF task. This finding, at first sight, might indicate that the allocentric encoding, encouraged in the subsequent ROTATE task, had no differential effect on performance. Alternatively, it is equally possible that allocentric encoding was used to a large extent in the EXECUTIVE-GOLF task, despite the fact that the viewpoint of the spatial array remained static. In support of this, the spatial display was constructed using a perspective drawing, which may have cued the patient to use an allocentric representation.

Allocentric memory in a real 3-D environment

A potential confound with the task described above is that, even though it is represented three-dimensionally, the subjects may solve the task using an egocentric framework, either by mentally rotating the image observed or by imagining themselves rotated with respect to the image (cf. Taube 1996). The patients use in studies we describe in this chapter are unimpaired in their mental rotation abilities. This was investigated using the Flags test for those individuals in the Feigenbaum *et al.* (1996) study. This test involves inspecting an exemplar flag in the normal plane and then deciding which, out of a series of rotated flags, matches the exemplar. Neither left or right TL groups were impaired on this task. We have also recently tested a further cohort of 20 left and 20 right TL patients on the Shepard and Metzler test (1971; involving matching representations of 3-D objects constructed by cuboid shapes) and the Ratcliffe 'little man test' (which requires the subject to decide in which hand a

(a)

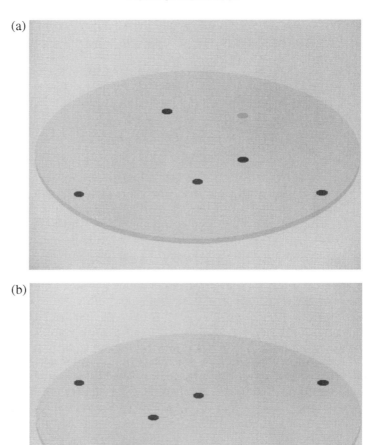

(b)

Fig. 14.6 The appearance of the ROTATE task on the VDU: (a) the initial arrangements of the spatial locations – the correct location turns from black to green temporarily
when touched (in this reproduction, the lighter shaded location); (b) these rotated
through 180° after the patient has discovered a correct location and is about to search
for another.

drawn manikin is holding a ball; the manikin can be facing towards or away,
be in the upright or downward facing position). No deficits were observed on
any of these tasks (Morris *et al.* in preparation).

However, remembering spatial locations on a VDU, in which the subject
remains static, may make rather different processing demands than when a

subject is moving around an environment. The spatial memory system may have developed to integrate whole body motion and spatial representation, as indicated by work with animals (Burgess and O'Keefe 1996). Accordingly, an allocentric spatial memory task was designed, sharing some of the same features of the Olton maze and also designed to test whether a putative spatial memory deficit could be dissociated from a more general impairment in episodic memory.

As indicated above, several theorists have suggested that spatial memory is not represented by a differentiated system, but the specialized *use* of an episodic memory system and, indeed, it is possible to model the involvement of the hippocampus in memory in the same way that a general system accounts for spatial memory (McClelland and Goddard 1996). This point has long been reflected in the 'working memory' model of hippocampal function, proposed by Olton *et al.* (1979), in which structures support the maintenance and manipulation of information that is pertinent to the present situation. This definition, developed to describe rodent memory, is very close to the notion of episodic memory, part of the declarative memory system described in humans (Squire 1992). It contrasts with information that is not dependent on the situation, and remains invariant across time. In terms of the radial arm maze, the distinction is between the memory requirements when different arms are baited between trials (Working) and when the same arms are baited (Reference).

In a study by Abrahams *et al.* (1997), we set out to distinguish between spatial mapping and working memory theories in humans, producing a human analogue of the rodent task designed by Jarrard and colleagues (Jarrard 1986). This task was again structurally analogous to the radial arm maze, as shown in Fig. 14.7, and now termed the BIN task. The subject is presented with an array of nine 'bins' arranged in a circle on a flat table top. In each trial, the experimenter places four objects in four of the bins, covering them up with the lids. The subject then has to walk slowly round the table and is distracted until a full minute has passed. They then have to point out the bins that have been filled with objects and also detect which objects have been hidden when shown an array of pictures of the objects mixed in with alternative ones. Thus, a feature of the design is that memory for the location is tested independently of recognition memory for the objects. To create the Working versus Reference comparison, two of the 'bins' are always used as locations across trials (Reference Locations), whilst two are constantly changed between trials (Working Memory). The same is true for the object, but independent of the locations used (creating Object Reference versus Object Working memory conditions). In summary, the task was structurally analogous to the Olton maze, and employing four main elements on a two factorial basis; spatial ('bin' location) and non-spatial (object) reference and working memory.

In this study a further group of patients with unilateral lesions specific to the hippocampal formation were included. These were pre-operative temporal lobe epilepsy patients who had epileptic foci emanating from the unilaterally damaged hippocampi, termed mesiotemporal lobe sclerosis (MTS) (in this

(a) (b)

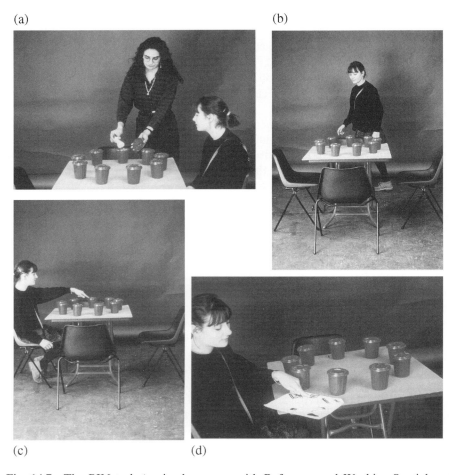

(c) (d)

Fig. 14.7 The BIN task (a nine-box maze with Reference and Working Spatial and Object memory test). (a) The experimenter (Dr. Sharon Abrahams) selects four to-be-remembered objects and hides them in four to-be-remembered containers. (b) The patient changes position relative to the apparatus, by moving to one of three other positions between the presentation and memory phases. (c) The patient points to the four previously selected containers (each of which has a hidden object). (d) The patient is presented with an object recognition picture booklet and points to the four hidden items.

case termed either left or right temporal lobe epilepsy patients; respectively, LTLE and RTLE). Post-operative pathology in such patients reveals atrophy and neuronal loss restricted to the hippocampal formation, the amygdala and uncus region (Babb and Brown 1987; Bruton 1988). The resulting four groups (14 LTLE; 16 RTLE; 24 left TL and 23 right TL) were compared to a matched control group.

The results from the study are shown in Fig. 14.8, expressed in terms of the number of errors made on each test. This shows a very consistent deficit in both the RTLE and right TL groups on both the Working and Reference Spatial Memory tasks. In other words, only those patients with right-sided pathology were impaired on spatial memory, but whether the locations varied between trials or remained same did not affect the overall pattern. With the Object Memory task, all four groups of patients were impaired, but only on the reference memory component.

This general pattern has since been replicated on a larger group of temporal lobe epilepsy patients (25 LTLE; 25 RTLE) (Abrahams *et al.* in press).

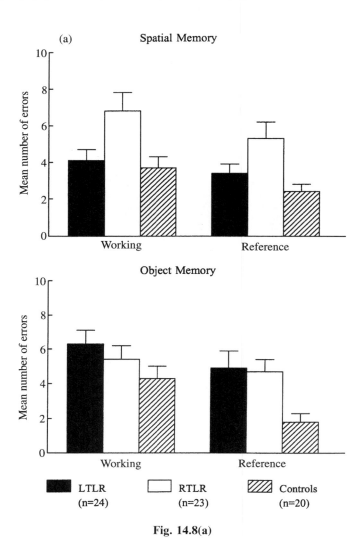

Fig. 14.8(a)

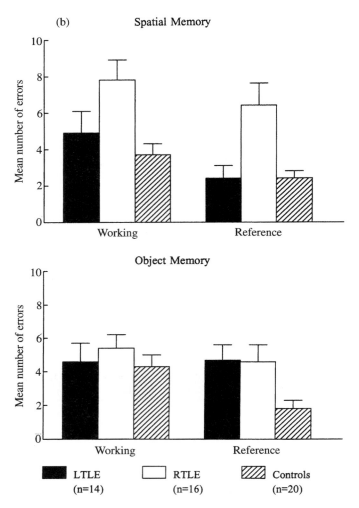

Fig. 14.8 (a) Temporal lobe resection groups (TLR). (*Above*) Performance on the two Spatial Memory components of the nine-box maze. (*Below*) Performance on the two Object Memory components of the task. Mean errors (summed over four trials) and standard error bars. (b) Temporal lobe epilepsy (TLE) group. (See (a) for details.)

The larger sample size enabled us also to explore whether the spatial working memory impairment was stable across trials. If the deficit was related to an impairment in encoding the context of the spatial locations, as could be predicted from the Olton *et al.* working memory theory, the impairment would increase each time the patient had to remember a new combination of spatial locations, with differential proactive interference from previous trials.

The study showed that there was no differential proactive interference effect, when comparing early (trials 1 and 2) to late trials (3 and 4) in the test. This adds further weight to the notion of a fixed spatial memory deficit, rather than one indirectly caused by difficulties in encoding context.

Additionally, a subgroup of this larger group were scanned using structural magnetic resonance imaging, with a volumetric analysis of the hippocampus, parahippocampal gyrus and remainder of temporal lobe (Abrahams *et al.* in press; see Fig. 14.9). The volumetric analysis involved delineating these regions across different coronal slices through the temporal lobes and then adding up the areas within the region to produce an estimate of volume. The volumetric analysis not only differentiated the two groups of patients (LTLE and RTLE), but significantly predicted the spatial memory deficit in those with reduced right hippocampal volume. In contrast, the volumetric analysis did not predict object memory impairment in either patient group.

Various conclusions can be drawn from these studies. First, the finding that the same pattern of deficit exists irrespective of whether the measure was working or reference memory and not related to proactive interference effects is evidence against the hippocampus being involved specifically in working memory. Perhaps the distinction between working and reference memory systems does not hold up for humans, as is also the case according to studies of rodents by Jarrard (1993). Second, the focal spatial memory deficit in the RTLE and right TL patients suggests the presence of a specialized spatial memory system, or at least, strong lateralization within the hemisphere non-dominant for language functioning. The LTLE and left TL patients showed no hint of an impairment suggesting that the lateralization is very pronounced. Third, the spatial memory deficit appears to dissociate from the object recognition memory deficit neuronally, since in the LTLE and left TL patients such a deficit was found in the absence of a spatial memory impairment. This deficit, not found in the working memory condition, may reflect the fact that the subjects were equally able to rehearse two items in memory temporarily, but the patient groups failed to learn the two permanent items and thus reduce their error score down to the control level.

14.5 Exploring allocentric memory using virtual reality

Whilst the design of the BIN task makes a mental rotation strategy much less likely, and 'involves' the subject in 3-D space, there is no way to ensure that other visual features or cues are not used to help remember the location of the hidden objects. In table-top or VDU presented tasks there is the opportunity for the subject to link spatial locations to non-specific cues in the environment. We used an immersive virtual reality system to control the visual input that the patient received. There were no directional cues, such as features in the room or the experimenter, since these were hidden from the patients. The visual input was provided by a head-mounted display and a Polhemus FasTrak

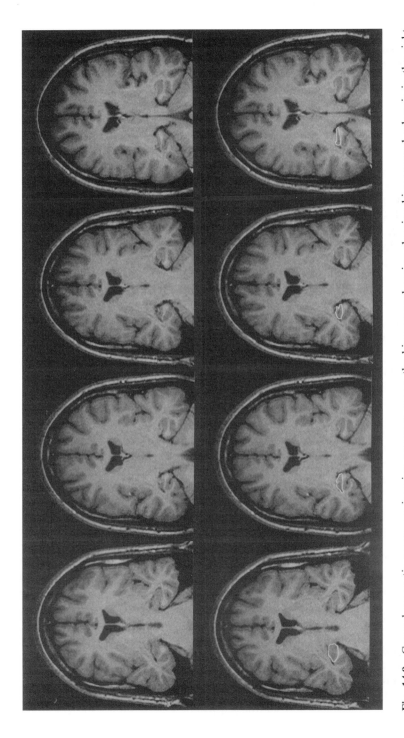

Fig. 14.9 Coronal magnetic resonance imaging sequence across the hippocampal region showing hippocampal sclerosis in the right hippocamus (top row in this picture) (1.5 tesla MRI with 5 mm slice thickness). The bottom row sequence illustrates the technique of tracing round the hippocampus using ANALYZE to obtain structural measurements. Additional measurements of the parahippocampal gyrus and rest of the temporal lobe were taken but are not illustrated here.

sensor was used to track the position and orientation of the subject's head. The World Tool Kit software package was used to construct the virtual environment and to maintain the appropriate image within the head mounted display. A virtual room was constructed in which the patient would perform the memory test, termed the *SHELL task* (Recce and Morris in prep.).

Figure 14.10 shows the layout for the *SHELL task* in which the patient is positioned in an artificial room (the Virtual Room; 2 × 2 m) with a central table (The Virtual Table). Around the rim of the table are arranged a number of 'shells'. The task is to walk round the Virtual Table, and to choose and look under the radially arranged shells until a blue cube is found. To inspect each shell, the subjects walks in front of it and instructs the examiner to 'lift' the shell. The lifting process is initiated by the experimenter using the keyboard (see Fig. 14.11). Each 'game' is composed of searches, and there are as many searches as there are shells. As in the EXECUTIVE-GOLF task the subject has to avoid lifting shells that have hidden the blue cube in a prior round of this game. The patient continues until the cube has been found under each of the shells. In order to prohibit the subject from using a simple search strategy,

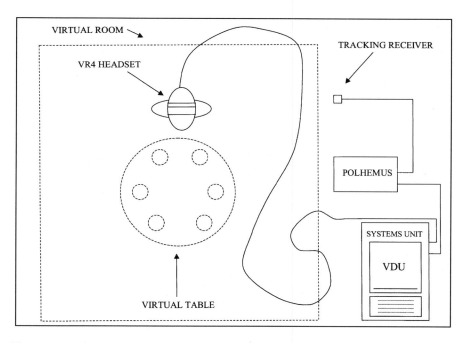

Fig. 14.10 The set-up for the Virtual Reality Shell Task. The Virtual Room is represented by the dashed lines, with the Virtual Table in the centre. The experiment is controlled through a microcomputer, which is connected to a receiver in order to track head position and the VR4 headset. The patient walks around the 'real room' whilst inside the Virtual Room.

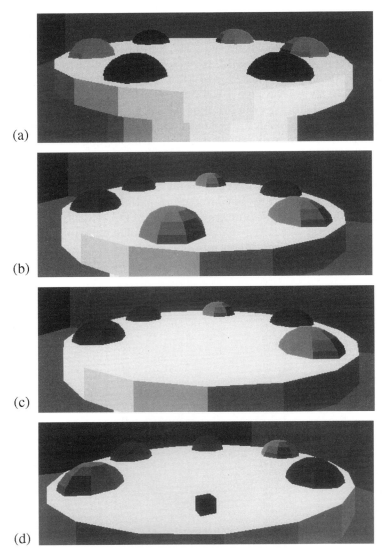

(a)

(b)

(c)

(d)

Fig. 14.11 A sequence of views for the patient through the VR4 headset. (a) The view when starting on a six-shell version of the task. The subject must choose which shell to 'try' but is limited in each search to those colour-coded green (in this black and white picture the shells are shaded more lightly). (b) The subject walks around the Virtual Table and stands in front of a shell in order to 'lift' it. (c) On lifting the shell, the subject sees that there is nothing underneath it and then will continue the search. (d) The subject moves to the right and lifts the next shell. This time a cube appears, signalling a successful search.

the subject can only lift a subset of the shells in any particular round. The shells that can be lifted are coloured green and those that cannot be lifted are coloured red (more lightly shaded in the black and white reproduction shown here).

Figure 14.11 shows an example layout and the different views of an individual subject traversing around the room to inspect a 'successful' shell. As previously, the task continues until the blue cube has been found in all locations. After two practice trials each subject was tested in four 'games' with four shells (4A, 4B, 4C and 4D) and three with six shells (6A, 6B, and 6C). For the four-shell task, only two shells can be inspected in any one search, whilst for the six shell game, three shells can be inspected. For each game, whilst the same shells were used at each level, the order of the 'correct' shells was different.

Altogether, 54 subjects were tested in the SHELL task, including 17 right TL patients, 19 left TL patients and 18 age and IQ score matched control subjects. One subject, a right TL patient, participated only in the four-shell variant of the task. The results for right and left TL groups versus controls are shown in Fig. 14.12. The performance is also compared to that computed if the subject searched at random.[1]

The last four-shell game (4C) was designed to check the subject's ability to follow the instructions, with the search paths deliberately set to minimize the possibility of error. In each round of this game one of the choices was always

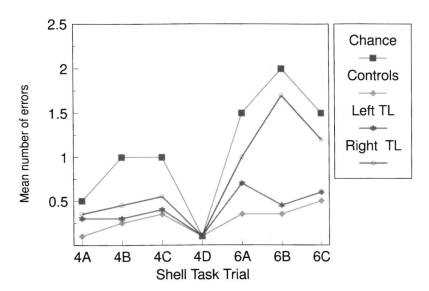

Fig. 14.12 Graph showing the performance of the three groups; left temporal lobectomy (left TL); right temporal lobectomy (right TL) and controls. Chance performance is given also for comparison (the chance performance level is based on an assumption outlined in the text). Data is given for each trial (Shell Games 4A to 6C).

the shell in which the blue cube had just been found. The results indicate that the subjects had no difficulties.

With four shells, the error rate is relatively low and the task does not discriminate between the groups. This was followed by the more demanding six-shell games, which clearly show a consistent deficit emerging in the right TL group. When the total score for the level 6 is considered, only the right TL patients show a significant impairment. By manipulating the target locations at level 6, it was also possible to differentiate between procedural mnemonic ability, as illustrated in Fig. 14.13 (Trial 6A) relating to the first level 6 problem (6A). For the first five searches, the memory load is low because the structure of the task provides a strong cue as to which shell to inspect. For example, on the second search, the next obvious shell is the one anticlockwise to the previously successful one. Up to the fifth search, the majority of all three groups (11 controls; 10 left TL; 12 right TL) chose exactly the same search paths as shown in Fig. 14.12), illustrating an approximate equal propensity to select the optimal sequence of moves. However, on the sixth search, the correct shell is not clearly guided by the structure of the task and the subject must pass at least one incorrect shell in order to reach the target. This point produced mnemonic errors, with at least one error made by three of the controls, five left TL and nine right TL patients.

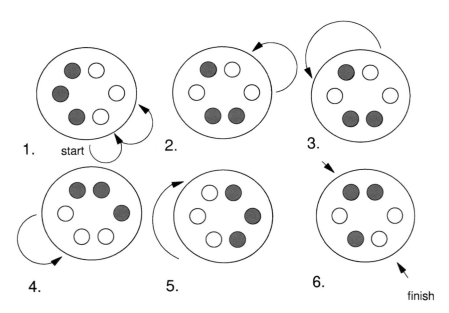

Fig. 14.13 Illustration of the strategy used by each patient on SHELL test 6A (see text for explanation). The shells colour-coded red are represented by *shaded circles*. The colour-coded green shells are represented by *open circles*. The arrows represent the paths of the patient as they search the shells.

In summary, this allocentric VR task revealed a selective deficit in the right TL group that is not easily accounted for by a mental rotation strategy or the patients having special difficulty in following the task procedure. Further development of this technique would enable the interaction between cue guidance and spatial mapping to be explored with more rigorous experimental control than is possible outside of the VR environment. Additionally, the virtual environments could be constructed with much larger spaces (e.g. a virtual park or field) that could be used to simulate the spatial orientation requirements in real life. In this way, spatial mapping could be explored in humans in 'naturalistic' settings, using longer time periods.

14.6 Discussion

Following on from previous investigations, there is ample evidence that the right temporal lobe is involved in spatial memory. This information has been gained largely from studying patients who have undergone unilateral temporal lobectomies (Smith 1989). The neurosurgical lesion, however, is very large and this makes it much more difficult to differentiate the critical structures in the same fashion as recent rodent or non-human primate studies. There are also severe clinical limitations on electrophysiological recording directly from mesiotemporal structures using extracellular electrodes, which have prevented developments in this field.

The studies conducted at the MNI suggest that 'large' right operations can cause more spatial memory impairment than those that are small, the distinction being based on whether the hippocampus had been spared completely or removal had not exceeded the pes. The difference in amount of tissue removed is not confined to the hippocampus, with the adjacent parahippocampal gyrus involved as well. In each case, however, the regions corresponding to the entorhinal and perirhinal cortex are removed. Likewise in the Maudsley/King's Neuroscience centre, variations in hippocampal removal associated with the *en bloc* resection will necessarily correlate with the amount of removal of the parahippocampal gyrus and the remaining temporal cortex. Despite this, the specific correlation between hippocampal removal and spatial memory impairment in the right TL group in the studies by Nunn *et al.* (1997*a,b*) are at least consistent with a more important role for the hippocampus.

Another approach, illustrated by the recent study by Abrahams *et al.* (in press) has been to investigate pre-operative temporal lobe epilepsy with hippocampal sclerosis. Measurement of the hippocampus, the parahippocampal gyrus and the ipsilateral temporal lobe could potentially provide a clue as to the relevant structure involved in spatial memory. In this case, hippocampal volume was shown to be clearly selectively reduced in patients with right epileptic foci. An additional point was that the extent of spatial memory deficit in these patients was as great as in those who had undergone unilateral temporal lobectomy. By inference, this might suggest that the additional removal of neocortex does not add anything by way of deficit and so again points towards the hippocampus as being the important structure. This is not quite so clear-cut because the status of the rest of temporal lobe in these patients may be suspect, magnetic resonance imaging structural measurements not reflecting more generalized changes in function across the lobe (mirroring a similar problem in studies of bilateral hippocampal damage due to anoxic brain injury). Despite this, in histopathological studies of patients with mesiotemporal lobe sclerosis (MTS), lesions tend to be restricted to the hippocampus and/or the amygdala (Bruton 1988). The most prominent areas of MTS tend to be CA1, CA3, CA4 regions of the hippocampus, the subiculum-prosubiculum and the fascia dentata (Babb and Brown 1987; Margerison and Corsellis 1966). The complications of concurrent intractible epilepsy should also be considered in this group, which may result in generalized memory and attentional impairment. Nevertheless, the presence of a selective deficit in the right temporal lobe epilepsy group and no deficit in the left group would argue against the non-specific cause for impairment.

Such observations can be compared to studies using non-human primates, which implicate the parahippocampal and perirhinal cortices in memory. For example, lesions of these latter regions, but sparing the hippocampus and amygdala, produce severe memory dysfunction (see Mishkin and Murray 1994; Murray 1996). In the LTLE patients the perirhinal cortex is intact and the parahippocampal gyrus shows much less neuronal damage than the hippocampus; but the unilateral temporal lobectomy removes both the perirhinal cortex and parahippocampal gyrus, without apparently increasing the degree of allocentric spatial memory impairment (Abrahams *et al.* in press). The critical role of the perirhinal cortex in primates thus is not necessarily supported in humans, although many further studies need to be conducted, for example, comparing patients pre- and post-operatively on such tests. Recently, Bohbot *et al.* (1997) have observed spatial memory deficits in patients with focal lesions in the right parahippocampal cortex. These were again neurosurgical lesions in patients with intractible epilepsy, so there is the possibility of additional hippocampal damage as well, complicating interpretation of this result.

The issue of localization in humans is greatly by helped by the advent of functional neuroimaging techniques (Maguire, Chapter 21), although these in turn have a different set of associated problems. If, for example, only a very small proportion of cells within a structure are active during spatial mapping, then this might not show up by measuring simply a haemodynamic response. If perfusion changes do occur, it is still not clear whether these reflect the mnemonic function of the brain tissue or are merely epiphenomena. It is likely that a combination of a functional neuroimaging approach and studying patients with specific brain lesions will be needed in the future to determine what are the critical structures involved.

The involvement of the right hippocampus in spatial memory in humans is inferred from these and previous studies. In humans, lateralization in the right hemisphere is consistent with the well known specialization of this hemisphere.

This finding prompts a further question as to whether lateralization of spatial memory is related to input into the system or the storage of spatial material. If spatial information arising from the product of right hemisphere processing can only enter the memory network predominately through the ipsilateral mesiotemporal lobe, then damage to this region would cause a deficit in spatial memory, irrespective of the site of final encoding. On the other hand, if the input was mainly bilateral, then spatial memory impairment would have to be caused by damaging the storage process directly and this would have to be lateralized in the right hemisphere. At the moment there are insufficient data to distinguish between the two possibilities, or whether lateralization of memory is caused by both mechanisms. One way of approaching this problem would be to investigate patients who have lesions cutting off the input to the right hippocampal formation; in this case if the deficit is in primary storage, there might not be a spatial memory impairment.

According to O'Keefe and Nadel's (1978) cognitive mapping hypothesis, in humans the right hippocampus specializes in the computation and storage of spatial information. This hypothesis, in its extreme form, has to be modified in the light of finding that right TL patients are impaired in their memories for other types of material, for example, object recognition and memory for faces. This suggests that the right hippocampal formation has a shared function, as has been argued in relation to the hippocampus in general in rodents (but on a bilateral basis) (Eichenbaum and Cohen 1992; Ono *et al*. 1991; Parkinson *et al*. 1988). Nevertheless, a consistent finding across the studies reviewed above is that the left TL patients are never impaired on spatial memory. Whilst the right hippocampal formation may not be exclusively involved in spatial memory, the latter is exclusively supported by the right hemisphere (see also Morris *et al*. 1996). A shared function could either indicate two systems using the same neuronal architecture or one system that can process different types of material. In humans, the dissociation between spatial and object memory (Nunn *et al*. 1998*a*) and between spatial and visual (Nunn *et al*. 1998*b*) may suggest in the first instance the former. The different types of memories at least show different accelerated rates of forgetting following brain lesions. Many computational models treat the hippocampus primarily as a memory system, but with the apparent specialization of the hippocampal system reflecting the computational characteristics (Gluck and Myers 1996; McClelland and Goddard 1996; Recce and Harris 1996; Treves and Rolls 1991). In relation to humans, such models would have to be constructed to predict differential forgetting rates across material specific memories in the context of a 'lesion' in the model.

The series of experiments described above progressed from those that required an egocentric representation (for example, the Nunn *et al*. (1998*a,b*) spatial locations tasks and the EXECUTIVE-GOLF task) to those that could be claimed to require predominately allocentric memory (the BIN and SHELL). This distinction was introduced because the spatial memory investigations in non-humans have focused on allocentric memory, with models such as the spatial mapping hypothesis specifically created in this context. This raises questions as to whether the spatial memory deficit observed in patients with mesiotemporal lobe lesions is any different, depending on whether an 'egocentric' or 'allocentric' task is used? A direct comparison, using 'egocentric' versus 'allocentric' as different conditions of the same task would help to answer this question. The patient samples across the different experiments described above overlap considerably, so some comparison can be made. Of note, the 'allocentric' tasks described above were more consistent in discriminating between the left and right TL group than the egocentric tasks, striking differences being observed using the BIN and SHELL tasks, in which the subject had to move around the spatial domain.

In summary, the findings are consistent with the general opinion expressed in many animal studies that proposed a large (but not exclusive) role of the hippocampus in spatial processing, but with the caveat of right lateralization. There may also be some indication of specialization in supporting allocentric memory, although more investigations in this area are needed. Perhaps virtual reality will provide the method for this type of exploration, where experimental control of the environment is much more rigorous that previously possible using 'real life' experimental methodology.

Endnotes

[1] 'Chance' was calculated with the assumption that the subject would not return to a shell just visited in any one search. In practice, this happened on three occasions only.

References

Abrahams, S., Pickering, A., Polkey, C. E. and Morris, R. G. (1997). Spatial memory deficits in patients with unilateral damage to the right hippocampal formation. Neuropsychologia, **35**, 11–24.

Abrahams, S., Pickering, A., Jarosz, J., Cox, T. and Morris, R. G. (In press). Spatial working memory impairment correlates with hippocampal sclerosis. *Brain and Cognition.*

Angeli, S. J., Murray, E. A. and Mishkin, M. (1993). Hippocampectomized monkeys can remember one place but not two. *Neuropsychologia*, **31**, 1021–30.

Babb, T. L. and Brown, W. J. (1987). Pathological findings in epilepsy. In *Surgical Treatment of the Epilepsies*, (ed., J. Engel Jr), pp. 511–40. Raven Press: New York.

Baddeley, A. D., Emslie, H. and Nimmo-Smith, I. (1994). *Doors and People: a Test of Visual and Verbal Recall and Recognition.* Bury St Edmunds, England: Thames Valley Test Company.

Bohbot, V., Kalina, M., Stepankova, J., Spackova, N., Petrides, M. and Nadel, N. (1997). Lesions to the right parahippocampal cortex cause navigational memory deficits in humans. *Neuroimage*, **5**(4), S626.

Brutton, C. J. (1988). *The Neuropathology of Temporal Lobe Epilepsy: Maudsley Monograph 31.* Oxford University Press, Oxford.

Burgess, N. and O'Keefe, J. (1996). Neuronal computations underlying the firing of place cells and their role in navigation. *Hippocampus*, **6**(6), 749–62.

Cave, C. B. and Squire, L. R. (1991). Equivalent impairment of spatial and nonspatial memory following damage to the human hippocampus. *Hippocampus*, **1**(3), 329–40.

Cohen, N. J. and Eichenbaum, H. (1993). Memory, amnesia and the hippocampal system. MIT press, Cambridge, MA.

Corkin, S. (1965). Tactually-guided maze learning in man: effects of unilateral and bilateral hippocampal lesions. *Neuropsychologia*, **3**, 339–51.

Correll, R. E. and Scoville, W. B. (1967). Significance of delay in the performance of monkeys with medial temporal lobe resection. *Experimental Brain Research*, **4**, 85–96.

Corsi, P. (1972). Human memory and the medial temporal region of the brain. Unpublished Ph.D. thesis, McGill University, Montreal.

De Renzi, E. (1982). *Disorder of Space Exploration and Cognition*. New York: Wiley.

Diamond, A., Zola-Morgan, S. and Squire, L. R. (1989). Successful performance by monkeys with lesions of the hippocampal formation on AB and object retrieval, two tasks that mark developmental changes in infant humans. *Behavioural Neurosciences*, **103**, 526–37.

Eichenbaum, H. O. and Cohen, N. J. (1992). The hippocampus: what does it do? *Behavioral and Neural Biology*, **57**(1), 2–36.

Falconer, M. A. (1971). In *Operative Surgery, Vol. 14*, (ed., V. Logue), pp. 142–9. Butterworths, London.

Farah, M. J., Hammond K. M., Levine, D. N. and Calvanio, R. (1988). Visual and spatial mental imagery: dissociable systems of representation. *Cognitive Psychology*, **20**, 439–92.

Feigenbaum, J. D., Polkey, C. E. and Morris, R. G. (1996). Deficits in spatial working memory after unilateral temporal lobectomy in man. *Neuropsychologia*, **34**, 163–76.

Feigenbaum, J. D. and Rolls, E. T. (1991). Allocentric and egocentric spatial information processing in the hippocampal formation of the behaving primate. *Psychobiology*, **19**(1), 21–40.

Gallistel, C. R. (1990). *The Organisation of Learning*. The MIT Press, Cambridge, UK.

Gluck, M. A. and Myers, C. E. (1996). Integrating behavioral and physiological models of hippocampal function. *Hippocampus*, **6**, 643–53.

Graydon, R., Nunn, J. and Morris, R. G. (in preparation). Lesion analysis of the unilateral temporal lobectomy and the relationship to memory function.

Gross, C. G. (1973) Visual functions of inferotemporal cortex. In *Handbook of Sensory Physiology, Vol. 7*, (ed., R. Jung), pp. 451–82. Springer-Verlag, Berlin.

Harris, K. D. and Recce, M. (1996). A biological simple thresholding strategy in an associative memory performs best. *Network: Computation in Neural Systems*, **7**, 741–56.

Jarrard, J. E. (1986). Selective hippocampal lesions and behaviour: implications for current research and theorizing. In *The Hippocampus, Vol. 4*, (ed., R. L. Isaacson and K. H. Pribram), pp. 93–126. Plenum, New York, NY.

Jarrard, J. E. (1993). On the role of the hippocampus in learning and memory in the rat. *Behavioral and Neural Biology*, **60**(1), 9–26.

Jones-Gotman, M. (1986). Memory for designs: the hippocampal contribution. *Neuropsychologia*, **24**, 193–203.

Margerison, J. H. and Corsellis, J. A. N. (1966). Epilepsy and the temporal lobes: a clinical electroencephalographic and neuropathological study of the brain in epilepsy with particular reference to the temporal lobes. *Brain*, **89**, 499–506.

Marr, D. (1969). Simple memory: a theory for archicortex. *Proceedings of the Royal Society London B*, **262**, 23–81.

Marr, D. (1971). Simple memory: a theory for archicortex. *Philosophical Transactions of the Royal Society London [Biology]*, **176**, 23–81.

MacAndrew, S. B. G. and Jones G. V. (1993). Spatial memory in amnesia: evidence from Korsakoff patients. *Cortex*, **29**, 235–49.

McClelland, J. L. and Goddard, N. H. (1996). Considerations arising from a complementary learning systems perspective on hippocampus and neocortex. *Hippocampus*, **6**, 654–65.

McNaughton, B. L. and Nadel, L. (1990). Hebb-Marr networks and the neurobiological representation of action in space. In *Neuroscience and Connectionist Theory*, (ed., M. A. Gluck and D. E. Rumelhart), pp. 1–64. Erlbaum, Hillsdale, NJ.

Milner, B. (1967). Brain mechanisms suggested by studies of the temporal lobes. In *Brain Mechanisms Underlying Speech and Language*, (ed., F. C. Darley), pp. 122–45. Grune and Stratton, New York.

Milner, B. (1968). Visually-guided maze learning in man: effects of bilateral hippocampal, bilateral frontal, and unilateral cerebral lesions. *Neuropsychologia*, 3, 317–38.

Miotto, E. C., Bullock, P., Polkey, C. E. and Morris, R. G. (1996). Spatial working memory in patients with frontal lobe lesions. *Cortex*, 32, 613–30.

Mishkin, M. and Murray, E. A. (1994). Stimulus recognition. *Current Opinions in Biology*, 200–6.

Morris, R. G. and Morton, N. (1995). The dissociation between visuospatial working memory and mental transformation. In *Broken Memories: Neuropsychological Case Studies*, (ed., R. Campbell and M. Conway), pp. 170–94. Blackwell, UK.

Morris, R. G., Abrahams, S. and Polkey C. E. (1995a). Recognition memory for words and faces following unilateral temporal lobectomy. *British Journal of Clinical Psychology*, 34, 571–6.

Morris, R. G., Abrahams, S., Polkey, C. E. and Baddeley, A. D. (1995b). Doors and people: visual and verbal memory after unilateral temporal lobectomy. *Neuropsychology*, 9, 464–9.

Morris, R. G., Pickering, A., Abrahams, S. and Feigenbaum, J. D. (1996). Space and the hippocampal formation in humans. *Brain Research Bulletin*, 40, 487–90.

Morris, R. G., Feigenbaum, J. D. and Polkey, C. F. (In preparation). Spatial manipulation and spatial working memory dissociate in patients with right unilateral temporal lobectomy.

Morris, R. G. M., Garrud, P., Rawlins, J. N. P. and O'Keefe, J. (1982). Place navigation in rats with hippocampal lesions. *Nature*, 297, 681–3.

Moser, E., Moser, M. B. and Andersen, P. (1993). Spatial learning impairment parallels the magnitude of dorsal hippocampal lesions, but is hardly present following ventral lesions. *Journal of Neuroscience*, 13(9), 3916–25.

Murray, E. A. (1996). What have ablation studies told us about the neural substrates of stimulus memory. *Seminars in Neuroscience*, 8, 13–22.

Nunn, J. A. and Hodges H. (1994). Review: cognitive deficits induced by global cerebral ischaemia: relationship to brain damage and reversal by transplants. *Behavioral Brain Research*, 65, 1–31.

Nunn, J. A., Le Peillet, E., Netto, C. A., Hodges, H., Gray, J. A. and Meldrum, B. S. (1994). Global ischaemia: hippocampal pathology and spatial deficits in the water maze. *Behavioral Brain Research*, 62, 41–54.

Nunn, J. A., Polkey, C. E. and Morris, R. G. (1998a). Differential spatial memory impairment after right temporal lobectomy demonstrated using temporal titration *Brain*, in press.

Nunn J. A., Polkey, C. E. and Morris, R. G. (1998b). Selective spatial rather than visual memory impairment after right unilateral temporal lobectomy. *Neuropsychologia*, in press.

O'Keefe, J. (1976). Place units in the hippocampus of the freely moving rat. *Experimental Neurology*, 51(1), 78–109.

O'Keefe, J. (1991). An allocentric spatial model for the hippocampal cognitive map. *Hippocampus*, 1, 230–5.

O'Keefe, J. and Burgess, N. (1996). Geometric determinants of the place fields of hippocampal neurons. *Nature*, 381, 425–8.

O'Keefe, J. and Nadel, L. (1978). *The Hippocampus as a Cognitive Map*. Clarendon Press, Oxford.

Olton, D. S., Walker, J. A. and Gage, H. (1978). Hippocampal connections and spatial discrimination. *Brain Research*, **139**, 295–308.

Olton, D. S., Becker, J. T. and Handelmann, G. E. (1979). Hippocampus, space and memory. *Behaviour and Brain Science*, **2**, 315–65.

Pavio, A. (1971). *Imagery and Verbal Processes*. Holt, Reinhart and Winston, New York.

Parkinson, J. K., Murray, E. A. and Mishkin, M. (1988). A selective mnemonic role for the hippocampus in monkeys: Memory for the location of objects. *Journal of Neuroscience*, 4159–67.

Petrides, M. (1985). Deficits on conditional associative-learning tasks after frontal- and temporal-lobe lesions in man. *Neuropsychologia*, **23**, 601–14.

Pigott, S. and Milner, B. (1993). Memory for different aspects of complex visual scenes after unilateral temporal- or frontal-lobe resection. *Neuropsychologia*, **31**, 1–15.

Polkey, C. E. (1987). Anterior temporal lobectomy at the Maudsley Hospital London. In *Surgical Treatment of the epilepsies* (ed. J. Engle Jr.), pp. 641–645. New York, Raver Press.

Rains, G. D. (1981). Aspects of memory in patients with temporal lobe lesions. Unpublished Ph.D. thesis, Cornell University, Ithaca.

Ratcliff, G. (1979). Spatial thought, mental rotation and the right cerebral hemisphere, *Neuropsychologia*, **17**, 49–54.

Recce, M. and Harris, K. D. (1996). Memory for place: a navigational model in support of Marr's theory of hippocampal function. *Hippocampus*, **6**, 735–48.

Recce, M. and Morris, R. G. (in preparation). Allocentric memory is impaired by right unilateral temporal lobectomy as indicated by headset virtual reality investigation. In preparation.

Rolls, E. T. (1996). A theory of hippocampal function in memory. *Hippocampus*, **6**(6), 601–20.

Shepard, R. N. and Metzler, J. (1971). Mental rotation of three-dimensional objects. *Science*, **171**, 701–3.

Shoqeirat, M. A. and Mayes, A. R. (1991). Disproportionate incidental spatial memory and recall deficits in amnesia. *Neuropsychologia*, **29**, 749–69.

Smith, M. L. (1989). Memory disorders associated with temporal-lobe lesions. In *Handbook of Neuropsychology, Vol. 3*, (ed., L. Squire), pp. 91–106. Elsevier Science Publishers, Oxford.

Smith, M. L. and Milner, B. (1981). The role of the right hippocampus in the recall of spatial location. *Neuropsychologia*, **19**, 781–95.

Smith, M. L. and Milner, B. (1989). Right hippocampal impairment in the recall of location: encoding deficit or rapid forgetting? *Neuropsychologia*, **27**, 71–82.

Squire, L. R. (1992). Memory and the hippocampus. A synthesis of findings with rats, monkeys, and humans. *Psychological Review*, **99**(2), 195–231.

Taube, J. S. (1996). Commentary on 'Space and the hippocampal formation in humans'. *Brain Research Bulletin*, **40**, 487–90.

Treves, A. and Rolls, E. T. (1991). What determines the capacity of autoassociative memories in the brain? *Network*, **2**, 371–97.

Ungerleider, L. G. and Mishkin, M. (1982). *Two cortical visual systems*. In *Analysis of Visual Behavior*, (ed., D. J. Ingle, M. A. Goodale and R. J. W. Mansfield), pp. 549–89. Cambridge, MA: MIT Press.

Visser, R. S. H. (1980). *Manual of the Complex Figure Test (CFT)*, 2nd edn. Lisse: Swets & Zeitlinger.

Wilson, M. A. and McNaughton, B. L. (1993). Dynamics of the hippocampal ensemble code for space. *Science*, **261**, 1055–8.

Zola-Morgan and Squire, L. R. (1985). Medial temporal lesions in monkeys impair memory on a variety of tasks sensitive to human amnesia. *Behavioral Neuroscience*, **9**, 22–34.

15

Hierarchical organization of cognitive memory

Mortimer Mishkin, Wendy A. Suzuki, David G. Gadian and Faraneh Vargha-Khadem

15.1 Introduction

Long-term cognitive memory, often referred to as declarative (Squire 1982) or propositional (Tulving 1993) memory, is critically dependent on the part of the medial temporal lobe that comprises the 'hippocampal system', a set of heavily interconnected structures consisting of the hippocampus and the underlying entorhinal, perirhinal and parahippocampal cortices. According to one functional view, the medial temporal hippocampal system contributes in a unitary fashion to cognitive memory ability, which includes both memory for specific events (episodic memory) and memory for factual information (semantic memory). This single-system, unitary-process view is based on results that suggest that the episodic and semantic memory impairments of amnesic patients with medial temporal-lobe damage vary together in a graded manner depending on the extent of damage to the hippocampal system as a whole (Rempel-Clower *et al.* 1996; Squire & Zola 1996). The importance of this cerebral region for both components of cognitive memory is exemplified by the well-studied amnesic patient H.M., who at the age of nearly 30 years underwent bilateral removal of the medial temporal lobe for relief of drug-resistant epilepsy (Scoville & Milner 1957). Extensive neuropsychological evaluation has shown that H.M. exhibits equally profound impairments for both facts (Gabrieli *et al.* 1988) and events (Scoville & Milner 1957; Milner *et al.* 1968); and a recent magnetic resonance imaging study confirmed that his cerebral excision included bilateral removal of the rostral half of the hippocampus, together with the entorhinal and part of the perirhinal cortices (Corkin *et al.* 1997).

According to an alternative functional view, the core defect in anterograde amnesia is the loss of episodic memory, in that the semantic memory of some amnesic patients appears to be relatively preserved (Kinsbourne & Wood 1975, 1982; Schacter & Tulving 1982; Wood *et al.* 1982). A particularly clear instance of such sparing was found in patient K.C., who also became densely amnesic at age 30, in his case after extensive brain injury, including bilateral medial temporal damage, sustained in a motorcycle accident. K.C. is unable to remember events for more than a few seconds; however, when tested for learning under conditions in which associative interference was held to a minimum, he was able to acquire a high level of factual information involving vocabulary items and to retain this new information for more than a year (Tulving *et al.* 1991; Hayman *et al.* 1993). The question of what brain damage might be responsible for such a dissociation of effects within cognitive memory has not yet been specifically addressed.

In this paper, evidence is presented that may help reconcile the two contending views described above. The evidence is based in part on behavioural and magnetic resonance imaging (MRI) data that were gathered recently in patients who became amnesic as a result of pathology incurred very early in life (Vargha-Khadem *et al.* 1997). These new findings, considered together with extant data on the neuroanatomy of the medial temporal hippocampal system as well as on the behavioural profiles of patients with adult-onset amnesia and of animals with selective medial temporal lesions, suggest the possibility that cognitive memory and its neural substrates are both organized hierarchically. Specifically, it is proposed as a working hypothesis that the cortices subjacent to the hippocampus are necessary for both episodic and semantic memory, whereas episodic memory (but not semantic) is critically dependent, in addition, on the stimulus processing provided by the hippocampus itself.

15.2 Neuroanatomy of the hippocampal system

To provide a framework for a discussion of the functional organization of the hippocampal system, this paper begins by briefly summarizing the anatomical organization of this region of the temporal lobe. It has long been known that the modality-specific cortical sensory processing areas in the monkey project in a stepwise and increasingly convergent manner onto the 'highest-order' association areas, including the prefrontal cortex, the cingulate cortex, the cortex in the dorsal bank of the superior temporal sulcus, and the hippocampus (Jones & Powell 1970). More recently, neuroanatomical studies focused on the hippocampus have begun to chart the precise pathways through which cortical sensory inputs activate this particular structure. A schematic diagram of these connections is shown in Fig. 15.1.

The diagram illustrates several important principles of organization. First, the hippocampal system receives a strong convergence of both modality-specific and polymodal input, rendering each component of the system a higher-order polymodal association area (Jones & Powell 1970; Van Hoesen & Pandya 1975*a,b*; Van Hoesen *et al.* 1975). Second, sensory information from widespread areas of the neocortical mantle enters the medial temporal lobe primarily via projections to the perirhinal and parahippocampal cortices. These areas provide the major cortical input to the entorhinal cortex; the entorhinal cortex, in turn, provides the major input to the hippocampus. The entorhinal cortex and hippocampus together constitute the 'hippocampal formation'.

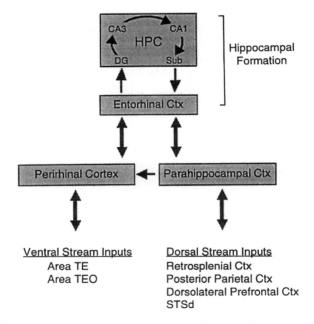

Fig 15.1 Schematic diagram of the connections of the medial temporal hippocampal system (filled boxes), depicting its hierarchical organization. The areas listed under ventral and dorsal streams are those providing the strongest inputs to the perirhinal and parahippocampal cortices, respectively. Abbreviations: CA1 and CA3, pyramidal-cell subfields of the hippocampus; Ctx, cortex; DG, dentate gyrus; HPC, hippocampus; STSd, dorsal bank of the superior temporal sulcus; Sub, subicular complex, including the subiculum, presubiculum and parasubiculum; TE and TEO, cortical subdivisions of Bonin & Bailey (1947).

Third, the perirhinal and parahippocampal cortices serve not only as the major port of entry into the hippocampal formation but also as its major cortical output, via dense, reciprocal projections. Thus the perirhinal and parahippocampal cortices constitute the major communication links between widespread areas of sensory cortex on the one hand and the hippocampal formation on the other.

Although all of the cortical areas in the medial temporal lobe receive convergent projections from multiple sensory modalities, these areas can be differentiated by their distinctive sources of input. These inputs can be broadly characterized as arising from cortical areas in the various modalities important for analysing stimulus quality (ventral processing streams), from cortical areas important for analysing stimulus location (dorsal processing streams), or from both. Thus, the perirhinal cortex is distinguished by its prominent projections from ventral processing streams, receiving nearly two-thirds of its cortical inputs from the adjacent ventral-stream visual areas, TE and TEO

(Suzuki & Amaral 1994*a*). Compared with the perirhinal cortex, the parahippo-campal cortex receives a far greater proportion of its inputs from dorsal-stream areas, including the posterior parietal cortex, the retrosplenial cortex, the dorso-lateral prefrontal cortex and the dorsal bank of the superior temporal sulcus (Martin-Elkins & Horel 1992; Suzuki & Amaral 1994*a*). Thus, whereas both the perirhinal and parahippocampal cortices receive projections from multiple sensory modalities, each is characterized by prominent ventral- and dorsal-stream inputs, respectively.

As already indicated, the entorhinal cortex receives most of its projections from the adjacent perirhinal and parahippocampal cortices, which provide approximately two-thirds of all entorhinal cortical inputs (Insausti *et al.* 1987). Consequently, within the hippocampal system, the entorhinal cortex serves as a second tier of convergence, a characterization that is also supported by an analysis of the laminar sources and terminations of the interconnections of this region. Specifically, both the perirhinal and parahippocampal cortices project to entorhinal cortex in a feedforward-like manner, whereas the latter recipro-cates these projections in a feedback-like manner (Suzuki & Amaral 1994*b*). Finally, the entorhinal cortex provides the strongest direct cortical projections to the hippocampus, via dense outputs terminating on the granule cells of the dentate gyrus.

The hierarchical pattern of medial temporal connections described above provides important clues to the mnemonic contributions of these areas. First, the differential patterns of cortical inputs to the perirhinal and parahippocam-pal cortices suggest that these two areas may be contributing to different aspects of memory. Whereas the parahippocampal cortex may participate primarily in memory for spatial location, the perirhinal cortex may serve mainly for memory of stimulus quality. Second, the further convergence of inputs from these two areas onto the entorhinal cortex, and subsequently onto the hippocampus, suggests that these latter areas may be specialized for forms of memory requiring the additional integration of sensory information that only they afford.

15.3 Findings in patients with early hippocampal damage

Although extremely valuable insights into the organization of memory have been gained from the study of amnesic patients, especially the distinction between cognitive memory and non-cognitive memory (e.g. procedural learn-ing, classical conditioning, priming), it has not yet been possible to evaluate the effects of subtotal medial temporal damage in relation to the episodic–semantic memory distinction outlined in the introduction. Most cases of human amnesia are not informative in this regard because their medial temporal pathology was either not selective or not well documented. Notable exceptions to this general-ization are three recent reports of amnesic patients in which postmortem histological analyses revealed medial temporal pathology limited largely to the hippocampus in each case (Zola-Morgan *et al.* 1986; Victor & Agamanolis 1990; Rempel-Clower *et al.* 1996). Importantly, these studies demonstrated for the first time that even such limited damage produces a clinically significant amnesia. Unfortunately, however, none of the above patients had been evaluated for possible differences in the degree to which their amnesia affected the episodic compared with the semantic components of cognitive memory.

A unique opportunity to assess the role of the hippocampus in memory has recently been provided by the discovery of three patients with amnesia due to hippocampal pathology sustained, in two of the cases, very early in life (a detailed description of the behavioural and MRI findings in all three cases is presented by Vargha-Khadem *et al.* (1997)). Briefly, each of the three patients developed pronounced memory impairment as a result of an anoxic–ischaemic episode associated in one case with difficult delivery at birth (Beth, now aged 14), in another with either premature birth or convulsions suffered at age 4 (Jon, now 19), and in the third with an accidental, toxic dose of theophylline, an anti-asthmatic, at age 9 (Kate, now 22). Memory impairments in Beth and Jon were not noted until they were about 5–6 years old, but in Kate they were evident immediately after her accidental drug dose.

Beth, Jon, and Kate were first examined neuropsychologically at the ages of 13, 16, and 19, respectively, at which time all three patients were found to have memory quotients on the Wechsler Memory Scale that fell about 20 points below the level predicted by their verbal IQs. Of the three, Jon has the highest verbal IQ (109), well within the average range, whereas Beth and Kate scored in the low-average range (82 and 86, respectively; Beth's relatively low IQ may be at least partly explained by the findings from MRI described below). Consistent with findings in patients with adult-onset amnesia, Beth, Jon, and Kate performed nearly at floor levels on all the delayed-recall tests of the Wechsler Memory Scale, as well as on other standard tests of delayed recall, while scoring well within normal limits on various standard tests of immediate memory.

Although the delayed-recall tasks on which the three patients were impaired do not explicitly measure episodic memory function, the symptom that initially brought each one of them to our attention was a pronounced memory loss for everyday events, the hallmark of an impairment in episodic memory. As reported by their parents, none of the three patients is well oriented in either place or time, can provide a reliable account of the day's activities, or can reliably remember messages, stories, visitors, appointments, etc. Indeed, their everyday-memory losses (which were confirmed with the Rivermead behavioural memory test (Wilson *et al.* 1985), a quantitative measure of event memory in a laboratory setting), are so severe that none of the patients can be left on his or her own for any extended period, much less hold a job or lead an independent life.

Yet, surprisingly, despite their disabling loss of episodic memory, all three patients have developed normal language and social competence, including conversational and interpersonal skills, and all were educated in mainstream schools. They have learned to read and write and have acquired new factual information at levels consistent with their verbal IQs rather than with predictions that might well have been made on the basis of their pronounced amnesic syndrome. The IQ levels themselves, as reflected, for example, in all three patients' fully normal scores on the Vocabulary, Information, and Comprehension subtests of the Wechsler Intelligence Scales, are a striking indication of their preserved ability to acquire factual knowledge in the face of early-onset amnesia. In sum, their social, linguistic, literacy, and intellectual attainments all seem to point to a disproportionate sparing of semantic compared with episodic memory.

The neuropathology in the three patients was assessed with quantitative magnetic resonance techniques (Jackson *et al.* 1993; Gadian *et al.* 1996; Van Paesschen *et al.* 1997), as well as through visual inspection of the scans. The quantitative measurements revealed that the hippocampi, which could be seen to be atrophic in each case, are reduced bilaterally to about 50 per cent (43, 50, and 61 per cent for Beth, Jon, and Kate, respectively) of the mean volume in normal subjects. Further, even the preserved hippocampal tissue is highly abnormal in each (as reflected by bilaterally elevated hippocampal T2 water values obtained with the T2-relaxometry method). Outside the hippocampus, the only detectable pathology in Jon and Kate was some diffuse abnormality in the right temporal lobe (as indicated by marginally abnormal ratios of the signal intensity for *N*-acetylaspartate to the sum of the signal intensities for choline-containing compounds and creatine + phosphocreatine, measured with magnetic resonance spectroscopy). This type of abnormality was not found in either temporal lobe in Beth, but visual inspection of her scans revealed increased T2-weighted signal intensity in the periventricular and peritrigonal white matter accompanied by a marked loss of this white matter, together with thinning of the corpus callosum. These extrahippocampal abnormalities in Beth could help account for her relatively low IQ.

Although the magnetic resonance findings suggest that the only abnormality all three patients have in common is bilateral pathology of the hippocampal formation, the possibility cannot be excluded that, in each case, some undetected pathology actually extends beyond the hippocampus into the underlying cortices. Indeed, some results to be described below raise questions about the integrity of the parahippocampal cortex in particular. Nevertheless, the evidence in all three patients suggesting relative sparing of semantic compared with episodic memory, and relative preservation of the medial temporal cortex as compared with the hippocampus, leads to the proposal that the cortex subjacent to the hippocampus may be sufficient to support their relatively spared semantic memory.

15.4 Comparison with studies of memory in monkeys

Additional results that are compatible with the foregoing proposal were obtained on a series of computerized recognition memory tasks that were administered to both the amnesic patients and 11 normal controls. The tasks included one-trial recognition for lists of words, non-words, familiar faces and unfamiliar faces; these tasks were similar in principle to measures of one-trial stimulus recognition widely used in studies on monkeys. Other tasks in the series assessed one-trial associative recognition for lists of paired items involving each of the materials described above, as well as multitrial associative recognition for lists of non-word pairs, face pairs, voice–face pairs, and object–place pairs. These tasks, too, have parallels with those used in monkeys (stimulus–stimulus association: Spiegler & Mishkin 1979; Murray & Mishkin 1985; Murray *et al*. 1993; and object–place association: Parkinson *et al*. 1988; Angeli *et al*. 1993). The great majority of the recognition tasks yielded results in the amnesic patients that are strikingly similar to those that have been obtained in monkeys with hippocampal lesions. For tasks requiring one-trial stimulus recognition, on which monkeys with hippocampal lesions exhibit little (Zola-Morgan *et al*. 1992, 1994) or no impairment (Murray & Mishkin 1996), the patients likewise were not significantly impaired. Again like monkeys with hippocampal lesions, the patients were not significantly impaired on recognition tasks involving either one-trial (Spiegler & Mishkin 1981) or multitrial (Murray & Mishkin 1985; Murray *et al*. 1993) stimulus–stimulus associations. In sharp contrast to these results are those from numerous studies in monkeys, which demonstrate that lesions of the cortex underlying the hippocampus, particularly lesions that include the perirhinal and entorhinal cortices, produce severe and long-lasting deficits in both item and associative recognition (Spiegler & Mishkin 1979; Murray & Mishkin 1986; Zola-Morgan *et al*. 1989, 1993; Meunier *et al*. 1993; Murray *et al*. 1993; Suzuki *et al*. 1993; Goulet & Murray 1995). The contrasting effects of the hippocampal and perirhinal–entorhinal lesions in monkeys strongly imply that the computerized tasks given to the patients would have revealed clear-cut deficits had the patients sustained a substantial amount of damage to the perirhinal–entorhinal complex.

Before considering the further implications of the recognition memory data, it is first necessary to consider a potential exception to the similarity of results obtained in the amnesic patients and in monkeys with hippocampal lesions. The one computerized task on which the patients showed a severe deficit, all three scoring far below all the control subjects, was the one requiring memory for object–place associations. Initially, this result too appeared to parallel an earlier finding in hippocampectomized monkeys, because such monkeys had exhibited severe impairment on an analogous task (Parkinson *et al*. 1988; Angeli *et al*. 1993). However, preliminary evidence from an ongoing study on the effects of separate lesions of the hippocampus and parahippocampal cortex (Malkova & Mishkin 1997) suggests that the object-location memory deficit in the monkeys studied earlier arose from damage to parahippocampal tissue, which had been removed in association with the hippocampectomy, rather than from removal of the hippocampus itself. If this preliminary interpretation is upheld, further investigations will be needed to resolve the discrepancy between the impairment in object-location memory in the amnesic patients and the lack of such an impairment in monkeys with selective hippocampal lesions. One possible resolution might be that the greater memory load in the human test compared with the one given to the animals (a list length of 20 object–place pairs compared with a list length of two such pairs) requires the spatial memory capacity of the hippocampus, which could well exceed that of the parahippocampal cortex. Alternatively, the impairment in the patients could reflect undisclosed damage to the parahippocampal cortex, consonant with the preliminary neurobehavioural evidence in monkeys as well as with the connectional evidence described in the section on neuroanatomy.

15.5 A hierarchy of neurocognitive memory processes

As already indicated, the patients' performance on the other, non-spatial, recognition tests corroborates the suggestion from the magnetic resonance findings that their perirhinal–entorhinal cortices, at least, are substantially spared. Further, in conjunction with their amnesic profile, the recognition data are consistent with the proposal that such partial preservation of their medial temporal cortices may be sufficient to support their semantic memory. It is important to point out that this proposal does not imply that the recognition tests measure semantic memory specifically; but neither do they measure only episodic memory. The distinction between these two types of mnemonic store refers to differences in their long-term contents, not to differences in the way those two types of contents were first acquired. Whenever a new item, association, or fact is being encoded for storage, that sensory information necessarily arrives in the form of an evolving event or episode rich in temporal, spatial, and other situational contexts, overlain with whatever mental and emotional experiences the subject brings to the event. How much of this abundant contextual information is retained in the long term largely determines to which category of cognitive memory the stored information should be assigned: to context-rich episodic memory or to context-free semantic memory.

The recognition memory tests may therefore more appropriately be viewed as measures of the basic sensory memory ability that is essential for the entry of information into both types of long-term store. Considered in this way, the neurobehavioural evidence in the patients suggests that, in the presence of a severely compromised hippocampus, the basic sensory memory functions served by the subjacent cortex are largely sufficient for entry of sensory information into context-free semantic memory but not into context-rich episodic memory, which must therefore require the additional information processing that is normally provided by the hippocampal circuit at the top of the hierarchy (see Fig. 15.1). The proposal is consistent with the anatomical evidence, which indicates progressively greater convergence, and presumably association, of sensory inputs as one ascends the hierarchy within the hippocampal system.

The proposal is also consistent with the notion that ontogenetic development of the semantic memory ability that underpins social, linguistic, and intellectual competence precedes development of, and may even also underpin, the ability to store and recollect earlier episodes (Tulving 1995). It is of interest in this connection that the amnesia in the two patients who had sustained hippocampal pathology very early in life did not become evident until they were 5–6 years old, long after they had acquired the social skills, speech and language, and factual knowledge that are normal for that age.

15.6 Implications for research

Despite its plausibility, the above proposal can only be considered a working hypothesis. The evidence for a behavioural dissociation in the amnesic patients with early hippocampal injury is largely based on the striking contrast between their episodic memory failures and semantic memory achievements in everyday life, that is, in situations that are difficult to compare directly. Additional evidence must therefore be gathered under controlled learning and retention conditions to determine whether the differences in their episodic and semantic memory are indeed greater than can be accommodated by a single-system, unitary-process view (Hamann & Squire 1995).

The applicability of the episodic–semantic memory distinction to the effects of brain injury in general, and of medial temporal damage in particular, has been much debated in the literature on late-onset amnesia, but thus far without a clear resolution (Glisky *et al.* 1986; McKoon *et al.* 1986; Shimamura & Squire 1989; Wood *et al.* 1989; Horner 1990; Ostergaard & Squire 1990; Tulving *et al.* 1991; Hayman *et al.* 1993; Hamann & Squire 1995). One possible explanation for the conflicting reports is that most of the previously studied patients had relatively unspecified or unselective pathology. According to the proposal being advanced here, a dissociation between the two components of cognitive memory can be expected only in cases where the hippocampus has been damaged selectively, the underlying cortices having remained largely intact. The correlative prediction is that extensive damage to the underlying cortices, which serve as the essential links between the sensory processing streams and the hippocampus, should produce severe impairment in both components of cognitive memory, whether or not the hippocampus itself is directly affected. The advent of quantitative magnetic resonance techniques, which are likely to be gradually refined and extended, will enable increasingly accurate assessment of the neuropathology in patients with amnesia and, consequently, examination of the predicted difference in outcome after the two types of damage.

Improved neuropathological assessment, together with the discovery that anoxic–ischaemic episodes early (Vargha-Khadem *et al.* 1997) as well as later (Zola-Morgan *et al.* 1986; Victor & Agamanolis 1990; Rempel-Clower *et al.* 1996) in life can lead to relatively selective hippocampal pathology, affords an opportunity to clarify the role of not only the lesion variable but also the variable of age at injury. The relative sparing of semantic memory in the patients studied here, two of whom incurred their hippocampal injury at a time when plasticity and compensatory potential are still at their peak, could well turn out to be greater than the sparing observed in patients who have sustained comparable damage in adulthood. Conversely, in other cognitive (e.g. intellectual) domains, the early onset of their amnesia may have disadvantaged them relative to those with late-onset amnesia, on the supposition that these other domains depend on cognitive memory ability far more for their initial development than for their later maintenance.

The possibility that cognitive memory is organized hierarchically also has implications for the search for an animal model of human amnesia. The amnesic symptoms in humans that are due to impairment in context-free semantic memory may be modelled in animals, at least in part, by the severe deficits in context-free associative memory that are produced by lesions of entorhinal, perirhinal, and parahippocampal cortices. However, an animal model must be considered incomplete unless those human amnesic symptoms that are due to an impairment in context-rich episodic memory are also reproduced. According to the present analysis, such symptoms are likely to be recognized in animals only if they are seen in the absence of a basic associative memory impairment, that is, only if they consist of deficits limited to context-rich associative memory due to selective hippocampal lesions.

Acknowledgements

The authors of the original report on the patients with early medial temporal pathology (Varga-Khadem *et al.* 1997) included K. E. Watkins, A. Connelly and W. Van Paesschen; we are indebted to all of them for their critical contributions to that study, on which this chapter leans so heavily. In addition, we thank A. Incisa della Rochetta, who helped design the computerized tests and collect the data on some of the control subjects.

References

Angeli, S. J., Murray, E. A. & Mishkin, M. 1993 Hippocampectomized monkeys can remember one place but not two. *Neuropsychologia* **31**, 1021–1030.

Bonin, G. V. & Bailey, P. 1947 *The neocortex of* Macaca mulatta. Urbana, IL: University of Illinois Press.

Corkin, S., Amaral, D. G., Gilberto Gonzalez, R., Johnson, K. A. & Hyman, B. T. 1997 H.M.'s medial temporal lobe lesion: findings from magnetic resonance imaging. *J. Neurosci.* **17**, 3964–3979.

Gabrieli, J. D. E., Cohen, N. J. & Corkin, S. 1988 The impaired learning of semantic knowledge following bilateral medial temporal-lobe resection. *Brain Cogn.* **7**, 157–177.

Gadian, D. G., Isaacs, E. B., Cross, H. J., Connelly, A., Jackson, G. D., King, M. D. *et al.* 1996 Lateralization of brain function in childhood revealed by magnetic resonance spectroscopy. *Neurology* **46**, 974–977.

Glisky, E. L., Schacter, D. L. & Tulving, E. 1986 Computer learning by memory-impaired patients: acquisition and retention of complex knowledge. *Neuropsychologia* **24**, 313–328.

Goulet, S. & Murray, E. A. 1995 Effects of lesion of either the amygdala or anterior rhinal cortex on crossmodal DNMS in rhesus macaques. *Soc. Neurosci. Abstr.* **21**, 566.

Hamann, S. B. & Squire, L. R. 1995 On the acquisition of new declarative knowledge in amnesia. *Behav. Neurosci.* **109**, 1027–1044.

Hayman, C. A. G., MacDonald, C. A. & Tulving, E. 1993 The role of repetition and associative interference in new semantic learning in amnesia: a case experiment. *J. Cogn. Neurosci.* **5**, 375–389.

Horner, M. D. 1990 Psychobiological evidence for the distinction between episodic and semantic memory. *Neuropsychol. Rev.* **1**, 281–321.

Insausti, R., Amaral, D. G. & Cowan, W. M. 1987 The entorhinal cortex of the monkey. II. Cortical afferents. *J. Comp. Neurol.* **264**, 356–395.

Jackson, G. D., Connelly, A., Duncan, J. S., Grunewald, R. A. & Gadian, D. G. 1993 Detection of hippocampal pathology in intractable partial epilepsy: increased sensitivity with quantitative magnetic resonance relaxometry. *Neurology* **43**, 1793–1799.

Jones, E. G. & Powell, T. P. S. 1970 An anatomical study of converging sensory pathways within the cerebral cortex of the monkey. *Brain* **93**, 793–820.

Kinsbourne, M. & Wood, F. 1975 Short-term memory processes and the amnesic syndrome. In *Short-term memory* (ed., D. Deutsch & J. A. Deutsch), pp. 258–291. New York: Academic Press.

Kinsbourne, M. & Wood, F. 1982 *Theoretical considerations regarding the episodic-semantic memory distinction* (ed., L. Cermak), pp. 194–212. Hillsdale, NJ: Erlbaun.

Malkova, L. & Mishkin, M. 1997 Memory for the location of objects after separate lesions of the hippocampus and parahippocampal cortex in rhesus monkeys. *Soc. Neurosci. Abstr.* **23**, 12.

Martin-Elkins, C. L. & Horel, J. A. 1992 Cortical afferents to behaviorally defined regions of the inferior temporal and parahippocampal gyri as demonstrated by WGA-HRP. *J. Comp. Neurol.* **321**, 177–192.

McKoon, G., Ratcliff, R. & Dell, G. S. 1986 A critical evaluation of the semantic-episodic distinction. *J. Exp. Psychol. Learn. Mem.* **12**, 295–306.

Meunier, M., Bachevalier, J., Mishkin, M. & Murray, E. A. 1993 Effects on visual recognition of combined and separate ablations of the entorhinal and perirhinal cortex in rhesus monkeys. *J. Neurosci.* **13**, 5418–5432.

Milner, B., Corkin, S. & Teuber, H. L. 1968 Further analysis of the hippocampal amnesia syndrome: 14-year follow-up study of H.M. *Neuropsychologia* **6**, 215–234.

Murray, E. A., Gaffan, D. & Mishkin, M. 1993 Neural substrates of visual stimulus-stimulus association in rhesus monkeys. *J. Neurosci.* **13**, 4549–4561.

Murray, E. A. & Mishkin, M. 1985 Amygdalectomy impairs crossmodal association in monkeys. *Science* **228**, 604–606.

Murray, E. A. & Mishkin, M. 1986 Visual recognition in monkeys following rhinal cortical ablations combined with either amygdalectomy or hippocampectomy. *J. Neurosci.* **6**, 1991–2003.

Murray, E. A. & Mishkin, M. 1996 40-minute visual recognition memory in rhesus monkeys with hippocampal lesions. *Soc. Neurosci. Abstr.* **22**, 281.

Ostergaard, A. & Squire, L. R. 1990 Childhood amnesia and distinctions between forms of memory: a comment on Wood, Brown, and Felton. *Brain Cogn.* **14**, 127–133.

Parkinson, J. K., Murray, E. A. & Mishkin, M. 1988 A selective mnemonic role for the hippocampus in monkeys: memory for the location of objects. *J. Neurosci.* **8**, 4159–4167.

Rempel-Clower, N. L., Zola, S. M., Squire, L. R. & Amaral, D. G. 1996 Three cases of enduring memory impairment after bilateral damage limited to the hippocampal formation. *J. Neurosci.* **16**, 5233–5255.

Schacter, D. L. & Tulving, E. 1982 Memory, amnesia, and the episodic/semantic distinction. In *Expression of knowledge* (ed., R. L. Isaacson & N. E. Spear), pp. 33–65. New York: Plenum Press.

Scoville, W. B. & Milner, B. 1957 Loss of recent memory after bilateral hippocampal lesions. *J. Neurol. Neurosurg. Psychiatr.* **20**, 11–21.

Shimamura, A. P. & Squire, L. R. 1989 Impaired priming of new associations in amnesia. *J. Exp. Psychol. Learn. Mem. Cogn.* **15**, 721–728.

Spiegler, B. J. & Mishkin, M. 1979 Associative memory severely impaired by combined amygdalo-hippocampal removals. *Soc. Neurosci. Abstr.* **5**, 323.

Spiegler, B. J. & Mishkin, M. 1981 Evidence for the sequential participation of inferior temporal cortex and amygdala in the acquisition of stimulus-reward associations. *Behav. Brain Res.* **3**, 303–317.

Squire, L. R. 1982 The neuropsychology of the human mind. *A. Rev. Neurosci.* **5**, 241–273.

Squire, L. R. & Zola, S. M. 1996 Structure and function of declarative and non-declarative memory systems. *Proc. Natn. Acad. Sci. USA* **93**, 13515–13522.

Suzuki, W. A., Zola-Morgan, S., Squire, L. R. & Amaral, D. G. 1993 Lesions of the perirhinal and parahippocampal cortices in the monkey produce long-lasting memory impairment in the visual and tactual modalities. *J. Neurosci.* **13**, 2430–2451.

Suzuki, W. A. & Amaral, D. G. 1994*a* Perirhinal and parahippocampal cortices of the macaque monkey: cortical afferents. *J. Comp. Neurol.* **350**, 497–533.

Suzuki, W. A. & Amaral, D. G. 1994*b* Topographic organization of the reciprocal connections between monkey entorhinal cortex and the perirhinal and parahippocampal cortices. *J. Neurosci.* **14**, 1856–1877.

Tulving, E. 1993 *Elements of episodic memory.* New York: Oxford University Press.

Tulving, E. 1995 Organization of memory: quo vadis? In *The cognitive neurosciences* (ed., M. S. Gazzaniga), pp. 839–847. Cambridge, MA: The MIT Press.

Tulving, E., Hayman, C. A. G. & MacDonald, C. A. 1991 Long-lasting perceptual priming and semantic learning in amnesia: a case experiment. *J. Exp. Psychol. Learn. Mem.* **17**, 595–617.

Van Hoesen, G. W. & Pandya, D. N. 1975*a* Some connections of the entorhinal (area 28) and perirhinal (area 35) cortices of the rhesus monkey. I. Temporal lobe afferents. *Brain Res.* **95**, 1–24.

Van Hoesen, G. W & Pandya, D. N. 1975*b* Some connections of the entorhinal (area 28) and perirhinal (area 35) cortices of the rhesus monkey. III. Efferent connections. *Brain Res.* **95**, 48–67.

Van Hoesen, G. W., Pandya, D. N. & Butters, N. 1975 Some connections of the entorhinal (area 28) and perirhinal (area 35) cortices of the rhesus monkey. II. Frontal lobe afferents. *Brain Res.* **95**, 25–38.

Van Paesschen, W., Connelly, A., King, M. D., Jackson, G. D. & Duncan, J. S. 1997 The spectrum of hippocampal sclerosis: a quantitative magnetic resonance imaging study. *Ann. Neurol.* **41**, 41–51.

Vargha-Khadem, F., Gadian, D. G., Watkins, K. E., Connelly, A., Van Paesschen, W. & Mishkin, M. 1997 Differential effects of early hippocampal pathology on episodic and semantic memory. *Science* **277**, 376–380.

Victor, M. & Agamanolis, D. 1990 Amnesia due to lesions confined to the hippocampus: a clinical-pathologic study. *J. Cogn. Neurosci.* **2**, 246–257.

Wilson, B., Cockburn, J. & Baddeley, A. 1985 *The Rivermead behavioral memory test.* Reading, UK: Thames Valley Test Company.

Wood, F., Ebert, V. & Kinsbourne, M. 1982 The episodic–semantic distinction in memory and amnesia: clinical and experimental observations. In *Human memory and amnesia* (ed. L. S. Cermak), pp. 167–193. New York: Erlbaum.

Wood, F. B., Brown, I. S. & Felton, R. H. 1989 Long-term follow-up of a childhood amnesic syndrome. *Brain Cogn.* **10**, 76–86.

Zola-Morgan, S., Squire, L. R. & Amaral, D. G. 1986 Human amnesia and the medial temporal region: enduring memory impairment following a bilateral lesion limited to field CA1 of the hippocampus. *J. Neurosci.* **6**, 2950–2967.

Zola-Morgan, S., Squire, L. R., Amaral, D. G. & Suzuki, W. A. 1989 Lesions of perirhinal and parahippocampal cortex that spare the amygdala and hippocampal formation produce severe memory impairment. *J. Neurosci.* **9**, 4355–4370.

Zola-Morgan, S., Squire, L. R., Clower, R. P. & Rempel, N. L. 1993 Damage to the perirhinal cortex exacerbates memory impairment following lesions to the hippocampal formation. *J. Neurosci.* **13**, 251–265.

Zola-Morgan, S., Squire, L. R. & Ramus, S. J. 1994 Severity of memory impairment in monkeys as a function of locus and extent of damage within the medial temporal lobe memory system. *Hippocampus* **4**, 483–495.

Zola-Morgan, S., Squire, L. R., Rempel, N. L., Clower, R. P. & Amaral, D. G. 1992 Enduring memory impairment in monkeys after ischemic damage to the hippocampus. *J. Neurosci.* **12**, 2582–2596.

Interactions between parietal and hippocampal systems in space and memory

This section deals with the functional interactions between hippocampal and parietal systems, following two main strands: that they form two parts of a memory system acting over different timescales or levels of abstraction, or that they form two parts of a spatial system acting on information in allocentric and egocentric frames of reference, respectively. These two strands are linked together in the final chapter by David Milner and colleagues.

The possible interaction between the hippocampus and neocortex in memory suggested by Marr (1971), such that information rapidly laid down in hippocampus is transferred to neocortex during sleep, is explored by Qin and colleagues by recording activity in both areas before and after sleep. Rolls reports on cells in monkey hippocampus that appear to encode the location at which the animal is looking, independent of its own location, or what the animal is looking at. This finding is used to provide a possible link between place cells in the rat and the episodic memory function ascribed to the hippocampus in humans. A neural network model is described that follows Marr's idea of the hippo-campus as an autoassociative memory and its interaction with cortex, and extends its level of quantitative analysis. Gaffan and Hornak argue that parietal neglect patients and temporal lobe amnesics have both perceptual and memory deficits for representations in egocentric frameworks.

Olsen describes how the allocentric and egocentric frames of reference provided by the hippocampal and parietal systems is complemented by object centred reference frames in the supplementary eye fields in monkeys. Berthoz examines the vestibular inputs to both parietal and hippocampal regions. He also uses functional imaging in humans to demonstrate parietal activation during saccadic eye movements to sequences of memorized locations and hippocampal activation during imagined movement along a previously walked route through Paris. The cooperation of both areas during large-scale navigation is hinted at by Maguire's functional imaging study in which taxi drivers describe routes generated from their long-term memory of London, showing hippocampal and parietal activation. In a more recent study, Maguire and colleagues have shown activation of the two regions to correlate with accuracy of navigation in a virtual reality environment. A neural network model of the hippocampal and parietal roles in allocentric and egocentric processing is described by Arbib in a synthesis of results from rats and monkeys. David Milner and colleagues examine the preserved spatial functions of a patient with damage to the ventral visual pathway. They conclude that the dorsal stream is responsible for short-term representation of locations in egocentric frameworks suitable for controlling actions, whereas the ventral stream, terminating in the hippocampus is for conscious perception of stimuli and providing allocentric representations more suitable for long term memory through not being dependent on the momentary orientation of the body and its parts.

16

Memory reprocessing in corticocortical and hippocampocortical neuronal ensembles

Yu-Lin Qin, Bruce L. McNaughton, William E. Skaggs and Carol A. Barnes

16.1 Introduction

The phenomenon of retrograde amnesia for certain kinds of information after temporal-lobe damage (Scoville & Milner 1957; Squire 1992) has led to the general hypothesis that the hippocampus somehow facilitates the reactivation of neocortical activity patterns during 'offline' periods such as sleep or quiet wakefulness, when the neocortex is not actively engaged in processing incoming data (Marr 1971). It is presumed that this reactivation somehow permits recently acquired information to become appropriately integrated into long-term memory. This could occur either if the hippocampus generated explicit, compact representations of the events themselves (Marr 1971; Squire 1992; McClelland *et al.* 1995), or if it merely generated a cognitive map (O'Keefe & Nadel 1978) that could also serve as a contextual code (Nadel *et al.* 1985; Teyler & Discenna 1986; McNaughton *et al.* 1996) for each event. Either of these sorts of codes could be associated with the pattern in the active neocortical modules at the time of the original experience. Because of the divergent, direct and indirect, return projections from hippocampus to neocortex (Amaral & Witter 1995) reactivation of the hippocampal component of the experience conceivably could reinstate the entire pattern of experience across the weakly interconnected neocortical network. The presumed attractor dynamics of the CA3 region of the hippocampus implies that reactivation of recent patterns in the hippocampus could arise either spontaneously (Shen & McNaughton 1997) or as a consequence of the reactivation of a subcomponent of the experience in the neocortex (Marr 1971) and subsequent pattern completion in the hippocampus. This general theory provides a framework for understanding the phenomenon of temporally graded retrograde amnesia after hippocampal damage. A minimal prediction of the theory is that, during offline periods, activity patterns corresponding to recent experiences should appear in both hippocampus and neocortex, and, moreover, that at any given time, the patterns in the two regions should be correlated with the same experience.

Three studies have provided neurophysiological evidence for memory reactivation within the hippocampus during sleep. If a rat is confined to the place field of a particular hippocampal place cell, the firing rate of that cell is increased during subsequent sleep (Pavlides & Winson 1989). More compellingly, if a rat is permitted to explore a larger environment during behaviour, so that many different place cells are activated, there is little change in the net firing rates of the corresponding place cells during subsequent slow-wave sleep, but a significant increase in the activity correlation between cell pairs whose activity had been correlated (by virtue of their place-field overlap) during behaviour (Wilson & McNaughton 1994). This could only occur if engrams, closely resembling the neuronal discharge patterns of prior experiences, were reactivated (Shen & McNaughton 1997). In addition to simple correlations, Skaggs & McNaughton (1996) have shown that the temporal biases in hippocampal cross-correlation functions persist from a period of behaviour into subsequent slow-wave sleep. Thus, information about the temporal sequence of events is also preserved and re-expressed in hippocampus.

Motivated by the theoretical considerations discussed above, the present study was designed to follow up on these observations by examining whether patterns of activity in the neocortex, and in hippocampal–neocortical relations, are replicated during sleep in a manner similar to that of intrahippocampal patterns. Some of the present results have previously been reported in abstract form (Qin *et al.* 1995, 1996).

16.2 Materials and methods

Subjects and behavioural procedures

Seven male F-344 rats, 10 months old (Harlan Sprague–Dawley; Indianapolis), were used. The rats were maintained at 85–90 per cent of their *ad libitum* body mass, under illumination from 0800 to 2000 h, and all recordings were conducted between 0800 h and 1400 h. During pretraining, the animals learned to shuttle back and forth in a linear alleyway for a food reward. After recovery from surgery, the rats were adapted to the recording headstage and learned to run for food reinforcement on one of two similar elevated-track mazes, 7.5 cm wide. One track (3 rats) was triangular (61 cm per side), and contained reward sites at the midpoint of each side. The other track (4 rats) was rectangular (87 cm × 36 cm), and contained two reward sites located at adjacent corners on the long axis. The long side opposite the reward locations was bordered by a plywood wall. Both tracks were located in the same central position in a moderately illuminated room, 3.7 m × 3.7 m, containing several prominent visual landmarks.

Recording sessions consisted of three phases: an initial period (S1) of sleep or quiet wakefulness lasting at least 20 min; a maze-running phase (M), during which the rats ran a minimum of 15 circuits of the maze without changing direction, and a second sleep phase (S2), also lasting at least 20 min. During the two sleep phases, the rats rested in a small bowl, which was placed on a pedestal about 20 cm above the maze. In these studies, the 'sleep' periods were defined by the animal's relatively motionless behaviour, and hippocampal electroencephalogram (EEG) exhibiting predominantly large irregular activity, typically preceded by periods of neocortical spindle activity. There was a small amount of rapid eye-movement (REM) sleep, as indicated by theta activity. No further effort was made to characterize the behavioural states during these episodes, which thus can be considered to comprise mostly slow-wave sleep plus a small amount of quiet wakefulness and REM sleep.

Surgery

All surgical procedures were carried out under deep sodium pentobarbital anaesthesia according to NIH guidelines. The stereotaxic surgery involved opening a craniotomy 2 mm in diameter in the right hemisphere over either the hindlimb sensorimotor region (Zilles (1985) area HL, 3.5 mm posterior and 2.0 mm lateral to bregma) or the posterior parietal area (Zilles (1985) area OC2 ml, 5.0 mm posterior and 3.0 mm lateral to bregma). The dura was retracted and the tip of the microdrive assembly (see below) was placed on the exposed cortex so that the probes penetrated about 100 μm into the cortex. The drive assembly was anchored in place by using dental acrylic supported by seven small jeweller's screws mounted in the skull.

Electrophysiological procedures

Recordings were made with a microdrive assembly containing 14 independently movable tetrodes. The construction of tetrode recording probes (McNaughton et al. 1983; Recce & O'Keefe 1989; Wilson & McNaughton 1993) and the multielectrode 'hyperdrive' assembly have been described in detail elsewhere (Gothard et al. 1996). Briefly, four HML-insulated Nichrome wires (HP Reid Co.), 14 μm in diameter, were twisted together and the end of the bundle was cut off at right angles with sharp scissors. Each tetrode was mounted in the guide cannula of one of the 14 microdrives on the assembly, and each wire was connected to a separate pin on a multichannel connector. The microdrives permitted each tetrode to be moved up or down independently of the others by turning a screw, with a full turn moving the electrode tip vertically by about 320 μm. The entire drive assembly weighed 12–14 g.

A 50 channel field effect transmitter (FET) headstage assembly was mounted on top of the hyperdrive during recording sessions. The headstage assembly included two arrays of infrared light-emitting diodes (LEDs) whose positions were monitored and sampled at 20 Hz to provide information on both head location and head orientation in the horizontal plane. The FET outputs were transmitted to the main amplifiers via a lightweight cable.

Electrophysiological data were collected by means of an array of eight 80486-based microcomputers with synchronized, programmable, event-timing clocks running at 10 kHz (Datawave Corporation). One of the probes was used as an EEG reference, placed near the hippocampal fissure. Another served as the indifferent reference electrode, located in the corpus callosum. The four channels of each of the remaining tetrodes were each amplified 2000–10 000 times (depending on the signal size), filtered between 600 Hz and 6 kHz, and digitized at 32 kHz per channel. An entire 1-ms sample of the waveforms of each action potential on the four tetrode channels was stored on disk, along with a time stamp code (0.1 ms resolution). In addition, the signals from one channel of each of several tetrodes was split off to a separate amplifier for EEG monitoring. EEG output on different channels was filtered with a bandpass of either 1–100 Hz or 1–3 kHz to permit simultaneous monitoring of hippocampal theta rhythm, sharp-waves and ripple activity as well as neocortical sleep spindles. Behavioural states were characterized as awake-theta, still-alert, slow-wave sleep, and REM sleep according to established behavioural and EEG criteria (Vanderwolf 1969; Winson 1977).

After surgery, the tetrode probes were advanced gradually, normally not more than 50–$200 \, \mu m \, d^{-1}$ depending on electrode location and the signal quality. During the first few recording sessions, all tetrodes were typically in the neocortex. About half of the probes were then gradually advanced to the CA1 layer of hippocampus to record hippocampal–neocortical interactions. Finally the remaining probes were advanced to CA1.

After recording, the animals were perfused transcardially with formalin, and the electrode tracks were verified histologically by using combined Nissl and myelin staining (Zilles 1985).

Unit isolation

Single units were isolated from the stored data by means of a visually guided, multidimensional cluster analysis method described by McNaughton *et al.* (1989). Only units that were considered well isolated were accepted for analysis. Although it is never possible to define precisely the degree of unit isolation, the tetrode method has been demonstrated to provide isolation that is substantially superior to that of other methods (McNaughton *et al.* 1983; Recce & O'Keefe 1989; Gray *et al.* 1995).

Analysis of spike-train interactions

The simple correlation between the spike trains of each pair of cells was used to describe the structure of the firing pattern of the recorded cells. For each pair of cells, the spike trains were divided into n 100 ms bins. If x_i and y_i denote the number of spikes fired by each cell in the ith bin, and $\bar{x}$ and $\bar{y}$ denote the mean numbers of spikes per bin, their rate-independent correlation coefficient is defined as:

$$r_{x,y} = \frac{\sum_{i=1}^{n}(x_i - \bar{x})(y_i - \bar{y})}{\sqrt{\sum_{i=1}^{n}(x_i - \bar{x})^2 \sum_{i=1}^{n}(y_i - \bar{y})^2}}. \qquad (16.1)$$

Within the hippocampus, in an animal performing a spatial task, the extent of positive correlation between the spike trains of two pyramidal cells is typically related to the overlap of their place fields. In the neocortex, for the types of task used in this study, pyramidal cells also tend to show spatially heterogeneous patterns of firing, because different locations are associated with different types of behaviour or reward contingency (McNaughton *et al*. 1994). Between hippocampal and neocortical cells, relatively strong correlations would be observed if the hippocampal place field was located at one of the regions where the behavioural correlate of the neocortical cell was strongly expressed. Examples of these effects are illustrated in Fig. 16.1.

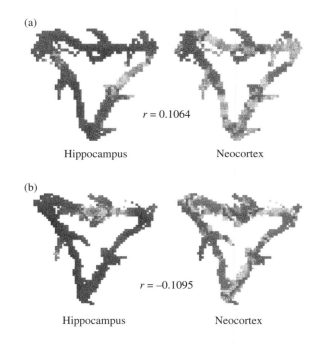

Fig. 16.1 Examples of spatial firing patterns for hippocampal and neocortical neurons, on the triangular track used for some of the experiments. (a) Activity patterns for two cells whose spike trains were positively correlated; (b) activity patterns for two cells with negative correlation. As this figure suggests, spatial firing patterns for cells from the neocortical regions examined here were always nearly symmetrical across the three sides of the triangle, whereas hippocampal pyramidal cells always showed spatially asymmetrical firing patterns. Firing rates are scaled independently in each plot, with red corresponding to the highest rates, and dark blue corresponding to zero.

Effects of experience on the activity correlations within and between anatomical structures

For each pair of cells in a data set, let Corr(s1), Corr(m) and Corr(s2) be their activity correlations in S1, M and S2, respectively. Thus, each pair of cells gives rise to a single point in a three-dimensional space. A data set containing N pairs of cells produces a cloud of N such points. The regression slope over all cell pairs between Corr(s1) and Corr(m) measures the similarity of neuron-ensemble firing patterns between phase S1 and phase M. A significant positive slope may reflect the rats' prior experience or the patterns of connections imposed by early developmental processes. The regression over all cell pairs between Corr(s2) and Corr(m) measures the similarity of neurone-ensemble firing patterns between phase S2 and phase M. The difference between Corr(s1) and Corr(s2) is taken to reflect the influence of the experience in phase M. If this is the case, then the magnitude and sign of this difference should be linearly related to the magnitude and sign of Corr(m).

Between-phase correlation coefficients were calculated on a within-session basis. If the numbers of neocortical and hippocampal cells recorded were n_c and n_h, respectively, then the numbers of pairwise activity correlations were $n_c(n_c - 1)/2$ within the neocortex, $n_h(n_h - 1)/2$ within the hippocampus, and $n_c n_h$ between regions. These pairwise correlations were calculated for each of phases S1, M, and S2 and were used to calculate Corr(s1, m) and Corr(s2, m). If a data set contained fewer than five cells in either hippocampus or neocortex, the corresponding within- and between-region correlations were excluded from the analysis.

Another way to determine whether there is an effect of experience on the activity pattern during sleep, one that cannot be predicted from the sleep before the experience, is to measure the strength of the linear relationship between variables Corr(m) and Corr(s2) after controlling for the effect of the variable Corr(s1). This is given by the partial correlation coefficient between Corr(m) and Corr(s2) controlling for Corr(s1), which is denoted as PCorr(m, s2|s1) (Kleinbaum *et al.* 1988):

$$\text{PCorr}(m, s2|s1) = \frac{\text{Corr}(m, s2) - \text{Corr}(s1, m)\text{Corr}(s1, s2)}{\sqrt{(1 - \text{Corr}(s1, m)^2)(1 - \text{Corr}(s1, s2)^2)}}. \tag{16.2}$$

Temporal bias of cross-correlation

For a pair of cells, whose binned firing rates are given by x_i and y_i, a measure of temporal ordering was calculated on the basis of their cross-correlation histogram (Skaggs & McNaughton 1996). As illustrated in Fig. 16.2, the temporal bias B for the cells was defined to be the difference between the

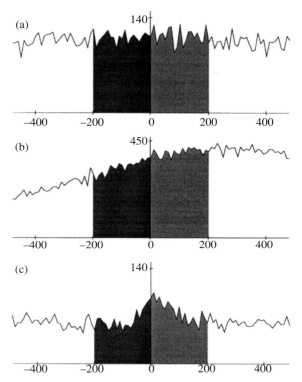

Fig. 16.2 Example of temporal bias for two neocortical cells. The three plots show cross-correlograms computed from data taken while the rat ran on a triangular track (Maze, b), during sleep beforehand (Sleep1, a), and during sleep afterwards (Sleep2, c). The measure of temporal bias is the difference between the light- and dark-shaded regions, i.e. the difference between the areas under the cross-correlograms for 200 ms after zero and 200 ms before zero. This example illustrates that the overall pattern of bias in the correlogram during Sleep2 resembles the bias during the Maze session more strongly than does the bias during Sleep1. As observed in the hippocampus (Skaggs & McNaughton 1996), there appears to be a compression of the peak in the correlogram during Sleep2 compared with Maze, suggesting an accelerated replay of sequence information; however, this aspect is not considered in detail here. Note that the count of spike pairs (ordinate) used 10 ms bins.

cross-correlation integrated over a T ms window after zero, and the cross-correlation integrated over a T ms window preceding zero. That is:

$$B_{x,y}(T) = \int_0^T r_{x,y}(t)\,\mathrm{d}t - \int_{-T}^0 r_{x,y}(t)\,\mathrm{d}t. \qquad (16.3)$$

For $t > 0$, $r_{x,y}(t)$ is the cross-correlation at lag t, defined as:

$$r_{x,y}(t) = \frac{\sum_{i=1}^{n-t}(x_i - \bar{x})(y_{i+t} - \bar{y})}{\sqrt{\sum_{i=1}^{n-t}(x_i - \bar{x})^2 \sum_{i=1+t}^{n}(y - \bar{y})^2}} \tag{16.4}$$

in which,

$$\bar{x} = \sum_{i=1}^{n-t} x_i/(n-t), \quad \bar{y} = \sum_{i=1+t}^{n} y_i/(n-t).$$

When $t < 0$, we have $r_{x,y}(t) = r_{y,x}(-t)$.

$B_{x,y}(t)$ is a normalized measure of the difference between the number of events in which a spike from cell x was followed within T ms by a spike from cell y, and the number of events in which a spike from cell y was followed within T ms by a spike from cell x. Following Skaggs & McNaughton (1996), for most analyses, T was taken as 200 ms.

16.3 Results

Neurones in the hippocampus were classified as pyramidal cells or inter-neurones according to standard criteria (Ranck 1973). In the present study, a fraction of neocortical cells (about 10%), diffusely scattered in depth, showed qualities similar to those of hippocampal interneurones, including short spike width, amplitude symmetry between negative and positive peaks, high overall firing rates (typically above 10 Hz), and regular discharge patterns. In accordance with several intracellular recording experiments (Connors et al. 1982; Connors & Gutnick 1990), these cells are considered likely to be interneurones, and are not considered further in the present report. It may be noted that none of the cells recorded from the neocortex in the present study was modulated by the hippocampal EEG theta rhythm.

Hippocampal pyramidal neurones typically exhibited spatially selective firing on the apparatus, as expected from many previous studies. As described previously (McNaughton et al. 1994), many neocortical cells in the regions recorded from here exhibited differential firing related to some component of the rat's behaviour or to the maze geometry itself. This inference is based on the fact that the spatial firing patterns exhibited symmetries that were correlated with the shape of the apparatus; no attempt was made in the present studies to characterize the basis of these correlates. Examples of behavioural correlates (based on the spatial distribution of firing rates) are illustrated in Fig. 16.1.

Based on 241 hippocampal and 568 neocortical cells, 5659 pairwise correlations were calculated in each of the S1, M and S2 phases, including 2762 neocortical cell pairs, 1982 hippocampal cell-pairs, and 915 hippocampal–neocortical cell pairs. When the data from all recording sessions were pooled, Corr(s2, m) was higher than Corr(s1, m), for all types of interaction. These data are illustrated in Fig. 16.3. Thus, for each type of interaction, the larger the correlation between any two cells on the maze, the greater was the increase in the correlation between the same two cells from S1 to S2 ($p < 0.0001$ for all three comparisons, paired t-test).

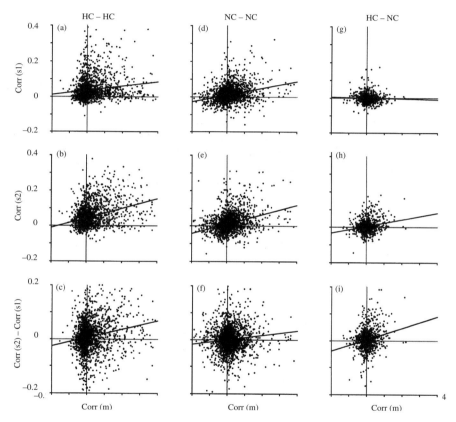

Fig. 16.3 Coherence between correlation on the maze and correlation during sleep, for different types of cell pair. Each point in a scatter plot represents one pair of simultaneously recorded neurons. The abscissa is the correlation of these neurones on the maze, Corr(m); the ordinate is their correlation during Sleep1 (Corr(s1); (a, d, g)), their correlation during Sleep2 (Corr(s2); (b, e, h)), or the difference between these correlations (Corr(s2) − Corr(s1); (c, f, i)). The *left* column (a, b, c) includes only pairs where both cells were recorded from the CA1 layer of the hippocampus; the *centre* column (d, e, f) only pairs of neurones both from the neocortex, and the *right* column (g, h, i) pairs with one cell each from the hippocampus and the neocortex. Each plot demonstrates a statistically significant positive correlation ($p < 0.001$), with the exception of (g) (hippocampus–neocortex for Sleep1 versus maze).

To confirm that this effect was not confined to a small number of data sets, partial regression analysis was conducted on each data set independently. Figure 16.4 shows the average correlations (over data sets) between Corr(s1) and Corr(m) and partial correlations between Corr(m) and Corr(s2) after controlling for Corr(s1).

For all comparisons, there was a significant ($p < 0.05$) overall effect of M on S2 after controlling for S1. For within-structure comparisons (NC and HC in Fig. 16.4), there were also significant relations between the cell–cell interactions on the maze and the corresponding interactions during S1 ($p < 0.05$); this result indicates that, within each structure, the interactions on the maze are partly predictable from the interactions that occur before the animal experiences the maze on the day in question. This was not true for the hippocampal–neocortical interaction (NC–HC, Fig. 16.3), for which the coherence between S1 and M was not significantly different from zero, but was significantly different from the other comparisons.

As reported previously by Skaggs & McNaughton (1996), the temporal bias in the interaction between hippocampal cell pairs is preserved between M and S2 more strongly than between M and S1. This finding was replicated in the current experiment, as shown in the left column of Fig. 16.5 ($p < 0.001$, paired *t*-test). Temporal bias for neocortical cell pairs significantly reflected the maze bias during both S1 and S2, but the degree of coherence was significantly enhanced during S2 relative to S1 ($p < 0.01$, paired *t*-test). For hippocampal–neocortical cell pairs, there was no significant correlation of bias during either S1 or S2 with bias during M and no significant difference between S1 and S2 in this correlation.

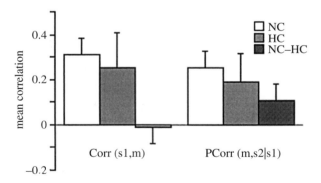

Fig. 16.4 Histograms of correlations and partial correlations between Maze, Sleep1 and Sleep2 for different types of cell pair, across data sets. (a) Mean correlations between Maze and Sleep1, for correlations between HC, NC, and HC–NC cell pairs. (b) Partial correlations of Maze with Sleep2, after the expected effect of correlation in Sleep1 has been subtracted. The error bars represent 95% confidence intervals. All correlations and partial correlations are significantly greater than zero ($p < 0.05$), except the correlation between Maze and Sleep1 for HC–NC cell pairs.

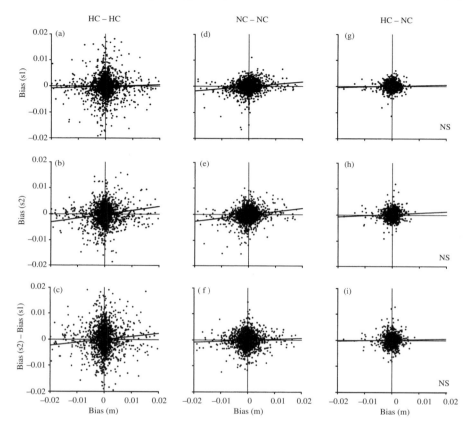

Fig. 16.5 Coherence between temporal bias on the maze and temporal bias during sleep, for different types of cell pair. Each point in a scatter plot represents one pair of simultaneously recorded neurons. The abscissa is the temporal bias of these neurons on the maze (Bias(m)); the ordinate is their bias during Sleep1 (Bias(s1); (a,d,g)), their bias during Sleep2 (Bias(s2); (b, e, h)), or the difference of these bias values (c, f, i). The *left* column (a, b, c) includes pairs where both cells were recorded from the CA1 layer of the hippocampus; the *centre* column (d, e, f) pairs of neurons both from the neocortex, and the *right* column (g, h, i) pairs with one cell each from the hippocampus and the neocortex. Each plot in the first two columns (a–f) demonstrates a statistically significant positive correlation ($p < 0.01$). None of the correlations for HC–NC pairs (g, h, i) is significant.

16.4 Discussion

The main finding of the present study is that, during periods of slow-wave sleep after an episode of spatially extended behaviour, patterns of neuronal correlation that were manifest during the behaviour re-emerge in neocortical and hippocampal circuits as well as in the interactions between these two areas.

For all three comparisons, the distribution of pairwise firing-rate correlations during sleep after the behaviour (S2) more strongly reflected the patterns observed during behaviour (M) than did the corresponding distributions recorded during sleep preceding behaviour (S1). The reactivation of patterns of correlation between hippocampus and neocortex is a necessary (but not sufficient) requirement of the theory that the hippocampus initiates and orchestrates the reactivation of traces of recent experience in neocortical circuits. Whether or not this is the case, this result indicates that, at a given moment, the patterns of activity in these two regions during sleep tend to reflect components of the same experience.

For within-area comparisons, there was also some correlation between S1 and M; this correlation indicates that patterns of network activity on the maze are related to patterns that occurred during sleep before-hand. This is to be expected for the posterior cortex, because many of these cells exhibit clear, mutually exclusive categories of behavioural correlates (e.g. left vs right turns (McNaughton *et al.* 1994)). This is presumably a reflection of previously established synaptic connectivity. It is also to be expected for within-hippocampus comparisons, because place fields are highly consistent from day to day in a given environment (Thompson & Best 1990), and the rats in the present study had substantial previous experience in the recording apparatus. Moreover, there is evidence to suggest that the possible patterns of place-field overlap are to some extent preconfigured within the hippocampal synaptic matrix (Hill 1978; Quirk *et al.* 1992; Kudrimoti *et al.* 1995; Gothard *et al.* 1996; McNaughton *et al.* 1996). On the other hand, if, as the evidence suggests, the hippocampus is primarily involved in providing a spatial coordinate representation, whereas the neocortical areas studied here are primarily involved in sensory–motor integration, there should be no strongly constrained set of preconfigured relations between the two regions. For example, it is *a priori* equally likely that the animal will turn right or left at location X. Thus, the fact that there was no strong relation between S1 and M in the patterns of correlation of hippocampal–neocortical pairs, but a significant relation between S2 and M, can be taken as evidence for a learning-related change in connection strengths in the direct or indirect pathways connecting these two regions. These changes apparently decayed within the *c.* 24-h time periods that separated recording sessions.

The decay of hippocampal–neocortical correlations appears to present some difficulty for the simple form of the consolidation theory, because the theory assumes that the enhanced connections should persist for a time period of weeks at least (in the rat). The effect might be explainable by a nonlinearity between the extent of reactivation in the hippocampus and the corresponding pattern in the neocortex, such that the observed reduction in intrahippocampal correlations from one day to the next (Wilson & McNaughton 1994; Skaggs & McNaughton 1996) leads to a greater reduction in hippocampal–neocortical correlations. This explanation assumes that the coherence seen in neocortex during S1 is due largely to stable patterns of connections in neocortex.

The present results also replicate the previous finding that some aspects of the temporal structure of hippocampal population activity in a spatial task are preserved during sleep afterwards (Skaggs & McNaughton 1996), and demonstrate that a similar effect occurs for neocortical cell pairs, but not for mixed hippocampal–neocortical pairs. This pattern of results is consistent with the prediction of the consolidation theory that information is transferred from the neocortex to the hippocampus during the waking state, and then replayed back to the neocortex from the hippocampus during sleep. Thus, temporal structure intrinsic to the hippocampus or neocortex should be replicated, but, because of the postulated change in the direction of information flow, the temporal relations between the two structures should be altered. For example, suppose that in waking, a pattern A–B–C of activity in neocortex gives rise, after a small delay, to a pattern A′–B′–C′ in the hippocampus; and that during sleep the same hippocampal pattern precedes the same neocortical pattern. Then we have the following scenario:

	Awake	Sleeping
NC:	A–B–C	A–B–C
HC:	A′–B′–C′	A′–B′–C′

The temporal relations are quite different in the two states, but a simple time-shift of the hippocampal pattern would bring them back into their original alignment. In reality, the patterns during sleep might also be subjected to a considerable temporal compression as well as to a time shift (August & Levy 1996; Skaggs & McNaughton 1996; Skaggs et al. 1996). These questions await further study.

An essential function of long-term memory is to construct, from past experience, internal representations of the world that permit adaptive generalization and appropriate responses to novel, or partly novel, situations. The development of such internal representations appears to require repeated interleaved exposure to exemplars of the categories to be formed, with small adjustments to the synapses on each trial (McClelland et al. 1995). Attempts to store new information all at once in such a memory lead to 'catastrophic interference' with items already stored (McClosky & Cohen 1989). Survival, however, often requires adding new items to the existing categorical structure, with only one or a few experiences. This leads to the idea of storage in a temporary buffer, followed by quasi-random reactivation during periods when the system is offline. The present findings, that memory traces are indeed reactivated during sleep both in the hippocampus and the neocortex, and that the patterns of correlation between these structures during sleep are consistent with prior behaviour, provide a key piece of evidence in support of this theory It still remains to be demonstrated, however, that the coherence of pattern reactivation across widely separated neocortical modules is dependent on an orchestrating flow of stored information from the hippocampal formation.

Acknowledgements

Supported by grants MH46823, MH01227 and the McDonnell and Pew Foundations. We thank M. Suster, K. Moore, L. Frank, R. D'Monte, J. Gerrard, K. Stengel, V. Pawlowski and Jie Wang for technical assistance with this project.

References

Amaral, D. G. & Witter, M. P. 1995 Hippocampal formation. In *The rat nervous system*, 2nd edn (ed., G. Paxinos), pp. 443–493. San Diego, CA: Academic Press.

August, D. A. & Levy, W. B. 1996 Temporal sequence compression by a hippocampal network model. In *INNS World Congress on Neural Networks*, pp. 1299–1304. Hillsdale, NJ: Lawrence Erlbaum.

Connors, B. W., Gutnick, M. J. & Prince, D. A. 1982 Electrophysiological properties of neocortical neurons *in vitro. J. Neurophys.* **48**, 1302–1320.

Connors, B. W. & Gutnick, M. J. 1990 Intrinsic firing patterns of diverse neocortical neurons. *Trends Neurosci.* **13**, 99–104.

Gothard, K. M., Skaggs, W. E., Moore, K. M. & McNaughton, B. L. 1996 Binding of hippocampal CA1 neural activity to multiple reference frames in a landmark-based navigation task. *J. Neurosci.* **16**, 823–835.

Gray, C. M., Maldonado, P. E., Wilson, M. A. & McNaughton, B. L. 1995 Tetrodes markedly improve the yield and reliability of multiple single-unit isolation from multi-unit recordings in cat striate cortex. *J. Neurosci. Meth.* **63**, 43–54.

Hill, A. J. 1978 First occurrence of hippocampal spatial firing in a new environment. *Expl Neurol.* **62**, 282–297.

Kleinbaum, D. G., Kupper, L. L. & Muller, K. E. 1988 *Applied regression analysis and other multivariable methods.* Belmont, CA: Duxbury Press.

Kudrimoti, H. S., McNaughton, B. L., Barnes, C. A. & Skaggs, W. E. 1995 Recent experience strengthens pre-existing correlations between hippocampal neurons during sleep. *Soc. Neurosci. Abstr.* **21**, 941.

Marr, D. 1971 Simple memory: a theory for archicortex. *Phil. Trans. R. Soc. Lond.* B **262**, 23–81.

McClelland, J. L., McNaughton, B. L. & O'Reilly, R. C. 1995 Why are there complementary learning systems in hippocampus and neocortex: insights from the successes and failures of connectionist models of learning and memory. *Psychol. Rev.* **5**, 245–286.

McClosky, M. & Cohen, N. J. 1989 Catastrophic interference in connectionist networks: the sequential learning problem. In *The psychology of learning and motivation* (ed., G. H. Bower), pp. 109–165. New York: Academic Press.

McNaughton, B. L., Barnes, C. A., Meltzer, J. & Sutherland, R. J. 1989 Hippocampal granule cells are necessary for normal spatial learning but not for spatially-selective pyramidal cell discharge. *Expl Brain Res.* **76**, 485–496.

McNaughton, B. L., Mizumori, S. J. Y., Barnes, C. A., Leonard, B. J., Marquis, M. & Green, E. J. 1994 Cortical representation of motion during spatial navigation in the rat. *Cerebr. Cortex* **4**, 27–39.

McNaughton, B. L., O'Keefe, J. & Barnes, C. A. 1983 The stereotrode: a new technique for simultaneous isolation of several single units in the central nervous system from multiple unit records. *J. Neurosci. Meth.* **8**, 391–397.

Nadel, L., Wilner, J. & Kurz, E. M. 1985 Cognitive maps and environmental context. In *Context and learning* (ed., P. D. B. A. Tomie), pp. 385–406. Hillsdale, NJ: Lawrence Erlbaum.

O'Keefe, J. & Nadel, L. 1978 *The hippocampus as a cognitive map*. Oxford: Clarendon Press.

Pavlides, C. & Winson, J. 1989 Influences of hippocampal place cell firing in the awake state on the activity of these cells during subsequent sleep episodes. *J. Neurosci.* **9**, 2907–2918.

Qin, Y.-L., McNaughton, B. L., Skaggs, W. E. & Barnes, C. A. 1995 Reactivation during sleep of cortico-cortical and hippocampo-cortical correlation states from preceding behaviour. *Soc. Neurosci. Abstr.* **21**, 941.

Qin, Y.-L., McNaughton, B. L., Skaggs, W. E., Barnes, C. A., Suster, M. S., Weaver, K. L. & Gerrard, J. L. 1996 Interaction between hippocampus and neocortex in the replay of temporal sequences during sleep. *Soc. Neurosci. Abstr.* **22**, 1872.

Quirk, G. J., Muller, R. U., Kubie, J. L. & Ranck, J. B. 1992 The positional firing properties of medial entorhinal neurons: description and comparison with hippocampal place cells. *J. Neurosci.* **12**, 1945–1963.

Ranck, J. B. Jr 1973 Studies on single neurons in dorsal hippocampal formation and septum in unrestrained rats. I. Behavioural correlates and firing repertoires. *Expl Neurol.* **41**, 461–531.

Recce, M. & O'Keefe, J. 1989 The tetrode: a new technique for multi-unit extracellular recording. *Soc. Neurosci. Abstr.* **19**, 1250.

Scoville, W. B. & Milner, B. 1957 Loss of recent memory after bilateral hippocampal lesions. *J. Neurol. Neurosurg. Psychiatr.* **20**, 11–21.

Shen, B. & McNaughton, B. L. 1997 Modeling the spontaneous reactivation of experience-specific hippocampal cell assemblies during sleep. *Hippocampus* **6**, 1–8.

Skaggs, W. E. & McNaughton, B. L. 1996 Replay of neuronal firing sequences in rat hippocampus during sleep following spatial experience. *Science* **271**, 1870–1873.

Skaggs, W. E., McNaughton, B. L., Wilson, M. A. & Barnes, C. A. 1996 Theta phase precession in hippocampal neuronal populations and the compression of temporal sequences. *Hippocampus* **6**, 149–172.

Squire, L. R. 1992 Memory and the hippocampus: a synthesis from findings with rats, monkeys, and humans. *Psychol. Rev.* **99**, 195–231.

Teyler, T. J. & Discenna, P. 1986 The hippocampal memory indexing theory. *Behav. Neurosci.* **100**, 147–154.

Thompson, L. T. & Best, P. J. 1990 Long-term stability of place-field activity of single units recorded from the dorsal hippocampus of freely behaving rats. *Brain Res.* **509**, 299–308.

Vanderwolf, C. H. 1969 Hippocampal electrical activity and voluntary movement in the rat. *EEG Clin. Neurophys.* **26**, 407–418.

Wilson, M. A. & McNaughton, B. L. 1993 Dynamics of the hippocampal ensemble code for space. *Science* **261**, 1055–1058.

Wilson, M. A. & McNaughton, B. L. 1994 Reactivation of hippocampal ensemble memories during sleep. *Science* **265**, 577–708.

Winson, J. & Abzug, C. 1977 Gating of neuronal transmission in the hippocampus: efficacy of transmission varies with behavioural state. *Science* **196**, 1223–1225.

Zilles, K. 1985 *The cortex of the rat*. Berlin: Springer.

17

The representation of space in the primate hippocampus, and its role in memory

Edmund T. Rolls

17.1 Introduction

The aims of this chapter are to consider how space is represented in the primate hippocampus, how this is related to the memory functions performed by the hippocampus, and how the hippocampus performs these functions. In addition to the evidence that is available from anatomical connections, the effects of lesions to the system, and recordings of the activity of single neurones in the system, neuronal network models of hippocampal function will also be discussed, as they have the promise of enabling one to understand what and how the hippocampus computes, and thus to understand the functions being performed by the hippocampus. The neurophysiological and brain lesion studies described have been performed (unless stated otherwise) with macaque monkeys in order to provide information as relevant as possible to understanding memory systems and amnesia in humans.

17.2 Damage to the hippocampal system and spatial function

Damage to the hippocampus or to some of its connections, such as the fornix in monkeys, produces deficits in learning about the places of objects and about the places where responses should be made. For example, macaques and humans with damage to the hippocampal formation or fornix are impaired in object–place memory tasks in which not only the objects seen, but where they were seen, must be remembered (Smith and Milner 1981; Gaffan and Saunders 1985; Parkinson *et al.* 1988). Such object–place tasks require a whole scene or snapshot-like memory in which spatial relations in a scene must be remembered (Gaffan 1994). Also, fornix lesions impair conditional left-right discrimination learning, in which the visual appearance of an object specifies whether a response is to be made to the left or the right (Rupniak and Gaffan 1987). A comparable deficit is found in humans (Petrides 1985). Fornix-sectioned monkeys are also impaired in learning on the basis of a spatial cue which object to choose (e.g. if two objects are on the left, choose object A, but if the two objects are on the right, choose object B) (Gaffan and Harrison 1989*a*).

Monkeys with fornix damage are also impaired in using information about their place in an environment. For example, Gaffan and Harrison (1989*b*) found learning impairments when which of two or more objects the monkey had to choose depended on the position of the monkey in the room.

17.3 Non-spatial aspects of the function of the hippocampus in primates: its role in memory

Damage to the perirhinal cortex, which receives from the high order association cortex and has connections to the hippocampus (see Fig. 17.1), accounts for the deficits in 'recognition' memory (i.e. for stimuli seen recently) produced by damage to this brain region (Zola-Morgan *et al*. 1989, 1994). Given that some topographic segregation is maintained in the afferents to the hippocampus through the perirhinal and parahippocampal cortices (Amaral and Witter 1989), it may be that these areas are able to subserve memory within one of these topographically separated areas, of, for example, visual object, or spatial, or olfactory information. In contrast, the final convergence afforded by the hippocampus into one network in CA3 (see Fig. 17.1) may be especially for an episodic memory typically involving arbitrary associations between any of the inputs to the hippocampus, e.g. spatial, visual object, olfactory, and auditory (see below). On the hypothesis described elsewhere (Rolls 1989*a–c*; Treves and Rolls 1994; Rolls 1996*a*; Rolls and Treves 1998) and summarized below that the hippocampus provides a neural network capable of storing a large number of different memories, deficits in memory tasks which require convergence from many different cortical processing streams might only be especially evident in studies with lesions restricted to the hippocampus proper when many different memories of this type must be stored and retrieved.

17.4 Relation between spatial and non-spatial aspects of hippocampal function and episodic memory

One way of relating the impairment of spatial processing to other aspects of hippocampal function is to note that this spatial processing involves a snapshot type of memory, in which one whole scene must be remembered. This memory may then be a special case of episodic memory, which involves an arbitrary association of a particular set of events which describe a past episode. Further, the non-spatial tasks impaired by damage to the hippocampal system may be impaired because they are tasks in which a memory of a particular episode or context rather than of a general rule is involved (Gaffan *et al*. 1984). Further, the deficit in paired associate learning in humans may be especially evident when this involves arbitrary associations between words, for example, window–lake.

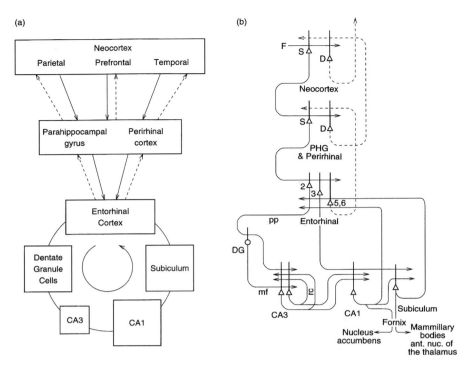

Fig. 17.1 Forward connections (*solid lines*) from areas of cerebral association neo-cortex via the parahippocampal gyrus and perirhinal cortex, and entorhinal cortex, to the hippocampus; and backprojections (*dashed lines*) via the hippocampal CA1 pyramidal cells, subiculum, and parahippocampal gyrus to the neocortex. There is great convergence in the forward connections down to the single network implemented in the CA3 pyramidal cells; and great divergence again in the backprojections. (a) Block diagram. (b) More detailed representation of some of the principal excitatory neurones in the pathways. Abbreviations: D, deep pyramidal cells; DG, dentate granule cells; F, forward inputs to areas of the association cortex from preceding cortical areas in the hierarchy; mf, mossy fibres; PHG, parahippocampal gyrus and perirhinal cortex; pp, perforant path; rc, recurrent collateral of the CA3 hippocampal pyramidal cells; S, superficial pyramidal cells; 2, pyramidal cells in layer 2 of the entorhinal cortex; 3, pyramidal cells in layer 3 of the entorhinal cortex. The thick lines above the cell bodies represent the dendrites.

I suggest that the reason why the hippocampus is used for the spatial and non-spatial types of memory described above, and the reason that makes these two types of memory so analogous, is that the hippocampus contains one stage, the CA3 stage, which acts as an autoassociation memory. (The structure, operation and properties of autoassociation memories in relation to hippo-campal function are described by Treves and Rolls (1994) and Rolls and Treves (1998).) It is suggested that an autoassociation memory implemented by the CA3 neurones equally enables whole (spatial) scenes or episodic memories to be formed, with a snapshot quality that depends on the arbitrary associations which can be made, and the short temporal window, which characterize, the synaptic modifiability in this system (see below and Rolls 1987, 1989*a,b*; Rolls and Treves 1998). The hypothesis is that the autoassociation memory enables arbitrary sets of concurrent activity, involving, for example, the spatial context where an episode occurred, the people present during the episode, and what was seen during the episode, to be associated together and stored as one event. Later recall of that episode from the hippocampus in response to a partial cue can then lead to reinstatement of the activity in the neocortex that was originally present during the episode. The theory we have developed shows how the episodic memory could be stored in the hippocampus, and later retrieved to the neocortex (see Section 17.6).

17.5 Systems level analysis of hippocampal function, including neuronal activity in the primate hippocampus

In order to understand how the hippocampus operates, we now turn to a systems level analysis in which we consider the connections of the hippocampus with the rest of the brain, and the activity of single neurones in the hippocampus when it is performing its normal function assessed by the effects of selective damage to the hippocampus described above.

Systems level anatomy

The primate hippocampus receives inputs via the entorhinal cortex (area 28) and the parahippocampal gyrus from many areas of the cerebral association cortex, including the parietal cortex, which is concerned with spatial functions, the visual and auditory temporal association cortical areas, and the frontal cortex (Van Hoesen 1982; Amaral 1987; Suzuki and Amaral 1994; see Rolls 1989*a,b*). In addition, the entorhinal cortex receives inputs from the amygdala. There are also subcortical inputs from, for example, the amygdala and septum. The hippocampus in turn projects back via the subiculum, entorhinal cortex, and parahippocampal gyrus (area TF-TH), to the cerebral cortical areas from which it receives inputs (Van Hoesen 1982), as well as to subcortical areas such as the mammillary bodies (see Fig. 17.1).

Systems level neurophysiology

The information processing being performed by the primate hippocampus while it is performing the functions for which lesion studies have shown it is needed, has been investigated in studies in which the activity of single hippocampal neurones has been analysed during the performance and learning of these (and related) spatial tasks.

Memory for the positions of responses and for the positions of stimuli in memory tasks

Watanabe and Niki (1985) have analysed hippocampal neuronal activity while monkeys performed a delayed spatial response task. In a delayed spatial response task, a stimulus is shown on, for example, the left, there is then a delay period, and after this the monkey can respond, by, for example, touching the left stimulus position. They reported that 6.4 per cent of hippocampal neurones responded differently while the monkey was remembering left as compared to right. The responses of these neurones could reflect preparation for the spatial response to be made, or they could reflect memory of the spatial position in which the stimulus was shown. To provide evidence on which was important, Cahusac, Miyashita and Rolls (1989) analysed hippocampal activity in this task, and in an object–place memory task. In the object–place memory task, the monkey was shown a sample stimulus in one position on a video screen, there was a delay of 2 s, and then the same or a different stimulus was shown in the same or in a different position. The monkey remembered the sample and its position, and if both matched the delayed stimulus, he licked to obtain fruit juice. Of the 600 neurones analysed in this task, 3.8 per cent responded differently for the different spatial positions, with some of these responding differentially during the sample presentation, some in the delay period, and some in the match period. Thus some hippocampal neurones (those differentially active in the sample or match periods) respond differently for stimuli shown in different positions in space, and some (those differentially active in the delay period) respond differently when the monkey is remembering different positions in space. In addition, some of the neurones responded to a combination of object and place information, in that they responded only to a novel object in a particular place. These neuronal responses were not due to any response being made or prepared by the monkey, for information about which behavioural response was required was not available until the match stimulus was shown. Cahusac et al. (1989) also found that the majority of the neurones that responded in the object–place memory task did not respond in the delayed spatial response task. Instead, a different population of neurones (5.7 per cent of the total) responded in the delayed spatial response task, with differential left–right responses in the sample, delay, or match periods. Thus this latter population of hippocampal neurones had activity that was related to the preparation for or initiation of a spatial response, which in the delayed response task could be encoded as soon as the sample stimulus was seen.

These recordings showed that there are some neurones in the primate hippocampus with activity that is related to the spatial position of stimuli or to the memory of the spatial position of stimuli (as shown in the object–place memory task), and that there are other neurones in the hippocampus with activity that is related not to the stimulus or the memory of the stimulus, but instead to the spatial response which the monkey is preparing and remembering (as shown in the delayed spatial response task). The recordings also showed that information about which visual stimulus was shown, and where it was shown, was combined onto some neurones in the primate hippocampus.

Object–place memory tasks

The responses of hippocampal neurones in primates with activity related to the place in which a stimulus is shown was further investigated using a serial multiple object–place memory task. The task required a memory for the position on a video monitor in which a given object had appeared previously (Rolls *et al*. 1989). This task was designed to allow a wider area of space to be tested than in the previous study, and was chosen also because memory of where objects had been seen previously in space was known to be disrupted by hippocampal damage (Gaffan and Saunders 1985; Gaffan 1987). In the task a visual image appeared in one of four or nine positions on a screen. If the stimulus had been seen in that position before, the monkey could lick to obtain fruit juice, but if the image had not appeared in that position before, the monkey had *not* to lick in order to *avoid* the taste of saline. Each image appeared in each position on the screen only twice: once as novel and once as familiar. The task thus required memory not only of which visual stimuli had been seen before, but of the positions in which they had been seen, and is an object–place memory task. It was found that 9 per cent of neurones recorded in the hippocampus and parahippocampal gyrus had spatial fields in this and related tasks, in that they responded whenever there was a stimulus in some but not in other positions on the screen. It was also found that 2.4 per cent of the neurones responded to a combination of spatial information and information about the object seen, in that they responded more the first time a particular image was seen in any position. Six of these neurones were found which showed this combination even more clearly, in that they, for example, responded only to some positions, and only provided that it was the first time that a particular stimulus had appeared there. Thus not only is spatial information processed by the primate hippocampus, but it can be combined as shown by the responses of single neurones with information about which stimuli have been seen before (Rolls *et al*. 1989).

The ability of the hippocampus to form such arbitrary associations of information probably originating from the parietal cortex about position in space with information originating from the temporal lobe about objects may be important for its role in memory. Moreover these findings provide neurophysiological support for the computational theory described here and elsewhere (Treves and Rolls 1994; Rolls and Treves 1998), according to which arbitrary associations should be formed onto single neurones in the hippocampus between signals originating in different parts of the cerebral cortex, e.g. about objects and about position in space.

An allocentric representation of space in the primate hippocampus

These studies show that some hippocampal neurones in primates have spatial fields. In order to investigate how space is represented in the hippocampus,

Feigenbaum and Rolls (1991) investigated whether the spatial fields use egocentric or some form of allocentric coordinates. This was investigated by finding a neurone with a space field, and then moving the monitor screen and the monkey relative to each other, and to different positions in the laboratory. For 10 per cent of the spatial neurones, the responses remained in the same position relative to the monkey's body axis when the screen was moved or the monkey was rotated or moved to a different position in the laboratory. These neurones thus represented space in egocentric coordinates. For 46 per cent of the spatial neurones analysed, the responses remained in the same position on the screen or in the room when the monkey was rotated or moved to a different position in the laboratory. These neurones thus represented space in allocentric coordinates. Evidence for two types of allocentric encoding was found. In the first type, the field was defined by its position on the monitor screen independently of the position of the monitor relative to the monkey's body axis and independently of the position of the monkey and the screen in the laboratory. These neurones were called 'frame of reference' allocentric, in that their fields were defined by the local frame provided by the monitor screen. The majority of the allocentric neurones responded in this way. In the second type of allocentric encoding, the field was defined by its position in the room, and was relatively independent of position relative to the monkey's body axis or to position on the monitor screen face. These neurones were called 'absolute' allocentric, in that their fields were defined by position in the room. These results provide evidence that in addition to neurones with egocentric spatial fields, which have also been found in other parts of the brain such as the parietal cortex (Sakata 1985; Andersen 1987), there are neurones in the primate hippocampal formation which encode space in allocentric coordinates.

Spatial view neurones in the primate hippocampus

In rats, place cells are found, which respond depending on the place where the rat is in a spatial environment (see McNaughton *et al*. 1983; O'Keefe 1984). In a first investigation to analyse whether such cells might be present in the primate hippocampus, Rolls and O'Mara (1993, 1995) recorded the responses of hippocampal cells when macaques were moved in a small chair or robot on wheels in a cue-controlled testing environment (a $2\,m \times 2\,m \times 2\,m$ chamber with matt black internal walls and floors). Tests were performed to determine whether cells might be found that could be described as 'place-related', i.e. firing differently when macaques are moved to different places in this environment; or according to the position in space at which the monkey is looking; or according to his 'head direction'. The most common type of cell responded to the part of space at which the monkeys were looking, independently of the place where the monkey was. These neurones were called 'view' neurones, and are similar to the space neurones described by Rolls *et al*. (1989), and Feigenbaum and Rolls (1991). (The main difference was that in the study of Rolls *et al*. (1989) and Feigenbaum and Rolls (1991), the allocentric representation was defined by where on a video monitor a stimulus was shown;

whereas view cells respond when the monkey looks at a particular part of a spatial environment.) Some of these view neurones had responses that depended on the proximity of the monkey to what was being viewed. Only one neurone had firing which appeared to depend on where the monkey was, and one on movement towards a particular place. Thus in this study the neuronal representation of space found in the primate hippocampus was shown to be defined primarily by the view of the environment, and not by the place where the monkey was (Rolls and O'Mara 1993, 1995). Ono et al. (1993) also performed studies on the representation of space in the primate hippocampus while the monkey was moved to different places in a room. They found that 13.4 per cent of hippocampal formation neurones fired more when the monkey was at some places than when at other places in the test area, and although some neurones responded more when the monkey was at some places than at others, it was not clear whether the responses of these neurones responded to the place where the monkey was independently of view, or whether the responses of place-like cells were view-dependent.

In rats, place cells fire best during active locomotion by the rat (Foster et al. 1989). To investigate whether place cells might be present in monkeys if active locomotion was being performed, in current experiments we recorded from single hippocampal neurones while monkeys move themselves round the test environment by walking (Rolls et al. 1995, 1997a, 1998; Robertson et al. 1998). Also, to bring out the responses of spatial cells in the primate hippocampus, we changed from the cue-controlled environment of Rolls and O'Mara (1995), which was matt black apart from four spatial cues, to the much richer environment of the open laboratory, within which the monkey has a 2.5×2.5 m area to walk. The position and head direction of the monkey are tracked continuously, and the eye position is recorded continuously with the search coil technique, so that we can measure exactly where the monkey is looking in the environment at all times. The responses of a hippocampal spatial view cell recorded in this environment is shown in Fig. 17.2. The firing rate of the cell is shown in Fig. 17.2a and 17.2b when the monkey was stationary at two different places in the environment and was looking at the spatial environment. The arrow shows the head direction of the monkey, which was fixed for the period of recording in which the firing rates were being measured in Fig. 17.2a and 17.2b. The cell only fired when the monkey was looking at a given part of the wall of the room (indicated approximately as the response field of the cell). The firing could not be due to the place where the monkey was, nor to the head direction of the monkey, both of which were different in Fig. 17.2a and 17.2b. Comparison of Fig. 17.2a and 17.2b shows that when the monkey was closer to the wall (Fig. 17.2a), the responsive region filled a larger part of the area visible to the monkey, as expected for a response field located on the wall of the room. (In the vertical direction, the area visible to the monkey may not have reached the centre of the response field, as shown in Fig. 17.2a and 17.2b.) In Fig. 17.2c, the firing rate of the same cell is shown when the monkey had been at many different places in the environment, looking in many different

(a)

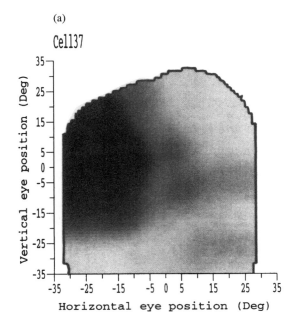

Cell 37

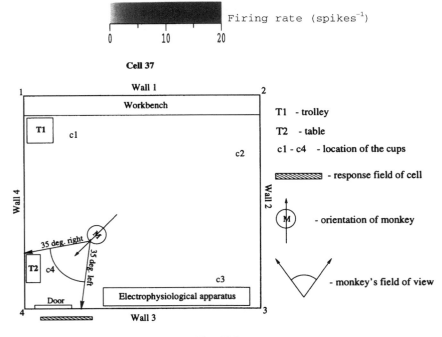

Fig. 17.2

(b)

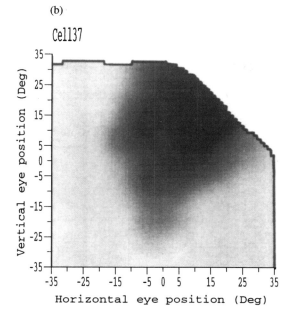

Cell 37

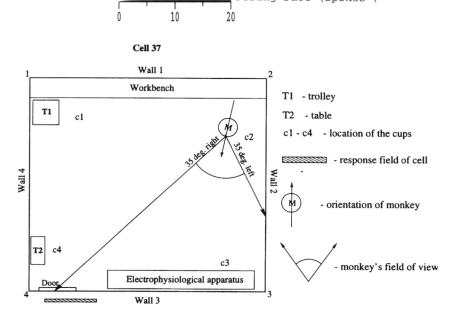

T1 - trolley

T2 - table

c1 - c4 - location of the cups

 - response field of cell

M - orientation of monkey

 - monkey's field of view

Fig. 17.2

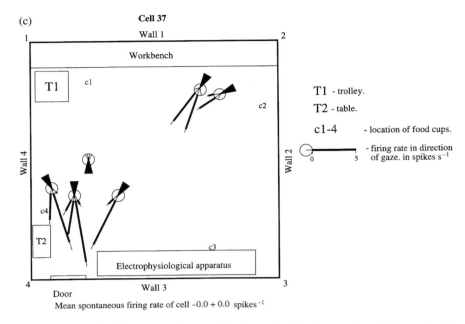

Fig. 17.2 (a) The firing rate of a spatial view cell with the monkey stationary in the environment, with its head direction indicated by the *arrow*, and moving its eyes to look at different parts of the environment. (b) Similar data when the monkey was at a different place in the environment, and with a different head direction. The cell increased its firing rate when the monkey looked at some parts of the environment (e.g. towards corner 4). The firing rate of the cell in spikes s^{-1} is indicated by the blackness of the diagram on the left (with the calibration bar in spikes s^{-1} shown below). The field of view sampled by the monkey is shown by the part of the firing rate grayscale plot which is contained by the black perimeter line. (c) A summary of the firing rates when the monkey was looking at different spatial views in the environment, from different places and with different head directions. The acute angle of the *solid triangle* indicates the head direction. The short lines within the circle indicate the view directions (binned with 17.5 degrees per bin) in which data were available. The bars outside the circle represent the mean firing rate (and the s.e.m.) of the cell when the monkey was looking in that direction; the absence of a bar outside the circle where data were available indicates a firing rate of 0 spikes s^{-1}. (From Rolls *et al.* 1997a.)

directions. Figure 17.2c also shows that the cell did not fire only when the monkey was at one place, and therefore cannot be described as a place cell. Instead the cell fired whenever the monkey looked at a certain part of the environment, which is termed the spatial view field of the neurone.

It was possible to repeat this type of experiment (with the monkey stationary) for 20 of the 40 cells analysed. In all 20 cases, the cells responded when the monkey was stationary but looking at and visually exploring the environment. In all 20 cases, it was shown, as in Fig. 17.2, that the cells could respond when the monkey was in different places in the environment, and that the critical factor in determining the firing rate of the cell was where in the environment the monkey was looking (Rolls *et al.* 1997*a*). The responses of a hippocampal cell with a spatial view field recorded during active locomotion are shown in Fig. 17.3a. The responses of these neurones when the monkey was exploring the spatial environment using eye movements but with the head and body still, were in all cases consistent with those measured during active locomotion (Rolls *et al.* 1997*a*).

In experiments of the type illustrated in Fig. 17.2, in which the head was placed at different positions and angles in the environment, it was possible to confirm that it was where the monkey was looking, and not the eye position in the head *per se*, nor the place where the monkey was located, nor the head direction, which accounted for the firing of these neurones (Georges-François *et al.* 1998). This series of experiments proved that the representation provided by these spatial view neurones was not egocentric (with respect to the head or body), but was instead allocentric, representing positions in space in world-based coordinates.

(a)   **Cell 26**

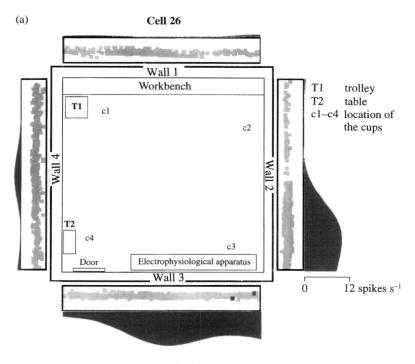

Fig. 17.3

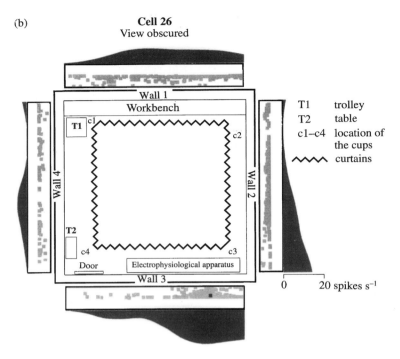

Fig. 17.3 (a) The spatial view field of a hippocampal pyramidal cell (number 26) during free exploration of the room. The firing rate of the cell (spikes s^{-1}) is shown for each wall in the graphs on the outside of the diagram. A spot on the set of four rectangles, each of which represents one of the walls of the room, indicates where on a wall the monkey had been looking every 67 ms during the 7-min recording session shown. The bottom of the wall is represented closest to the centre of the diagram. (b) For the same cell the firing rate is shown when the monkey walked in the room with all the visual details of the four walls obscured by ceiling-to-floor black curtains. (From Rolls *et al*. 1997*a*.)

In further experiments on these spatial view neurones, it was shown that their responses reflected quite an abstract representation of space, in that if the visual details of the view were completely obscured by black curtains, then many of the neurones could still respond when the monkey looked towards where the view had been (e.g. Fig. 17.3b, cell AV057) (Robertson *et al*. 1998). This is an impressive result, for it shows that the responses of these neurones can be produced by any combinations of head direction and eye position commands made by the monkey, which together result in the monkey looking towards a given position in space, even when the monkey cannot actually see that position in space. It was further possible to demonstrate a memory component to this representation, by placing the room in darkness (with, in addition, black curtains completely obscuring all views of the testing environment), and showing that at least some of these neurones still responded (though with smaller selectivity) when the monkey was rotated to face towards the view to which the view neurone being recorded normally responded. These neurones were certainly influenced by visual inputs, in that the spatial view fields often slipped by a small amount and might become less selective when the curtains were drawn closed and the room was in darkness (see, for example, Fig. 17.3b). These properties were typical for cells in the hippocampal CA1 region and in the parahippocampal gyrus. Additional evidence that visual inputs are important in defining the responses of spatial view neurones is that for CA3 pyramidal cells, obscuring the view details produced a considerable reduction in the neuronal response (to on average 19 per cent of the response with the spatial environment visible) (Robertson et al. 1998). This reduction in the firing of the CA3 cells reflects the reduction in the visual sensory drive or recall cue to a CA3 memory system. Even the recall by autoassociation thought to be present in the CA3 system is insufficient to produce full recall with the incomplete input. However, with an additional association stage of synapses implemented in the Schaffer collateral connections from the CA3 to the CA1 cells, further retrieval would occur by a pattern association effect, resulting in better firing of the CA1 than the CA3 cells (see Robertson et al. 1998). Another factor that could contribute to the better responses of CA1 cells when the spatial view is obscured is the direct perforant path input to the CA1 cells, which may provide additional input to the CA1 cells (see further Rolls and Treves 1998).

The spatial view field of the cells shown in Figs 17.2 and 17.3, and of many others, occupies a part of space that is typically about as large as half to all of one of the walls of the testing room. Each cell has a different spatial view to which it responds. Thus over a population of many such neurones, these partly overlapping view fields represent rather precise information about the part of space being viewed, as confirmed by an information theoretic approach, which shows that an independent contribution is made by each of the cells in an ensemble to representing allocentric space (Rolls et al. 1998). This shows that the number of different spatial views that can be represented by these spatial view neurones increases approximately exponentially with the number of neurones in the ensemble, a very powerful type of representation with many computationally attractive properties (Rolls and Treves 1998).

Many view (or 'space' or 'spatial view') cells have been found in this series of experiments (Rolls et al. 1997a, 1998; Robertson et al. 1998). (The current number of spatial view cells is 40.) No place cells have been found that responded based on where the monkey was, and not on where he was looking in the environment. These cells in the primate hippocampus are thus unlike place cells found in the rat (O'Keefe 1979; Muller et al. 1991). Primates, with their highly developed visual and eye movement control systems, can explore and remember information about what is present at places in the environment without having to visit those places. Such view cells in primates would thus be useful as part of a memory system, in that they would provide a representation of a part of space that would not depend on exactly where the monkey was, and which could be associated with items that might be present in those spatial locations. An example of the utility of such a representation in monkeys might be in enabling a monkey to remember where it had seen ripe fruit. The representations of space provided by hippocampal view-responsive neurones may thus be useful in forming memories of spatial environments (for example, of where an object such as ripe fruit has been seen, and of where the monkey is as defined by seen views). The representations of space provided by hippocampal view-responsive neurones may also, together with whole-body motion cells, be useful in remembering trajectories through environments, of use, for example, in short-range spatial navigation (O'Mara et al. 1994).

The representation of space in the rat hippocampus, which is of the place where the rat is, may be related to the fact that with a much less developed visual system than the primate, the rat's representation of space may be defined more by the olfactory and tactile as well as distant visual cues present, and may thus tend to reflect the place where the rat is. Although the representation of space in rats therefore may be in some ways analogous to the representation of space in the primate hippocampus, the difference does have implications for theories of hippocampal function. In rats, the presence of place cells has led to theories that the rat hippocampus is a spatial cognitive map, and can perform spatial computations to implement navigation through spatial environments (O'Keefe and Nadel 1978; O'Keefe 1991; Burgees et al. 1994). The details of such navigational theories could not apply in any direct way to what is found in the primate hippocampus. Instead, what is applicable to both the primate and rat hippocampal recordings is that hippocampal neurones contain a representation of space (for the rat, primarily where the rat is, and for the primate, primarily of positions 'out there' in space), which is a suitable representation for an episodic memory system. In primates, this would enable one to remember, for example, where an object was seen. In rats, it might enable memories to be formed of where particular objects (e.g. defined by olfactory, tactile and taste inputs) were found. Thus at least in primates, and possibly also in rats, the neuronal representation of space in the primate hippocampus may be appropriate for forming memories of events (which usually have a spatial component). Such memories would be useful for spatial navigation, for which according to the present hypothesis the hippocampus would implement the memory component but not the spatial computation component.

Responses to whole body motion in the primate hippocampus

Another type of cell found in the primate hippocampus responds to whole body motion (O'Mara et al. 1994). For example, some cells respond when the monkey is rotated about the vertical axis. By occluding the visual field, it was possible to show that in some cases the response of these cells required visual input. For other cells, visual input was not required, and it is likely that such cells responded on the basis of vestibular inputs. Some cells were found that responded to a combination of body motion and view or place. In some cases these neurones respond to linear motion, in others to axial rotation ($N=43$). In some cases these neurones require visual input for their responses; in other cases the neurones appear to be driven by vestibular inputs. Some cells responded to a combination of movement together with either a particular local view seen by the monkey ($N=2$) or a particular place towards which the monkey is moving ($N=1$). These whole-body motion cells may be useful in a memory system for remembering trajectories through environments, of use for example in short range spatial navigation (O'Mara et al. 1994).

Neurones related to learning associations between visual stimuli and spatial responses

In another type of task for which the primate hippocampus is needed, conditional spatial response learning, in which the monkeys had to learn which spatial response to make to different stimuli, i.e. to acquire associations between visual stimuli and spatial responses, 14 per cent of hippocampal neurones responded to particular combinations of stimuli and responses (Miyashita et al. 1989). The firing of these neurones could not be accounted for by the motor requirements of the task, nor wholly by the stimulus aspects of the task, as demonstrated by testing their firing in related visual discrimination tasks. These results showed that single hippocampal neurones respond to combinations of the visual stimuli and the spatial responses with which they must become associated in conditional response tasks, and are consistent with the computational theory described above, according to which part of the mechanism of this learning involves associations between visual stimuli and spatial responses learned by single hippocampal neurones.

In a following study, it was found that during such conditional spatial response learning, 22 per cent of this type of neurone analysed in the hippocampus and parahippocampal gyrus altered their responses so that their activity, which was initially equal to the two new stimuli, became progressively differential to the two stimuli when the monkey learned to make different responses to the two stimuli (Cahusac et al. 1993). These changes occurred for different neurones just before, at, or just after the time when the monkey learned the correct response to make to the stimuli, and are consistent with the hypothesis that when new associations between objects and places (in this case for responses) are learned, some hippocampal neurones learn to respond to the new associations that are required to solve the task.

Recognition memory tasks

Although it appears that recognition memory tasks can be performed using the perirhinal cortex without the hippocampus (Zola-Morgan et al. 1989), the perirhinal cortex does provide afferents to the hippocampus (see Fig. 17.1). Consistent with this connectivity, it has been found that in the macaque hippocampus, some neurones do respond differently to novel and familiar stimuli in a serial recognition memory task, with those that did respond differentially typically responding more to novel than to familiar visual stimuli (Rolls *et al.* 1993). It was notable that the proportion of hippocampal neurones that responded in this way was small, 2.3 per cent. It is suggested that because a visual recognition memory task does not require arbitrary associations to be made between representations in different modalities, the learning required may be performed in the perirhinal cortex, a region before complete mixing of inputs to the hippocampal system occurs (see Fig. 17.1). In contrast, the hippocampus proper, and particularly the single network in CA3 (see Fig. 17.1), may be especially important when arbitrary associations between events originating in different parts of the cerebral neocortex must be made, for the CA3 may implement a single network in which such arbitrary conjunctions can be detected and learned (see Fig. 17.1 and below).

17.6 The computational significance of the functional architecture of the hippocampus

Given the systems level hypothesis about what the hippocampus performs, and the neurophysiological evidence about what is represented in the primate hippocampus, the next step is to consider how using its internal connectivity and synaptic modifiability (see Rolls 1996b), the hippocampus could store and retrieve many memories, and how retrieval within the hippocampus could lead to retrieval of the activity in the neocortex that was present during the original learning of the episode. To develop understanding of how this is achieved, we have developed a computational theory of the operation of the hippocampus (see Rolls 1987, 1989a–c, 1990a,b; Treves and Rolls 1991, 1992, 1994; Rolls and Treves 1998). Some key aspects of the theory, which addresses especially the systems-level anatomy, neurophysiology, and lesion effects in primates to make it relevant to understanding hippocampal function in humans, are outlined next. It is noted at the outset that given the very different neurophysiology of the primate and the rat hippocampus, any theory based on rat place cells and their role in spatial computation is not likely to be directly applicable to primates including humans.

Hippocampal circuitry (see Fig. 17.1)

Projections from the entorhinal cortex reach the granule cells (of which there are 10^6 in the rat) in the dentate gyrus (DG) via the perforant path (pp). The granule cells project to CA3 cells via the mossy fibres (MF), which provide a *sparse* but possibly powerful connection to the 3×10^5 CA3 pyramidal cells in the rat. Each CA3 cell receives approximately 50 mossy fibre inputs, so that the sparseness of this connectivity is thus 0.005 per cent. By contrast, there are many more—possibly weaker–direct perforant path inputs onto each CA3 cell, in the rat of the order of 4×10^3. The largest number of synapses (about

1.2×10^4 in the rat) on the dendrites of CA3 pyramidal cells is, however, provided by the (recurrent) axon collaterals of CA3 cells themselves (rc). It is remarkable that the recurrent collaterals are distributed to other CA3 cells throughout the hippocampus (Amaral and Witter 1989; Amaral et al. 1990; Ishizuka et al. 1990), so that effectively the CA3 system provides a single network, with a connectivity of approximately 2 per cent between the different CA3 neurones given that the connections are bilateral.

CA3 as an autoassociation memory

One key hypothesis is that the CA3 recurrent collateral network provides a single autoassociation network. This would allow any combination of inputs originating from any of the neocortical areas providing afferents to the hippocampal formation to be associated together. It is because there is effectively a single network that arbitrary associations can be made. The system would act as a single network even if there is some spatial gradient in the CA3–CA3 connection, probability as a function of the distance between the CA3 cells. This would provide for an episodic memory. In the context of the hippocampal spatial view cells, one part of the memory might be the spatial position, another might be the sight of an object, and these could become associated together in an object–place memory. Later, the full memory (e.g. of where the object was located) could be recalled from part of it (e.g. from the object used as a retrieval cue). Such a memory would be useful to spatial computation, but would not itself perform spatial computation.

Some advances made to address the biological plausibility of this system (or more generically of any system in the brain with modifiable recurrent collateral connections) are as follows. We have extended previous formal models of auto-associative memory (see Amit 1989) by analysing a network with graded response units, so as to represent more realistically the continuously variable rates at which neurones fire, and with incomplete connectivity (Treves 1990; Treves and Rolls 1991). The analysis shows how the system operates (in terms, for example, of its capacity) with a sparse representation (with, for example, only some neurones active), or in a general case with an exponential distribution of firing rates, and with diluted recurrent connectivity (e.g. with 5 per cent connectivity). We have shown by simulation that such a system operates as predicted even with asymmetrically diluted connectivity (if neurone 1 connects to neurone 2, neurone 2 may not connect to 1) (Simmen et al. 1996b). We have also highlighted by simulation of both a single autoassociation network (Rolls et al. 1997b) and of much of the circuitry shown in Fig. 17.1 (Rolls 1995a) the fact that for such a system to store a large number of different memories, there is a high cost to be paid for using graded firing, and a considerable advantage to keeping the firing of the CA3 neurones with a relatively binary firing rate distribution (i.e. low rates generally, with only a few high rates). The implications of this for the actual firing rate distribution of primate hippocampal CA3 neurones are being explored (Rolls et al. 1998).

Another issue addressed is how rapidly such an autoassociation system, if implemented with biologically plausible components, will perform its recall. A discrete-state autoassociation (Hopfield) network may take 8–15 iterations for full recall, which if an iteration time in the brain were in the order of 15 ms, would be much too slow. If, however, the system is analysed and simulated with integrate-and-fire neurones (and neurones with thresholds that are kept close to the firing point), then information can be exchanged between the neurones even within one synaptic time constant, and the whole system settles into recall in a time of the order of 2–3 synaptic time constants, i.e. within a time of the order of 30 ms (Treves 1993; Simmen *et al.* 1996*a*; Treves *et al.* 1997; Rolls and Treves 1998, Appendix 5). This is an important issue in the speed of brain computation (Rolls and Treves 1998).

Another issue addressed is how in a biologically plausible autoassociation network, new patterns to be learned (rather than the effects of the recurrent collateral connections that are used for recall) are made to dominate the activity of the firing during learning. Using a quantitative analysis, we have suggested that the mossy fibre input to the CA3 neurones may perform this effect during learning, and that during recall, the perforant path input to the CA3 network provides the recall cue (Treves and Rolls 1992, 1994; Rolls and Treves 1998). We have also shown how the dentate granule cells could act as a competitive network to enhance storage in the CA3 network by performing expansion recording, producing a sparse and relatively orthogonal set of representations as input to the CA3 network (Rolls 1989*a–c*; Treves and Rolls 1992; Rolls and Treves 1998).

Recall and backprojection pathways

Another issue addressed quantitatively is how information stored in the hippocampus (whether for the intermediate or the long term, see Rolls 1996*a*) could be recalled to activate the correct neurones for that memory back in the neocortex, using backprojections, and starting with the CA1 cells (see Fig. 17.1). We have shown that the recall operation in such a multistage pathway is analytically very similar to that at each iteration in an autoassociation network, with the number of backprojecting connections to any neurone in the back-projection pathway being the leading term in defining how many different memories can be retrieved (Treves and Rolls 1994). This provides a quantitative basis for understanding why in the cerebral cortex there are as many backprojecting as forward-projecting connections between any two cortical areas adjacent in an information processing stream (Rolls 1989*a–b*, 1996*a*; Treves and Rolls 1994; Rolls and Treves 1998). Once recall has been produced in the cerebral cortex, it would then be in a position to use the information to initiate action, or to use the recalled episodic information to contribute to the formation of new structured semantic memories (see Rolls 1989*a–c*; Treves and Rolls 1994; McClelland *et al.* 1995; Rolls and Treves 1998).

17.7 Conclusion

A computational theory of the hippocampus, which has as a key feature the ability to implement an autoassociation memory using the CA3 pyramidal cells, has been proposed. It is proposed that the hippocampus is involved in both spatial and episodic memory as a result of its ability to form arbitrary associations between input stimuli, so that whole spatial scenes or all the events that comprise a single episodic memory can be associated together. Recordings from single neurones in the primate hippocampus are consistent with the theory that inputs to the hippocampus, originating from different parts of the cerebral cortex, are brought together onto single neurones within the hippocampus, and that synaptic modifications within the hippocampus implement the associations.

It is only by analysing the responses of single neurones (or ensembles of single neurones) that it is possible to define what is represented in a part of the brain such as the hippocampus, and how it is represented. Showing by imaging that a brain area is active in a particular task does not provide a full description of what is represented in a brain area. Such studies do not show that, for example, there is an allocentric representation of space 'out there' that is accessed either by looking at the particular location in space, or by rotating the head and moving the eyes to any combination that will result in looking towards that location in space when the view details are made invisible. Nor can such studies show that, for example, other neurones in the hippocampus can be activated either by vestibular cues, or for other neurones by optical flow cues, or for other neurons by either cue to a particular whole body motion. Analyses at the neuronal level are thus essential because they provide clear evidence about what is being represented in a brain structure, and are also especially relevant to understanding how a part of the brain operates, because they show what information is being exchanged between the computing elements of the brain (Rolls and Treves 1998).

Acknowledgements

The author has worked on some of the experiments and neuronal network modelling described here with A. Berthoz, P. M. B. Cahusac, J. D. Feigenbaum, D. Foster, P. Georges-François, R. P. Kesner, Y. Miyashita, H. Niki, S. Panzeri, R. Robertson and A. Treves, and their collaboration is sincerely acknowledged. Discussions with David G. Amaral of the Salk Institute, La Jolla, were also much appreciated. This research was supported by the Medical Research Council, PG8513790, and by a grant from the Human Frontier Science Program.

References

Amaral, D. G. (1987). Memory: anatomical organization of candidate brain regions. In *Handbook of physiology, Section I, The nervous system Vol. V, Higher functions of the brain, Part 2* (ed., V. B. Mountcastle), Ch. 7, pp. 211–94. American Physiological Society, Washington, D.C.

Amaral, D. G. and Witter, M. P. (1989). The three-dimensional organization of the hippocampal formation: a review of anatomical data. *Neuroscience*, **31**, 571–91.

Amaral, D. G., Ishizuka, N., and Claiborne, B. (1990). Neurones, numbers and the hippocampal network. *Progress in Brain Research*, **83**, 1–11.

Amit, D. J. (1989). *Modeling brain function. The world of attractor neural networks.* Cambridge University Press.

Andersen, R. A. (1987). Inferior parietal lobule function in spatial perception and visuomotor integration. In *Handbook of physiology, Section I, The nervous system. Vol. V, Higher functions of the brain, Part 2* (ed., V. B. Mountcastle), Ch. 7, pp. 483–518. American Physiological Society, Washington, D.C.

Bolhuis, J. J., Stewart, C. A., and Forrest, E. M. (1994). Retrograde amnesia and memory reactivation in rats with ibotenate lesions to the hippocampus or subiculum. *Quarterly Journal of Experimental Psychology*, **47**B, 129–50.

Burgess, N., Recce, M., and O'Keefe, J. (1994). A model of hippocampal function. *Neural Networks*, **7**, 1065–81.

Cahusac, P. M. B., Miyashita, Y., and Rolls, E. T. (1989). Responses of hippocampal formation neurons in the monkey related to delayed spatial response and object–place memory tasks. *Behavioural Brain Research*, **33**, 229–40.

Cahusac, P. M. B., Rolls, E. T., Miyashita, Y., and Niki, H. (1993). Modification of the responses of hippocampal neurons in the monkey during the learning of a conditional spatial response task. *Hippocampus*, **3**, 29–42.

Conquet, F., Bashir, Z. I., Davies, C. H., Daniel, H., Ferragutl, F., Bordl, F. *et al.* (1994). Motor deficit and impairment of synaptic plasticity in mice lacking mGluR1. *Nature*, **372**, 237–43.

Feigenbaum, J. D. and Rolls, E. T. (1991). Allocentric and egocentric spatial information processing in the hippocampal formation of the behaving primate. *Psychobiology*, **19**, 21–40.

Foster, T. C., Castro, C. A., and McNaughton, B. L. (1989). Spatial selectivity of rat hippocampal neurons: dependence on preparedness for movement. *Science*, **244**, 1580–82.

Gaffan, D. (1987). Amnesia, personal memory and the hippocampus: experimental neuropsychological studies in monkeys. In *Cognitive neurochemistry* (ed., S. M. Stahl, S. D. Iversen, and E. C. Goodman), pp. 46–56. Oxford University Press.

Gaffan, D. (1994). Scene-specific memory for objects: a model of episodic memory impairment in monkeys with fornix transection. *Journal of Cognitive Neuroscience*, **6**, 305–20.

Gaffan, D. and Harrison, S. (1989*a*). A comparison of the effects of fornix section and sulcus principals ablation upon spatial learning by monkeys. *Behavioural Brain Research*, **31**, 207–20.

Gaffan, D. and Harrison, S. (1989*b*). Place memory and scene memory: effects of fornix transection in the monkey. *Experimental Brain Research*, **74**, 202–12.

Gaffan, D. and Saunders, R. C. (1985). Running recognition of configural stimuli by fornix transacted monkeys. *Quarterly Journal of Experimental Psychology*, **37**B, 61–71.

Gaffan, D., Saunders, R. C., Gaffan, E. A., Harrison, S., Shields, C., and Owen, M. J. (1984). Effects of fornix transaction upon associative memory in monkeys: role of the hippocampus in learned action. *Quarterly Journal of Experimental Psychology*, **26**B, 173–221.

Georges–François, P., Rolls, E. T., and Robertson, R. G. (1998). Spatial view cells in the primate hippocampus: allocentric view not head direction or eye position or place, in preparation.

Ishizuka, N., Weber, J., and Amaral, D. G. (1990). Organization of intrahippocampal projections originating from CA3 pyramidal cells in the rat. *Journal of Comparative Neurology*, **295**, 580–623.

McNaughton, B. L., Barnes, C. A., and O'Keefe, J. (1983). The contributions of position, direction, and velocity to single unit activity in the hippocampus of freely-moving rats. *Experimental Brain Research*, **52**, 41–9.

McClelland, J. J., McNaughton, B. L., and O'Reilly, R. C. (1995). Why there are complementary learning systems in the hippocampus and neocortex: insights from the successes and failures of connectionist models of learning and memory. *Psychological Review*, **102**, 419–57.

Miyashita, Y., Rolls, E. T., Cahusac, P. M. B., Niki, H., and Feigenbaum, J. D. (1989). Activity of hippocampal neurons in the monkey related to a conditional spatial response task. *Journal of Neurophysiology*, **61**, 669–78.

Morris, R. G. M. (1989). Does synaptic plasticity play a role in information storage in the vertebrate brain? In *Parallel distributed processing* (ed., R. G. M. Morris), Ch. 11, pp. 248–85. Oxford University Press.

Muller, R. U., Kubie, J. L., Bostock, F. M., Taube, J. S., and Quirk, G. J. (1991). Spatial firing correlates of neurons in the hippocampal formation of freely moving rats. In *Brain and space* (ed., J. Paillard), pp. 296–33. Oxford University Press.

O'Keefe, J. (1979). A review of the hippocampal place cells. *Progress in Neurobiology*, **13**, 419–39.

O'Keefe, J. (1984). Spatial memory within and without the hippocampal system. In *Neurobiology of the hippocampus* (ed., W. Seifert), Ch. 20, pp. 375–403. Academic Press, London.

O'Keefe, J. (1991). The hippocampal cognitive map and navigational strategies. In *Brain and space* (ed., J. Paillard), Ch. 16, pp. 296–33. Oxford University Press.

O'Keefe, J. and Nadel, L. (1978). *The hippocampus as a cognitive map*. Clarendon Press, Oxford.

O'Mara, S. M., Rolls, E. T., Berthoz, A., and Kesner, R. P. (1994). Neurons responding to whole-body motion in the primate hippocampus. *Journal of Neuroscience*, **14**, 6511–23.

Ono, T., Tamura, R., Nishijo, H., and Nakamura, K. (1993). Neural mechanisms of recognition and memory in the limbic system. In *Brain mechanisms of perception and memory: from neuron to behavior* (ed., T. Ono, L. R. Squire, M. E. Raichle, D. I. Perrett and M. Fukuda), Ch. 19, pp. 330–55. Oxford University Press, New York.

Parkinson, J. K., Murray, E. A., and Mishkin, M. (1988). A selective mnemonic role for the hippocampus in monkeys: memory for the location of objects. *Journal of Neuroscience*, **8**, 4059–67.

Petrides, M. (1985). Deficits on conditional associative-learning tasks after frontal- and temporal-lobe lesions in man. *Neuropsychologia*, **23**, 601–14.

Robertson, R. G., Rolls, E. T., and Georges-François, P. (1998). Spatial view cells in the primate hippocampus: effects of removal of view details. *Journal of Neurophysiology*, **79**, 1145–56.

Rolls, E. T. (1987). Information representation, processing and storage in the brain: analysis at the single neuron level. In *The neural and molecular bases of learning* (ed., J.-P. Changeux and M. Konishi), pp. 503–40. Wiley, Chichester.

Rolls, E. T. (1989*a*). Functions of neuronal networks in the hippocampus and neocortex in memory. In *Neural models of plasticity: experimental and theoretical approaches* (ed., J. H. Byrne and W. O. Berry), Ch. 13, pp. 240–65. Academic Press, San Diego.

Rolls, E. T. (1989*b*). The representation and storage of information in neuronal networks in the primate cerebral cortex and hippocampus. In *The computing neuron* (ed., R. Durbin, C. Miall and G. Mitchison), Ch. 8, pp. 125–59. Addison-Wesley, Wokingham, England.

Rolls, E. T. (1989c). Functions of neuronal networks in the hippocampus and cerebral cortex in memory. In *Models of brain function* (ed., R. M. J. Cotterill), pp. 15–33. Cambridge University Press.

Rolls, E. T. (1990a). Functions of the primate hippocampus in spatial processing and memory. In *Neurobiology of comparative cognition* (ed., D. S. Olton and R. P. Kesner), Ch. 12, pp. 339–62. L. Erlbaum, Hillsdale, N.J.

Rolls, E. T. (1990b). Functions of neuronal networks in the hippocampus and of backprojections in the cerebral cortex in memory. In *Brain organization and memory: cells, systems and circuits* (ed., J. L. McGaugh, N. M. Weinberger and G. Lynch), Ch. 9, pp. 184–210. Oxford University Press: New York.

Rolls, E. T. (1991). Functions of the primate hippocampus in spatial and non-spatial memory. *Hippocampus*, **1**, 258–61.

Rolls, E. T. (1992). Neurophysiological mechanisms underlying face processing within and beyond the temporal cortical visual areas. *Philosophical Transactions of the Royal Society*, **335**, 11–21.

Rolls, E. T. (1994). Brain mechanisms for invariant visual recognition and learning. *Behavioural Processes*, **33**, 113–38.

Rolls, E. T. (1995a). A model of the operation of the hippocampus and entorhinal cortex in memory. *International Journal of Neural Systems*, **6**, Supplement, 51–70.

Rolls, E. T. (1995b). Learning mechanisms in the temporal lobe visual cortex. *Behavioural Brain Research*, **66**, 177–85.

Rolls, E. T. (1996a). A theory of hippocampal function in memory. *Hippocampus*, **6**, 601–20.

Rolls, E. T. (1996b). Roles of long term potentiation and long term depression in neuronal network operations in the brain. In *Cortical plasticity: LTP and LTD* (ed., M. S. Fazeli and G. L. Collingridge), Ch. 11, pp. 223–50. Bios, Oxford.

Rolls, E. T., Cahusac, P. M. B., Feigenbaum, J. D., and Miyashita, Y. (1993). Responses of single neurons in the hippocampus of the macaque related to recognition memory. *Experimental Brain Research*, **93**, 299–306.

Rolls, E. T. and O'Mara, S. (1993). Neurophysiological and theoretical analysis of how the hippocampus functions in memory. In *Brain mechanisms of perception and memory: from neuron to behavior* (ed., T. Ono, L. R. Squire, M. E. Raichle, D. I. Perrett and M. Fukuda), Ch. 17, pp. 276–300. Oxford University Press, New York.

Rolls, E. T. and O'Mara S. M. (1995). View-responsive neurons in the primate hippocampal complex. *Hippocampus*, **5**, 409–24.

Rolls, E. T. and Treves, A. (1990). The relative advantages of sparse versus distributed encoding for associative neuronal networks in the brain. *Network*, **1**, 407–421.

Rolls, E. T. and Treves, A. (1998). *Neural networks and brain function*. Oxford University Press, Oxford.

Rolls, E. T., Miyashita, Y., Cahusac, P. M. B., Kesner, R. P., Niki, H., Feigenbaum, J. et al. (1989). Hippocampal neurons in the monkey with activity related to the place in which a stimulus is shown. *Journal of Neuroscience*, **9**, 1835–45.

Rolls, E. T., Robertson, R. G., and Georges-François, P. (1995). The representation of space in the primate hippocampus. *Society for Neuroscience Abstracts*, **21**, 586.10.

Rolls, E. T., Robertson, R. G., and Georges-François, P. (1997a). Spatial view cells in the primate hippocampus. *European Journal of Neuroscience*, **9**, 1789–94.

Rolls, E. T., Treves, A., Foster, D., and Perez-Vicente, C. (1997b). Simulation studies of the CA3 hippocampal subfield modelled as an attractor neural network. *Neural Networks*, **10**, 1559–69.

Rolls, E. T., Treves, A., Robertson, R. G., Georges-François, P., and Panzeri, S. (1998). Information about spatial view in an ensemble of primate hippocampal cells. *Journal of Neurophysiology*, **79**, 1797–1813.

Rupniak, N. M. J. and Gaffan, D. (1987). Monkey hippocampus and learning about spatially directed movements. *Journal of Neuroscience*, **7**, 2331–7.

Sakata, H. (1985). The parietal association cortex: neurophysiology. In *The scientific basis of clinical neurology* (ed., M. Swash and C. Kennard), Ch. 16, pp. 225–36. Churchill Livingstone, London.

Salmon, D. P., Zola-Morgan, S., and Squire, L. R. (1985). Retrograde amnesia following combined hippocampus-amygdala lesions in monkeys. *Psychobiology*, **15**, 37–47.

Sanders, H. I. and Warrington, E. K. (1971). Memory for remote events in amnesic patients. *Brain*, **94**, 661–8.

Simmen, M. W., Rolls, E. T., and Treves, A. (1996*a*). On the dynamics of a network of spiking neurons. In *Computations and Neuronal Systems: Proceedings of CNS95*, (ed., F. H. Eekman and J. M. Bower). Kluwer: Boston.

Simmen, M. W., Treves, A., and Rolls, E. T. (1996*b*). Pattern retrieval in threshold-linear associative nets. *Network*, **7**, 109–22.

Smith, M. L. and Milner, B. (1981). The role of the right hippocampus in the recall of spatial location. *Neuropsychologia*, **19**, 781–93.

Squire, L. R. (1992). Memory and the hippocampus: a synthesis from findings with rats, monkeys and humans. *Psychological Review*, **99**, 195–231.

Squire, L. R. and Knowlton, B. J. (1994). Memory, hippocampus, and brain systems. In *The cognitive neurosciences* (ed., M. Gazzaniga), Ch. 53, pp. 825–37. MIT Press, Cambridge, Mass.

Squire, L. R., Shimamura, A. P., and Amaral, D. G. (1989). Memory and the hippocampus. In *Neural models of plasticity: theoretical and empirical approaches* (ed., J. Byrne and W. O. Berry), Ch. 12, pp. 208–39. Academic Press, New York.

Suzuki, W. and Amaral, D. G. (1994). Topographic organisation of the reciprocal connections between the monkey entorhinal cortex and the perirhinal and parahippocampal cortices. *Journal of Neuroscience*, **14**, 1856–77.

Treves, A. (1990). Graded-response neurons and information encodings in autoassociative memories. *Physical Review*, **42**, 2418–30.

Treves, A. (1993). Mean-field analysis of neuronal spike dynamics. *Network*, **4**, 259–84.

Treves, A. and Rolls, E. T. (1991). What determines the capacity of autoassociative memories in the brain? *Network*, **2**, 371–97.

Treves, A. and Rolls, E. T. (1992). Computational constraints suggest the need for two distinct input systems to the hippocampal CA3 network. *Hippocampus*, **2**, 189–99.

Treves. A. and Rolls, E. T. (1994). A computational analysis of the role of the hippocampus in memory. *Hippocampus*, **4**, 374–91.

Treves, A., Rolls, E. T., and Simmen, M. (1997). Time for retrieval in recurrent associative memories. *Physica D*, **107**, 392–400.

Van Hoesen, G. W. (1982). The parahippocampal gyrus. New observations regarding its cortical connections in the monkey. *Trends in Neurosciences*, **5**, 345–50.

Wallis, G. and Rolls, E. T. (1997). Invariant face and object recognition in the visual system. *Progress in Neurobiology*, **51**, 167–94.

Watanabe, T. and Niki, H. (1985). Hippocampal unit activity and delayed response in the monkey. *Brain Research*, **325**, 241–54.

Zola-Morgan, S. and Squire, L. R. (1990). The primate hippocampal formation: evidence for a time-limited role in memory storage. *Science*, **250**, 288–90.

Zola-Morgan, S., Squire, L. R., and Amaral, D. G. (1986). Human amnesia and the medial temporal region: enduring memory impairment following a bilateral lesion limited to field CA1 of the hippocampus. *Journal of Neuroscience*, **6**, 2950–7.

Zola-Morgan, S., Squire, L. R., Amaral, D. G., and Suzuki, W. A. (1989). Lesions of perirhinal and parahippocampal cortex that spare the amygdala and hippocampal formation produce severe memory impairment. *Journal of Neuroscience*, **9**, 4355–70.

Zola-Morgan, S., Squire, L. R., and Ramus, S. J. (1994). Severity of memory impairment in monkeys as a function of locus and extent of damage within the medial temporal lobe memory system. *Hippocampus*, **4**, 483–94.

18

Amnesia and neglect: beyond the Delay–Brion system and the Hebb synapse

David Gaffan and Julia Hornak

18.1 Introduction

This volume offers a rare opportunity to consider the hippocampus, and its role in the explanation of memory and amnesia, in a broad context including other brain structures and other clinical disorders, as the abstract above indicates. To cover these topics in a short space does not allow full consideration of all the relevant evidence. Instead, a short review of the most important points in each topic is given.

18.2 Does hippocampal damage in humans cause amnesia?

It is now widely accepted that human amnesia after surgical removal of the medial temporal lobe (Scoville & Milner 1957) cannot be ascribed to the hippocampus alone, because many other structures involved in these removals, such as the amygdala and the perirhinal cortex, have important functions of their own in memory. There is less complete consensus, however, about the assessment of two other sources of clinical evidence: amnesia after ischaemic–anoxic hippocampal damage, and after surgical damage to the fornix.

Delay & Brion (1969) published sections of the brain of a patient who had developed severe amnesia postcomitially. The only area of cell death was in the CA1 field of the hippocampus bilaterally. Similar selective damage was seen by Zola-Morgan *et al.* (1986) in a patient who developed mild amnesia after an anoxic incident. Warrington & Duchen (1992) reported a patient who developed severe amnesia after the unilateral surgical removal of one medial temporal lobe, a removal that did not cause amnesia in many other similar patients. Post-mortem histological analysis revealed discrete sclerosis in area CA1 in the temporal lobe contralateral to the surgical removal. These cases appear to show that bilateral damage to the CA1 field of the hippocampus can be sufficient to cause severe amnesia. However, the area of functional disorder after anoxic damage may be wider than the area of cell death. Bachevalier & Mishkin (1989) investigated the effects in monkeys of ischaemia experimentally induced by bilateral occlusion of the posterior cerebral artery. Some of the monkeys had cell death only in area CA1 of the hippocampus and had severe impairments in visual recognition memory, similar in severity to the same impairment in Warrington & Duchen's patient. However, the memory impairment in these monkeys was much more severe than that which was produced, in other monkeys, by surgical removal of the whole hippo-campus bilaterally. The most likely explanation of these findings is that anoxia produces more widespread functional disorders than those that result in cell death, perhaps axonal damage for example. Therefore, the severe amnesia seen in the patients of Delay & Brion (1969) and Warrington & Duchen (1992) may result from undisclosed damage outside the hippocampus.

Damage or complete section of the fornix is a risk in the surgical removal of colloid cysts from the third ventricle inferior to the fornix, and patients with fornix lesions show memory disorder (for a review see Gaffan & Gaffan 1991). Furthermore, the severity of memory disorder after colloid-cyst removal is correlated with the amount of destruction to the fornix, not with other variables such as the route of surgical approach (McMackin et al. 1995). These patients show impairments in some kinds of episodic memory, the memory for discrete personally experienced events. Their memory impairments are revealed in the standard clinical tests of delayed reproduction of the Rey figure and in delayed recall of a story (the 'logical memory' test in the Wechsler memory scale). Furthermore, their impairments in everyday life are clinically significant and require a sheltered lifestyle. Nevertheless, these patients do not suffer from amnesia in the full clinical sense of that term. For example, they score in the normal range on the Warrington Recognition Memory Test. It may be asked whether the relatively mild amnesia seen in these patients results from the fact that the hippocampus itself is intact although the fornix is damaged or destroyed. Evidence from animals gives no support to such a possibility, however. Discrete lesions of the hippocampus in monkeys produce a less severe effect than surgical transection of the fornix in the same animals (O'Boyle et al. 1993). Thus, the implication from the colloid-cyst patients is that the hippocampus–fornix system facilitates the normal performance of human episodic memory in some way, but is not essential for some other kinds of memory that are impaired in the clinical amnesic syndrome.

Amnesic patients frequently have lesions in the mamillary nuclei; the well-known hypothesis put forward by Delay & Brion (1969) was that amnesia is caused by any bilateral interruption of a connected system of structures including the hippocampus, fornix and mamillary nuclei. However, because the main pathway into the mamillary nuclei is the fornix, it is difficult to see how the effects of a lesion in the mamillary nuclei could be more severe than the effects of fornix transection. Evidence from monkeys (reviewed below) indicates that the effects of discrete lesions in the mamillary nuclei are similar to the effects of fornix transection. Thus, given that fornix transection in humans does not cause severe amnesia, it is difficult to believe that mamillary nuclei lesions alone are sufficient to do so. Furthermore, amnesic patients with neuronal death in the mamillary nuclei frequently or always have additional neuronal death elsewhere, and the inflammatory disease process in Wernicke–Korsakoff pathology may, like anoxia or ischaemia, produce dysfunction more widespread than that which reveals itself in cell death, particularly by interfering with axonal conduction (Victor *et al*. 1971, p. 157).

In conclusion, the effects of discrete hippocampal or mamillary damage in man are not known with any certainty. The effects of fornix transection are to impair episodic memory without producing a full amnesic syndrome.

18.3 Scene memory: a functional connection between human episodic memory and animal spatial memory

It is widely accepted that discrete damage to the hippocampus or fornix in animals leads to impairments in spatial memory. What exactly is meant by 'spatial memory' is not so clear, however. The cognitive-map hypothesis of O'Keefe & Nadel (1978) is only one possible account of the cognitive abilities that underlie tests of spatial memory in animals. An alternative possibility has recently been developed from experiments with monkeys. This idea, beginning with Gaffan & Harrison (1989), is that monkeys have a snapshot-like memory, that is, a memory of the objects in a complex scene and their spatial relations to each other from the point of view of the witness. Tasks that require such a snapshot-like memory were impaired by fornix transection, while other tasks that required the monkeys to learn about places in the world objectively defined were not (Gaffan & Harrison 1989). Recently these experiments have been extended to investigate the relationship between snapshot spatial memory and episodic memory. O'Keefe & Nadel (1978, pp. 390 onwards) put forward the idea that human memory frequently relies on spatio-temporal context. However, human episodic memory frequently involves the reconstruction in memory of the subjectively witnessed scene in which a discrete personally experienced event took place, rather than the objective place in the world. If you remember a conversation with a friend, what comes out of your memory, subjectively, is not simply the words but the whole event, the room in which the conversation took place as viewed from the place where you were sitting. In this way episodic memory differs from general knowledge, because in general knowledge facts are retrieved that are not set in any specific scene. More technically, analysis of sources of interference in long-term memory suggests that retrieval of the background or scene in which some target event took place facilitates the accurate retrieval of the target event itself; importantly, this facilitation only occurs where different target events have taken place in different background scenes (Gaffan 1992, 1994*b*). Thus, the very poor performance of the patients with fornix damage in delayed story recall could represent an impairment in the subjectively familiar process of reconstructing the scene of a past conversation with a friend. Now the spatial learning impairments of animals with fornix damage are also seen in tasks where memory of a whole scene is potentially relevant. In spatial recognition memory, for example, in which rats and monkeys with fornix section have equivalent impairments (Markowska *et al*. 1989; Murray *et al*. 1989), memory of going left or going right on a previous trial can be facilitated by remembering spatial relations among any or all of a large number of objects in the scene of the trial. In object–reward association learning in the Wisconsin General Test Apparatus, by contrast, in which monkeys with fornix transection perform perfectly normally (Moss *et al*. 1981), all the objects are presented in a constant identical back-ground scene; therefore, remembering whether an individual object was rewarded or not on a previous trial cannot be facilitated by remembering the scene in which that event took place. Thus, a common feature of the tasks in which fornix transection was known to produce an impairment (episodic memory in humans, and 'spatial' tasks in animals) was that memory of whole scenes, as opposed to memory of discrete objects independent of their setting, could facilitate their performance. This common feature suggested that the fornix might subserve a single common function, scene memory, both in animals and in humans.

To test this idea, scene memory was investigated in the monkey in a task that was not a spatial memory task (Gaffan 1994*b*). Artificially created fore-ground objects were presented on artificially created back-grounds. Each scene was unique, both in its foreground objects and in its background. The task for the monkeys was to learn which of the foreground objects in each scene produced reward. Fornix transection produced a severe impairment in this task. Note that the task is similar to human memory for a discrete event, involving some object situated in a particular place in a particular background. The importance of scene memory as opposed to memory for objects in themselves, independent of their setting, was demonstrated in a control experiment where the monkeys learned whether foreground objects were rewarded or not, but the backgrounds were not uniquely linked to individual objects. For example, object A might be consistently rewarded, but every time it was presented it was set in a new background that had never been seen before. Monkeys with fornix transection learned normally in this control object-only condition. The main task, the scene memory or object-in-background task, has subsequently been given to groups of monkeys with other experi-mental lesions. One main purpose of these studies was to test the validity of the Delay–Brion hypothesis as to the functional unity of the hippocampus–fornix–mamillary system. The predictions of this hypothesis were verified. Lesions of the mamillary nuclei or of the anterior thalamic nuclei (which receive the main output of the mamillary nuclei through the mamillothalamic tract, and form a subsequent stage of the Delay–Brion system) produced quantitatively similar impairments of scene memory quantitatively similar to that produced by fornix transection; furthermore, as the hypothesis of functional unity requires, the combination of two lesions within the system (fornix transection plus mamillary nuclei lesion) produced no more severe an impairment than that which was produced by either of these lesions alone

(Parker & Gaffan 1997a,b). Thus, although the interpretation of amnesic pathology put forward by Delay & Brion (1969) needs to be substantially modified because discrete lesions in the Delay–Brion system do not produce severe amnesia (Section 18.2), nevertheless the functional unity that Delay & Brion suggested does apply to the specialized function of this system in scene memory.

18.4 Multiple distinct functional specializations in the temporal lobe

The unique role of the perirhinal cortex in object memory was first suggested by the electrophysiological findings of Brown et al. (1987) and the cooling studies of Horel et al. (1987), and it was first conclusively verified by the selective ablation experiments carried out by Meunier et al. (1990, 1993). Subsequently the behavioural effects of selective lesions of the perirhinal cortex or of the perirhinal plus entorhinal cortex ('rhinal cortex') was investigated in greater detail by Gaffan & Murray (1992), Murray et al. (1993), Eacott et al. (1994), Buckley et al. (1997) and Buckley & Gaffan (1997). To summarize these studies, it is clear that the perirhinal cortex is involved in memory for individual objects whether assessed by recognition memory for multiple objects, by configural learning or associative learning about objects, or by the ability to identify a familiar object in a new scene. Scene memory (Section 18.3) requires information about object identity to be put together with information about the spatial relations of the objects. As this account predicts, scene memory is severely impaired by disconnecting the fornix from the perirhinal cortex (Gaffan & Parker 1996). Nevertheless, the role of the perirhinal cortex can be differentiated quite clearly from the role of the fornix, as shown by double-dissociation experiments. In a simple spatial learning task involving only two identical objects, fornix transection produced a severe impairment but monkeys with perirhinal cortex ablations were normal; the relative severity of impairment of these two groups was reversed (double dissociation) in a visual recognition memory task involving many different objects (Gaffan 1994a). Thus, the roles of the perirhinal cortex and the fornix can be distinguished from each other qualitatively, even though in many memory tasks (such as the scene memory task) both play a part. Therefore, it is wrong to think of different memory impairments, produced by different temporal-lobe lesions, as reflecting simply a quantitative gradation of severity of impairment in a single memory system, as suggested by Squire & Zola-Morgan (1991). Severe amnesia after medial temporal lesions in humans, for example in surgical cases (Scoville & Milner 1957), is best thought of as resulting from combined damage to at least three functionally different structures: the hippocampus, the perirhinal cortex and the amygdala. The effects of amygdala lesions on memory can be doubly dissociated from the effects both of perirhinal cortex lesions and of fornix transection (Gaffan 1994a).

Yet further specializations of function have been shown within the macaque temporal lobe. The effects of perirhinal cortical lesions on visual memory are quite clearly qualitatively different from the effects of lesions in the adjacent visual cortex of the middle temporal gyrus. Lesions of the middle temporal gyrus impaired colour discrimination much more than object memory, but perirhinal cortex lesions impaired object memory more than did middle temporal gyrus lesions while leaving colour discrimination quite unaffected (Buckley *et al*. 1997).

These specializations suggest a loosely hierarchical arrangement of function in the temporal lobe. Visual features of objects, such as colour, are analysed in the neocortex of the middle and inferior temporal gyri; this information about isolated features can then be put together, and combined with non-visual object qualities, in the perirhinal cortex to form coherent representations of individual objects. Information about individual objects can then be combined in the hippocampus with spatial information, derived from both visual and non-visual modalities, to represent a spatially organized scene of foreground and background objects. Since a witnessed 'scene' is represented perceptually by the total exteroceptive information available to the observer at any one moment, the hippocampus is necessarily at the top of this loose hierarchy. The specializations of function within all these cortical areas of the temporal lobe are derived hodologically, that is by the nature of the afferent information that each cortical area receives (Gaffan 1996), rather than from specialized types of processing as is suggested by the cognitive-map hypothesis of hippocampal function (O'Keefe & Nadel 1978) or by many other once popular hypotheses of hippocampal function. Further, consistent with this hodological account of functional localization, the plasticity of what we think of as perceptual cortical areas, in perceptual learning, is not fundamentally different from the plasticity of what we think of as memory areas (Gaffan 1996).

18.5 Neglect and memory

Retrieval of spatially organized memories is disordered in neglect patients (Bisiach *et al*. 1979; Meador *et al*. 1987). For example, when a neglect patient was asked to describe from memory the street in which his home was situated, one side or the other of the street was omitted from the description, depending on the direction in which the patient imagined himself to be facing (Meador *et al*. 1987). A deeper understanding of neglect, therefore, should add to our understanding of memory for spatially organized complex scenes. The evidence reviewed in Section 18.3 above indicates that the hippocampus–fornix system is involved in just this kind of memory retrieval, the reconstruction from memory of a familiar scene such as one's home street. Why should this process fail unilaterally in a neglect patient?

Hornak (1992, 1995) put forward a representational explanation of visual neglect. In this view, the disordered retrieval from long-term memory in neglect is only one sign of a much broader deficit: neglect patients 'have a poor internal representation of space to the left of their current direction of gaze' (Hornak 1995, p. 323). Eye-movement recordings showed that when neglect patients inspected incomplete drawings, such as their own attempt to copy a drawing of a butterfly, they consistently failed to fixate the missing parts of the drawings. Similarly, when inspecting complete drawings of symmetrical objects, they never fixated the left half. When inspecting asymmetrical objects that could not be identified from the right half alone, however, the patients did fixate the left half, showing that their neglect did not simply reflect an oculomotor impairment. These disorders could not be explained by perceptual disorders in the left visual field of neglect patients, because patients without neglect but with hemianopia accurately made saccades into parts of drawings that lay in their blind field at the beginning of the saccade.

The representational hypothesis of neglect implies that not only the perceptual analysis of current retinal input, but also the retrieval of visual memory, is organized in a retinotopic fashion. If so, then visual neglect should be produced by depriving one hemisphere of all visual input, so that visual memories can no longer be laid down or retrieved in that hemisphere. We (Gaffan & Hornak 1997) tested this prediction in the monkey by combining unilateral optic-tract section with forebrain commissurotomy (section of the corpus callosum and anterior commissure), thus disconnecting one hemisphere from both halves of the retinas. These animals showed neglect in a visual search task, whereas animals with hemianopia alone did not. Furthermore, monkeys with cortical ablations in the parietal lobe and frontal eye field did not show neglect, although monkeys with lesions in the white matter inferior to the intraparietal sulcus did.

These findings, both from patients and from monkeys, imply that memory retrieval is retinotopically organized. Cortical cells that show retinotopically organized responses lie, of course, in visual cortical areas that are usually thought of as being perceptual in function. However, it is an over-simplification to think that the function of the visual cortex is vision. Rather, we suggest that the function of the visual cortex is to maintain a representation of the visible world, based not only on analysis of the current retinal input but also on memory. The influence of the Delay–Brion system on retrieval of scene memory is mediated, according to this view, by widespread influences on cortical areas that are thought of as perceptual in function. Delay & Brion themselves suggested that the output of the anterior thalamus in their system was conveyed to the cingulate cortex, the final proposed step in their system; however, Parker & Gaffan (1997a) showed that cingulate-cortex lesions do not produce the predicted effect on scene memory, and reviewed evidence that the anterior thalamus projects to widespread cortical areas, not to the cingulate cortex alone.

18.6 Hemiamnesia

If visual memories are retrieved retinotopically, as the data from neglect indicate, then one should expect that each temporal lobe should be relatively more involved in memories that relate to the contralateral visual hemifield than in those that relate to the ipsilateral visual hemifield. Hornak *et al*. (1997) tested this prediction in patients who had received unilateral partial surgical removals of the medial temporal lobe, including the amygdala and hippocampus in most cases, for the relief of epilepsy. Recognition of tachistoscopically presented half-scenes was markedly superior in the hemifield ipsilateral to the temporal lobe removal, irrespective of the side of the removal.

These patients do not have any known perceptual impairments in the parts of the visual field that were used for the half-scene memory tests. Nevertheless, one is tempted to ask whether hemiamnesia, i.e. the lateralized memory impairment shown by these patients, is secondary to some subtle, as yet undiscovered perceptual impairment. This question is less interesting than it seems, however. According to the interpretations put forward in Section 18.4, the functional specialization of memory systems derives from the afferent information that they receive, and both perceptual and memory systems show plasticity. Thus memory impairments may quite generally go along with some subtle perceptual impairments. Certainly, lesions in the rhinal cortex, which produce profound impairments in object memory, also produce some impairments in non-delayed matching judgments about objects (Eacott *et al*. 1994). It would not be surprising if future work were to reveal that a bilateral fornix lesion, for example, produces some subtle perceptual disorder in the processing of scene information (although, because different scenes can only be presented successively, not simultaneously, one can envisage that it might be logically very difficult to distinguish a perceptual from a memory disorder in the processing of scene information). If it turns out that patients with unilateral medial temporal-lobe removals have some subtle perceptual deficit in processing half-scenes contralateral to their removal—for which there is no evidence as yet—then presumably it would also be true that patients who are amnesic as a result of bilateral medial temporal damage would show the same subtle perceptual deficit bilaterally. The classification of a disorder as 'perceptual' or 'mnemonic' is not of fundamental importance.

18.7 The Hebb synapse, the cognitive map and temporal contiguity

The original, purely psychological specification of the cognitive-map hypothesis by Tolman (1932) dealt with maze learning in rats. The proposal was that, with experience of running through a maze, rats built up a map-like knowledge of the connected parts of the maze. Thus, a rat put in the start box of the maze could by a chain of association retrieve an 'expectancy of the specific character of the terminal parts of the maze' (Tolman 1932, p. 134). Behavioural evidence leaves no doubt that rats can retrieve such an expectancy (Gaffan & Gowling 1984) but it remains an open question whether this is the only mechanism or even the most important mechanism at work in maze learning by rats (the expectancy effects revealed in Gaffan & Gowling's experiment were statistically significant, but small). One of the alternative explanations to Tolman's is Hull's (1943) proposal that the animal's choices at all the choice-points in a maze, even those that are spatially distant from the goal box, can be directly associated with the primary reward that is ultimately discovered in the goal box. Hull's proposal requires that events can be directly associated with each other even when quite considerable temporal delays, of the order of tens of seconds, intervene between the two events to be associated. Tolman's proposal, on the other hand, allows spatially and temporally distant events to be associated with each other indirectly by a chain of mediating associations, each of which links parts of the maze that are perceived simultaneously or with millisecond delays.

There is thus an alliance between the cognitive-map explanation of maze learning and the Hebb-synapse model of associative learning (Hebb 1949, p. 62) according to which association formation takes place by the strengthening of a synaptic connection when action potentials are virtually simultaneous in the pre- and the postsynaptic cell. Long-term potentiation has been frequently proposed as a mechanism of associative learning that realizes the Hebb-synapse model (Brown *et al.* 1990) but behavioural pharmacological studies do not support the idea that long-term potentiation underlies associative learning (Saucier & Cain 1995; Gutnikov & Gaffan 1996; Hoelscher *et al.* 1997; but see Morris & Frey, Chapter 12). It is therefore appropriate to reassess the evidence for the role of temporal contiguity in associative learning, because the assumed necessity of temporal contiguity underlies so much theory and experiment, not only in the hippocampus but more broadly in the almost universal acceptance of the Hebb-synapse model of associative learning.

There is no doubt that animals can learn not only spatial but also non-spatial tasks when there is, operationally speaking, a temporal delay between the animal's choice and the reward that is dependent on that choice (Wolfe 1934; Perin 1943), but an experiment by Grice (1948) has been widely accepted as showing that delayed choice–reward associative learning can only proceed if it is mediated by two separate associations that are each between temporally contiguous events, that is, between the choice and a secondary reinforcer and between the secondary reinforcer and primary reward. Grice argued that when the mediation of secondary reinforcement was eliminated then associative learning showed a sharp gradient of temporal delay, such that a delay of 500 ms between choice and reward was enough to retard dramatically the rate of associative learning, by comparison with zero delay. In view of the importance of this issue to modern neurobiological investigations of the mechanism of associative learning based on the Hebb synapse model, Gutnikov *et al.* (1997; S. A. Gutnikov & D. Gaffan, unpublished results) decided to reinvestigate the temporal gradient of associative learning.

In the first experiment (Gutnikov *et al.* 1997) monkeys chose between two visual patterns on a screen by touching one. Immediately upon the animal's choice, both patterns disappeared. Then, either immediately (zero delay) or after a delay of 500 or 1000 ms, an audible food reward was delivered if the pattern chosen had been the correct one. The animals learned several sets of such associative learning 'problems' with ten new problems (pairs of new visual patterns) in each set. The learning curves were indistinguishable in the three delay conditions, all showing rapid learning.

Subsequently we investigated the effect of a filled delay, in which monkeys learned reward associations to a series of sequentially presented visual patterns. For example, an animal faced a choice between two patterns, say A and D. If A was chosen then immediately both A and D disappeared and A was replaced by B; 1250 ms later, B was replaced by C; after a further 1250 ms, by now 2.5 s after the animal's choice, C disappeared and food reward was delivered. Similarly, if D was chosen then A and D disappeared, D was replaced by E for 1250 ms, then E by F for 1250 ms, but, because D was the wrong choice, no food reward was delivered. Monkeys easily learned to choose the correct pattern (A in the example) in sets of ten problems of this kind. Furthermore, transfer tests showed that the animals learned about all three stimuli in each sequence; for example, having learned the sequence A–B–C reward they chose B or C if B or C was then presented as a choice stimulus.

In learning such sequences there are three different possible kinds of association to be formed.

1. The monkey could associate each visual pattern with the 'specific character' (in Tolman's sense, above) of the events that form each sequence. This is a cognitive-map explanation. The animal could look at A and retrieve the knowledge that A if chosen is followed by B, B by C, and C by reward. There is no doubt that monkeys can form visual–visual associations between successively presented patterns, albeit rather slowly (Murray *et al.* 1993), but the question at issue is whether they do so in the present task.
2. The monkey could learn by associations involving conditioned reinforcement. According to this explanation, A is associated not with the 'specific character' of B, and so on; rather, the animal learns only that A is followed by a predictor (a tertiary reinforcer) of a predictor (a secondary reinforcer) of food. This is a Grice-like explanation.
3. The animal could associate A directly with food, despite the temporal delay and the other intervening patterns. This is a Hull-like explanation.

These three possibilities can be distinguished by including some problems that share a common path to the ultimate outcome (a procedure similar in principle to Grice's). For example, the monkey chooses between G and J, and a choice of G produces the sequence H–I–food, whereas a choice of J produces (instead of K–L–no food, as in the standard procedure) the sequence H–I–no food. The common path H–I rules out both mechanisms (1) and (2) in the list above, leaving only (3). Monkeys learned the common-path problems G–H–I versus J–H–I just as easily as they did the standard problems A–B–C versus D–E–F. Thus, they showed direct visual–reward associative learning across a delay even when the delay was filled with other visual stimuli and those intervening stimuli were themselves attended to and learned about, as the transfer tests showed.

These findings appear to rule out a model of associative learning by simultaneous depolarizations. The pattern of action potentials in visual association cortex that encodes the perception of A must necessarily be replaced by a different pattern to encode the perceptions of B and then C. These patterns of action potentials cannot all be simultaneous with the pattern that represents the delivery of food reward. One might argue that at least some cells might still encode a 'shadow' of A even when C is perceived. However, visual objects have a distributed representation in the visual association cortex, and the discriminability of objects depends critically on the number of cells taking part in the representation (Rolls *et al.* 1997). In keeping with this concept, the effects of a partial ablation of visual association cortex on visual associative learning can be modelled by a reduction in the number of cells taking part in a distributed representation of the stimuli (Gaffan *et al.* 1986). Therefore, if the number of cells encoding the shadow is much smaller than the number of cells encoding the actual perception, then associative learning should be much slower with the shadows, which was not observed.

These experiments should be followed up to see whether similar direct associations between temporally noncontiguous events underlie maze learning by rats. At least in visual–reward associative learning in the primate brain, however, the code in which a predictive event enters into associative memory-trace formation (that is, the form in which the predictor is encoded at the time the event to be predicted occurs) cannot be action potentials. Rather, that code must consist of some long-lasting consequence of action potentials. To suggest what the code might be would be premature, but it is encouraging to note that electrophysiological studies have already begun to identify intracellular processes other than action potentials by which temporally discontiguous events can be integrated at the single-cell level (Batchelor & Garthwaite 1997).

18.8 General conclusions

The hippocampus is important for scene memory and this is required for normal performance (both in monkeys and in people) in non-spatial episodic memory and in spatial memory tasks. However, damage to the hippocampus–fornix–mamillary system is not sufficient to explain the full range of deficits in the human amnesic syndrome. Even within the realm of scene memory, the hippocampus is only one of the structures involved in a retrieval process which, as the data from neglect and hemiamnesia show, involves posterior retinotopically organized cortical areas that have previously been thought to have a perceptual function only. Furthermore, associative learning between temporally non-contiguous events shows that the brain mechanism of associative learning allows far greater temporal integration than is provided for in the Hebb-synapse model of association formation, which has been widely accepted as the basis of learning within the hippocampus and elsewhere. In conclusion, therefore, the primate brain encompasses widespread and powerful memory mechanisms which will be poorly understood if theory and experimentation continue to concentrate too much, as they have in the past, on the hippocampus and the Hebb synapse.

References

Bachevalier, J. & Mishkin, M. 1989 Mnemonic and neuropathological effects of occluding the posterior cerebral artery in *Macaca mulatta*. *Neuropsychologia* **27**, 83–105.

Batchelor, A. M. & Garthwaite, J. 1997 Frequency detection and temporally dispersed synaptic signal association through a metabotropic glutamate receptor pathway. *Nature* **385**, 74–77.

Bisiach, E., Luzzatti, C. & Perani, D. 1979 Unilateral neglect, representational schema and consciousness. *Brain* **102**, 609–618.

Brown, M. W., Wilson, F. A. W. & Riches, I. P. 1987 Neuronal evidence that inferomedial temporal cortex is more important than hippocampus in certain processes underlying recognition memory. *Brain Res.* **409**, 158–162.

Brown, T. H., Kairiss, E. W. & Keenan, C. L. 1990 Hebbian synapses: biophysical mechanisms and algorithms. *A. Rev. Neurosci.* **13**, 475–511.

Buckley, M. J. & Gaffan, D. 1997 Visual discrimination learning is impaired following perirhinal cortex ablation. *Behav. Neurosci.* **11**, 67–475.

Buckley, M. J., Murray, E. A. & Gaffan, D. 1997 A functional double-dissociation between two inferior temporal cortical areas: perirhinal cortex vs middle temporal gyrus. *J. Neurophysiol.* **97**, 587–598.

Delay, J. & Brion, S. 1969 *Le syndrome de Korsakoff*. Paris: Masson.

Eacott, M. J., Gaffan, D. & Murray, E. A. 1994 Preserved recognition memory for small sets, and impaired stimulus identification for large sets, following rhinal cortex ablation in monkeys. *Eur. J. Neurosci.* **6**, 1466–1478.

Gaffan, D. 1992 Amnesia for complex naturalistic scenes and for objects following fornix transection in the Rhesus monkey. *Eur. J. Neurosci.* **4**, 381–388.

Gaffan, D. 1994a Dissociated effects of perirhinal cortex ablation, fornix transection and amygdalectomy: evidence for multiple memory systems in the primate temporal lobe. *Expl Brain Res.* **99**, 411–422.

Gaffan, D. 1994b Scene-specific memory for objects: a model of episodic memory impairment in monkeys with fornix transection. *J. Cogn. Neurosci.* **6**, 305–320.

Gaffan, D. 1996 Associative and perceptual learning and the concept of memory systems. *Cogn. Brain Res.* **5**, 69–80.

Gaffan, D. & Gaffan, E. A. 1991 Amnesia in man following transection of the fornix: a review. *Brain* **114**, 2611–2618.

Gaffan, D. & Gowling, E. A. 1984 Recall of the goal box in latent learning and latent discrimination. *Q. J. Exp. Psychol. B* **36**, 39–51.

Gaffan, D. & Harrison, S. 1987 Amygdalectomy and disconnection in visual learning for auditory secondary reinforcement by monkeys. *J. Neurosci.* **7**, 2285–2292.

Gaffan, D. & Hornak, J. 1997 Visual neglect in the monkey: representation and disconnection. *Brain.* **120**, 1647–1657.

Gaffan, D. & Murray, E. A. 1992 Monkeys (*Macaca fascicularis*) with rhinal cortex ablations succeed in object discrimination learning despite 24-hr intertrial intervals and fail at matching to sample despite double sample presentations. *Behav. Neurosci.* **106**, 30–38.

Gaffan, D. & Parker, A. 1996 Interaction of perirhinal cortex with the fornix-fimbria: memory for objects and object-in-place memory. *J. Neurosci.* **16**, 5864–5869.

Gaffan, D., Harrison, S. & Gaffan, E. A. 1986 Visual identification following inferotemporal ablation in the monkey. *Q. J. Exp. Psychol.* **B38**, 530.

Grice, G. R. 1948 The relation of secondary reinforcement to delayed reward in visual discrimination learning. *J. Exp. Psychol.* **38**, 1–16.

Gutnikov, S. A. & Gaffan, D. 1996 Systemic NMDA receptor antagonist CGP 40116 does not impair memory acquisition but protects against NMDA neurotoxicity in Rhesus monkeys. *J. Neurosci.* **16**, 4041–4045.

Gutnikov, S. A., Ma, Y., Buckley, M. J. & Gaffan, D. 1997 Monkeys can associate visual stimuli with reward delayed by 1 second even after perirhinal cortex ablation, uncinate fascicle section or amygdalectomy. *Behav. Brain Res.* **87**, 85–96.

Hebb, D. O. 1949 *Organization of behavior*. New York: Wiley.

Hoelscher, C., McGlinchey, L., Anwyl, R. & Rowan, M. J. 1997 HFS-induced long-term potentiation and LFS-induced depotentiation in area CA1 of the hippocampus are not good models for learning. *Psychopharmacology* **130**, 174–182.

Horel, J. A., Pytko-Joiner, D. E.,Voytko, M. L. & Salsbury, K. 1987 The performance of visual tasks while segments of the inferotemporal cortex are suppressed by cold. *Behav. Brain Res.* **23**, 29–42.

Hornak, J. 1992 Ocular exploration in the dark by patients with visual neglect. *Neuropsychologia* **30**, 547–552.

Hornak, J. 1995 Perceptual completion in patients with drawing neglect: eye-movement and tachistoscopic investigation. *Neuropsychologia* **33**, 305–325.

Hornak, J., Oxbury, S., Oxbury, J., Iversen, S. D. & Gaffan, D. 1997 Hemifield-specific visual recognition memory impairments in patients with unilateral temporal lobe removals. *Neuropsychologia* **35**, 1311–1315.

Hull, C. L. 1943 *Principles of behaviour*. New York: Appleton–Century–Crofts.

Markowska, A. L., Olton, D. S., Murray, E. A. & Gaffan, D. 1989 A comparative analysis of the role of the fornix and cingulate cortex in memory: rats. *Expl Brain Res.* **74**, 187–201.

Mc Mackin, D., Cockburn, J., Anslow, P. & Gaffan, D. 1995 Correlation of fornix damage with memory impairment in six cases of colloid cyst removal. *Acta Neurochir.* **135**, 12–18.

Meador, K. J., Loring, D. W., Bowes, D. & Heilman, K. M. 1987 Remote memory and neglect syndrome. *Neurology* **37**, 522–526.

Meunier, M., Murray, E. A., Bachevalier, J. & Mishkin, M. 1990 Effects of perirhinal cortical lesions on visual recognition memory in Rhesus monkeys. *Soc. Neurosci. Abstr.* **16**, 616.

Meunier, M., Bachevalier, J., Mishkin, M. & Murray, E. A. 1993 Effects on visual recognition of combined and separate ablations of entorhinal and perirhinal cortex in rhesus monkeys. *J. Neurosci.* **13**, 5418–5432.

Moss, M., Mahut, H. & Zola-Morgan, S. 1981 Concurrent discrimination learning of monkeys after hippocampal, entorhinal or fornix lesions. *J. Neurosci.* **1**, 227–240.

Murray, E. A., Davidson, M., Gaffan, D., Olton, D. S. & Suomi, S. J. 1989 Effects of fornix transection and cingulate cortical ablation on spatial memory in Rhesus monkeys. *Expl Brain Res.* **74**, 173–186.

Murray, E. A., Gaffan, D. & Mishkin, M. 1993 Neural substrates of visual stimulus–stimulus association in rhesus monkeys. *J. Neurosci.* **13**, 4549–4561.

O'Boyle, V. J., Murray, E. A. & Mishkin, M. 1993 Effects of excitotoxic amygdalo-hippocampal lesions on visual recognition in rhesus monkeys. *Soc. Neurosci. Abstr.* **19**, 438.

O'Keefe, J. & Nadel, L. 1978 *The hippocampus as a cognitive map*. Oxford University Press.

Parker, A. & Gaffan, D. 1997*a* The effect of anterior thalamic and cingulate cortex lesions on object-in-place memory in monkeys. *Neuropsychologia* **35**, 1093–1102.

Parker, A. & Gaffan, D. 1997*b* Mamillary body lesions in monkeys impair object-in-place memory: functional unity of the fornix-mamillary system. *J. Cogn. Neurosci.* **9**, 512–521.

Perin, C. T. 1943 A quantitative investigation of the delay-of-reinforcement gradient. *J. Exp. Psychol.* **32**, 37–51.

Rolls, E. T., Treves, A. & Tovee, M. J. 1997 The representational capacity of the distributed encoding of information provided by populations of neurons in primate temporal visual cortex. *Expl Brain Res.* **114**, 149–162.

Saucier, D. & Cain, D. P. 1995 Spatial learning without NMDA receptor-dependent long-term potentiation. *Nature* **378**, 186–189.

Scoville, W. B. & Milner, B. 1957 Loss of recent memory after bilateral hippocampal lesions. *J. Neurol. Neurosurg. Psychiatr.* **20**, 11–21.

Squire, L. R. & Zola-Morgan, S. 1991 The medial temporal lobe memory system. *Science* **253**, 1380–1386.

Tolman, E. C. 1932 *Purposive behavior in animals and men*. New York: Century.

Victor, M., Adams, R. D. & Collins, G. H. 1971 *The Wernicke–Korsakoff syndrome*. Philadelphia: F. A. Davis.

Warrington, E. K. & Duchen, L. W. 1992 A re-appraisal of a case of persistent global amnesia following right temporal lobectomy: a clinico-pathological study. *Neuropsychologia* **30**, 437–450.

Wolfe, J. B. 1934 The effect of delayed reward upon learning in the white rat. *J. Comp. Psychol.* **17**, 1–21.

Zola-Morgan, S., Squire, L. R. & Amaral, D. G. 1986 Human amnesia and the medial temporal region: enduring memory impairment following a bilateral lesion limited to field CA1 of the hippocampus. *J. Neurosci.* **6**, 2950–2967.

19

Representation of allocentric space in the monkey frontal lobe

Carl R. Olson, Sonya N. Gettner and Leon Tremblay

19.1 Introduction

In discussions of how the brain represents space, it is common to make a contrast between environment-centred spatial information (encoded in the hippocampal system to be used in the service of spatial orientation) and body-centred spatial information (encoded in the parietal cortex to be used in the service of action and attention). However, this distinction, while fundamental, is not exhaustive. There is a third form of spatial information of great importance for cognition and behaviour in humans, namely, information about the locations of things relative to other things: of parts relative to an object and of objects relative to each other. Object-centred spatial information is allocentric in that it concerns locations defined relative to an external reference frame, but this reference frame, rather than encompassing the environment at large, is confined to the micro-environment of a particular object. Object-centred spatial judgments come into play in numerous situations including: when we direct actions to a particular location, as defined relative to an object; when we make judgments about topology, as in characterizing a closed curve as a knot; and when, in reading a word, we take into account the relative locations of the letters.

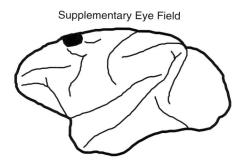

Fig. 19.1 Location of the supplementary eye field in a lateral view of the macaque left hemisphere with the frontal pole pointing to the left.

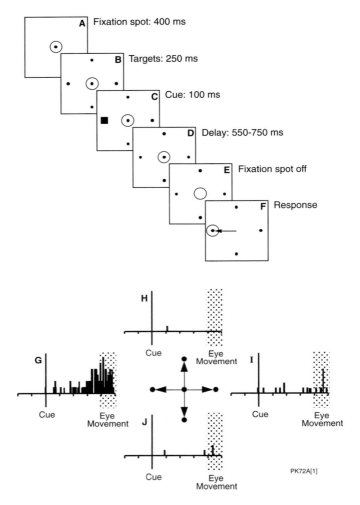

Fig. 19.2 Neurones were tested for oculocentric direction selectivity by monitoring their activity while monkeys performed the task summarized in the panels (A–F). These panels represent the screen in front of the monkey during successive epochs of a single trial. The centre of the circle in each panel indicates the monkey's direction of gaze. The *arrow* indicates the direction of the monkey's saccadic eye movement. All of the other items are patterns visible to the monkey. (A) A white fixation spot appeared at the centre of the screen and the monkey achieved foveal fixation. (B) Four potential targets appeared at 20° eccentricity. (C) A white cue flashed on one target. (D) During an ensuing delay period of variable length, the monkey was required to remember which target had been marked by the cue. (E) The fixation spot was extinguished. (F) The monkey responded by making an eye movement to the target cued earlier in the trial. (G–J) show data from an SEF neurone exhibiting leftward oculocentric direction selectivity in this task. Tick marks demarcate 200-ms intervals. In forming average histograms, data from successive trials were aligned on the time of onset of the cue. The

Recently has there been significant progress in understanding the neural representation of object-centred space. This progress has come in part from studies based on single-neurone recording in the cerebral cortex of monkeys trained to make eye movements to locations defined relative to reference objects (Gettner and Olson 1997; Olson and Gettner 1995, 1996a,b; Olson and Tremblay 1997). The essential finding is that neurones in the supplementary eye field (SEF, Fig. 19.1), a premotor area in the frontal lobe, fire when the monkey is planning to make eye movements to specific object-centred locations, with individual neurones exhibiting selectivity for different locations. They do so regardless of the visual features of the reference object and independently of whether the monkey is selecting the target by an object-centred rule. The aim of this chapter is to summarize the results of the key experiments and to consider the significance of these results for our understanding of brain mechanisms underlying spatial awareness.

19.2 Background: oculocentric direction selectivity in the supplementary eye field

Since its discovery more than 10 years ago, the SEF has generally been viewed as a motor area involved in the control of eye movements (Schlag and Schlag-Rey 1985). The identification of the area as 'supplementary' was suggested by the fact that the SEF is adjacent to the supplementary motor area (SMA) and captures the idea that the SEF is an oculomotor extension of the SMA. In accord with this view, most single-neurone recording studies of the SEF have focused on very simple tasks in which the size and direction of eye movements are varied, but no special demands are placed on spatial cognition beyond the need to identify the retinal locations of the small spots commonly used as eye-movement targets. During the performance of such tasks, SEF neurones fire when the monkey is preparing or executing saccadic eye movements and exhibit direction selectivity (Schall 1991; Schlag and Schlag-Rey 1987).

We recorded from SEF neurones during performance of a standard task requiring the monkey to make memory-guided eye movements to targets located at 20° eccentricity above, below, to the right of and to the left of the fixation point (Olson and Gettner 1995). The main stages of a single representative trial lasting around 1.5 s are summarized in Fig. 19.2A–F. The staggered panels in this figure represent the display on the screen in front of the monkey

---

delay between presentation of the cue and onset of the eye movement varied from trial to trial both because of random variation in the interval before the signal to move and because of variability in the behavioral reaction time. The *stippled bar* indicates the range of times of eye-movement onset. Note that firing ramped up during the delay and response periods when the eye movement was to the left (G) but not when it was in other directions (H–J).

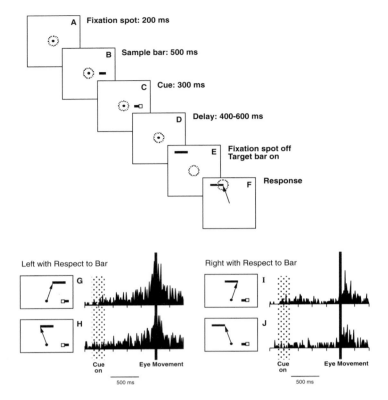

Fig. 19.3 Neurones were tested for object-centred direction selectivity by monitoring their activity while the monkey performed the task summarized in panels (A–F). These panels represent the screen in front of the monkey during successive epochs of a single trial. The centre of each circle indicates the monkey's direction of gaze during the corresponding trial epoch and the *arrow* indicates the direction of the eye movement. All other items are patterns visible to the monkey. (A) A white fixation spot appeared at the centre of the screen and the monkey achieved foveal fixation. (B) A horizontal sample bar appeared in the visual field lateral to the fixation spot. (C) A white cue flashed on one end of the sample bar. (D) During an ensuing delay period of variable length, the monkey was required to remember whether the right or left end of the sample bar had been marked by the cue. (E) The fixation spot was extinguished and a horizontal target bar simultaneously appeared in the upper visual field. (F) The monkey responded by making an eye movement to the end of the target bar corresponding to the cued end of the sample bar. (G–J) Show data collected from an SEF neurone during performance of this task. Each panel represents the location of the sample bar, the location of the cue, the location of target bar and the oculocentric direction of the eye movement for one trial condition. Each histogram represents neuronal firing rate as a function of time during successfully completed trials for the condition indicated to its left. Data from successive trials are aligned on the time of onset of the eye movement (*vertical line*). The time of onset of the cue (*vertical stippled bar*) varied across trials due both to variability in the behavioural reaction time and to randomization of the interval between cue-onset and target-onset. Firing depended primarily on the direction of the

during successive stages of the trial. In each panel, a circle indicates the monkey's direction of gaze. While the monkey maintained fixation on a central spot (panel A), four potential targets were presented (panel B) and one of the targets was cued (panel C). The monkey was then required to maintain central fixation during a delay period (panel D) at the end of which the fixation spot was extinguished (panel E), whereupon the monkey made an eye movement rapidly and directly to the previously cued target (panel F). SEF neurones typically fire during the delay period between presentation of the cue and offset of the fixation spot and may in addition fire a burst at the time of the eye movement. For example, the neurone in Fig. 19.2 fired almost exclusively before and during leftward eye movements (histogram G).

19.3 A new approach: object-centred direction selectivity

The directional preferences of SEF neurones have commonly been regarded as 'oculocentric' or 'orbital' insofar as they appear to concern the movement of the eye in the orbit. However, in a monkey with head fixed, a neurone with a leftward directional preference could be firing for movements to the left as defined relative to numerous reference frames, including ones centred on the eye, the head, the body, the screen or the room. It seems plausible that SEF neurones might encode directional information relative to a comparatively abstract reference frame because the SEF is connected to a family of cortical areas of fairly high order, including frontal, cingulate and parietal areas (Huerta and Kaas 1990). Accordingly, we carried out an experiment to determine whether SEF neurones are selective for the object-centred directions of eye movements (Olson and Gettner 1995).

   To induce monkeys to make eye movements to locations defined with respect to a reference object, we used the task diagrammed in Fig. 19.3A–F. The staggered panels in this figure represent the display on the screen in front of the monkey at successive stages during a single trial; the circle in each panel indicates the monkey's direction of gaze at the corresponding stage of the trial. The monkey began each trial by fixating a central spot (panel A). While he maintained central fixation, a sample bar was presented (panel B) and a cue spot was flashed briefly on one end of the sample bar (panel C). A delay period ensued during which the monkey was required to remember the instruction conveyed by the sample-cue display while maintaining central fixation (panel D). Finally, two events occurred simultaneously: the central spot was extinguished and a target bar appeared (panel E). The monkey's task at this point was to

---

eye movement relative to the bar (leftward in G–H; rightward in I–J) and not on its direction relative to the orbit (rightward in G and I; leftward in H and J). Note that conditions (G) and (I) are matched for both the retinal location of the cue and the oculocentric direction of the eye movement, as are conditions (H) and (J). Figure adapted from Olson & Gettner 1995.

make an eye movement rapidly and directly to the end of the target bar corresponding to the cued end of the sample bar (panel F). In the example of Fig. 19.3A–F, the right end of the sample bar was cued (panel C) and the eye movement was directed to the right end of the target bar (panel F).

In order to dissociate the direction of the eye movement as defined with respect to the bar from other task variables that might influence neuronal activity, we allowed three factors to vary independently across trials. These factors were the location of the sample bar, the location of the target bar, and object-centred direction. Varying these factors permitted a complete dissociation between the object-centred direction of the eye movement, on one hand, and the retinal location of the cue and oculocentric direction of the eye movement, on the other hand.

We monitored the activity of 29 SEF neurones during performance of this task and found, in a majority, clear evidence for object-centred direction selectivity. Data demonstrating object-centred direction selectivity in one neurone are shown in Fig. 19.3G–H. Each of the four histograms in this figure represents the neurone's average firing rate as a function of time during trials conforming to a particular condition identified by the inset to the left of the histogram. The upper histograms represent activity during a pair of conditions which differed only with respect to the object-centred direction of the eye movement, being identical with respect to the retinal location of the cue and the orbital direction of the eye movement. Likewise, the bottom histograms are a matched pair. It is evident that activity before and during eye movements to the left end of the target bar (left histograms) was greater than activity before and during eye movements to the right end of the target bar (right histograms).

To quantify these effects, we carried out an analysis of variance on data from each neurone, assessing the dependence of neuronal activity on the direction of the eye movement as defined (a) with respect to the target (right or left end of bar) and (b) with respect to the orbit (up and to the right or up and to the left). Separate analyses were carried out on activity occurring during:

(1) a delay epoch 500-ms long, terminating with onset of the target;
(2) a preparation epoch extending from onset of the target to initiation of the eye movement; and
(3) a response epoch extending from initiation of the eye movement to a point in time 100 ms after its termination.

We found that the rate of firing depended significantly ($P < 0.05$) on bar-centred direction, either as a main effect or as an interaction effect between object-centred and orbital direction, in 23/29 neurones.

These results indicate that neurones in the SEF have object-centred preferences defined with respect to the horizontal axis. However, object-centred spatial awareness is expressed with respect to axes at all orientations. For example, we are able to distinguish between lower-case 'b' and 'p' on the basis of the disposition of their elements with respect to the vertical axis. If object-centred direction selectivity in the SEF were indeed related to the general function of object-centred spatial awareness, then we would expect SEF neurones to exhibit selectivity for locations as defined relative to non-horizontal axes.

To test this expectation, we carried out additional experiments in two monkeys trained to perform the object-centred task with either horizontal or vertical bars as reference objects. On each trial, a sample bar was presented at either vertical or horizontal orientation; one end was cued; a delay ensued; a target bar then was presented at the same orientation; finally, after a further delay, the monkey was required to make an eye movement to the end of the target bar corresponding to the cued end of the sample bar. The conditions critical for analysis were those in which the cued end of the sample bar (right, left, top or bottom) and the corresponding end of the target bar fell at an identical location, thus permitting us to hold constant the factors of the cue's retinal location and the eye's direction of movement in the orbit while assessing the effect of object-centred direction.

Upon analysis of data from 65 neurones in two monkeys, we found that they exhibited horizontal (right vs. left) and vertical (top vs. bottom) selectivity with equivalent frequency (14/65 horizontal only, 16/65 vertical only, 11/65 both). For the 41 neurones exhibiting significant selectivity with respect to either axis, we estimated the best direction by summing a horizontal vector weighted by the strength of the horizontal directional signal and a vertical vector weighted by the strength of the vertical directional signal. For example, if a neurone's mean firing frequency had been $10\,\text{spikes}\,\text{s}^{-1}$ greater for bar-left than for bar-right conditions and $10\,\text{spikes}\,\text{s}^{-1}$ greater for bar-top than for bar-bottom conditions, then we would have computed its best direction as 45° up and to the left. The resultant vectors were distributed fairly evenly around the clock.

19.4 SEF neurones combine object-centred and oculocentric signals

The question of whether individual SEF neurones carry both oculocentric and object-centred signals is of interest from a theoretical point of view because the answer may cast light on how neural networks responsible for object-centred behaviour carry out the underlying computations. This fact is emphasized by a recent modelling study demonstrating that neural networks containing hidden units selective for specific conjunctions of oculocentric and object-centred location are capable of generating object-centred eye movements (Deneve and Pouget 1998). In this section, we first will describe findings clarifying how individual neurons in the SEF combine object-centred and oculocentric signals and then will consider how these findings relate to the model.

Our first approach was to collect data from a series of neurones using both the standard task to characterize oculocentric direction selectivity and the horizontal-bar task to characterize object-centred direction selectivity

(Olson and Gettner 1995). We found that neurones exhibiting object-centred direction selectivity in the horizontal-bar task often exhibited oculocentric direction selectivity in the standard task. Further, there was a significant correlation between preferred horizontal directions in the two tasks. Neurones firing most strongly during leftward (or rightward) eye movements in the standard task tended to fire most strongly during eye movements to the left (or right) end of the bar in the bar task. We carried out a further analysis to test the possibility that neurones with upward oculocentric preferred directions in the standard task would preferentially express object-centred direction selectivity in the horizontal bar task (in which bars were always presented in the upper visual field). We found that neurones with upward preferred directions were no more likely than others to exhibit object-centred direction selectivity. These general points are evident in data from a single neurone studied in both tasks, as shown in Fig. 19.2G–J and Fig. 19.4G–J. In the standard task, this neurone fired vigorously before leftward eye movements (Fig. 19.2G) and was virtually silent during upward eye movements (Fig. 19.2H). In contrast, in the bar task, it fired vigorously during upward eye movements to the left end of the bar (Fig. 19.4G–H).

The general finding that the same neurone can express oculocentric direction selectivity in the standard task and object-centred direction selectivity in the bar task might be interpreted in at least three ways.

1. SEF neurones carry both oculocentric and object-centred signals.
2. SEF neurones carry solely object-centred signals. Signals interpreted as oculocentric in the standard task actually encode direction as referred to a default reference object, for example, the central fixation point or the screen as a whole.
3. SEF neurones carry solely oculocentric signals. In the bar task, the instruction to make an eye movement to the left (or right) end of the target bar induces the monkey to prepare, during the delay period, to make an eye movement to the left (or right) in the orbit, even though, across the full set of trial conditions, there is no correlation between bar-centred direction and oculocentric direction.

To tease apart these possibilities, we used a variant of the original bar task in which oculocentric and object-centred signals could be distinguished (Fig. 19.4A–F). This was like the original bar task except in that when the target bar came on (panel E) the central fixation spot was not extinguished and the monkey was required to maintain central fixation. The important feature of this task was that during the delay period following onset of the target bar, both the oculocentric direction and the object-centred direction of the impending eye movement were determined. We wished to know whether, during this period, neural activity would reflect object-centred direction alone, oculocentric direction alone, or a combination of the two. We found that neurones carried

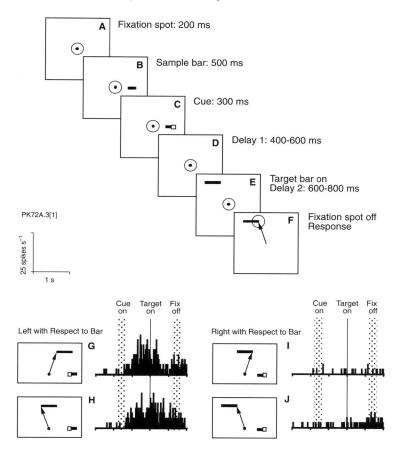

Fig. 19.4 The bar task with two delays was used to assess combined selectivity for object-centred and oculocentric direction. (A–F) Represent the screen in front of the monkey during successive epochs of a single trial. This task differed from the standard bar task (Fig. 19.3) in that the central fixation spot remained on following the appearance of the target bar (E). The monkey was required to maintain central fixation until offset of the fixation spot at the end of the second delay period (F). (G–J) Show data collected from an SEF neurone during performance of this task. Data from successive trials are aligned on the time of onset of the target bar (*vertical line*). The time of onset of the cue (*lef vertical stippled bar*) and the time of offset of the fixation spot (*right vertical stippled bar*) varied across trials due to randomization of the delay intervals. During delay 1, firing was greater on bar-left trials (G and H) than on bar-right trials (I and J). During delay 2, bar-centred direction selectivity persisted, but there was an added influence of oculocentric direction, whereby firing was greater when the eye moved up and to the left than when it moved up and to the right (H vs. G and J vs. I). Conventions as in Fig. 19.3.

both kinds of signal. Out of 73 neurones, six showed main effects for both object-centred and oculocentric direction, 12 showed significant interaction effects, and one showed both main effects and an interaction effect. An example of combined object-centred and oculocentric selectivity is shown in Fig. 19.4G–J. During the first delay period, prior to onset of the target, this neurone fired vigorously on bar-left trials (panels G and H). After onset of the target bar, it continued to exhibit bar-left selectivity (activity was stronger under conditions G and H than under conditions I and J) but it also fired more strongly when the impending eye movement was up and to the left vs. up and to the right (H vs. G; J vs. I). These results support the first scenario described above: individual SEF neurones carry both object-centred and oculocentric signals.

Deneve and Pouget (1998) have recently described a network, capable of generating object-centred eye movements, in which the hidden units carry both object-centred and oculocentric signals. Their network can produce eye movements to the intrinsic right or left side of an object tilted at any orientation. However, because the essential features of the network are apparent in the restricted case of an upright object, we will consider only this case. Each unit in the SEF-like hidden layer possesses a restricted oculocentric motor field: when it is active it produces an eye movement of a particular size and direction. Each hidden unit also receives two kinds of input—a command and a visual signal—which interact multiplicatively. The command input arises either from an object-left command line (in half of the hidden units) or from an object-right command line (in the other half). The visual input arises from a visual unit with the properties (a) that it has a restricted visual receptive field matching the hidden unit's oculocentric motor field and (b) that it is active when a particular side of an object, matching the hidden unit's command-line input, is in its receptive field. For example, a hidden unit with an object-left command-line input and with a motor field in the upper right quadrant would receive its visual input from a visual unit selective for the left side of an object and having a receptive field in the upper right quadrant. Gated on by the object-left command-line, this neurone would produce an eye movement into the upper right quadrant in response to the presence of an object at a location such that its left end is in the upper right quadrant. Thus each hidden unit encodes a particular combination of object-centred and oculocentric direction and the entire population provides even coverage of the family of possible combinations.

Because the SEF-like hidden units in their network carry a mixture of object-centred and oculocentric signals, Deneve and Pouget consider that the 'representation' of object-centred space is neither 'explicit' nor 'invariant'. However, like SEF neurones, the units in their model do carry object-centred signals, which are 'explicit'—in the sense that activity is overtly different during eye movements to the right and left ends of the bar—and 'invariant'—in the sense that a given unit's object-centred preference is constant over the full range of oculocentric directions for which it is active. The Deneve–Pouget model diverges from the SEF primarily in the fact that oculocentric and object-centred signals interact strictly multiplicatively in the model, whereas, in the SEF, their interaction is partially additive. This has the concrete consequence that a hidden unit in the model is not active during an eye movement to the preferred end of a bar if the eye movement is outside the unit's oculocentric motor field, whereas an SEF neurone may still exhibit object-centred direction selectivity under this condition (cf. Figs 19.2G–J and 19.4G–J). Whether this discrepancy is merely one of degree or reflects a different modes of processing in the SEF and in the model remains to be worked out through future work on both fronts.

19.5 Object-centred signals do not depend on the visual features of the object

Do object-centred directional signals contain purely spatial information or, alternatively, are they influenced by the nature of the object to which spatial judgments are referred? To answer this question, we carried out additional experiments in which the visual features of the stimuli were manipulated. Two experiments, one in which we changed the nature of the instructional cue and another in which we changed the nature of the target object, will be described in this section.

In early variants of the bar task, the instructional cue was a spot flashed on the right or left end of the sample bar. The configuration of the display (a cue spot on the left or right end of sample bar) covaried with the object-centred direction of the eye movement. Neuronal activity dependent on bar-centred direction thus could plausibly be interpreted either as a visual memory signal (selective for the display of the cue spot on the left or right end of the sample bar) or as a correlate of the monkey's intention to make an eye movement to the left or right end of the target bar. To select between these interpretations, we trained monkeys to perform a variant of the bar task using coloured squares as cues (blue instructing a bar-left response and yellow instructing a bar-right response). This differed from previous versions of the bar task in that, when the sample bar would have come on, a small 'location marker' spot appeared, and, when the cue would have flashed on the right or left end of the sample bar, a coloured square flashed in direct superimposition on the location marker. We recorded from 21 neurones during performance of tasks differing only in the use of coloured vs. configurational cues. Upon carrying out an analysis of variance on data from each neurone, we found that activity depended significantly on the object-centred direction of the eye movement in a majority of the tested neurones. Moreover, the preferred object-centred direction, as observed during the use of colour cues, was always the same as in tasks using configurational cues. Eleven neurones exhibited significant dependence on object-centred direction both in the task with coloured cues and in a task identical except in that the cues were configurational. In all 11 neurones, the preferred bar-centred direction was identical across both tasks (six neurones favoured bar-right and five favoured bar-left). We conclude that neuronal activity is related to the bar-centred direction of the impending eye movement rather than to the visual attributes of the cues.

We have also assessed the impact of the visual features of the target bar. In particular, we have asked whether it is necessary that directions be referred to a single coherent object (a bar) rather than to a more complex display (a pair of dots defining the ends of a virtual bar). This comparison was motivated in part by neuropsychological evidence suggesting that the processing of coherent objects and arrays may be carried out by distinct sets of brain areas. First, some patients with neglect show different error patterns when bisecting solid horizontal bars and virtual bars defined by pairs of dots. Second, within-object and within-array aspects of neglect are dissociable. Some patients, in copying drawings, neglect the leftmost of two flowers only when they are united into a single object by a common stem (Marshall and Halligan 1993). Further, a few patients have been described in whom the side affected by neglect differs for objects and arrays (Humphreys and Riddoch 1994, 1995). When presented with a written word and required to read it (treating it as a unitary object) they neglect its left half. When presented with the same word and required to spell it out (treating each letter as a separate object) they neglect letters on the right.

In light of these findings, we decided to ask whether the object-centred signals carried by SEF neurones are specific to judging locations on a physically continuous object, or are also present during the judgment of array-relative locations (Olson and Tremblay 1997). We trained monkeys to perform a task in which, on interleaved trials, the reference image was either a continuous horizontal bar (as in the standard task) or a pair of dots separated horizontally by a distance equal to the length of the continuous bar. On 'object' trials, both the sample image and the target image were continuous bars, whereas, on 'array' trials, each was an array of two dots. An analysis of variance on data from 143 neurones in two monkeys, carried out to determine whether neuronal activity during the delay and response periods was significantly dependent on relative direction (rightward vs. leftward) and type of reference image (bar vs. array), revealed that selectivity to relative location was affected only to a minor degree by the type of reference image. Among neurones exhibiting dependence on relative direction (more than half of the sample) a majority exhibited no interaction effect traceable to object-type. Moreover, in those neurones in which a significant interaction effect was present, the most common form of interaction was a change in the strength (but not the sign) of the directional signal as a function of whether the reference image was a bar or a pair of dots.

We conclude that SEF neurones encode relative locations not only within physically continuous objects but also within arrays. However it must be noted that the array of two dots used in this experiment defines a 'virtual' bar, in the same way that a constellation of stars defines a meaningful shape, by a bottom-up gestalt-based process. It would be of interest to determine whether neuronal signals reflecting relative direction are still present in a task where the reference image lacks gestalt unity and is selected out from the background strictly by a top-down process. For example, one might train monkeys to select between the two rightmost dots in a four-dot horizontal array, so as to ask whether bar-left neurons (as identified in the standard task) are active during targeting of the leftmost of the two relevant dots (despite the fact that even this dot occupies a position to the right of center in the four-dot array).

19.6 Object-centred direction selectivity is automatic

Object-centred direction selectivity might arise only under conditions requiring the monkey to choose responses on the basis of object-centred spatial judgments. Alternatively, it might occur under conditions in which the monkey simply happens to look at one end or the other of a bar, without following an object-centred instruction. To distinguish between these possibilities, we recorded from SEF neurones during performance of a task in which monkeys made visually guided eye movements to spots that only incidentally were superimposed on the ends of bars (Fig. 19.5). Interleaved trials were of two types: 'spot + bar' trials (panels A–E) and 'spot only' trials (panels A′–E′). In each 'spot + bar' trial, a bar appeared in isolation for 500 ms (panel B), then a spot was presented on one end of it (panel C). During the remainder of the trial, both the bar and the spot remained on. The monkey was required to maintain central fixation until the fixation light was turned off (panel D) and then to make an eye movement to the target spot (panel E). The monkey could perform this task correctly without ever taking note of the existence of the bar. 'Spot only' trials were identical except in that a bar never appeared (panels A′–E′). These trials were included to characterize orbital direction selectivity in the absence of bars and to provide a baseline against which to assess the effects of the bars. Data from a neurone studied while the monkey performed this task are shown in Fig. 19.5F–J. This neurone displayed preparatory activity during the period between appearance of the target spot and initiation of the eye movement. On 'spot only' trials, it fired most strongly before rightward eye movements (Fig. 19.5F–H). On trials in which the target was superimposed on a bar, the firing rate was enhanced when the spot was on the right end of a bar (panel I) and was reduced when the spot was on the left end of a bar (panel J). Statistically significant dependence on bar-centred direction was present in 24 out of 45 neurones tested by this procedure. It thus appears that SEF neurones manifest bar-centred direction selectivity, even when the monkey is performing a task that is not dependent on the use of bar-centred information. However, this conclusion is provisional. Because the monkey was trained to perform other tasks requiring the use of bar-centred information, it is possible that he actively attended to the bar-relative location of the spot in this task, despite not having to use the information. To resolve this issue it will be necessary to carry out the same test in monkeys not trained on any task requiring the active use of bar-centred information.

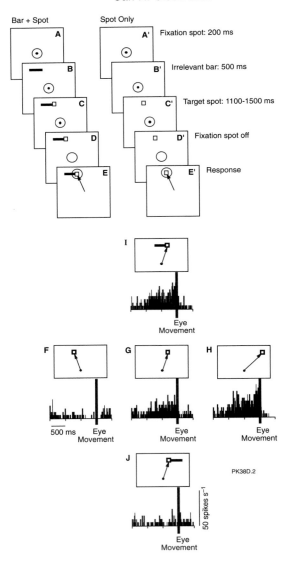

Fig. 19.5 The bar task with an irrelevant bar was used to determine whether bar-centred direction depended on the monkey's using object-centred information to select the target. (A–E) and (A'–E') Represent the screen in front of the monkey during successive epochs of 'spot + bar' and 'spot only' trials, respectively. Note, in 'spot + bar' trials that, although the spot is superimposed on the end of the bar, the monkey need not register the presence of the bar in order to make a correct response (an eye movement directly to the spot). (F–J) Show data from a SEF neurone exhibiting, in the context of this task, both rightward object-centred direction selectivity (I vs. J) and rightward oculocentric direction selectivity (F–H). Conventions as in Fig. 19.3. Figure adapted from Olson and Gettner 1995.

A further experiment has added additional weight to the notion that SEF neurones automatically encode object-centred locations. In this experiment, we recorded from neurones while the monkey performed a task requiring him to select the rightmost or leftmost of a pair of dots on the basis of colour rather than location. We then analysed the data to determine whether SEF neurones continued to encode object-centred locations, which were not relevant for target selection, and, conversely, whether they encoded colours, which were relevant. The sequence of events in a representative colour trial is summarized in Fig. 19.6A–G. A sample array first came on, consisting of two white dots, which defined the ends of a virtual bar (B); then a coloured cue (red or green) flashed on the array's right or left end (C); then, after a delay, a target array appeared, consisting of one red dot and one green dot (E); finally, upon offset of the fixation spot (F), the monkey was required to make an eye movement to the target element corresponding in colour to the cue (G). Across trials, the sample array could appear at either the rightward or leftward screen location,

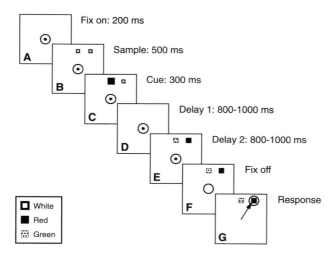

Fig. 19.6 A task with a colour rule was used to assess whether neuronal activity continued to encode the object-centred direction of the target, even when the monkey was selecting the target on the basis of its colour rather than object-centred location. (A–G) Show a representative trial. Following onset of a two-dot sample array (B), a red or green cue was flashed on the right or left array element (C). A delay ensued (D). Then the target array appeared, consisting of one red and one green dot (E). The monkey had to wait until offset of the fixation light (F) to make an eye movement to the target dot corresponding in colour to the cue regardless of its location (G). Conventions as in Fig. 19.3.

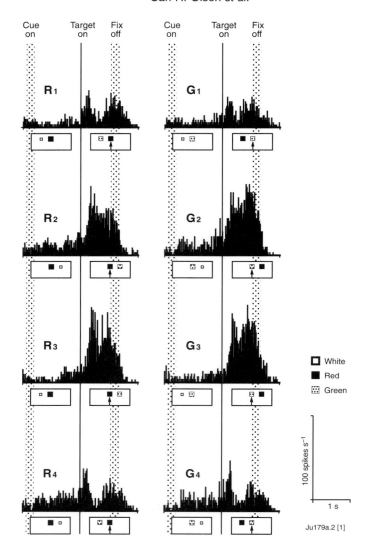

Fig. 19.7 Data collected from an SEF neurone in the context of the colour task with a red cue (R1–R4) or green cue (G1–G4). Conditions R1–R4 are matched with G1–G4 for cue location and target location, differing only with respect to the colour of the cue and target. Each histogram was formed by aligning data from successive trials on onset of the target. The box under the *left half* of each histogram shows the cue superimposed on one element of the sample array (the larger, *shaded square* is the cue; the smaller, *white square* is the remaining element of the sample array). The box under the *right half* of each histogram shows an eye movement (*arrow*) directed to one element of the target array. For example, in condition R1, the sample array appeared in the left visual field, a red cue was presented on its right end, the target array, consisting of a green dot on the left and a red dot on the right, appeared in the right visual field, and the monkey

and the same was true of the target array. The cue could appear on either end of the sample array and the target dot could appear on either end of the target array, and there was no correlation across trials between the location of the cue and the location of the target. For example, in the representative trial of Fig. 19.6A–G, the red cue flashed on the left end of the sample array whereas the dot of corresponding colour was on the right end of the target array (we refer to the 50% of trials with such locational mismatch as 'incongruent' trials).

The results of this experiment were very clear-cut. SEF neurones encoded the cue's array-relative location (during the first delay period, following cue presentation) and the target spot's array-relative location (during the second delay period, following onset of the target array). On 'incongruent' colour trials, there was actually a reversal of activity between the first and second delay periods: a bar-left neurone might fire strongly following presentation of the red (or green) cue on the sample array's left end and then grow silent following onset of a target array containing a red (or green) dot on its right end. The negligible influence of colour (red vs. green) on neuronal activity during colour trials was all the more striking because the monkey had to remember and use colour information in order to perform the task successfully. An example demonstrating these points is presented in Fig. 19.7. This neurone fired at virtually identical rates during trials when the cue and target were red (R1–R4) and when they were green (G1–G4). During the first delay period, it fired more strongly when the cue had been presented at the array-left location (R2, R4, G2 and G4). During the second delay period, it fired more strongly when the target was at the array-left location (R2, R3, G2 and G3). The trial conditions presented in Fig. 19.7 are a subset in which the location of the cue was constant (immediately above fixation) and the oculocentric direction of the response was constant (straight upward). The observed differences in firing rate thus cannot be ascribed to the oculocentric location of the cue or direction of the response. Across this subset of conditions, the location of the array relative to the screen did covary with the location of the cue or target relative to the array. However, data from additional conditions (not shown) established that the rate of firing of the neurone depended on the location of the cue or target relative to its array, not on the location of the array relative to the screen, except during a period immediately following target-onset, when presentation of the target in the left visual field elicited a brief burst (R1, R4, G1 and G4),

---

made an eye movement to the red dot. The conditions shown in this figure are a subset selected to hold constant the location of the cue (directly above the fixation point) and the physical direction of the eye movement (straight up). Note that the neurone fired more strongly following presentation of the cue on the left of the sample (before 'target on') and when the target spot was on the left of the target array (after 'target on'), regardless of the colour of cue and target and regardless of the fact that the monkey was selecting the target that matched the cue in colour, not location. Conventions as in Fig. 19.3.

whereas presentation in the right visual field did not (R2, R3, G2 and G3). We confirmed these observations by carrying out an analysis of variance on data from 74 neurones, with colour and object-centred direction as factors. Whereas more than half of the tested neurones showed a significant effect of object-centred direction, only a few were significantly influenced by colour. We conclude that neurones in the SEF specialize in representing the object-centred location of the target. The fact that they are specialized for the representation of spatial information is evident in the dual observations (a) that they represent object-centred location even when the monkey is not following an object-centred rule and (b) that they do not represent other stimulus variables even when these are highly relevant for task performance.

19.7 Possible functions of object-centred direction selectivity

The general conclusion arising from the experiments described above is that neurones in the supplementary eye field (SEF) carry object-centred spatial information, firing selectively before eye movements to the left (or right) end of a reference object regardless of the location of the object or its particular visual features and even regardless of whether or not the monkey is using an object-centred rule. We strongly suspect that the property of object-centred spatial selectivity is not unique to the SEF and that the fact of its not having been observed in other brain areas is simply a result of its not having been looked for. The SEF may well be just one station in a distributed cortical system dedicated to the processing of spatial information as defined relative to multiple reference frames including object-centred ones. Through its connections with other cortical areas, the SEF may contribute to several different important behavioural and cognitive processes.

Scanning of natural scenes

Directing eye movements to particular locations as defined relative to a reference object may seem to be a highly artificial activity of little use outside the laboratory. However, there are at least two kinds of situation in which it might be adaptive to fixate a location not marked by visible local contrast and therefore of necessity defined only by its relation to other elements visible in the scene. First, one might make an eye movement to a point known to contain informative features that are currently not discriminable because of limits on extrafoveal acuity. For example, subjects reading printed text tend to make saccades to the left of centre of the next word in the fixation sequence, a within-word location yielding maximal processing efficiency (Vitu *et al.* 1990). Second, one might make a saccade to a blank region at which it is anticipated that something will soon appear. Humans and monkeys do make spontaneous anticipatory saccades (Miyashita *et al.* 1996; Ross *et al.* 1994). There has been no formal study demonstrating that these are object-centred, but it is clear that in some cases they must be. For example, when monkeys or humans look at the region on a blank screen where they expect a stimulus to appear, they are probably guided in selecting a fixation point by the contours of the screen.

Attention

Making an eye movement to a target is inevitably accompanied by directing attention to it; moreover, the functions of oculomotor control and attention may well be mediated by an overlapping set of neural structures (Rizzolatti *et al.* 1994). Thus it is possible that the object-centred activity of SEF neurones is related to the selection of targets for attention and not just for eye movements. The idea that neurones mediating attention have object-centred spatial selectivity is compatible with the fact that some aftereffects of attention are specific to the object- or array-relative location at which a stimulus previously appeared (Gibson & Egeth 1994; Maljkovic & Nakayama 1996). Furthermore, there is neuropsychological evidence indicating that separate brain systems may mediate object-right and object-left attention. Patients with left hemispatial neglect arising from right parietal lobe injury tend to neglect the left half of an object or array even when it is in the right visual field (Arguin and Bub 1993; De Renzi *et al.* 1989; Làdavas *et al.* 1990, 1994; Posner *et al.* 1987; Young *et al.* 1992) or is rotated in the viewing plane so as to bring the left side to the top or bottom or right as defined with respect to the retina (Behrmann and Tipper 1994; Driver *et al.* 1994; Tipper and Behrmann 1996; Young *et al.* 1992). It is reasonable to speculate that object-centred neglect, as observed in these cases, has arisen from the loss of neurones with object-left spatial selectivity. However, the data allow other interpretations. In particular, right-hemisphere injury might give rise to a decline in the efficiency of attention, with the deficit growing worse gradientally from the right to the left side of the visual field. The gradiental model, like the object-centred model, can account for both the translation invariance and rotation invariance of object-centred neglect. A gradiental mechanism could produce translation-invariant object-left neglect by conferring a visual-field-wide advantage on any object's right half as compared to its left half, if there were a competition for attention between the two halves (Làdavas *et al.* 1990; Pouget and Sejnowski 1996). A gradiental mechanism could also produce rotation-invariant object-left neglect if patients mentally rotated images to upright orientation before the stage of competitive interaction between the right and left halves (Buxbaum *et al.* 1996).

Recognition

The idea that object-centred representations form a basis for visual object recognition was proposed in a general form by Marr and Nishihara (1978) and has been developed further in the geon-based model of Biederman (1987). These authors envision, as an early and automatic step in recognition of an object, the decomposition of the image into three-dimensional structural components (geons), the locations and orientations of which are expressed relative to a three-dimensional reference frame centred on and oriented with respect to the object itself. In an extreme form of such a model, any image of a given object, regardless of its size and orientation should give rise to an identical central representation, up to the point where information is lost due to self-occlusion. There is modest electrophysiological support for this notion, insofar as many inferotemporal neurones respond selectively to the image of a preferred object regardless of the retinal location of the image (Lueschow *et al.* 1994; Tovee *et al.* 1994) and a few neurones remain selective across changes in orientation (Hasselmo *et al.* 1989; Perrett *et al.* 1991). Moreover, it has been argued that some neurones in area V4 are selective for the presence of a preferred feature at a preferred object-centred (or, at least, attention-centred) location (Connor *et al.* 1996). However, the view that recognition is carried out on three-dimensional object-centred structural representations has been called into question, at least for certain classes of objects, by the demonstration that humans and monkeys (Logothetis and Pauls 1995; Logothetis *et al.* 1994) as well as inferotemporal neurons (Logothetis and Pauls 1995) recognize particular views of objects rather than their three-dimensional structures. Even if recognition is based on structural representations, it is unlikely that the SEF contributes to these representations because SEF neurones are selective for object-centred locations and not for particular objects or features.

Appreciation of structure

We can appreciate the structure of a visible object independently of recognizing it. For example, shown an entirely novel curve in three dimensions, we can make judgments concerning topological attributes such as whether it forms a knot. Likewise, we can distinguish possible from impossible figures. Our ability to carry out these tasks attests to our capacity for forming structural representations of visible objects. Appreciation of any reasonably complicated structure must involve analyzing the parts of the object serially, through shifts of gaze or attention, and building up a composite description in working memory. Neurones in the SEF might contribute to forming structural representations, insofar as they mediate directing gaze or attention to particular object-centred locations. However, it seems unlikely that they contribute to holding the representations in working memory, because they lack selectivity for particular objects or features.

Acknowledgments

We acknowledge support for C.R.O. from NSF (IBN 9312763) and NIH (RO1 NS27287; RO1 EY11506) and for S.N.G. from NIH (1 F32 NS09452) and the McDonnell-Pew Program in Cognitive Neuroscience. We thank J. McClelland for helpful comments.

References

Arguin, M. and Bub, D. N. (1993). Evidence for an independent stimulus-centered spatial reference frame from a case of visual hemineglect. *Cortex*, **29**, 349–57.

Behrmann, M. and Tipper, S. P. (1994). Object-based attentional mechanisms: evidence from patients with unilateral neglect. In *Attention and Performance XV*, (ed., C. Umiltà and M. Moscovitch), pp. 351–375. MIT Press, Cambridge, Massachusetts.

Biederman, I. (1987). Recognition-by-components: a theory of human image understanding. *Psychological Review*, **94**, 115–47.

Buxbaum, L. J., Coslett, H. B., Montgomery, M. W. and Farah, M. J. (1996). Mental rotation may underlie apparent object-based neglect. *Neropsychologia*, **34**, 113–26.

Connor, C. E., Gallant, J. L., Preddie, D. C., and Van Essen, D. C. (1996). Responses in area V4 depend on the spatial relationship between stimulus and attention. *Journal of Neurophysiology*, **75**, 1306–8.

Deneve, S. and Pouget, A. (1998). Neural basis of object-centred representations. In *Advances in Neural Information Processing Systems 10*, (ed., M. I. Jordan, M. J. Keams and S. A. Solla), pp. 24–30. MIT. Press, Cambridge, Massachusetts.

De Renzi, E., Gentilini, M., Faglioni, P. and Barbieri, C. (1989). Attentional shift towards the rightmost stimuli in patients with left visual neglect. *Cortex*, **25**, 231–7.

Driver, J., Baylis, G. C., Goodrich, S. J. and Rafal, R. D. (1994). Axis-based neglect of visual shapes. *Neuropsychologia*, **32**, 1353–65.

Gettner, S. N. and Olson, C. R. (1997). Object-centered direction selectivity in macaque supplementary eye field is expressed with respect to multiple axes. *Society for Neuroscience* (Abstracts), **23**, 17.

Gibson, B. S. and Egeth, H. (1994). Inhibition of return to object-based and environment-based locations. *Perception and Psychophysics*, **55**, 323–39.

Hasselmo, M. E., Rolls, E. T., Baylis, G. C. and Nalwa, V. (1989) Object-centered encoding by face-selective neurons in the cortex of the superior temporal sulcus of the monkey. *Experimental Brain Research*, **75**, 417–29.

Huerta, M. F. and Kaas, J. H. (1990). Supplementary eye field as defined by cortical microstimulation: connections in macaques. *Journal of Comparative Neurology*, **293**, 299–330.

Humphreys, G. W. and Riddoch, M. J. (1994). Attention to within-object and between-object spatial representations: multiple sites for visual selection. *Cognitive Neuropsychology*, **11**, 207–41.

Humphreys, G. W. and Riddoch, M. J. (1995). Separate coding of space within and between objects: evidence from unilateral visual neglect. *Cognitive Neuropsychology*, **12**, 283–311

Làdavas, E., Petronio, A. and Umiltà, C. (1990). The deployment of visual attention in the intact field of hemineglect patients. *Cortex*, **26**, 307–17.

Làdavas, E., Farnè, A., Carletti, M. and Zeloni, G. (1994). Neglect determined by the relative location of responses. *Brain*, **117**, 705–14.

Logothetis, N. K. and Pauls, J. (1995). Psychophysical and physiological evidence for viewer-centered object representations in the primate. *Cerebral Cortex*, **3**, 270–88.

Logothetis, N. K., Pauls, J., Bülthoff, H. H. and Poggio, T. (1994). View-dependent object recognition by monkeys. *Current Biology*, **4**, 401–14.

Lueschow, A., Miller, E. K. and Desimone, R. (1994). Inferior temporal mechanisms for invariant object recognition. *Cerebral Cortex*, **5**, 523–31.

Maljkovic, V. and Nakayama, K. (1996). Priming of pop-out: II. role of position. *Perception and Psychophysics*, **58**, 977–91.

Marr, D. and Nishihara, H. K. (1978). Representation and recognition of the spatial organization of three-dimensional shapes. *Proceedings of the Royal Society, London*, B, **200**, 269–94.

Marshall, J. C. and Halligan, P. W. (1993). Visuo-spatial neglect: a new copying test to assess perceptual parsing. *Journal of Neurology*, **240**, 37–40.

Miyashita, K., Rand, M. K., Miyachi, S. and Hikosaka, O. (1996). Anticipatory saccades in sequential procedural learning in monkeys. *Journal of Neurophysiology*, **76**, 1361–6.

Olson, C. R. and Gettner, S. N. (1995). Object-centered direction selectivity in the macaque supplementary eye field. *Science*, **269**, 985–8.

Olson, C. R. and Gettner, S. N. (1996a). Brain representation of object-centred space. *Current Opinion in Neurobiology*, **6**, 165–70.

Olson, C. R. and Gettner, S. N. (1996b). Representation of object-centered space in the primate frontal lobe. *Cognitive Brain Research*, **5**, 147–56.

Olson, C. R. and Tremblay, L. (1997). What vs. where in macaque supplementary eye field. *Society for Neuroscience* (Abstracts), **23**, 17.

Perrett, D. I., Oram, M. W., Harries, M. H., Bevan, R., Hietanen, J. K., Benson, P. J. et al. (1991). Viewer-centred and object-centred coding of heads in the macaque temporal cortex. *Experimental Brain Research*, **86**, 159–73.

Pouget A. and Sejnowski, T. J. (1996). A model of spatial representations in parietal cortex explains hemineglect. In *Advances in Neural Information Processing Systems 8*, (ed. D. S. Touretzky, M. C. Mozer and M. E. Hasselmo), pp. 10–16). MIT Press, Cambridge, Massachusetts.

Posner, M. I., Walker, J. A., Friedrich, F. A. and Rafal, R. D. (1987). How do the parietal lobes direct covert attention? *Neuropsychologia*, **25**, 135–45.

Rizzolatti, G., Riggio, L. and Sheliga, B. M. (1994). Space and selective attention. In *Attention and Performance XV*, (ed., C. Umiltà and M. Moscovitch), pp. 231–265. MIT Press, Cambridge, Massachusetts.

Ross, R. G., Radant, A. D., Young, D. A. and Hommer, D. W. (1994). Saccadic eye movements in normal children from 8 to 15 years of age: a developmental study of visuospatial attention. *Journal of Autism and Developmental Disorders*, **24**, 413–31.

Schall, J. D. (1991). Neuronal activity related to visually guided saccadic eye movements in the supplementary motor area of rhesus monkeys. *Journal of Neurophysiology*, **66**, 530–58.

Schlag, J. and Schlag-Rey, M. (1985). Unit activity related to spontaneous saccades in the frontal dorsomedial cortex of the monkey. *Brain Research*, **58**, 208-11.

Schlag, J. and Schlag-Rey, M. (1987). Evidence for a supplementary eye field. *Journal of Neurophysiology*, **57**, 179–200.

Tipper, S. P. and Behrmann, M. (1996). Object-centered not scene-based visual neglect. *Journal of Experimental Psychology: Human Perception and Performance*, **22**, 1261–78.

Tovee, M. J., Rolls, E. T. and Azzopardi, P. (1994). Translation invariance in the responses to faces of single neurons in the temporal visual cortical areas of the alert monkey. *Journal of Neurophysiology*, 1049–60.

Vitu, F., O'Regan, J. K. and Mittau, M. (1990). Optimal landing position in reading isolated words and printed text. *Perception and Psychophysics*, **47**, 583–600.

Young, A. W., Hellawell, D. J. and Welch, J. (1992). Neglect and visual recognition. *Brain*, **115**, 51–71.

20

Hippocampal and parietal contribution to topokinetic and topographic memory

Alain Berthoz

20.1 Introduction

The purpose of this paper is to address the question of a particular aspect of spatial memory: the memory of self-produced movement in a spatial environment. The mathematician H. Poincaré wrote: 'To localise a point in space is to imagine the movement necessary to reach it' (Poincaré 1970, p. 67). By this statement he proposed a dynamic theory of spatial memory very different from the current theories, which suppose that, because there are 'place cells' in the hippocampus, or because spatial coordinates seem to be represented in the parietal cortex, the brain codes space on static 'topographical maps' (O'Keefe & Nadel 1978; Anderson 1995). Indeed, most studies concerning spatial memory have considered visual representational memory in static object recognition and recall processes (Smith & Milner 1981; Mishkin *et al*. 1983). In addition, most studies of the neural basis of spatial memory have been based on types of mental exploration of the environment that adopt a 'survey' type of strategy, although dissociations between route and topographical memory have been found (Incisa della Rocchetta *et al*. 1996). In the field of visual exploration, alternative hypotheses have been proposed (Droulez & Berthoz 1990, 1991; Colby *et al*. 1995), which promote the idea that the brain is using some dynamic processes to reprsent space and to control either executed or imagined movements. In addition, it is proposed that during whole-body motion and the so-called 'path integration' process, movement itself (rather than, or in addition to, distance) is stored in a way that is not yet known: it has recently been shown, by using a mobile robot on which subjects could be transported passively and subsequently asked to reproduce their linear displacement, that displacement memory seems to involve dynamic storge of movement patterns based on multisensory cues (Berthoz *et al*. 1995), an idea that is in accordance with the general view that internally simulated action is a fundamental element of perception and spatial memory (Berthoz 1997).

This paper reviews some recent experimental results concerning the problem of which cortical areas are involved in the storage and retrieval of movement in memory, with a particular reference to the parietal cortex and hippocampus.

The author is interested in self-generated movements, such as those produced during eye movements or a locomotor trajectory, which involve not only the memory of visual objects or space but also vestibular memory and the memory of idiothetic cues and motor actions.

First, some previous findings concerning memorized eye movements are recalled; these findings demonstrated that the parietal cortex is involved in memorized sequences of saccades, together with the frontal lobe, although it is not involved in spontaneous self-paced saccades in darkness or in imagined saccades.

Second, experiments are reviewed concerning the contribution of the vestibular system to spatial memory during whole-body rotation in 'vestibular contingent memory saccades', tasks that reflect the memory of a passively imposed whole-body motion (Bloomberg et al. 1988; Israël & Berthoz 1989). The present paper concentrates on passively induced whole-body rotation.

Third, the problem of topographical memory is considered. Some recent results concerning the memory of previously learned spatial locomotor routes are also reviewed.

20.2 Contribution of the parietal cortex to the memory of sequences of saccadic eye movements to visual targets

Eye saccades are an interesting model for studying the involvement of the parietal cortex in memory. The contribution of the parietal cortex to visually evoked saccades has been extensively reviewed (Thier & Karnath 1997; see also Anderson, Chapter 5). In a series of experiments with the use of positron emission tomography (PET), regional cerebral blood flow (rCBF) was measured in human subjects during self-generated saccades in total darkness. Three distinct paradigms were used.

Subjects were first asked to perform self-paced horizontal saccades in total darkness (Petit et al. 1993). Three main cortical areas were found to be activated: the frontal eye field (FEF), which is located in the precentral gyrus; the supplementary eye field (SEF); and the median cingulate gyrus. No activation of the parietal cortex was seen in this case. The same three areas were activated when the subjects were asked to perform imaginary self-paced saccades in total darkness (Lang et al. 1994).

The subjects were then asked to perform, from memory and in total darkness, a sequence of five prelearned visually guided saccades (Israël et al. 1993a; Petit et al. 1996a). In the baseline condition subjects were asked to relax, eyes open in darkness (REST). In the first active condition subjects were asked to execute self-paced voluntary horizontal saccades as in the previous sets of experiments (SAC). In the third condition the subjects were shown a set of five successive positions of light-emitting diodes (LEDs) on a horizontal bar a few minutes before the scan and were asked to make saccades to these five visual targets (SEQ). The targets were placed at 0, 5, 10 and 15° on each side of the primary position but were chosen randomly for each session. The subject was shown these targets five times to allow learning of the sequence. As the subject had to return to the centre, the total number of saccades in a sequence was in fact six. Horizontal electro-oculography was measured to assess that subjects were performing the task. Standard SPM and hierarchical multiscale detection (HMSD) analyses were performed on the blood-flow measurements.

Subtraction between the SEQ and SAC conditions revealed that the parietal cortex was activated during the recall of the sequence of memorized saccades. The repetition in total darkness of the prelearned sequence of horizontal saccades led to a bilateral increase in activation at the depth of the intraparietal sulcus, extending towards both the lateral and the medial superior parietal cortex, i.e. the superior parietal gyrus and precuneus, respectively (Fig. 20.1). Activation of the intraparietal sulcus has been previously shown in monkeys; the role of this structure in the planning of visually guided saccades has been suggested (Barash *et al.* 1991; Anderson, Chapter 5) but this was the first evidence in humans for an involvement of this structure in internally generated saccades from memory (see also the review by Pierrot-Deseilligny *et al.* (1995)).

Activation of the superior parietal sulcus during this memory task has to be related to numerous recently found activations of this structure. This point will not be discussed here, as it has been extensively reviewed (Petit *et al.* 1996*b*). Activation of the precuneus could be related to the generally accepted role of this area in the recall of visual scenes (Fletcher *et al.* 1995).

These results suggest that the parietal cortex is indeed involved in the recall of visually guided saccades and in the organization of saccade sequences from memory. It should be noted that this function is probably performed in conjunction with the superior frontal sulcus, which was found to be activated in the SEQ task and not in the other tasks. A bilateral activation was found at the depth of the superior frontal sulcus; the activated area overlaps areas 6 and 8 and this overlap makes the designation of prefrontal of premotor difficult. However, this area was clearly distinct from the FEF. Several recent PET studies have found superior frontal activation during memorized spatial tasks requiring spatial memory. This area does therefore seem to belong to the dorsal stream involved in spatial processing and may be particularly important in the memory component of the task described here (Haxby *et al.* 1994; Courtney *et al.* 1996).

20.3 Contribution of the parietal cortex to vestibular memory

The problem of path integration: is distance coded and memorized separately from direction?

Animals, including humans, have been shown to have a remarkable sense of direction and a propensity for navigation and 'path integration' which allow them to return to the initial location of their travels. The basic mechanisms

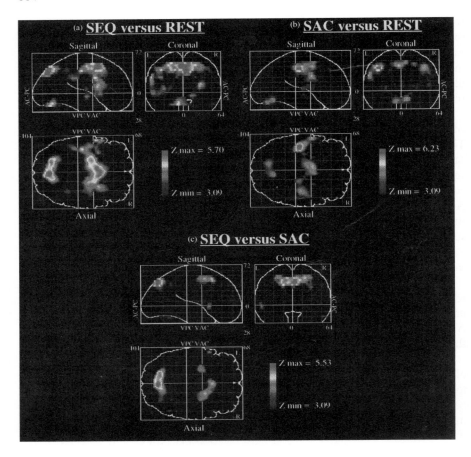

Fig. 20.1 Brain areas activated during the reproduction of a previously learned sequence of saccades. PET scan recordings of the brain areas activated during the execution of saccades in total darkness (see text). Three conditions are compared: the execution of self-paced saccades without any memory task (SAC), the execution of previously learned sequences of saccades to remembered visual targets (SEQ), and rest (REST). Statistical parametric maps are shown for three comparisons: (a) SEQ versus REST; (b) SAC versus REST; (c) SEQ versus SAC. Voxels significant at the given threshold of $p < 0.001$ (Z score > 3.09), uncorrected for multiple comparisons, are displaced on single sagittal, coronal, and axial projections of the brain. The spatial location of each activated area can be established by comparing its position in the three views. AC–PC, anterior commissure–posterior commissure; R, right. (From Petit *et al.* 1996*a*.)

underlying navigation and homing have long been questioned, for example with homing pigeons as a fruitful model and paradigm. It is, however, probable that navigation and path integration are subserved by a large variety of mechanisms according to the specific species and the particular type of travel (navigation across the planet by a bird is a totally different problem from homing behaviour or memory of a locomotor path). All these capacities, however, draw upon brain mechanisms for spatial cognition and spatial memory.

The contribution of the vestibular system to the orientation and localization of the body in space after a displacement, in animals and humans, has also long been suggested (Beritoff 1965; Potegal 1982). Beritoff was the first to report that animals (cats and dogs) can return blindfolded to their starting position after they have been passively transported. Because accurate performance in this task was only achieved in animals with an intact vestibular system, he concluded that the vestibular organs are required for navigation in the dark. He also observed that deaf–mute children with lesioned labyrinths could not, when blindfolded, retrace the route along which they had been taken, whereas normal children were perfectly able to do so. This result was confirmed in rats by Miller *et al.* (1983), who observed a degradation of the performance after vestibular lesion. These results have been reviewed by Wiener & Berthoz (1993).

Quantitative experiments concerning the capacity to compute actual displacement during passive whole-body motion on the basis of vestibular signals in humans were later reported (Mergner *et al.* 1983; Young 1984; Metcalfe & Gresty 1992; Schweigart *et al.* 1993). In addition, psychophysical measurements of the relative contribution of proprioceptive and vestibular input for the detection of head and/or trunk rotation have recently been described. Finally, several studies in humans have shown that the brain can estimate and memorize the travelled path solely from vestibular information, not only from angular but also from linear motion (Berthoz *et al.* 1987, 1995; Israël & Berthoz 1989; Israël *et al.* 1993*b*).

During locomotion, it has been demonstrated that human subjects can reach a previously seen visual target on the floor several metres away with eyes closed (Thomson 1983). These results, confirmed by several groups, indicate that information about step length, derived from proprioceptive or outflow motor command signals as well as from vestibular signals, could contribute to the updating of the mental representation of the subject's location in space and allow for path integration (Mittelstaedt & Glasauer 1991; Glasauer *et al.* 1994). Patients with a vestibular deficit could perform without error the simple task of walking in a straight path to a previously seen target a few metres away (Glasauer *et al.* 1994) but accumulated errors when asked to perform a triangular or rectangular path composed of successive turns, and also if they were asked to locomote through a previously seen circular trajectory (Takei *et al.* 1997). It seemed that the main deficit in these two tasks was a directional error, as the total distance seemed to be unimpaired. This points to a definite contribution of the vestibular system to the detection of *direction*, whereas *distance* could be coded by the motor and proprioceptive system.

The hypothesis discussed in this paper is that vestibular patients have a specific deficit of the head-direction cell system. This deficit leads to a deficit in the ability to store direction; in the absence of vision or in the presence of conflicting visual cues, it also leads to a deficit in the evaluation of direction.

The term 'integration' could therefore correspond to several different processes:

(1) spatial integration over the whole travelled trajectory, i.e. the computation of the travelled distance by cumulating successive positions along the path, a method that can be achieved, for example, by counting or measuring the steps during locomotion;
(2) time integration of the velocity of acceleration signals generated during self-motion, for instance the inertial vestibular signals;
(3) multisensory integration of all the messages delivered during self-motion, including its duration.

These three interpretations are not mutually exclusive.

To understand the respective contributions of these different sensory systems to path integration, the vestibular projections to the cerebral cortex and hippocampus are first decided below. The deficits in a vestibular memory task of patients with focal cortical lesions are then examined.

Vestibular projections to the parietal cortex and hippocampus

Recent work by Grüsser and others in the monkey (Grüsser *et al*. 1990*a,b*, 1991; Gulyás & Roland 1994) and from PET studies (Vallar *et al*. 1990; Bottini *et al*. 1994) in humans have confirmed the existence of an area in the parietoinsular cortex that is involved in the processing of multisensory, and particularly vesibular, cues about head motion in space. This parietoinsular vestibular cortex (PIVC) is probably the essential station in the transmission of ascending vestibular information from the vestibular nuclei, through the sensory thalamus, to the cortical areas involved in the elaboration of spatial cues, which are now identified as areas 6, 3a, 2v, T3 and 7a in the monkey. The same areas project to the vestibular nuclei in the monkey Ventre & Faugier-Grimaud 1988; Faugier-Grimaud & Ventre 1989; Akbarian *et al*. 1993; Guldin *et al*. 1993).

Vestibular signals may also reach the cerebral cortex and the hippocampus through a second route. A head direction cell system has been discovered by Ranck (1984) and Taube *et al*. (1990). Further studies (Sharp *et al*. 1995; Taube 1995) have revealed that a second route (other than the PIVC route) from the vestibular nuclei through the anterior thalamus, the mamillary bodies and the subiculum could reach the hippocampus after receiving visual environmental information from the parietal cortex, and contribute to the reconstruction at this level of spatial localization and movement detection.

To gain insight into the contribution of the vestibular system to cortical functions a further study has been made of the vestibular activated areas by using both caloric and galvanic stimulation. Brain activity has been recorded by functional magnetic resonance imaging (fMRI) of the whole brain.

Caloric stimulation was applied to seven subjects by injection of cold water to the left ear and compared with a rest condition (Lobel *et al*. 1996).

The activated areas were the left temporoparietal junction (probably the PIVC), the postcentral gyrus, the premotor cortex, the insular cortex, the posterior middle temporal gyrus, the inferior parietal lobule, the frontal cortex, the anterior cingulate gyrus and the hippocampal gyrus. On the right side these areas were also activated, but more rarely. This list does contain several of the areas already found in other PET studies; however, the activation of the hippocampus had not been reported previously.

To verify the activation of the hippocampus by vestibular stimulation, as had been predicted by previous results obtained in the monkey (O'Mara *et al*. 1997) and in the rat (Gavrilov *et al*. 1995; Wiener *et al*. 1995), this region was investigated specifically in a dedicated campaign (Vitte *et al*. 1996). Cold water was injected into the right ear during a visual fixation task and the results were compared with visual fixation alone. Ipsilateral activation of the hippocampal formation (including the subiculum) was found in eight subjects and in three of those subjects three times or each subject. This activation may result from an indirect activation of the hippocampus, either through the PIVC or through the head-direction cell system, which is thought to carry vestibular information about horizontal head rotation to the hippocampus via the thalamus and pre- or post-subiculum.

More recently, this experiment has been repeated with bipolar, binaural galvanic stimulation of the labyrinth in six subjects (Lobel *et al*. 1996). This stimulation consisted of a sinusoidal current of frequency 1 Hz and maximum intensity 2–3.5 mA applied for 30 s. The stimulation induced an illusion of pendular rotation of the body in the frontal plane (the subject lying in the MRI apparatus) and torsional eye movements, which were not measured. This is the first successful attempt to use galvanic stimulation in fMRI studies. Two sets of experiments were performed. Rest and stimulation were first compared. During stimulation no control task was given to the subjects. Galvanic stimulation was then superimposed on this simple motor task. In the first set bilateral activation of the insula, inferior frontal gyrus and inferior precentral gyrus and left activation of the medial frontal gyrus was observed in more than four subjects. In three subjects or fewer, activations of the inferior parietal lobule, superior temporal gyrus, and postcentral gyrus were found. These results confirm the previous identification of vestibular cortical areas but, in addition, indicate new areas in the frontal and hippocampal regions.

A recent direct electrophysiological study has confirmed the existence of additional areas involved in vestibular processing at short latency (Baudonniére *et al*. 1997). Activation by electrical stimulation of the vestibular nerve pre-operatively in patients undergoing vestibular surgery evoked field potentials in five main areas: the ipsilateral temporoparietal region or so-called parieto-insular vestibular cortex, the controlateral posteroparietal cortex and inferior parietal lobule, the controlateral supplementary motor area and possibly its specialized subarea for eye movements (the supplementary eye field in the dorsomedial frontal cortex), an ipsilateral prefrontal area, and finally ventro-medial prefrontal areas known to have connections with the limbic system.

These data give some indication as to the areas of the cortex in which one may find deficits in tasks involving the contribution of the vestibular system to perception, memory, or the control of movement. This knowledge has been used to study the deficits of vestibular memory about self-motion in patients with focal cortical lesions. These results are briefly reviewed in the next section.

The vestibular memory contingent saccade task

To study the role of several cortical areas in vestibular memory, a new psychophysical test of passive body-rotation estimation, the 'vestibular memory contingent saccade' (VMCS) paradigm, has been used (Bloomberg et al. 1988). The seated subject is first presented with an earth-fixed visual target and is then rotated by turning the chair about its swivel base (oriented along the earth-vertical axis). During the rotation, the subject has to fixate another target, which remains at a fixed position with respect to the head (head-fixed target), to suppress the vestibulo-ocular reflex (VOR). After a delay of about 2 s, the subject is required to make a saccade toward the 'memorized' earth-fixed target, in complete darkness. The results showed that humans can correctly match the amplitude of a preceding head rotation with a voluntary ocular saccade of equal but opposite amplitude (Fig. 20.2). The amplitude of a passive body rotation in darkness can therefore be correctly estimated by the brain; this information can also be adequately stored, and further retrieved and used by the oculomotor system. This is also true for rotations in different planes of three-dimensional space (Israël et al. 1993c).

In experiment (Israël et al. 1991) the duration of vestibular information storage was studied in greater detail by using delays of less than 20 s, as well as 1 and 5 min. The results showed that the amplitude of a passive rotation detected by the vestibular system can be accurately memorized for as long as 5 min (Fig. 20.3). At such long delays, however, smaller rotation angles (less than 20°) are overestimated (i.e. lead to an undershoot).

From these results the involvement of the hippocampus and cortical structures (frontal and parietal lobes) in the representation of self-rotation detected by the vestibular system (Berthoz 1989) was inferred. Further research aimed to discover which areas of the cortex were particularly important in the VMCS. Those areas of the cortex that are activated during saccade generation, or that have been suggested to be involved either in visuospatial delay tasks and working memory or in the processing of vestibular signals, were chosen.

Deficits in the vestibular memory tasks in patients with cortical and hippocampal lesions

The working hypothesis was that lesions in two areas of the brain would account for the main deficits in the VMCS task. These areas were:

(1) the prefrontal cortex because of its known involvement in 'visual representational memory' (Goldman-Rakic 1987; Quintana & Fuster 1993) and

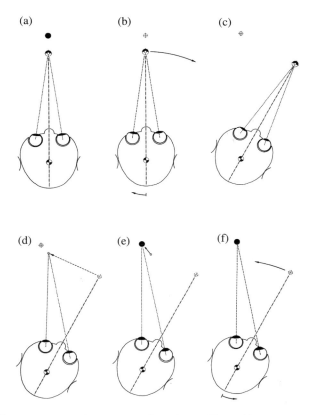

Fig. 20.2 The memory contingent saccade task. (a) The subject, seated on a turntable, views two targets: a head-fixed and an earth-fixed target. (b) The subject is passively rotated in darkness, only viewing the head-fixed target, and is asked to remember the location of the earth-fixed target. The only information available to the subject about the rotation is derived from the horizontal semicircular canal. (c) The subject is still and views the head-fixed target for a few seconds to let the vestibular effects decrease. (d) The head-fixed target is turned off and the subject has to remember the location of the previously seen earth-fixed target in total darkness. (e) The subject makes a saccade to the remembered target in total darkness. Then the light is turned on and the subject makes a corrective saccade if the saccade in darkness was not of the appropriate amplitude. (f) The turntable is returned to the initial position for control.

which it is proposed should be also involved in what is here called 'vestibular representational motion memory'; and

(2) the parietoinsular cortex.

The vestibular memory contingent saccade task was applied to 24 neurological patients with various cortical lesions and to 18 age-matched control subjects (Israël *et al*. 1992, 1995; Pierrot-Deseilligny *et al*. 1993) (Fig. 20.4).

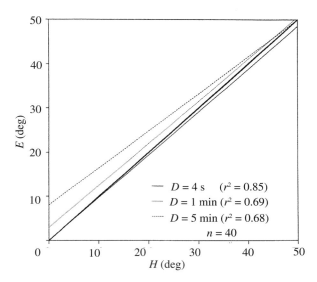

Fig. 20.3 The memory contingent saccade can be executed with a delay. Three regression lines between the amplitude of the vestibular memory contingent eye saccade (*E*) and head rotation (*H*) when the subject was asked to wait with a delay of 4 s, 1 min and 5 min, respectively. In this form the task becomes a form of delay task well suited to test spatial memory of a passive whole-body rotation. (From Israël *et al*. 1991.)

Anticipation and latency, direction errors and accuracy of the first saccade, stability of eye position in darkness, and final eye position were quantified. Patients were divided into small groups with lesions affecting the following cortical areas: left or right frontal eye field (FEF), left or right prefrontal cortex (area 46 of Brodmann) (PFC), left supplementary eye field (SEF), left or right posterior parietal cortex (PPC) and right parieto-temporal cortex (PTC) (i.e. the vestibular cortex). There were some abnormalities in the results of the right FEF group, concerning anticipation, direction errors and latency of the first saccade, but no differences from controls in the accuracy of the first saccade or of the final eye position. Results in the left FEF group were normal. Accuracy of the first saccade was bilaterally impaired in the SEF group. Final eye position was also inaccurate in the SEF group. In both PFC groups, significant and generally bilateral abnormalities existed for all parameters tested.

Parietal lesions

The only deficit that was found in patients with PPC lesions was a slightly increased percentage of anticipated responses in the right PPC group. In the monkey the PPC is involved in spatial attention and integration (Barash *et al*. 1991; Duhamel *et al*. 1992; Anderson 1995; Colby *et al*. 1995). PPC cells receive direct projections from different cortical visual areas and have eye and head position gain fields; some of them also receive vestibular information (Kawano *et al*. 1980, 1984).

(a)

(b)

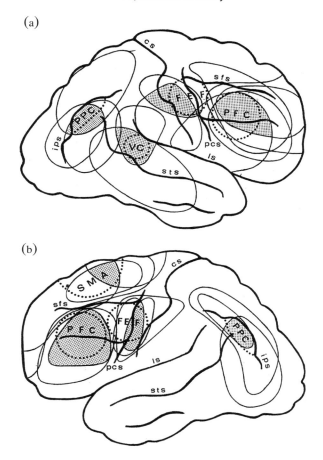

Fig. 20.4 Location of the lesions of patients who were tested with the vestibular memory contingent saccade task. PPC, posterior parietal cortex; FEF, frontal eye field; SEF, supplementary eye field; PFC, prefrontal cortex; VC, vestibular cortex. Deficits in the task were mainly found in patients with lesions of the PFC, VC, or SEF. CS, PS, SFS, PCS, LS, STS indicate, respectively, the central, intraparietal, sylvian, precentral, lateral, and superior temporal sulci. (From Israël *et al.* 1995.)

The parietal cortex is clearly involved in the control of visual memory-guided saccades. In a previous study in patients with parietal lesions, performance of a similar vestibular-driven paradigm was markedly impaired (Tropper *et al.* 1990). The exact limits of the lesions, which were much larger than those of the patients in the present study, were not indicated, thus reducing the validity of any comparison between the two studies.

Finally, the absence of marked deficits in the results of the present study after PPC lesions suggests that the PPC is not crucial for this paradigm. Vestibular integration probably takes place elsewhere.

Parietotemporal cortex lesions

The right PTC group was found to be deficient in the spatial aspects of saccade performance, showing a decrease in first saccade accuracy, an increase in direction errors, and a decrease in the duration during which eye position in darkness was accurate to within 50 per cent. The fact that the right PTC group was markedly impaired reflects the vestibular input of the task. Although this result was expected, or our knowledge this is the first behavioural demonstration, together with the observation of deficits in the perception of the subjective vertical (Brandt *et al.* 1994), that the PTC is the probable equivalent in humans to the parietoinsular vestibular cortex in the monkey. Despite the difficulty of extrapolating from monkey to human cortex, because PPC lesions did not result in impairment in the present study, it is suggested that vestibular processing is carried out in the PTC or in a nearby area, and the integrated information sent directly to the frontal lobe. This answers the third question about the relative contribution of the PPC and PTC in this vestibular-guided task: the PPC is not crucial in the control of such a task.

These results suggest that:

(1) the PFC is involved in the memorization of saccade goals, probably encoded in spatiotopic coordinates since PFC patients were impaired in both vestibular- and visual-memory guided tasks;

(2) the SEF, but not the FEF, is involved in the control of accuracy of these vestibular-derived goal-directed saccades, whereas the reversed pattern of results was found for the visual-derived saccades; and

(3) the PTC (i.e. the vestibular cortex), but not the PPC, is involved in the control of vestibular memory-guided saccades, the reverse pattern again being found for visually derived saccades.

This represents two different cortical networks, with only the PFC in common. The network found here the VMCS paradigm may be specific to the vestibular input, or else could be a pathway used for all non-retinotopic (craniotopic and spatiotopic) saccades, as the SEF has been found to be involved in sequences of visual memory-guided saccades, i.e. visual-derived saccades encoded in craniotopic coordinates (Gaymard *et al.* 1990, 1993).

In conclusion, a new network is here suggested for the cortical control of vestibular memory-guided saccades, which, although still speculative, is different from that of visual memory-guided saccades (Israël *et al.* 1995): the cortical pathway involved in the control of vestibular-guided saccades includes the PTC, which could be involved in the integration of vestibular and other sensory information to reconstruct head movement in space. Patients with PPC lesions showed impairment in the visual memory-guided saccade task, but not in the vestibular-guided saccade task (Pierrot-Deseilligny *et al.* 1993). The PTC would then play in the vestibular task a role similar to that played by the PPC in the visual task. After integration, vestibular information could be sent to and stored in the PFC, where 'spatial' memory could be organized. The vestibular saccade could then be triggered by the SEF, via the superior colliculus (SC) rather than by the FEF in visual memory-guided saccades, as it has recently been shown that additional channels beside those coursing through the FEF and SC are utilized to access the saccade generator of the brainstem: patients with FEF lesions exhibited impairment in the visual memory-guided saccade task, but not in the vestibular-guided saccade task, whereas the contrary was observed for patients with SEF lesions, who were impaired in the vestibular but not in the visual task. Therefore, the networks corresponding to these two tasks could both pass through the PFC, which would store the processed (integrated) information and select the next step.

The role of the hippocampus in vestibular memory

Given that vestibular stimulation can activate the hippocampal regions in humans, it would be interesting to see whether the VMCS task is impaired in hippocampal patients. This was not tested. A recent report indicates, however, that patients with hippocampal lesions show deficits in sequences of visually guided memory saccades (Müri et al. 1994) and Wiest et al. (1996) have found a clear deficit in a whole-body return task. They exposed ten patients with temporal-lobe epilepsy and unilateral hippocampal atrophy and ten age-matched controls to random rotational displacemnets away from the centre position in darkness. They required them to perform the whole-body return task (Metcalfe & Gresty 1992). They found a hypometry in the return angle towards the side ipsilateral to the lesion. The question remains, however, open to furture investigation.

20.4 Mental navigation along memorized routes

The neurobiological mechanisms of spatial navigation have been studied extensively in rodents. However, very little is known concerning the cerebral structures involved in the memory of routes in primates and humans.

In primates, only two research groups have reported data concerning the activity in the hippocampus and related structures during navigation or spatial tasks. T. Ono and his collaborators (Tamura et al. 1992a,b), in the hippocampus of the monkey, have found neurones that were activated when the animal was moving actively or passively to a given location in the room. These cells therefore had properties similar to those of place cells. In addition, some of these neurones were activated when a task (visual object recognition, motor task) was performed at a given location in the room: an association was made between task and place. This group has also suggested that hippocampal neurones are influenced by the meaning of the object–place association for the monkey (either reward or punishment). E. T. Rolls has recently proposed that in the hippocampus and parahippocampus of the monkey there is a diversity of cells; some were called view cells and were activated when the animal was paying attention to an object at a particular location in space (Miyashita *et al*. 1989; Rolls 1991). Given that he did not find any place cells, he concluded that the primate hippocampus was coding objects in place in allocentric coordinates. Recently, he has discovered cells that are activated when the animal is looking at a particular place in a cue control room independently of the location of the animal in the room. These cells have been named 'space cells'. They seem to code an area of space 'out there' in allocentric coordinates independently of where the animal is. It is important to note that these cells seem to keep some of their properties in total darkness and therefore have an activity related to memorized object-in-place location. However, nothing is known of the exact processing occurring in the hippocampus of the monkey that gives rise to this type of coding.

In humans, several strategies can be used to remember topographic routes, for example, if one tries to recall the route from home to office or laboratory. The brain can use a survey strategy and try to imagine a map of the environment and mentally visualize the route on this map. This neural basis for this survey type of strategy has been studied in humans (Mellet *et al*. 1995). On the other hand, subjects can try to remember the sequence of turns and walks in relation to visual landmarks and eventually to other cues or actions associated with the route. This type of memory can be subserved by several types of cognitive strategies (Amorim *et al*. 1997).

A clear dissociation has been found between these different strategies in patients with brain lesions. Several studies have demonstrated impairment in topographic memory, and a dissociation has been claimed between the ability to recognize familiar landmarks (Whiteley & Warrington 1978; Incisa della Rocchetta *et al*. 1996), sometimes leaving the capacity to describe well-known routes relatively intact, and the ability to describe routes with recognition landmarks relatively unaffected (Pallis 1955; Paterson 1994). Sometimes patients can also describe routes and recognize landmarks but they still lose their way because landmarks no longer convey directional information (Hécaen *et al*. 1980). The hippocampus is not necessarily the only area involved in these spatial memory deficits: Habib (1987), for instance, has shown that lesions in patients with topographic memory loss were restricted to the parahippocampus and the subiculum but did not extend to the hippocampus. By contrast, patient R. B., who had a severe anterograde amnesia following selective damage to the hippocampus, did not report getting lost in his neighbourhood (Zola-Morgan *et al*. 1986).

The patient studied by Incisa della Rocchetta *et al*. (1996) had a severe deficit in describing familiar routes in her environment but no difficulty in identifying countries from outline maps and in naming a city within a country when it was identified by a dot. Both episodic and semantic memory were impaired in this patient. The suggestion is that this patient has a specific deficit for category-specific knowledge of inanimate objects (hills, buildings, etc.). There seems to be a specific coding of topographic objects distinct from other classes of object; there could also be a separation between the objects that require locomotion to reach them, and other objects.

One should therefore be careful before ascribing to any particular area of the cortex a crucial role in spatial memory. It seems more likely that this function is distributed over several areas, each making a distinct contribution. For example, the frontal cortex seems to be involved in visual spatial memory (Courtney *et al.* 1996) and in mental recall of complex environments (Guariglia *et al.* 1993).

It therefore seemed interesting to explore the areas of the brain involving recall of an actual locomotor route, mostly in view of the difficulty encountered by other investigators in activating the hippocampus. The brain structures activated during a mental navigation task, in which the emphasis was put on memory of self-motion associated with visual landmark recall during route navigation, were therefore investigated.

The details of the experiments are given by Ghaem *et al.* (1997) and the main features of this task are therefore only summarized here. Subjects were driven to a totally unfamiliar urban environment and were asked to walk along a previously selected route in the city of about 800 m in length (Fig. 20.5). The subjects walked three times along the route and were asked to remember the route and in particular seven prominent visual landmarks (tower, petrol station, telephone box, etc.). The first two times the subject was guided by the experimenter and the third time the subject walked under supervision. Time of locomotion recorded. The day after this learning session and 4–6 h before PET acquisition, the subjects executed two tasks, which were repeated in the PET apparatus.

MSR task

In this mental simulation of routes the subject was instructed verbally to indicate the name of two landmarks, chosen by the experimenter, between which he or she was supposed to walk mentally. The subject pressed a button upon the mental arrival to the final landmark and the sequence was repeated with another set of two landmarks. This also allowed the mental locomotion time to be measured and compared with the previously recorded actual time in the real environment.

VIL task

In this visual recall task the subject was instructed to mentally visualize a landmark and keep it in memory upon hearing its name through the earphones.

Results

The results indicated that there was a strong correlation between the time taken to 'walk' mentally between two segments and the real time of locomotion

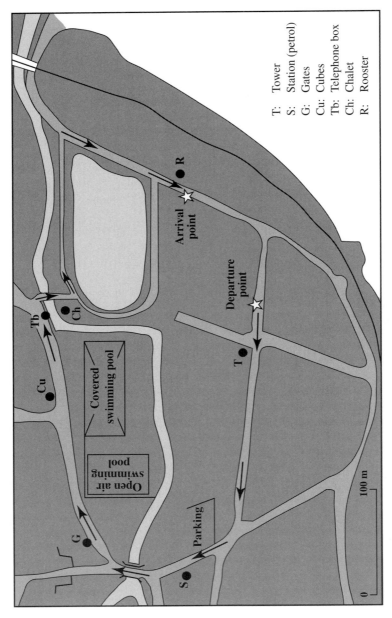

Fig. 20.5 The map of the trajectory of the subjects in the city of Orsay (see text for further details). Subjects were conducted to the departure point and walked with eyes open along the path, which was divided into seven segments. Each of the segments was marked by a prominent landmark, which the subjects were asked to remember. When laying in the PET scan they had to remember their walk. This procedure was aimed at giving them a 'route' type of memory of the path.

in the city during both the training session ($r = 0.99$, $p = 0.0003$) and the PET session ($r = 0.92$, $p = 0.024$), suggesting that subjects were doing the required task. The following main areas were activated during these tasks when compared with the rest condition.

MSR task: there was bilateral activation of the dorsolateral cortex, the posterior hippocampal areas, the posterior cingulate gyrus, the supplementary motor area, the right middle hippocampal areas, the left precuneus, the middle occipital gyrus, the fusiform gyrus and the lateral premotor area. VIL task: there was bilateral activation of the middle hippocampal regions, the left inferior temporal gyrus, the left posterior hippocampal regions, the precentral gyrus and the right posterior cingulate gyrus. When these two conditions were subtracted (MSR minus VIL) activation of only the left hippocampal regions, precuneus and insula was observed.

Discussion

The activation of the right hippocampal areas is important: this is the first time that the hippocampus has been shown to be activated in a navigation task (three reports were presented simultaneously: Aguirre et al. 1996; Maguire et al. 1996; and Ghaem et al. 1996. It is coherent with the literature on the effects of lesions, which show a dominance of the right hippocampus in spatial deficits. There is a definite difference in the location of these activations (middle, posterior, anterior) within the hippocampal formation. However, the resolution of the PET images is not sufficient for a definition of the precise part of the hippocampal formation activated during this task. It is hoped that current work in which the experiment has been repeated will allow more detailed description of the exact areas involved.

A surprising result was the activation of the left hippocampus and the fact that it was the only side activated after the MRS minus VIL subtraction. This is in contrast with the current view attributing to the left hippocampus a major role in the processing of verbal material. One explanation could be that in these experiments the instructions for the mental route task were given verbally. However, the instructions to recall a visual landmark in the VIL condition were also verbal and the two effects may have subtracted from each other. It is proposed that there is a potential involvement of the left hippocampus in the combination of visuospatial and body-position information, which is important for navigation. The activation of the insula may be related to the fact that subjects had to remember the turns of their body during the memorized locomotory task. Activation of the insula has been found during tasks requiring mental repositioning of the body with respect to external objects (Bonda et al. 1995). One may therefore, as do Ghaem et al. (1997), suggest that there may be two subsystems involved in the processing of spatial memory and that the left hippocampus could be particularly involved when memories including the relation between whole-body movements and the environment have to be recalled.

20.5 Conclusion

These three studies confirm the idea that there is a class of spatial memory, which I propose to call 'topokinetic' memory, which involves several brain structures (parietal and parietoinsular cortex, insula, cingulate cortex, hippocampal formation, dorsolateral frontal cortex, etc.) involved in the processing of self-generated eye or locomotor movements. It seems that the design of tasks requiring the recall of some previously generated movements is important if one wants to study spatial memory in relation to real physiological functions and not to artificial tasks based upon the wrong idea that the brain is essentially designed to process visual information and not first of all action involving self generated movement which will be detected by a combination of visual, vestibular and idiothetic cues together with efferent copies from motor commands. New paradigms have therefore still to be designed to study this problem adequately and understand the contribution of each of these areas to the memory of movement.

References

Aguirre, G. K., Detre, J. A., Alsop, D. C. & D'Esposito, M. 1996 The parahippocampus subserves topographical learning in man. *Cerebr. Cortex* **6**, 823–829.

Akbarian, S., Grüsser, O. J. & Guldin, W. O. 1993 Corticofugal projections to the vestibular nuclei in squirrel monkeys: further evidence of multiple cortical vestibular fields. *J. Comp. Neurol.* **332**, 89–104.

Amorim, M. A., Glasauer, S., Corpinot, K. & Berthoz, A. 1997 Updating an object's orientation and location during non visual navigation: a comparison between two processing modes. *Percept. Psychophys.*, **59**, 404–418.

Andersen, R. A. 1995 Encoding of intention and spatial location in the posterior parietal cortex. *Cerebr. Cortex* **5**, 457–469.

Barash, S., Bracewell, R., Fogassi, L., Gnadt, J. W. & Andersen, R. A. 1991 Saccade related activity in the lateral intraparietal area. I. Temporal properties: comparison with area 7a. *J. Neurophysiol.* **66**, 1095–1108.

Baudonnière, P. M., de Waele, C., Tran Ba Huy, P. & Vidal, P. P 1997. Réponses évoquées vestibulaires avant et après neurectomie vestibulaire unilaterale chez l'homme. In *Le Cortex Vestibulaire*. (Ed. Colland, *et al.*). Ipsen.

Beritoff, J. S. 1965 *Neural mechanisms of higher vertebrate behavior*. New York: Little, Brown & Co.

Berthoz, A. 1989 Cooṗration et substitution entre le système saccadique et les réflexes d'origine vestibulaires: faut-il réviser la notion de reflexe? *Rev. Neurol.* **145**, 513–526.

Berthoz, A. 1997 *Le sens do mouvement* (O. Jacob). Paris:

Berthoz, A., Israël, I., Georges-François, P., Grasso, R. & Tsuzuku, T. 1995 Spatial memory of body linear displacement: What is being stored? *Science* **269**, 95–98.

Berthoz, A., Israël, I., Vieville, T. & Zee, D. S. 1987 Linear head displacement measured by the otoliths can be reproduced though the saccadic system. *Neurosci. Lett.* **82**, 285–290.

Bloomberg, J., Melvill Jones, G., Segal, B., McFarlane, S. & Soul, J. 1988 Vestibular contingent voluntary saccades based on cognitive estimates of remebered vestibular information. *Adv. Oto-Rhino-Laryngol.* **40**, 71–75.

Bonda, E., Petrides, M., Frey, S. & Evans, A. 1995 Neural correlates of mental transformations of the body-in-space. *Proc. Natn. Acad. Sci. USA* **92**, 11180–11184.

Bottini, G., Sterzi, R., Paulelscu, E., Vallar, G., Cappa, S., Erminio, F., Passingham, R. E., Frith, C. D. & Frackowiack, R. S. J. 1994 Identification of the central vestibular projections in man: a positron emission tomography activation study. *Expl. Brain Res.* **99**, 164–169.

Brandt, T., Dieterich, M. & Danek, A. 1994 Vestibular cortex lesion affect the perception of verticality. *Annls Neurol.* **35**, 403–412.

Colby, C. L., Duhamel, J. R. & Goldberg, M. E. 1995 Oculocentric spatial representation in parietal cortex. *Cerebr. Cortex* **5**, 470–481.

Courtney, S. M., Ungerleider, L. G., Keil, K. & Haxby, J. V. 1996 Object and spatial visual working memory activate separate neural systems in the human cortex. *Cerebr. Cortex* **6**, 39–49.

Droulex, J. & Berthoz, A. 1991 The concept of dynamic memory in sensorimotor control. In *Motor control: concepts and issues* (ed. D. R. Humphrey & J. R. Freund), pp. 137–161. Chichester, UK: Wiley.

Droulez, J. & Berthoz, A. 1991 A neural network model of sensoritopic maps with predictive short term memory properties. *Proc. Natn. Acad. Sci. USA* **88**, 9653–9657.

Duhamel, J.-R., Colby, C. L. & Goldberg, M. E. 1992 The updating of the representation of visual space in parietal cortex by intended eye movements. *Science* **255**, 90–92.

Faugier-Grimaud, S. & Ventre, J. 1989 Anatomic connections of inferior parietal cortex (area 7) with subcortical structures related to vestibular-ocular function in a monkey (*Macaca fascicularis*). *J. Comp. Neurol.* **280**, 1–14.

Fletcher, P. C., Frith, C. D., Grasby, P. M., Shallice, T., Frackowiak, R. S. J. & Dolan, R. J. 1995 The mind's eye-precuneus activation in memory related imagery. *Neuro-Image* **2**, 195–200.

Gavrilov, V. V., Wiener, S. I. & Berthoz, A. 1995 Enhanced hippocampal theta EEG during whole body rotations in awake restrained rats. *Neurosci. Lett.* **197**, 239–241.

Gaymard, B., Pierrot-Deseilligny, C. & Rivaud, S. 1990 Impairment of sequences of memory-guided saccades after supplementary motor area lesions. *Annls Neurol.* **28**, 622–626.

Gaymard, B., Rivaud, S. & Pierrot-Deseilligny, C. 1993 Role of the left and right supplementary motor areas in memory-guided saccade sequences. *Annls Neurol.* **34**, 404–406.

Ghaem, O., Mellet, E., Crivello, F., Tzourio, N., Mazoyer, B., Berthoz, A. & Denis, M. 1996 Functional anatomy of mental stimulation of memorized routes. *NeuroImage* **3**, S249.

Ghaem, O., Mellet, E., Crivello, F., Tzourio, N., Mazoyer, B, Berthoz, A. & Denis, M. 1997 Mental navigation along memorized routes activates the hippocampus, precuneus, and insula. *Neuroreport* **8**(3), 739–744.

Glasauer, S., Amorim, M. A., Vitte, E. & Berthoz, A. 1994 Goal directed linear locomotion in normal and labyrinthine defective subjects. *Expl Brain Res.* **98**, 323–335.

Goldman-Rakic, P. 1987 Circuitry of primate prefrontal cortex and regulation of behavior by representational memory. In *Handbook of physiology: the nervous system*, vol. 5 (ed., V. B. Mountcastle, F. Plum & D. R. Humphrey), pp. 373–417. Bethesda, MD: American Physiological Society.

Grüsser, O. J., Guldin, W., Harris, L., Lefèbre, J. C. & Pause, M. 1991 Cortical representation of head-in-space movement and some psychophysical experiments on head movement. In *The head–neck sensorimotor system* (ed., A. Berthoz, W. Graf & P. P. Vidal), pp. 497–509. Oxford University Press.

Grüsser, O. J., Pause, M. & Schreiter, U. 1990*a* Localisation and responses of neurones in the parieto-insular vestibular cortex of awake monkeys (*Macaca fascicularis*). *J. Physiol.* **430**, 537–557.

Grüsser, O. J., Pause, M. & Schreiter, U. 1990*b* Vestibular neurons in the parieto-insular cortex of monkeys (*Macaca fascicularis*): visual and neck receptor responses. *J. Physiol.* **430**, 559–583.

Guariglia, C., Padovani, A., Pantano, P. & Pizzamiglio, L. 1993 Unilateral neglect restricted to visual imagery. *Nature* **364**, 235–237.

Guldin, W. O., Mirring, S. & Grüsser, O.-J. 1993 Connections from the neocortex to the vestibular brain stem nuclei in the common marmoset. *Neuroreport* **5**, 113–116.

Gulyás, B. & Roland, P. E. 1994 Binocular disparity discrimination in human cerebral cortex: Functional anatomy by positron emission tomography. *Proc. Natn. Acad. Sci. USA* **91**, 1239–1243.

Habib, M. 1987 Pure topographical disorientation: a definition and anatomical basis. *Cortex* **23**, 73–85.

Haxby, J. V., Hotwitz, B., Ungerleider, L. G., Maisog, J. M., Pietrini, P. & Grady, C. L. 1994 The functional organisation of the human extrastriate cortex: a PET-rCBF study of selective attention to faces and locations. *J. Neurosci.* **14**, 6336–6353.

Hécaen, H., Tzortzis, C. & Rondot, P. 1980 Loss of topographical memory with learning deficits. *Cortex* **16**, 525–542.

Incisa della Rocchetta, A., Cipolotti, L. & Warrington, K. 1996 Topographical disorientation: selective impairement of locomotor space? *Cortex* **32**, 727–735.

Israël, I., André-Deshays, C., Charade, O., Berthoz, A., Popov C. & Lipsitz, M. 1993*a* Gaze control in microgravity. II. Sequences of saccades towards memorized visual targets. *J. Vest. Res.* **3**, 345–360.

Israël, I., & Berthoz, A. 1989 Contribution of the otoliths to the calculation of linear deplacement. *J. Neurophysiol.* **62**, 247–263.

Israël, I., Chapuis, N., Glasauer, S., Charade, O. & Berthoz, A. 1993*b* Estimation of passive linear whole body displacement in humans. *J. Neurophysiol.* **70**, 1270–1273.

Israël, I., Fetter, M. & Koenig, E. 1993*c* Vestibular perception of passive whole body rotation about the horizontal and vertical axes in humans: goal directed vestibulo-ocular reflex and vestibular memory contingent saccades. *Expl Brain Res.* **96**, 335–346.

Israël, I., Rivaud, S., Berthoz, A. & Pierrot-Deseilligny, C. 1992 Cortical control of vestibular memory-guided saccades. *Annls NY Acad. Sci.* **656**, 472–484.

Israël, I., Rivaud, S., Gaymard, B., Berthoz, A. & Pierrot-Deseilligny, C. 1995 Cortical control of vestibular-guided saccades in man. *Brain* **118**, 1169–1183.

Israël, I., Rivaud, S., Pierrot-Deseilligny, P. & Berthoz, A. 1991 'Delayed VOR': an assessment of vestibular memory for self motion. In *Tutorials in motor neuroscience* (ed., J. Requin & J. Stelmach), pp. 599–607. Dordrecht: Kluwer.

Kawano, K., Sasaki, M. & Yamashita, M. 1980 Vestibular input to visual tracking neurons in the posterior parietal association cortex of the monkey. *Neurosci Lett.* **17**, 55–60.

Kawano, K., Sasaki, M. & Yamashita, M. 1984 Response properties of neurons in posterior parietal cortex of monkey during visual-vestibular stimulation. *J. Neurophysiol.* **51**, 340–351.

Lang, W., Petit, L., Hölliger, P, Pietrzyck, U., Tzourio, N., Mazoyer, B. & Berthoz, A. 1994 A positron emission tomography study of oculomotor imagery. *Neuroreport* **5**, 921–924.

Lobel, E., Le Bihan, D., Leroy-Willig, A. *et al.* 1996 Searching for the vestibular cortex with functional MRI. (Abstract). *NeuroImage* **3**, S351.

Maguire, H., Frackowiak, R. & Frith, C. 1996. *NeuroImage* **3**, S589.

Mellet, E., Tzourio, N., Denis, M. & Mazoyer, B. 1995 A positron emission tomography study of visual and mental exploration *J. Cogn. Neurosci.* **7**, 433–445.

Mergner, T., Nardi, G. L., Becker, W. & Deecke, L. 1983 The role of canal-neck interaction for the perception of horizontal trunk and head rotation. *Expl Brain Res.* **49**, 198–208.

Metcalfe, T. & Gresty, M. 1992 Self controlled reorienting movements in response to rotational displacements in normal subjects and patients with labyrinthine diseases. In *Sensing and controlling motion* (ed. B. Cohen, D. L. Tomko, & F. E. Guedry), pp. 695–698. New York Academy of Sciences.

Miller, S., Potegal, M. & Abraham, L. 1983 Vestibular involvement in a passive transport and return task. *Physiol. Psychol.* **11**, 1–10.

Mishkin, M., Ungerleider, L. G. & Macko, K. A. 1983 Object vision and spatial vision: two cortical pathways. *Trends Neurol. Sci.* **6**, 414–417.

Mittelstaedt, M. L. & Glasauer, S. 1991 Idiothetic navigation in gerbils and humans. *Zool. J. Physiol.* **95**, 427–435.

Miyashita, Y., Rolls, E. T., Cahusac, P. M. B., Niki, H. & Feigenbaum, J. D. 1989 Activity of hippocampal neurons in the monkey related to a conditional spatial response task. *J. Neurophysiol.* **61**, 669–678.

Müri, R. M., Rivaud, S., Timsit, S., Cornu, P. & Pierrot–Deseilligny, C. 1994 The role of the right medial temporal lobe in the control of memory-guided saccades. *Expl Brain Res.* **101**, 165–168.

O'Keefe, J. & Nadel, L. 1978 *The hippocampus as a cognitive map.* Oxford: Clarendon Press.

O'Mara, S. M., Rolls, E. T., Berthoz, A. & Kesner, R. P. 1997 Neurons responding to whole body motion in the primate hippocampus. *J. Neurosci.* **14**, 6511–6523.

Pallis, C. A. 1955 Impaired identification of faces and places with agnosia for colors. *J. Neurol. Neurosurg. Psychiatr.* **18**, 218–224.

Paterson, A. 1994 A case of topographical disorientation associated with a unilateral cerebral lesion. *Brain* **68**, 188–212.

Petit, L., Orssaud, C., Tzourio, N., Crivello, F., Berthoz, A. & Mazoyer, B. 1996*a* Functional anatomy of a prelearned sequence of horizontal saccades in man. *J. Neurosci.* **16**, 3714–3726.

Petit, L., Orssaud, C., Tzourio, N., Mazoyer, B. & Berthoz, A. 1996*b* Superior parietal lobule involvment in the representation of visual space: a review. In *Parietal lobe contributions to orientation in 3D space* (ed., P. Thier & O. Karnath), pp. 77–91. Berlin: Springer.

Petit, L., Orssaud, C., Tzourio, N., Salamon, G., Mazoyer, B. & Berthoz, A. 1993 PET study of voluntary saccadic eye movements in humans: basal ganglia-thalamocortical system and cingulate cortex involvement. *J. Neurophysiol.* **69**, 1009–1017.

Pierrot-Deseilligny, C., Israël, I., Berthoz, A., Rivaud, S. & Gaymard, B. 1993 Role of the different frontal lobe areas in the control of the horizontal component of memory-guided saccades in man. *Expl Brain Res.* **95**, 166–171.

Pierrot-Deseilligny, C., Rivaud, S., Gaymard, B., Müri, R. & Vermersch, A.-I. 1995 Cortical control of saccades. *Annls Neurol.* **37**, 557–567.

Poincaré, H. 1970 *La valeur de la science.* Paris: Flammarion.

Potegal, M. 1982 Vestibular and neostriatal contribution to spatial orientation. In *Spatial abilities. Devetopment and physiological foundations* (ed., Potegal), pp. 361–387. New York: Academic Press.

Quintana, J. & Fuster, J. M. 1993 Spatial and temporal factors in the role of prefrontal and parietal cortex in visuomotor integration. *Cerebr. Cortex* **3**, 122–132.

Quintana, J. & Fuster, J. M. 1993 Spatial and temporal factors in the role of prefrontal and parietal cortex in visuomotor integration. *Cerebr. Cortex* **3**, 122–132.

Ranck, J. B. 1984 Head-direction cells in the deep layers of the dorsal presubiculum in freely moving rats. *Soc. Neurosci. Abstr.* **10**, 599.

Rolls, E. T. 1991 Functions of the primate hippocampus in spatial and non-spatial memory. *Hippocampus* **1**, 258–261.

Schweigart, G., Heimbrand, S., Mergner, T. & Becker, W. 1993 Perception of horizontal head and trunk rotation: modification of neck input following loss of vestibular function. *Expl Brain Res.* **95**, 533–546.

Sharp, P. E., Blair, H. T., Etkin, D. & Tzanetos, D. B. 1995 Influences of vestibular and visual motion information on the spatial firing patterns of hippocampal place cells. *J. Neurosci.* **15**, 173–189.

Smith, M. L. & Milner, B. 1981 The role of the right hippocampus in the recall of spatial location. *Neuropsychologia* **19**, 781–793.

Takei, Y., Grasso, R., Amorim, M. A. & Berthoz, A. 1997 Circular trajectory formation during blind locomotion. A test for path integration and motor memory. *Exp. Brain Res.* **115**, 361–368.

Tamura, R., Ono, T., Fukuda, M. & Nakamura, K. 1992*a* Spatial responsiveness of monkey hippocampal neurons to various visual and auditory stimuli. *Hippocampus* **2**, 307–322.

Tamura, R., Ono, T., Fukuda, M. & Nishijo, H. 1992*b* Monkey hippocampal neuron response to complex sensory stimulation during object discrimination. *Hippocampus* **2**, 287–306.

Taube, J. S. 1995 Head direction cells recorded in the anterior thalamic nuclei of freely moving rats. *J. Neurosci.* **15**, 70–86.

Taube, J. S., Muller, R. U. & Ranck, J. B. Jr 1990 Head-direction cells recorded from the postsubiculum in freely moving rats. I. Description and quantitative analysis. *J. Neurosci.* **10**, 420–435.

Thier, P. & Karnath, O. 1997 *Parietal lobe contribution to orientation in 3D space*. Berlin: Springer.

Thomson, J. 1983 Is continuous visual monitoring necessary in visually guided locomotion? *J. Exp. Psychol.* **9**(3), 427–443.

Tropper, J., Melvill Jones, G., Bloomberg, J. & Fadlallah, H. 1990 Vestibular perceptual deficits in patients with parietal lobe lesions: a preliminary study. *Acta Otolaryngol.* **111**(48), 528–533.

Vallar, G., Sterzi, R., Bottini, G., Cappa, S. & Rusconi, M. L. 1990 Temporary remisssion of left hemianesthesia after vestibular stimulation. A sensory neglect phenomenon. *Cortex* **26**, 123–131.

Ventre, J. & Faugier-Grimaud, S. 1988 Projections of the temporo-parietal cortex on vestibular complex in the macaque monkey. *Expl Brain Res.* **72**, 653–658.

Vitte, E., Derosier, C., Caritu, Y, Berthoz, A., Hasboun, D. & Soulié, D. 1996 Activation of the hippocampal formation by vestibular stimulation: a functional magnetic resonance imaging study. *Expl Brain Res.* **112**, 523–526.

Whiteley, A. M. & Warrington, E. K. 1978 Selective impairment of topographical memory: a single case study. *J. Neurol. Neurosurg. Psychiatr.* **41**, 575–578.

Wiener, S. I. & Berthoz, A. 1993 Forebrain structures mediating the vestibular contribution during navigation. In *Multisensory control of movement* (ed., A. Berthoz), pp. 427–455. Oxford University Press.

Wiener, S. I., Korshunov, V. A., Garcia, R. & Berthoz, A. 1995 Inertial, substratal and landmark cue control of hippocampal CAl place cell activity. *Eur. J. Neurosci.* **7**, 2206–2219.

Wiest, G., Baumgartner, C., Deecke, L., Olbrich, A., Steinhof, N. & Müller, C. 1996 Effects of hippocampal lesions on vestibular memory in whole body rotation. *J. Vest. Res.* **6**, 4S, S17.

Young, L. 1984 Perception of the body in space. In *Handbook of physiology: the nervous system III. Sensory processes* pp. 978–1023. Bethesda, MD: American Physiological Society.

Zola-Morgan, S., Squire, L. R. & Amaral, D. G. 1986 Human amnesia and the medial temporal region: enduring memory impairement following a bilateral lesion limited to field CAl of the hippocampus. *J. Neurosci.* **6**, 2950–2967.

21

Hippocampal and parietal involvement in human topographical memory: evidence from functional neuroimaging

Eleanor A. Maguire

21.1 Introduction

The ability of humans to orient and navigate successfully in the large-scale spatially-extended environments that constitute the real-world is commonly referred to as topographical orientation. Way-finding is complex and not a unitary process; there are many aspects to it including attentional, perceptual and mnestic components. Topographical disorientation, therefore, can occur because of disturbance to one or more component processes. Occasionally cases of topographical disorientation are reported and are typically described in terms of perceptual or mnestic difficulties, such as perceptual disturbance where there is an agnosia for landmarks and buildings even in well-known surroundings, often found in association with prosopagnosia (Patterson and Zangwill 1944; Landis *et al.* 1986); or a topographical memory disturbance, where buildings and landmarks can be recognized and recalled, but the memory for their place in space and spatial relationships is dysfunctional (DeRenzi *et al.* 1977; Habib and Sirigu 1987; Bottini *et al.* 1990; Maguire *et al.* 1996*a*). Some general conclusions about the neural basis of topographical orientation systems can be drawn from the patient literature. Damage to several brain regions can produce topographic deficits of one sort or another. These include the posterior parietal lobe, the occipital lobe, hippocampal formation and parahippocampal gyrus. However, the dearth of relatively pure cases of topographical disorientation and the mixed picture of deficits typically present in many of the reported cases leave questions about the neural instantiation of topographical orientation remaining to be answered. More distinct conclusions about memory for the spatial layouts of environments are possible from work with animals, particularly rodents, where the hippocampus has been found to have a significant role in processing spatial information which is independent of the location or orientation of a navigating animal, i.e. processing spatial information in an allocentric frame of reference. The hippocampus has been proposed to maintain a cognitive map of the spatial layout of learned environments (O'Keefe and Nadel 1978), and complex spike cells within the rat hippocampus have been found to exhibit spatially localised firing (O'Keefe and Dostrovsky 1971).

Functional neuroimaging provides the opportunity to explore cognitive processes *in vivo* in neurologically intact humans. Here I will describe how positron emission tomography (PET) in particular has extended our understanding of the neural basis of topographical memory. Several questions will be addressed: What brain regions are involved in the learning of a spatially extended environment? What distinct functions might the various regions perform in the context of topographic learning? Similar questions are asked about the retrieval of previously learned environmental information. In addition, are the brain regions subserving topographical memory processes common also to those serving non-topographical memory. Currently there have been a limited number of functional neuroimaging studies examining topographical memory. This is not surprising given the restrictive environment of brain scanners and the complexity of the cognitive processing engendered by environmental cognition. Examining topographical memory or way-finding in this context necessitates the use of novel stimuli in order to simulate exploration and navigation in as naturalistic a manner as possible.

21.2 Topographical learning

Findings

Four functional neuro imaging studies of topographical learning and their findings will be briefly reviewed, with subsequent discussion of the broader issues surrounding these results.

Maguire *et al.* (1996*b*) used PET to measure regional cerebral blood flow (rCBF) while subjects watched and memorized film footage depicting, in one case, navigation in an urban area (topographical memory), while in another the film footage to be remembered was of a similar urban area but the camera was stationary while people, cars and such moved past (non-topographical memory). On the basis of viewing the second film, therefore, it was not possible to construct an internal spatial map of the environment but the tasks were comparable in terms of demands on memory. When changes in rCBF associated with non-topographical memory encoding were subtracted from the changes in rCBF associated with topographical memory, focal and significantly increased activation of the medial parietal region, the parahippocampal cortex and hippocampus on the right and the parahippocampal cortex on the left resulted (see Fig. 21.1). However, comparison of the activity during the non-topographical memory condition with control tasks revealed patterns of activation that, notably, did not include the medial temporal region. Such comparisons revealed activation of the middle occipital gyrus (area 19), the cuneus and bilateral activation of the middle frontal gyri. Aguirre and colleagues (1996) used

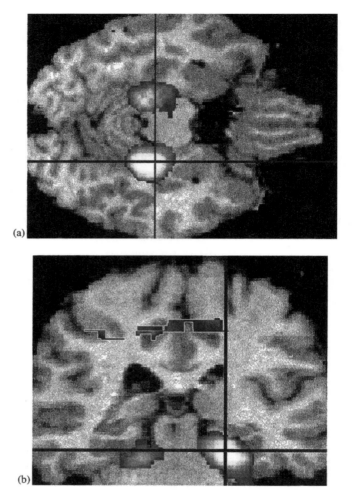

Fig. 21.1 Statistical parametric map (SPM) showing the location of increases in cerebral blood flow in (a) transverse and (b) coronal sections, while subjects watched film footage of navigation through a town (topographical memory) compared to a non-navigation memory condition. Superimposed on to a template magnetic resonance image (MRI) at the level of the peak activation in the right hippocampal region. Areas activated in this comparison: parahippocampal cortex and hippocampus on the right, with activation of the parahippocampal gyrus on the left, and the medial parietal lobe (data from Maguire *et al*. 1996*b*).

functional magnetic resonance imaging (fMRI) and a computer simulation of a maze-like environment with objects located in it to examine topographical learning. They too report activation of the parahippocampus, medial parietal region and posterior cingulate cortex associated with encoding of the maze.

Maguire *et al.* (1998*a*) developed an interactive means of assessing navigation—'the use of computer simulated environments that subjects could navigate through by their own volition. The purpose of this study was to extend the investigation of the topographical memory acquisition process beyond previous studies by examining its neural substrates, where environmental inputs were more specifically identifiable (i.e. the presence or absence of landmarks). They scanned different sets of subjects during topographical learning under different manipulations of the simulated environment. In one study, the environment had five corridors off a central area, an object placed in each room, and each area had different textures and colours. Compared to control tasks, the exploration and learning of this environment was associated with activation in occipito-temporal regions, posterior cingulate cortex, medial parietal regions and also the right parahippocampal gyrus. In a further study the environment was plain and empty where the rooms in the environment were only discriminable by shape, with no objects present. Compared to control tasks the learning of the environment without objects was associated with occipito-temporal activity, posterior cingulate cortex and medial parietal activation but no activity in medial temporal regions. Comparison of the two studies revealed the difference was in the right parahippocampal gyrus for objects in the environment. Interestingly, the hippocampus proper was not activated with either environment. This is perhaps because the environments were too simplistic and required no increase in hippocampal activity in order to process the spatial layout.

Implications

Based on the findings of these four experiments, a quite consistent pattern of brain activations is observed in association with topographical learning. Not surprisingly, compared to low-level baseline tasks, striate and extrastriate regions are involved, the other elements of the network being medial parietal and occipitotemporal areas, posterior cingulate cortex, the parahippocampal gyrus, and the right hippocampal formation. This is compatible with patient findings where lesions in all of these brain areas have been implicated at one time or another in topographical disorientation.

It would seem that the processing of environmental space in humans, as in rats, relies on hippocampal formation involvement. This is congruent with the patient findings alluded to previously (Habib and Sirigu 1987; Maguire *et al.* 1996*a*). The hippocampal formation is not consistently activated in functional imaging studies of episodic memory, although damage to this area is known to give rise to amnesia (Scoville and Milner 1957; Mayes 1988). It has been speculated that perhaps the lack of hippocampal activation in such studies is because the task-associated activity of the hippocampus is of a magnitude beyond the sensitivity of the PET camera. However, this is clearly not the case given its activation in the first study described here (Maguire *et al.* 1996*b*) and its activation in other functional imaging studies (e.g. Vandenberghe *et al.* 1996).

A more likely explanation is that the hippocampus maintains a level of continuous activity throughout tasks, experimental and control, so that in effect its activity is cancelled out during many cognitive subtractions. However, tasks such as the film viewing of naturalistic navigation with the processing demand to represent complex large-scale space, may activate the hippocampus beyond its normal level. Two of the studies involving simulated or virtual reality environments (Aguirre *et al.* 1996; Maguire *et al.* 1998a, experiment 1), while associated with increased activity in the parahippocampal cortex, did not demonstrate changes in activity in the hippocampus proper. It may be that the normal level of hippocampal activity was enough to support the demands of these tasks, which, while attempting to simulate real environments, did not embrace the true complexities and richness of the real-world designed as they were in a maze-like way.

Cognitive models of environmental learning commonly describe predictable stages in the development of allocentric representations of large-scale space (Siegal and White 1975). Typically, a significant role is ascribed to distinctive features or landmarks as the initial anchor points of topographical memory formation, and there is empirical support for the importance of landmarks in facilitating spatial and route-learning tasks (Allen *et al.* 1978; Garling *et al.* 1982; Presson 1987; Tlauka and Wilson 1994). In the Maguire *et al.* (1998a) studies, the purpose of comparing the encoding of the virtual environment with object/landmarks present with an environment with no objects was to pinpoint what areas might be specifically interested in object-in-place encoding in large-scale space. The finding that the parahippocampal gyrus is significantly involved in the encoding of an environment within which salient objects are located accords with their distinct role in cognitive models of environmental learning. It further provides evidence that the parahippocampal gyrus provides the neural substrate for landmark/object-in-place encoding within the larger system for topographical learning in humans. Further evidence for this is reported by Owen *et al.* (1996) and Milner *et al.* (Chapter 13) in this volume.

Increased activity in the medial parietal lobe (the precuneus), is commonly reported in functional imaging memory studies (Grasby *et al.* 1993; Fletcher *et al.* 1995a; Buckner *et al.* 1996). This has been interpreted as being associated with the retrieval of visual imagery in episodic memory. Fletcher *et al.* (1995b) confirmed this in a study where the recall of imageable word pairs, but not non-imageable word pairs, was associated with significant activation of the medial parietal region. All functional neuroimaging studies of topographical memory encoding report the medial parietal region as active. Activity in this region may relate to the construction of an internal representation of large-scale environments, and seems compatible with the role of the medial parietal cortex in imagery. Additional information on the role of this region in the context of way-finding has been reported in a study of topographical memory retrieval (Maguire *et al.* 1997)—discussed below.

The posterior cingulate cortex is also an active region during topographical learning. Cammalleri *et al.* (1996) report a case of topographical disorientation in a patient following a lesion to the right caudal cingulate cortex. Sutherland *et al.* (1988) found that rats with aspiration of the posterior cingulate cortex were impaired on swimming to a place in space using distal cues. Vogt *et al.* (1992) suggest that the posterior cingulate may contribute to spatial orientation because of its anatomical interposition between parietal regions and the parahippocampal gyrus. They propose that the posterior cingulate may participate in the transformation from a parietal (egocentric) frame of reference to a parahippocampal system based on an allocentric frame of reference. The activation of the medial parietal cortex, posterior cingulate and parahippocampal gyrus during exploration of the environment may be evidence of this spatial orientation pathway.

Verbal episodic memory encoding in functional imaging studies is typically associated with activation of the left dorsolateral prefrontal cortex and the medial parietal region but not the medial temporal region (Shallice *et al.* 1994; Fletcher *et al.* 1995*a*). This pattern of activation was indeed observed with the non-topographic memory encoding in the Maguire *et al.* (1996*b*) study. Notably, the activations in all cases associated with topographical learning are in the posterior brain, and even relative to very low-level baseline tasks, such as watching a screen change colour, no increased activation of the prefrontal cortices is observed. Interestingly, case reports of patients where topographical disorientation is the primary deficit are most consistently reported following posterior brain lesions. The ability to navigate in large-scale space is one humans share with a multitude of other species. Many species with a smaller relative area of prefrontal cortex than humans (e.g. birds) are able to navigate successfully, suggesting that perhaps other more posterior brain areas are most involved in such abilities. Other work has found that it is the size of the hippocampus relative to the size of the telencephalon that varies according to whether spatial skills are critical to survival. For example, in food-storing birds the hippocampus is reported as larger than species who cache food to a lesser extent (Sherry *et al.* 1992; Hampton *et al.* 1995). It is, of course, possible that frontal regions get recruited into topographical memory encoding under circumstances that have not yet been examined in functional neuro imaging studies, or perhaps become more active during topographical memory retrieval—as we shall see below.

21.3 Topographical memory retrieval

Findings

The retrieval or use of topographic information is of two types. The first are those recently formed memories which may still retain a specific spatiotemporal reference, and be therefore classified as episodic in nature (Tulving 1983). Such memory retrieval may conceivably still involve a degree of active encoding if knowledge of the spatial layout of the environment is still being verified or consolidated. Aguirre *et al.* (1996) scanned subjects while they navigated to specific objects within a computer-simulated environment after they had learned it. They report the activation of the same network of regions during retrieval as encoding, including the parahippocampal gyrus and pre-cuneus. Ghaem *et al.* (1997) got subjects to learn a short route and then scanned them as they imagined walking along the route. They report activation of the posterior cingulate, precuneus and bilateral hippocampal/parahippo-campal region (see also Berthoz, Chapter 20).

Most behaviour, however, takes place in environments with which we are very familiar and knowledge of their spatial layout has entered the domain of general facts about the world often referred to as semantic memory. The neural substrates of topographical memories of long-standing (i.e. over several years) have been examined in a study by Maguire *et al.* (1997). The aim of this study was primarily to test subjects on their knowledge of complex routes (and not simple maze-like environments of the simulated type), where all subjects could be tested on the same stimuli and with a high level of retrieval success, where there was no encoding of new environmental information during the performance of the tasks. This study also assessed the retrieval of landmark knowledge *per se*, where such knowledge was not confounded by location information about position within a large-scale spatial layout. This was achieved by using a task where famous landmarks were known, but their large-scale spatial context was not (i.e. never been visited). This study also examined topographical memory (landmarks/spatial layouts) and also non-topographic semantic memory retrieval to ascertain if common brain regions subserve semantic memory irrespective of memory type. In order to examine well-established topographical memory, subjects were all licensed London taxi drivers of many years experience. Official London taxi drivers must train for approximately 3 years, passing stringent examinations of spatial knowledge before receiving a licence. Subjects overtly recalled the relevant memories during PET scanning.

Comparison of the activity during the routes recall task with that during the landmark recall revealed activation of the medial parietal lobe, the posterior cingulate cortex, the parahippocampal gyrus, and activation also of the right hippocampal formation (see Fig. 21.2). The landmarks task compared to baseline also resulted in activation of the posterior cingulate cortex, the medial parietal lobe and occipito-temporal regions including the parahippocampal gyrus. In this case, however, there was no activation of the hippocampus. In comparison with a baseline task, the recall of non-topographical memory, in this case plots from very familiar famous films, activated left frontal regions and the left middle temporal gyrus. Topographical routes recall and the recall of the plots of familiar famous films involve the recall of memories in a specific temporal sequence. When these two tasks with implicit sequences were com-pared to tasks where the memory recall had no inherent sequence—landmark recall and the recall of freeze-frames from familiar famous films—the brain region most active in the sequencing tasks was bilateral medial parietal cortex.

z = – 8mm   z = – 6mm   z = – 4mm

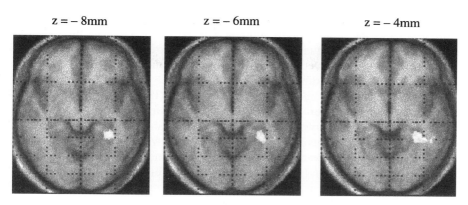

Fig. 21.2 Activation in the right hippocampal region during the comparison between recall of routes around London by taxi drivers and the recall of famous landmarks. Located here on adjacent transverse sections of the averaged MRI scan of the eleven taxi drivers at the level of peak activation in the right hippocampal region (data from Maguire *et al.* 1997).

Implications

It appears that both topographical learning and recall (from episodic or semantic memory) have broadly the same network of brain regions as their neural substrate. Thus, for topographical memory at least, the distinction between episodic and semantic memory appears to have no anatomical basis. The right hippocampus is clearly involved in processing spatial layouts over long as well as short time-courses, and participates in both the encoding and the retrieval of topographical memory.

Both landmarks and routes activated occipitotemporal regions, posterior cingulate gyrus, medial parietal areas and the parahippocampal gyrus. The involvement of many of the same brain regions, both dorsal and ventral, in routes and landmark memory indicates that the topographical memory system may be primed to receive relevant topographical information even when the landmarks have no context within large-scale space. It was noted previously that topographical learning was associated with different brain regions than those involved in non-topographical episodic memory encoding. The use of familiar film plots as stimuli in the Maguire *et al.* (1997) study engaged subjects in memory recall at a similar level and with broadly similar characteristics as the routes task—such as the recall of information in a specific temporal sequence (i.e. progression along a route or progression of a storyline). Except for cerebellar activity, recall of film plots was associated with different brain regions to those activated during the routes task. Most activity was left-sided and there was no activation of occipitotemporal or medial temporal regions when compared to the baseline. However, the recall of film plots resulted in activation of the left inferior frontal gyrus. In this case, topographical memory for large-scale space was clearly not recalled via this mechanism and, as with topographical learning, caused increased neuronal activity in the posterior brain. It might be argued that thorough familiarity with an environment diminishes the need to recruit frontal regions for planning or strategizing for the purposes of way-finding.

The taxi-driver study and that of Maguire *et al.* (1996*b*), where activation of the hippocampus proper during topographical learning was also recorded, contrast with the other two topographical memory studies (Aguirre *et al.* 1996; Maguire *et al.* 1998), where hippocampal activation was not found. These latter two studies employed computer-simulated environments, while the taxi study and that of Maguire *et al.* (1996*b*) involved memory for real-world environments. Real environments are more complex than the simulations used to date and involve the potential for using many routes to navigate to a goal, as reflected in the task put before the taxi drivers to find the shortest route to the destination. The recruitment of the hippocampus when real-world environments are involved may reflect its role in higher level spatial manipulation and decision-making.

Recent evidence to support this has come from work by Maguire *et al.* (1998*b*), where subjects were scanned using PET while they performed retrieval tasks in a complex computer-simulated town, which they had spent some time learning prior to scanning. Subjects either found their way to specified destinations in the town using their internal representation built up during learning, or followed a trial of arrows through the town, which did not require the use of topographical memory but controlled for movement and optical flow. Subjects' behavioural performances, as well as changes in cerebral perfusion during scanning, were recorded and analysed. There was activation of the right hippocampus when comparison was made between reaching a destination successfully compared with the activity when following the trail of arrows. In addition, there was a significant correlation between blood flow changes in the right hippocampus and right inferior parietal cortex and accuracy of navigation—the more accurate the path taken to the goal place the more active the right hippocampus in particular. This result is consistent with the idea that the right hippocampus in humans provides an allocentric representation of space which enables direct navigation, while the right inferior parietal cortex is involved in generating the appropriate egocentric body-turns.

Movement through the environment was assessed by comparing rCBF while following arrows with a static scenes task—this showed activation of the medial parietal region and the right inferior parietal cortex. The activation of these areas may be associated with egocentric movement and the related optical flow (DeJong *et al.* 1994), without any requirement for memory consistent with the view that one of the functions of the posterior parietal region includes spatial processing within a body-centred frame of reference (see Anderson, and Karnath, Chapters 3 and 5). Speed of movement through the environment was correlated with activity in the basal ganglia in the region of the right caudate nucleus. Left frontal cortex activation was apparent when successful navigation was compared to following arrows or compared to unsuccessful navigation.

Interestingly, navigation requiring detours—where direct routes were precluded by closing some of the doors/blocking roads—compared to direct way-finding also revealed left frontal activation. These frontal activations are consistent with the view of a role for this region in planning, in this case spatial planning, and decision making (Shallice 1982).

21.4 Comment

Most human spatial behaviour takes place in large-scale spatially-extended environments. This requires the ability to recall points in space which cannot be perceived simultaneously in one field of view. This ability, common to most animals, is subserved in humans by a network of brain regions. Functional neuroimaging studies are beginning to reveal this network of brain regions, illuminating the patient lesion findings where cases of topographical disorientation result from insults to various and disparate brain regions. The parallels with animal work, in terms of the involvement of the hippocampus in the mapping of space, are also clear. Once topographical information is acquired, the neuroanatomy that supports its use and retrieval is very similar to those used in its acquisition. Functional neuroimaging is also starting to reveal the distinct contributions of various elements of the topographical learning system: the posterior parietal region in temporal sequencing and in egocentric movement through the environment, regions of the frontal cortex when planning in less familiar environments is required, the basal ganglia in motoric aspects of way-finding, and the parahippocampal gyrus for supporting object-in-place associations. Most crucially, functional neuroimaging has allowed us to observe that the right hippocampus in humans provides an allocentric representation of space which, with the help of the right inferior parietal cortex, enables direct and accurate navigation. The precise inputs and outputs of a human navigation network remain to be specified, as do the functions in this context of other regions known to be involved in memory—such as the left hippocampus. Functional neuroimaging offers us a means to pursue many of the outstanding issues in understanding the neural implementation of navigation.

Acknowledgements

Support from The Wellcome Trust is gratefully acknowledged. Thanks to my collaborator on all studies, Chris Frith; and to collaborators on the virtual reality work, John O'Keefe, Neil Burgess and Jim Donnett.

References

Aguirre, G. K., Detre, J. A., Alsop, D. C. and D'Esposito, M. 1996 The parahippocampus subserves topographical learning in man. *Cerebral Cortex* **6**, 823–9.

Allen, G. L., Siegal, A. W. and Rosinski, R. R. 1978 The role of perceptual context in structuring spatial knowledge. *Journal of Experimental Psychology: Human Learning and Memory* **4**, 617–30.

Bottini, G., Cappa S. and Sterzi, R. 1990 Topographic disorientation—a case report. *Neuropsychologia* **28**, 309–12.

Buckner, R. L., Raichle, M. E., Miezin, F. M. and Petersen, S. E. 1996 Medial parietal (precuneus) activation during episodic memory retrieval: one area that is involved and one that isn't. *NeuroImage*, **3**, S533.

Cammalleri, M., Gangitano, M., D'Amelio, M., Raieli, V., Raimondo, D. and Camarda, R. 1996 Transient topographical amnesia and cingulate cortex damage: a case report. *Neuropsychologia* **34**, 321–6.

De Jong, B. M., Shipp, S., Skidmore, B., Frackowiak, R. S. J. and Zeki, S. 1994 The cerebral activity related to the visual perception of forward motion in depth. *Brain* **117**, 1039–54.

De Renzi E., Faglioni, P. and Villa, P. 1977 Topographical amnesia. *Journal of Neurology, Neurosurgery and Psychiatry* **40**, 498–505.

Fletcher, P. C., Frith, C. D., Grasby, P. M., Shallice, T., Frackowiak, R. S. J. and Dolan, R. J. 1995a Brain systems for encoding and retrieval of auditory-verbal memory. *Brain* **118**, 401–16.

Fletcher, P. C., Frith, C. D., Baker, S. C., Shallice, T., Frackowiak, R. S. J. and Dolan, R. J. 1995b The mind's eye—precuneus activation in memory-related imagery. *Neuroimage* **2**, 195–200.

Garling, T., Book, A. and Ergenzen, N. 1982 Memory for the spatial layout of the physical environment: differential rates of acquisition of different types of information. *Scandinavian Journal of Psychology* **23**, 23–35.

Ghaem, O., Mellet, E., Crivello, F., Tzourio, N., Mazoyer, B., Berthoz, A. *et al.* 1997 Mental navigation along memorized routes activates the hippocampus, precuneus, and insula. *NeuroReport* **8**, 739–44.

Grasby, P. M., Frith, C. D., Friston, K. J., Bench, C. Frackowiak, R. S. J. and Dolan, R. J. 1993 Functional mapping of brain areas implicated in auditory–verbal memory function. *Brain* **116**, 1–20.

Habib, M. and Sirigu, A. 1987 Pure topographical disorientation: a definition and anatomical basis. *Cortex* **23**, 73–85.

Hampton, R. R., Sherry, D. F., Shettleworth, S. J., Khurgel, M. and Ivy, G. 1995 Hippocampal volume and food-storing behavior are related in parids. *Brain, Behavior and Evolution* **45**, 54–61.

Landis, T., Cummings, J. L. Benson, D. F. and Palmer, E. P. 1986 Loss of topographical familiarity: an environmental agnosia. *Archives of Neurology* **43**, 132–6.

Maguire, E. A., Burke, T., Phillips, J. and Staunton, H. 1996a Topographical disorientation following unilateral temporal lobe lesions in humans. *Neuropsychologia* **34**, 993–1001.

Maguire, E. A., Frackowiak, R. S. J. and Frith, C. D. 1996b Learning to find your way —a role for the human hippocampal region. *Proceedings of the Royal Society of London. Series B, Biological Sciences* **263**, 1745–50.

Maguire E. A., Frackowiak, R. S. J. and Frith, C. D. 1997 Recalling routes around London: activation of the right hippocampus in taxi drivers. *Journal of Neuroscience* **17**, 7103–10.

Maguire, E. A., Frith, C. D., Burgess, N., Donnett, J. G. and O'Keefe, J. 1998a Knowing where things are: parahippocampal involvement in encoding object locations in virtual large-scale space. *Journal of Cognitive Neuroscience* **10**, 61–76.

Maguire, E. A., Burgess, N., Donnett, J. G., Frackowiak, R. S. J., Frith, C. D. and O'Keefe, J. 1998b Knowing where and getting there: a human navigation network. *Science* **280**, 921–924.

Mayes, A. R. 1988 *Human Organic Memory Disorders*. Cambridge: Cambridge University Press.

O'Keefe, J. and Dostrovsky, J. 1971 The hippocampus as a spatial map: preliminary evidence from unit activity in the freely-moving rat. *Brain Research* **34**, 171–5.

O'Keefe, J. and Nadel, L. 1978 *The Hippocampus as a Cognitive Map*. Oxford: Clarendon Press.

Owen, A. M., Milner, B., Petrides, M. and Evans, A. C. 1996 A specific role for the right parahippocampal gyrus in the retrieval of object-location: a positron emission tomography study. *Journal of Cognitive Neuroscience* **8**, 588–602.

Patterson, A. and Zangwill, O. L. 1944 Disorders of visual space perception associated with lesions of the right cerebral hemisphere. *Brain* **67**, 331–58.

Presson, C. C. 1987 The development of landmarks in spatial memory: the role of differential experience. *Journal of Experimental Child Psychology* **44**, 317–34.

Scoville, W. B. and Milner, B. 1957 Loss of recent memory after bilateral hippocampal lesions. *Journal of Neurology, Neurosurgery and Psychiatry* **20**, 11–21.

Shallice, T. 1982 Specific impairments of planning. *Philosophical Transactions of the Royal Society London, Series B* **298**, 199–209.

Shallice, T., Fletcher, P. C., Frith, C. D., Grasby, P., Frackowiak, R. S. J. and Dolan, R. J. 1994 Brain regions associated with acquisition and retrieval of verbal episodic memory. *Nature* **368**, 633–5.

Sherry, D. F., Jacobs, L. F. and Gaulin, S. J. 1992 Spatial memory and adaptive specialization of the hippocampus. *Trends in Neurosciences* **15**, 298–303.

Siegal, A. W. and White, S. H. 1975 The development of spatial representation of large-scale environments. In *Advances in Child Development and Behavior* (*Vol. 10*) pp. 9–55. (ed., H.W. Reese), New York: Academic Press.

Sutherland, R. J., Whishaw, I. Q. and Kolb, B. 1988 Contributions of the cingulate cortex to two forms of spatial learning and memory. *Journal of Neuroscience* **8**, 1863–72.

Tlauka, M. and Wilson, P. N. 1994 The effect of landmarks on route-learning in a computer-simulated environment. *Journal of Environmental Psychology* **14**, 305–13.

Tulving, E. 1983 *Elements of Episodic Memory*. Oxford: Clarendon Press.

Vandenberghe, R., Price, C., Wise, R., Josephs, O. and Frackowiak, R. S. J. 1996 Functional anatomy of a common semantic system for words and pictures. *Nature* **383**, 254–6.

Vogt, B. A., Finch, D. M. and Olson, C. R. 1992 Functional heterogeneity in cingulate cortex: the anterior executive and posterior evaluative regions. *Cerebral Cortex* **2**, 435–43.

22

Parietal cortex and hippocampus: from visual affordances to the world graph

Michael A. Arbib

22.1 Introduction

The present paper is based on Arbib (1997), extended in Section 22.3 to provide a sampling of results from Guazzelli *et al.* (1998).

Gibson (1966) observed that the pattern of *optic flow*, the movement of features across the retina from moment to moment, contains valuable information that could be used to guide navigation through the environment without prior recognition of objects. We adopt Gibson's term '*affordances*' for parameters for motor interactions signalled by sensory cues without the necessary intervention of 'high-level processes' of object recognition. Neurological data relate human parietal function not only to impairment of a variety of affordances but also to impairment of 'cognitive maps'. Bilateral parietal lobe damage often yields 'global spatial disorientation' (Kase *et al.* 1977), a symptom complex which involves the three systems whose parietal roles are modelled in this paper: the control of eye movements; the control of the grasping of objects; and the use of 'cognitive maps' in navigation. Some of these deficits can also be seen in relatively pure isolated form.

In short, the parietal cortex is a complex system involved in a great diversity of subfunctions. More specifically, the inferior parietal lobule (IPL) of the parietal cortex in monkey receives visual inputs from occipito-temporal areas, as well as from the visual field periphery of V3 and V2 (Baizer *et al.* 1991). IPL is functionally subdivided into several areas buried in the intraparietal sulcus, including the *lateral* (LIP), *ventral* (VIP) and *anterior* (AIP) *intraparietal areas*, as well as areas 7a and 7b, and the *secondary somatosensory area* (SII). These areas have specific sensory–motor functions, including those for saccadic eye movements (LIP), ocular fixation (7a), reaching (VIP and 7b) and grasping (AIP). A similar modular organization is seen in the motor sector of the frontal lobe.

We will outline biologically-based neural network models for the role of LIP in remapping during a double saccade task; and for the interactions of AIP with premotor cortex during the control of grasping. We thus demonstrate how visual areas of posterior parietal cortex process the affordances, such as those involved in looking and grasping; other areas may be involved in more 'purely visual' functions, such as shape extraction and motion extraction.

Many data suggest that rats:

(1) have associative memory for complex stimulus configurations;
(2) can encode the spatial effect of their own movements; and
(3) are able to form sequences of actions to go from a starting location to a goal.

In other words, rats are assumed to have a *cognitive map* (Tolman 1948). To understand this notion, we must distinguish *egocentric* representations from *allocentric* representations. The former, based on the organism's current view of the world, are appropriate for looking, reaching, grasping and locomotion, with respect to directly perceptible features of the landscape. The latter can be understood in terms of a subway map of a city. Such a map is not drawn from the viewpoint of any rider, but nonetheless sets out the spatial relations between different stations, lines that link them, and the junctions between these lines.

O'Keefe and Nadel (1978) distinguished two paradigms for navigation, one based on maps and the other based on routes, and proposed that independent neural systems exist in the brain to support these two types of navigation. They called these systems the *locale* system for map-based navigation and the *taxon* (behavioural orientation) system for route navigation. Our concern is not only to model these systems, but also to analyse their interaction, and the role of motivation in their execution. The taxon system is based on egocentric spatial information, which can be viewed as sets of guidance and orientation cues.

Arbib and Lieblich (1977; see also Lieblich and Arbib 1982) have represented the cognitive map as a graph, i.e. a set of nodes, some of which are connected by edges, with nodes corresponding to a recognizable situation in the animal's world (cf. the stations on a subway map), and with each edge representing a path from a recognizable situation to the next. This 'world graph' (WG) is constructed so that the organism has the ability to move from one point to another in a fashion determined by both cognitive knowledge and motivational states. The WG theory can be used to analyse how the brain can encode the sequences of actions required to pass from one spatial representation to another and, likewise, how an animal builds up a model of the world around it in such a way that, when under the influence of a particular drive, it can find its way to a location where it has learned that the drive will be reduced.

22.2 Parietal cortex and affordances in monkey

Parietal cortex and dynamic remapping of saccade targets

Dominey and Arbib (1992) modelled the interaction of various brain regions in the execution of voluntary saccades in primates. Here, we focus on the putative role of LIP in the double saccade experiment: the monkey is seated in a primate chair with its head fixed and eyes free to move. Illuminated fixation points and saccade targets are presented on a visual screen in front of the primate, which has been trained not to move its eye while the fixation point remains on. In the *double saccade task*, following offset of the initial fixation point (F), targets A and B are successively presented in less than the time required to initiate the first saccade. Reward is contingent on successive saccades from F to A and then to B. In the double saccade, target B is not visible during or after the saccade to A. Thus, the representation of target B in a motor error map must be remapped to represent where B would appear were it still visible after the saccade to A. The double saccade task, then, is used to study the dynamic remapping of target representations to compensate for intervening movements.

Mays and Sparks (1980) detected a class of 'quasi-visual' (QV) cells in the intermediate layers of the superior colliculus that, prior to the second saccade in the double saccade task, were active *in loci* related to the second saccade, even though a visual stimulus with this retinal error did not appear in the receptive field of these cells. However, it appears that the QV property is not intrinsic to SC, but instead depends on a prominent direct projection from LIP (Lynch *et al.* 1985). Indeed, Gnadt and Andersen (1988) found 'QV-like' cells in LIP that code for the second eye movement, though a visual stimulus never falls in the cells' receptive field; while Goldberg and Bruce (1990) found similar cells in the frontal eye fields (FEF). Where does this dynamic remapping occur? It may well be computed 'independently' in several regions, with the regions interconnected to calibrate their computations. However, Dominey and Arbib (1992) hypothesize that the primary remapping occurs in LIP, and model LIP by two connected arrays of cells, PP, which is driven by retinal input and PPqv (posterior parietal cells with QV-like activity), which drives both SCqv and FEFvis to yield the dynamic remapping in these regions.

To model the shifting activity in an array of QV-like cells, Droulez and Berthoz (1990) used an eye velocity signal to shift a 'mountain' of activity on a two-dimensional map of motor error. To date, a representation of eye velocity has not been recorded in posterior parietal cortex. Dominey and Arbib (1992) thus developed an alternative model, which uses two eye position signals, one a delayed version of the other, as the input for dynamic remapping. The difference between the two position signals is used to modulate two types of interneurones. Type 'r' neurones implement *recurrent* self-excitation of the PPqv cells when the eye position signals are equal, which is reduced when the eyes are moving. Type 'S' interneurones gate the lateral *shift* of activation between neighbouring cells as a function of the difference between the two position inputs. In a leftward saccade, the difference between the delayed signal and the original signal (calculated by S) is positive, so activity shifts from left to right.

The model also involves a projection from PP to PPqv, which ensures that when retinal input is available, it will eventually predominate over the 'memory map'. This allows the brain to combine stored, updated target information with current visual input.

Parietal cortex and object grasping

In monkeys trained to grasp objects requiring different types of grip, about half of the AIP neurones related to hand movements fired almost exclusively during one type of grip, with precision grip being the most represented grip type (Taira *et al*. 1990; Sakata *et al*. 1992). Some cells demonstrated specificity toward the size of the object to be grasped; and some cells demonstrated independence from the size of the object. A small number of cells showed modulation based upon the object's position and/or orientation in space. In summary, we say that the visual responses of these cells provide a distributed code for affordances for grasping. Most neurones in AIP also show phasic activity related to the motor behaviour. The identifiable phases in the paradigm used by Sakata to study these cells are: set (*key phase*), preshape, enclose, hold (*object* phase), and ungrasp. Cells participate in varying degrees during different phases of the movement, but are usually most highly active during the preshape and enclose phases of movement. Very importantly, once a cell becomes active, it typically remains active until the object is released.

The area of monkey agranular frontal cortex involved in grasping is called F5 (Rizzolatti *et al*. 1988) and forms the rostral part of inferior area 6. Its main anatomical connections are with AIP and the hand field of the precentral motor area (Muakkassa and Strick 1979; Matelli *et al*. 1985). Rizzolatti *et al*. (1988) described various classes of F5 neurones, which discharge during specific hand movements (e.g. grasping, holding, tearing, manipulating). The largest class is related to grasping. The temporal relations between neurone discharge and grasping movements vary among neurones.

We now outline the FARS (Fagg–Arbib–Rizzolatti–Sakata) model of the grasping process, implemented in terms of simplified but biologically plausible neural networks (Fagg and Arbib 1998). For example, given visual input from an object, AIP computes—according to the model—the affordances corresponding to the various ways in which it may be grasped (as distinct from recognizing *what* the object is). The corresponding set of grasps is passed to F5. As a function of task or other information, F5 selects one of the specified grasps, and is responsible for unfolding the grasp in time. F5 activity is broadcast back to AIP, strengthening the affordance that corresponds to the selected grasp. Motor responses in AIP are explained as corollary discharges from F5, and AIP provides an *active memory* for the grasp, which is continuously updated. This is similar to the *dynamic remapping* mechanism we saw in our study of saccades, in which motor efference copies updated a map of targets of potential eye movements.

The location of target objects is represented in VIP (Colby *et al*. 1993), using a broadly-tuned population code. This affordance is passed to F4, which represents the arm goal position. Since grasp programming affects arm movements, the model modulates F4 with information from AIP specific to the affordance/grasp pair selected by the AIP/F5 system.

A neighbouring region, the *posterior intraparietal area* (PIP), codes object-centred information (Sakata, personal communication) concerning different shapes presented to the monkey. In the model, PIP codes the shape and size of the object to be grasped. An affordance derived from PIP maps an object configuration to one possible grasp for that object. Castiello *et al.* (1991) studied impaired grasping in a patient (AT) with a lesion impairing the pathway V1 → PP, and found evidence for a mapping from object identity to affordances that is effective whenever the nature of the object merits such a mapping. The model thus includes a corresponding path PIP → IT → AIP.

Figure 22.1 outlines the interaction between AIP and F5 populations during execution of the Sakata paradigm. Three AIP units are shown: a visual-related cell, which recognizes objects that require a precision pinch; a motor-related cell of the same type; and a visual-related cell, which recognizes objects requiring power grasps. Each F5 unit shown fires during a different phase of the program. At each program phase, the state is reported back to the AIP motor-type population. The full model also includes the role of SII in creating

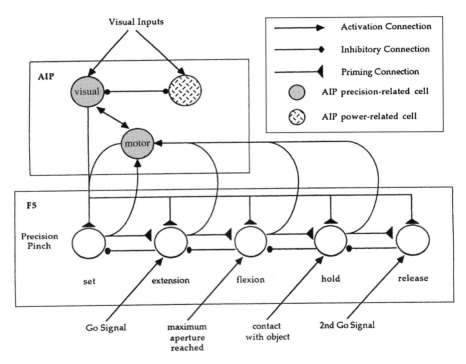

Fig. 22.1 FARS model of interaction between AIP and F5 populations (*circles*) during execution of the preshape/grasp/hold program. Activity within F5 cascades from left to right as the program is executed. Each phase primes the next phase (which must await further activation to control motor output) and inhibits the preceding phase. At each program phase, the state is reported back to the AIP motor-type population.

and monitoring haptic expectations, the role of dorsal premotor cortex (F2) in the association of arbitrary stimuli with motor program preparation, and the role of area 46 as a working memory in tasks requiring information to be held during a delay period. However, these details (and the presentation of simulation results) are beyond the scope of the present paper. We do stress, however, the circuitry controlling F5 programs in the model is more complex than is shown in Fig. 22.1: the *effective connections* between program states are not coded within F5 but are managed by the combined action of pre-SMA (F6) and the basal ganglia (BG).

In summary, the FARS model introduces not only the affordances for grasping in AIP but also those for reaching in VIP. It also shows that parietal areas need not be restricted to computing affordances—PIP extracts object shape and size information that is as useful to IT's object recognition as it is to AIP's determination of affordances. We have also moved from the 'self-contained' study of a parietal region accorded LIP in the Dominey–Arbib model of dynamic remapping of saccades to a 'cooperative computation' model of AIP in which its computation of visual affordances is complemented by corollary discharge from F5, which in the model is hypothesized to resolve multiple potential grasps by information on task constraints (from F6), working memory (from area 46) and instruction stimuli (from F2). As a result, AIP can function as an active memory in which a set of affordances, not all of which need be activated by visual input, are updated as the plan of action unfolds. IT gives a broadly-tuned coarse code for affordances when object knowledge is appropriate for this, and when visual input to AIP is available, AIP can refine or replace IT input with a more finely-tuned coarse code for affordances. Finally, action generally involves plans that take advantage of, but are not wholly driven by, current affordances and the FARS model thus addresses the role of pre-SMA and BG in sequence management.

22.3 Affordances, world graphs and navigation

Although addressing data from rat neurophysiology, the model of the role of the rat parietal cortex and hippocampus in navigation, to be described in this section, is strongly motivated by data from primate neurophysiology, whose implications for analogous properties of the rat brain have yet to be tested.

Cognitive maps and the hippocampus

To use a road map, we must locate (the representations of) where we are and where we want to go, and then find a path that we can use as we navigate towards our goal. We use the term '*cognitive map*' for a mental map together with these processes for using it. Thus the 'place cells' found in rat hippocampal CA3 and CA1 (O'Keefe and Dostrovsky 1971) provide only a 'you are here' signal, not a full cognitive map. Moreover, a given place cell will have a 'place field' in a highly familiar environment with up to 70 per cent probability. This suggests that the hippocampus is dynamically tuned to a 'chart' of the current locale, rather than providing a complete 'atlas' with a different place cell for every place in the rat's 'entire world'. This suggest two alternatives (at least):

1. The different 'charts' are stored elsewhere, and must be 'reinstalled' in the hippocampus as dictated by the current task and environment.
2. The cells of the hippocampus receive inputs encoding task and environment, which determine how sensory cues are used to activate a neural representation of the animal's locale.

   In either case, we see that these 'charts' are highly labile. Noting the importance of parietal systems in representing the personal space of humans, we seek to understand cognitive maps in a framework that embraces parietal cortex as well as hippocampus.

   Although some hippocampal cells fire when rats drink water or approach water sources (Ranck 1973), O'Keefe and Conway (1978) did not find the role of food or water to be markedly different from other cues that identify the location of a place field. Eichenbaum *et al.* (1987) recorded from rats repetitively performing a sequence of behaviours in a single odor-discrimination paradigm, and found *goal-approach cells*, which fired selectively during specific movements, such as approach to the odor port or to the reward cup. Despite these and related findings, there is still no evidence that hippocampus proper can simultaneously encode the rat's current location and the goal of current navigation.

Hippocampal–parietal interactions in navigation

McNaughton *et al.* (1989) found cells in the rat posterior parietal cortex with location specificity that were dependent on visual input for their activation. These cells had 40 per cent responses discriminating whether the animal was turning left, turning right, or moving forward (we call these MLC cells). Some cells required a conjunction of movement and location(e.g. one parietal cell fired more for a right turn at the western arm of a cross-maze than for a right turn at the eastern arm, and these firings were far greater than for all left turns. Another parietal cell fired for left turns at the centre of the maze but not for left turns at the ends of the arms, or for any right turns) Turn-direction information was varied, with a given cell responding to a particular subset of vestibular input, neck and trunk proprioception, visual field motion, and (possibly) efference copy from motor commands.

   McNaughton and Nadel (1990) offered a model of rat navigation with four components (Fig. 22.2a):

1. B, a spatio-sensory input.
2. A, in the hippocampus, provides a place representation.

3. L, posited to be parietal, outputs a movement representation.

4. AL, provides a place/movement representation, by means of the parietal MLC cells.

In the model, A both transforms visual input from B into place cell activity, and responds to input from AL by transforming the neural code of (prior place, movement) into that for the place where the rat will be after the movement. But this model becomes untenable since MLC cells are *not* place/movement cells in the sense of 'place' in 'place cells' (Examples of such a cell's 'place/movement field' are 'left turn at end of arm' or 'move ahead along arm'.)

To proceed, we pursue analogies with monkey parietal cortex. We first *hypothesize* (for future experimental testing) that the parietal cortex of the rat *also* contains *affordance cells* for locomotion and navigation, akin to those documented in the monkey for reaching and grasping. Figure 22.2b thus has the cells in AL (parietal cortex) code for affordances, and includes a direct link from B to AL that is absent in Fig. 22.2a. Since 'grip affordance cells' in AIP project to 'grip premotor cells' in premotor region F5, we postulate analogously (Fig. 22.2b) that L is premotor and driven by AL. Once again, the current place is encoded in A, but we now posit that movement information from L enables A to compute the correct transformation from current place to next place. In either model, then, the loop via AL can, in the absence of sensory input, update the place representation in A, with the cycle continuing until errors in this *expectation* accumulate excessively.

Figure 22.2b also adds links from brain areas involved in goals and motivation—the navigation of a hungry rat is different from that of a sated rat. In analogy to the monkey, it posits (without further analysis) that interactions between prefrontal cortex and basal ganglia *choose* the rat's next movement on the basis of its current position relative to its goal. We shall say more of this when we discuss our model of rat navigation.

We now return to the MLC cells. Some fire prior to the rat's execution of a turn, and correspond to the affordance cells of Fig. 22.2b, but others do not fire until the turn commences. These, then, are not signaling affordances, and we now describe a supplementary circuit (Paul Rothemund, USC term paper, Spring 1996), which includes our model of these cells. To ground this circuit, we turn to reports from the *monkey* literature of neurones, which detect optic flow and have traces similar to those for MLC cells whose responses start at the initiation of a turn. These include MST neurones selective for expansion, contraction and rotation (Graziao *et al.* 1994). Rotation-sensitive (RS) neurones of the posterior parietal association cortex which, unlike MST neurones which seem specific for rotation in a fronto-parallel plane, were mostly sensitive to rotation in depth (Sakata *et al.* 1994).

A neurone responding to a focus of expansion could seem to code for straight ahead and a neurone encoding translational flow or rotation in depth could code for a turn. Some of the MLC cells, which fire at a turn, require head

Michael A. Arbib

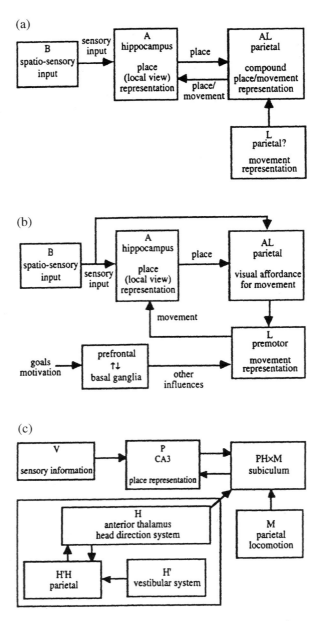

Fig. 22.2 (a) A systems view of the role of the hippocampus in spatially guided navigation (adapted from McNaughton and Nadel 1990). (b) A recasting of the systems view of (a), which makes explicit that the parietal cortex provides 'affordances' rather than explicit place information (Arbib *et al.* 1997). (c) The McNaughton *et al.* (1996) systems level view of the role of the hippocampus in navigation, redrawn from the perspective of (a).

orientation in addition to visual input. We suggest that 'parietal left turn' neurones combine input from an 'MST left turn neurone' with vestibular input, efference copy, or somatosensory input. Such a 'parietal left turn' neurone can thus function in the dark, but does not code place as well as movement. A neurone that does code for a 'place specific left turn' might be constructed from a 'parietal left turn' neurone and hippocampal input. We postulate that, though based on monkey data, this circuitry will (with different anatomical loci) be instantiated in rat brain as well.

McNaughton *et al.* (1996) have proposed a new systems-level model, which incorporates head direction information in the implementation of an angular path-integrator module. Note that head direction here is *not* absolute but is established with respect to sensory, e.g. visual, cues. It can be maintained moderately well if the animal moves in the dark, but will be changed if the sensory cues are rearranged. Figure 22.2c presents this model redrawn to emphasize its similarity to Fig. 22.2a. Box PH × M, previously P × M and assumed to be parietal, is now assumed to be implemented by the subiculum, based on the report by Sharp and Green (1994) that some cells in the subiculum and dorsal presubiculum have broad, but significant, directional tuning in situations where directionality is absent from hippocampal cells.

McNaughton *et al.* (1996) view head direction as a point on a circle centred on the rat, and assign each head-direction cell a location on this circle. This head-direction ring (H) has local Gaussian excitatory connections from a cell to its neighbours. Another layer of neurones (H′H) receives information about the current location from H and information about rotational motion from the vestibular system and other sources of such information (H′). These cells encode the interaction between current location and the sign of rotation and feed this information to cells on the appropriate side of the current focus of activity in the direction circle. Cells with these response properties have been observed in the rat posterior cortex (Chen *et al.* 1994*a,b*). The posterior cortex is now assumed to implement the H′H system, which is almost identical with the dynamic remapping module postulated for LIP in the Dominey–Arbib model described before.

Taxon and locale systems: an affordance is not a map

As mentioned before, O'Keefe and Nadel (1978) have distinguished the *taxon* (*behavioural orientation*) *system* for route navigation (a '*taxis*' is an organism's response to a stimulus by movement in a particular direction), and the *locale system* for map-based navigation, and proposed that the locale system resides in the hippocampus. We have already qualified the latter assertion, showing how the hippocampus may function as *part of* a cognitive map. Here we want to relate taxis to the notion of an affordance. Just as a rat may have basic taxes for approaching food or avoiding a bright light, say, so does it have a wider repertoire of affordances for possible actions associated with the immediate sensing of its environment. Such affordances include 'go straight ahead' for visual sighting of a corridor, 'hide' for a dark hole, 'eat' for food as sensed generically, 'drink' similarly, and the various turns afforded by, for example, the sight of the end of the corridor) Since the rat's behaviour also depends on odor cues, we should add 'olfactory affordances', but relevant data are sparse.

O'Keefe (1983) has found that both normal and fornix-lesioned rats can learn to solve a simple T-maze in the absence of any consistent environmental cues other than the T-shape of the maze. If anything, lesioned animals learned this problem faster than normals. All this suggests that without the hippocampus, the rat uses a pure orientation cue; whereas with the hippocampus, there is competition and cooperation between the orientation cue and the cue provided by the map-based system.

After criterion was reached on turns to a specific arm of the T-maze, probe trials with an eight-arm radial maze were interspersed with the usual T-trials. Control and fornix-lesioned animals consistently chose the side to which they were trained on the T-maze. However, when in the eight-arm radial maze, many animals did not choose the 90° arm but preferred either the 45° or the 135° arm, suggesting that the rats solved the T-maze by learning to rotate within an egocentric orientation system at the choice point (the maze junction) through approximately 90° (O'Keefe 1983). This led to the hypothesis of an orientation vector being stored in the animal's brain(with the actual turn depending on environmental cues to determine the appropriate movement most consonant with the encoded orientation)

With the short intertrial intervals used in this study (approximately 1 min), well-trained lesioned rats readily learned to reverse the T-maze habit. During reversal, every third trial was a probe with the eight-arm radial maze to assess the position of the orientation vector at that stage of learning. Fornix-lesioned animals showed a steady, incremental shift in the direction of the orientation vector from the original quadrant through straight ahead and into the new reversal quadrant. If observed only in the T-maze, the shift from the incorrect to the correct arm of the T-maze was relatively abrupt. However, as mentioned above, the orientation bias gradually swings from the direction of the originally rewarded turn through straight ahead and over the reversed turn when behaviour is observed in the eight-arm radial maze (Fig. 22.5a).

The behaviour of control rats during reversal training was different. Although performance on the T-maze proceeded in roughly the same pattern as in the lesioned rats, the underlying orientation vector of the group did not shift in a smooth fashion but jumped around. Examination of the individual curves also failed to reveal any systematic shifts (Fig. 22.8a).

Strongly motivated by these results, we developed two models of the rat navigational system/ The first, our TAM model of the rat's Taxon–Affordances system, explains data on the behaviour of fornix-lesioned animals. The second, our World Graph (WG) model, explains data on the behaviour of control rats and is also used for the study of cognitive maps(Together, these models shed light on the interactions between the taxon and locale systems and allow us to explain motivated spatial behaviour.) In order to describe both models, however, we first consider the notion of motivation, and its implementation as a motivational schema with a dual role: setting current goals and providing reinforcement for learning in TAM and in the WG model.

Motivation

A motivational system is required to select goals to be pursued and to organize the animal's commerce with appropriate goal objects. The hypothalamus has been divided into functionally related circuitry (subsystems) for eating, drinking, sex and temperature regulation (Swanson and Mogenson 1981). The hypothalamus can then be assumed to be the basic motivation-related neural circuitry. In the systems level model of Fig. 22.2, goals and motivational information are passed to the prefrontal cortex and basal ganglia. These are considered to form a 'potential field' planner in the sense that food, for example, is coded as an attractant field if the animal is hungry.

So far, most models of spatial learning and navigation do not incorporate the role of motivation into their computation. By contrast, the WG theory posits a set $d_1, d_2, \ldots, d_k$ of discrete drives to control the animal's behaviour. At time t, each drive d_i in $(d_1, \ldots, d_k)$ has a value $d_i(t)$. The idea is that an appetitive drive spontaneously increases with time towards d_{max}, while aversive drives are reduced towards 0, both according to a factor a_d intrinsic to the animal. An additional increase occurs if an incentive $I(d, x, t)$ is present such as the aroma of food in the case of hunger. Drive reduction $a(d, x, t)$ takes place in the presence of some substrate—ingestion of water reduces the thirst drive. If the animal is at the place it recognizes as being node x at time t, and the value of drive d at that time is $d(t)$, then the value of d for the animal at time $t+1$ will be:

$$d(t+1) = d(t) + a_d|d_{max} - d(t)| - a(d, x, t)|d(t)| + I(d, x, t)|d_{max} - d(t)|. \quad (22.1)$$

This is the drive dynamics incorporated into the motivational schema.

Moreover, our motivational schema is not only involved in setting current goals for navigation; it is also involved in providing reinforcement for learning. Midbrain dopamine systems are crucially involved in motivational processes underlying the learning and execution of goal-directed behaviour. Various studies have found that dopamine neurones in monkeys are uniformly activated by unpredicted appetitive stimuli, such as food and liquid rewards (Apicella et al. 1992; Schultz et al. 1995; Mirenowicz and Schultz 1996), and conditioned reward-predicting stimuli (for reward neurones in rats, see Lavoie and Mizumori 1994; Wiener 1993). Schultz et al. (1995) have hypothesized that dopamine neurones may mediate the role of unexpected rewards to bring about learning.

In the present work, reward information is used to learn *expectations* of future reinforcements. Furthermore, the motivational schema implements the idea that the amount of reward is dependent on the current motivational state of the animal. If the rat is extremely hungry, the presence of food might be

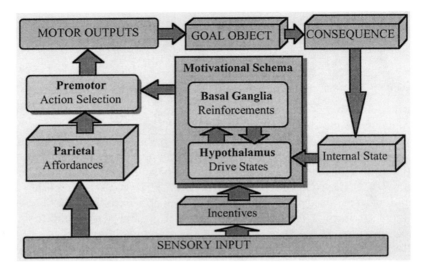

Fig. 22.3 Assemblage of TAM components. Parietal affordances, motivational information and drive-related stimuli are combined in the premotor cortex, where the selection of the next movement takes place.

very rewarding, but if not, it will be less rewarding. In this way, the influence of a reward $r(t)$ in TAM and the WG model will depend on the value of the animal's current dominant drive $d(t)$ (the maximum drive amongst all drives at a particular time, t), its corresponding maximum value, and the actual drive reduction, according to:

$$r(t) = \frac{d(t)}{d_{max}} a(d, x, t). \tag{22.2}$$

In this way, reward will bring about learning in TAM and the WG model depending on the animal's current motivational state. On the other hand, if the rat reaches the end of a corridor and does not find food, the drive reduction factor $a(d, x, t)$ is set equal to -0.1 times the normal value $a^*(d, x)$ it would have if food were present, and the motivational schema uses the above formula to generate a negative value of $r(t)$, a frustration factor, that will cause unlearning in TAM and in the WG model.

TAM: the taxon–affordances model

Our taxon–affordances model (TAM) is implemented by a reinterpretation of the Arbib and House (1987) model of frog detour behaviour. In this model, each prey object was represented by a peak of excitation coarsely coded across a population, while barriers to movement were encoded by inhibition whose extent was closely linked to the retinotopic extent of each barrier. The resultant sum of excitation was passed through a winner-takes-all circuit to yield the choice of movement direction. In TAM, however, the behavioural orientation system is implemented by replacing the direction of the prey (frog) by the direction of the orientation vector (rat), while the barriers correspond to directions in which no arm of the maze is visible, i.e. the presence of an obstacle or wall constrains the possible movements of the animal. Visible arms are encoded by the use of excitatory fields, since this seemed to accord with the idea of affordances, e.g. go straight if an opening exists.

Figure 22.3 shows the assemblage of TAM components. Sensory input provides the system with incentives and current affordances, as well as the sensing of drive relevant stimuli, like food. Parietal affordances, motivational information, and drive-related stimuli are then combined in the premotor cortex, where the selection of the next movement takes place. The premotor cortex is then considered to be the neural substrate of our action selection schema.

Recall the forementioned discussion of reversal of the T-maze habit in normal and fornix-lesioned rats. From the relatively smooth changing of the orientation vector shown by the fornix-lesioned animals, one might expect that, in their case, only the cells close to the preferred behavioural direction are excited, and that learning 'marches' this peak, called 'rewardness expectation' in the present work, from the old to the new preferred direction. However, the peak in our model does not actually march. Rather, it is the mean of two peaks that moves (Fig. 22.4). During reversal of the T-maze, the reinforcement learning rule, implemented in the present model by the use of temporal differences in an actor-critic architecture (Barto *et al*. 1983; Barto 1994; Sutton 1988), will 'unlearn' $-90°$ (turn to the left in the T-junction), by reducing the peak there, while at the same time 'building' a new peak at the new direction of $+90°$ (turn to the right in the T-junction). If the old reinforcement peak has 'mass' $p(t)$ and the new reinforcement peak has 'mass' $q(t)$, then as $p(t)$ declines toward zero, while $q(t)$ increases steadily from zero, the centre of mass, the animal's rewardness expectation:

$$\frac{(-90)p(t)+90q(t)}{p(t)+q(t)}, \tag{22.3}$$

will progress from -90 to $+90$.

The finding of food, besides reducing the hunger level, is also used as the only rewarding event by the reinforcement learning rule. In this case, the $r(t)$ value, supplied by the motivational schema, is used as the reinforcement signal. On the other hand, if the rat reaches the end of a corridor and does not find food, the frustration factor $u(t)$, also supplied by the motivational schema, is used by the reinforcement rule as a punishment signal. In TAM, reinforcement learning is used as a way of learning expectations of future reinforcement associated with state/action pairs, e.g. the expectation associated with turning left at the T-junction is increased if the rat finds food at the end of the left arm.

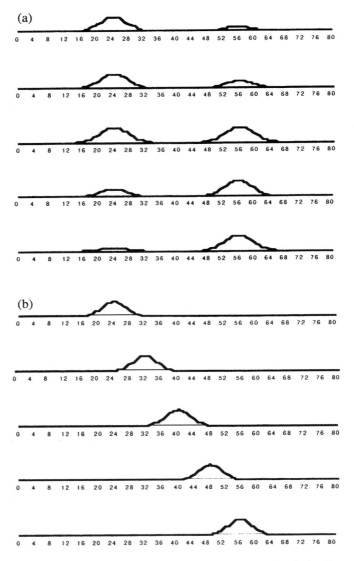

Fig. 22.4 (a) Peaks of reinforcement activity during reversal of the T-maze. Each activity bump (computed from the reinforcement weight, w) represents a previously reinforced action associated with the current state. The activity bump on the left is in fact decreasing. However, due to a normalization process used to generate the activity plots, it appears to decrease only when the activity bump in the right passes it in magnitude. Activity plots are depicted in intervals of four trials, approximately. (b) Marching from left to right of the rewardness expectation activity, $RE(i, t)$. Each activity bump represents the coarse coded centre of mass of its correspondent (from *top* to *bottom*) peaks of activity displayed in (a), where the maximum values of the left and right bumps are q and p, respectively.

The reinforcement learning system tries to influence the behaviour of the rat to maximize the sum of the reinforcement that will be received over time.

The decision to turn to a certain angle (the orientation vector) is given by a winner-takes-all process performed over the integration of fields produced by the available affordances (AF), drive relevant stimuli (ST), e.g. food if sensed, and rewardness expectation (RE), which contains an associated noise factor, $noise\_re$. In our model, then, the total input I_{in} to the action selection schema becomes:

$$I_{in}(i,t) = AF(i,t) + ST(i,t) + (RE(i,t) + noise\_re),\tag{22.4}$$

where i varies from 1 to N, the length of our population of cells in every linear array.

Under the influence of the rewardness expectation activity, the animal's turn will then be the available direction closest to that encoded by the 'centre of mass' of the neural activity in its reinforcement field, as shown in Fig. 22.4a. In this way, during reversal, the animal will march the peak from left to right (Fig. 22.4b).

The simulation results (Fig. 22.5b) replicate the data obtained by O'Keefe (1983) with fornix-lesioned animals (Fig. 22.5a). In Fig. 22.5, the top graphs show that the shift from the incorrect to the correct arm of the T-maze is reasonably abrupt in real and simulated rats; the bottom graphs show that the orientation bias gradually swings from the direction of the originally rewarded turn through

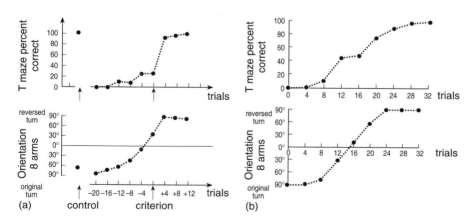

Fig. 22.5 *Top graphs*: percentage of correct choices on the T-maze task. *Bottom graphs*: choice of arm in the radial maze task. (a) The performance of six rats with fornix lesions during reversal on a T-maze. Each graph was obtained by averaging the graphs of the individual animals backwards and forwards from the beginning of the criterion run. Extracted from O'Keefe (1983). (b) The performance of 10 TAM simulated rats during reversal on a T-maze. The bottom graph was obtained by computing the medians amongst animals and trials (four by four). The top graph was obtained by averaging the performance of each animal over periods of four trials.

straight ahead and over to the reversed turn. We stress however that we see the orientation vector as, in this case, representing the mean of two peaks of activity.

For O'Keefe (1983), the fact that the shift in behaviour on the T-maze occurs around the point that the orientation bias crosses the midline suggests that the former is caused by the latter. The same shift in behaviour can also be observed in the data gathered from simulated animals. However, the rats in O'Keefe's experiment did go to the right side of the maze (a few times) even before the orientation vector had crossed the midline (Fig. 22.5a). In our simulations, the rat showed the same behaviour, but this behaviour actually accelerated the march of the reinforcement peak towards the right. Based on this, we prefer to assume that the shift in behaviour and the shift in the orientation vector are tightly related to each other in a mutually causal relationship.

The world graph model

The world graph model is strongly attached to the WG theory, which gives the model many of its features. In order to describe the WG model, we first describe the kinds of inputs presented to it, how these are processed, and how these inputs are finally incorporated into the model dynamics.

The WG model receives three kinds of inputs. These are given by three different systems the place layer, the motivational schema, and the action selection schema. The WG model is composed of three distinct layers (Fig. 22.6). The first layer contains coarse coded representations of the current sensory stimuli. This layer comprises four different perceptual schemas, which are responsible for coding head direction, walls, and landmarks (bearings and distances), respectively. Perceptual schemas incorporate 'what' and 'where' information, the kind of information assumed to be extracted by the parietal and infero-temporal cortices (Mishkin et al. 1983; Kolb et al. 1994) to represent the perception of environmental landmarks and maze walls. In this model, perceptual schemas, like affordances, employ coarse coding in a linear one-dimensional array of cells to represent pertinent sensory input.

In the WG model, two distinct perceptual schemas are responsible for presenting landmark information to the network: one to code landmark bearing and the other to code landmark distance. However, since the experiments here are landmark-free, the importance of landmarks for navigation and their further WG modelling will be described in another paper.

Walls are also responsible for the formation of the rat's local view. O'Keefe and Burgess (1996) show place cells responsive to the walls of a box environment that modify their place fields in relation to different configurations of the environment. Muller et al. (1987) observed that, in some cases, place cells had a crescent-shaped field that was assumed to be related to the arena wall. In the WG model, if the wall is close to the rat (less than a body length in the current implementation), it will be represented in the 'wall perceptual schema'.

Cells that show a unimodal tuning to head direction independent of location and relative to a 'compass direction' have been reported in several areas of the

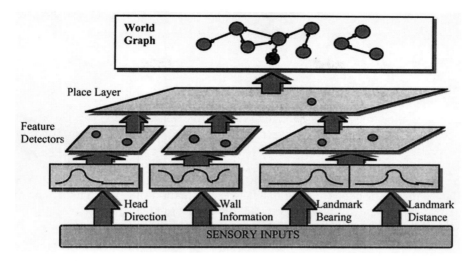

Fig. 22.6 The WG model components. Sensory inputs are coarse coded over linear arrays of cells, our perceptual schemas. These send information to feature detector layers, where the information is contrast-enhanced by a competitive process. The set of feature detector winners are, in turn, used by the Place Layer to determine the current place. Current place information is then used by the World Graph layer to determine its current active node, or, conversely, to determine if a new node must be created. In the current implementation, the World Graph is non-neural, and is represented as nodes connected by edges. Edges are directional and this is represented by a little circle attached to the nodes they point to. The currently active node is darker than the other nodes and has an × inside. In case of more than one landmark, new landmark feature detectors and perceptual schemas are added to the model for each landmark.

rat brain, including the postsubiculum (Taube *et al.* 1990a,b) and the posterior parietal cortex (PPC) (Chen *et al.* 1994a,b). Head direction cells provide the animal with an internal representation of the direction of its motion. This information, like the other perceptual inputs in the WG model, will be coarse coded as a bump of activity over a linear array of cells, the head direction perceptual schema.

Each perceptual schema projects in turn to its respective feature detector layer. Each of these layers are organized in a two dimensional matrix. Each node in the perceptual schema connects to all nodes in its corresponding feature detector layer, i.e. the two are fully connected. The feature detector units then interact through a local competition mechanism to contrast–enhance the incoming activity pattern, i.e. a neurone in a feature detector layer produces a non-zero output (G_j) if and only if it is the most active neurone within a neighbourhood. The adjustments to the connection weights between any pair of perceptual schema-feature detector layers are done using a normalized Hebbian learning algorithm. This ensures that the same set of feature detectors is activated by increasing the connection strength from active units (V_i) in the perceptual schema to active feature detectors, thereby increasing their response level the next time. This rule is captured in the following connection strength update equation:

$$\Delta w_{ij} = \alpha V_i G_j w_{ij}, \tag{22.5}$$

where Δw_{ij} is the change to the connection strength w_{ij} and α is the learning rate parameter.

Placed atop the feature detector layers is the Place Layer. This layer will keep track of the feature detector winners and will activate a different place/node if the set of winners that becomes active in the feature detector layers does not activate any previously activated node in the place layer. (The matching of winners is based on a pre-determined threshold.) In the WG theory there is a node for each distinct place/situation the animal experiences. This is implemented in the WG model by a functional layer, called the World Graph layer, placed above the Place Layer. In this way, for each 'new' set of feature detector winners, a 'new' node is activated in the place layer and, consequently, a node x is created in the world graph layer of the WG model.

In the WG theory, there is an edge from node x to node x' in the graph for each distinct and direct path the animal has traversed between a place it recognizes as x and a place it recognizes as x'. This is implemented in the WG model as a link between two nodes of the World Graph layer. If, for example, a node x is currently active at time t, but by deciding to move towards north the animal activates a 'different' set of feature detectors and so a distinct node x' in the world graph at time $t+1$, a link will be created from node x to node x'. Appended to each link/edge will be sensorimotor features associated with the corresponding movement/path. In the current model, these features consist of a motor efference copy (e.g. movement towards north) supplied to the world graph via a feedback connection from the action selection schema.

Edge information allows the animal to perform goal-oriented behaviours. As in TAM, the WG model learns expectations of future reward by the use of temporal differences learning in an actor–critic architecture (Barto *et al.* 1983; Barto 1994; Sutton 1988). In the WG model, however, expectations of future reinforcement are associated with pairs of nodes/edges, and not with state/ actions as is the case in TAM. For this reason, when a particular node of the world graph is active and, for example, the simulated animal is hungry, all it needs to do is to select the edge containing the biggest hunger reduction expectation and follow its direction towards the node it points to. In the WG model, each drive will have a drive reduction expectation value associated to it. In this way, if the rat is thirsty, it will not base the next node selection on hunger reduction expectations, but on thirst reduction expectations.

The integrated model: TAM and the WG model working together

The integrated model, TAM–WG, joins together TAM (Fig. 22.3) and the WG model (Fig. 22.6). The result is depicted in Fig. 22.7.

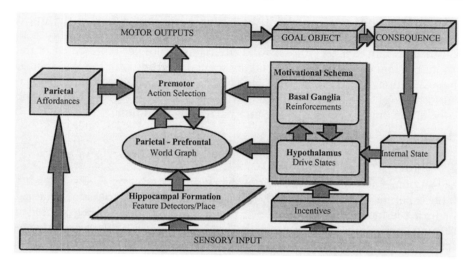

Fig. 22.7 Integrated TAM–WG model of rat navigation.

In TAM–WG, the decision to turn to a certain angle (the orientation vector) is given by a winner-takes-all process performed over the integration of fields produced by the available affordances (*AF*), drive relevant stimuli (*ST*), rewardness expectation (*RE*), map information from the world graph (*MI*), and a curiosity level (*CL*)—to be described below. *MI*, as well as *RE*, contains an associated noise factor, *noise_mi*. If a node x is active in the world graph, there will be expectations associated to each edge coming from node x. Since associated to each edge is the direction it points to, a peak of activity with the magnitude of the expectation associated to that node/edge pair will be coarse coded over a linear array of neurons in the location respective to the edge's direction. In TAM–WG, then, the total input I_{in} to the action selection schema becomes:

$$I_{in}(i,t) = AF(i,t) + ST(i,t) + (RE(i,t) + noise\_re)$$

$$+ (MI(i,t) + noise\_mi) + CL(i,t). \qquad (22.6)$$

Eventually, the selected motor outputs will enable the system to reach the goal object. When a selected action is executed, it will produce consequences in the animal's internal state and in the way it perceives the world (cf. the action–perception cycle, Arbib 1972). The internal state will alter the drive levels, which will in turn influence the selection of the next node in the world graph, and so on.

A crucial aspect of the WG theory and of the TAM–WG model is that an animal may go to places that are not yet represented in its world graph. To see how this occurs, we must clarify what is meant by a node x' immediately adjacent to a node x. Certainly, if there is an edge from x to x' in the world graph, then x' is immediately adjacent to x. However, the WG theory also considers as adjacent to x those world situations x' not yet represented in the graph, but that can be reached by taking some path from x. In the WG model, these situations will have a value attached to them, which can be seen as a 'curiosity level' attached to the unknown. The curiosity level is based on the value of the animal's biggest drive at a particular given time.

Experiments and results

As mentioned above, the behaviour of the control rats during reversal training in the experiments reported by O'Keefe (1983) was different from that obtained for fornix-lesioned animals. Although performance on the T-maze proceeded in roughly the same pattern as in the lesioned rats, the underlying orientation vector of the group did not shift in a smooth fashion but jumped around. Examination of the individual curves failed to reveal any systematic shifts (Fig. 22.8a). O'Keefe (1983) concluded that the reversal performance of the controls was not based solely on a shift in their orientation system but also on the rat's use of its hippocampal cognitive mapping system. He also assumed that this system can operate on the basis of the shape of the maze, since no landmarks were available during the task.

Figure 22.8b shows the performance of 10 TAM–WG simulated rats. Like O'Keefe's rats, our 'control rats' did not show any systematic shifts in behaviour.

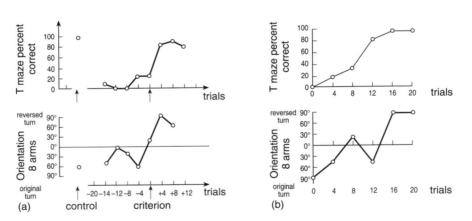

Fig. 22.8 (a) The performance of four control rats during reversal on a T-maze. Each graph was obtained by averaging the graphs of the individual animals backwards and forwards from the beginning of the criterion run. Extracted from O'Keefe (1983). (b) The performance of 10 TAM–WG 'rats' during reversal on a T-maze. The bottom graph was obtained by computing the medians amongst animals and trials (four by four). The top graph was obtained by averaging the performance of each animal over periods of four trials.

They randomly chose different arms to orient to when in the dais of the radial maze. However, by analysing the simulation results, we saw that the orientation vector given by the rewardness expectation signal shifts from the left quadrant to the right quadrant, just as in the TAM simulated animals.

In the present situation, however, when the simulated rat is learning to go to the left arm, the rewardness expectation signal given by TAM and the expectation of future reinforcement given by the world graph will coincide. In this case, the simulated rat will learn to go to the left consistently and will eventually meet the criterion once the combined expectation is bigger than noise. In fact, the animal will tend not to go to the right arm once it is represented in the rat's world graph, since the simulated rat already 'knows' that food was not found at that particular arm (there are no expectations of future reinforcement associated with any node/edge pair leading to the right arm). In this case, the rat's curiosity level for the right arm is decreased.

During reversal of the T-maze, the expectations of future reinforcement for the left arm will decrease continuously, since the absence of food is coded as a frustrating event by the reinforcement learning rule. When the combined expectation activity given by TAM and the world graph is smaller than the curiosity level, the TAM–WG simulated rat will persist in going to the left arm in the T-maze, but not in the radial arm maze. Since its curiosity level for the extra available arms is bigger than the one for the right and left arms, the rat will start to explore the arms not yet represented in its world graph. Once the combined expectation is smaller than noise, the rat will visit the right arm in the T-maze and will continuously create a peak of activity in the world graph and in TAM for the right arm. Since in the beginning the peak for the right arm is smaller than the combined curiosity and noise levels, the rat will still tend to choose arms randomly in the eight-arm maze. Although shifting steadily, the rewardness

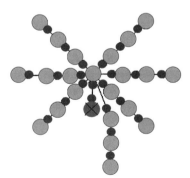

Fig. 22.9 World graph formed by the WG model after completion of the reversal T-maze task. The shape of the graph reflects the topology of the eight-arm radial maze. In the figure, the world graph is represented as nodes connected by edges. Edges are directional and this is represented by a little circle attached to the nodes they point to. The currently active node is darker than the other nodes and has an × inside.

expectation activity in this case is too small to influence the behaviour of the animal. The slow increase of activity in TAM can be explained due to a difference in the eligibility decay traces in the two systems. While the expectations in the world graph obey a fast-learning/fast-decay principle, expectations of future reinforcement in TAM obey a slow-learning/slow-decay mechanism.

The world graph constructed by a typical simulation of TAM–WG is depicted in Fig. 22.9. This figure was taken after the simulated rat finished the reversal task. It is easy to see in the figure that the world graph formed for the T-maze is contained in the world graph formed for the eight-arm radial maze. The node in the centre of the graph represents the T-junction and the dais of the radial arm maze. In fact, in the experiments conducted by O'Keefe (1983), the animals are always tested in the same eight-arm radial maze. However, for each T-trial five arms are pulled away from the centre so that the remaining three arms form the T-maze (there is no reason to think the animals do not recognize the dais of the maze for the T and radial maze conditions as the same place). During the simulated experiments, the animals were always placed in the same starting position in the south arm for the T and the eight-arm radial maze. The world graph depicted in Fig. 22.9 has also three nodes for each arm visited, with the exception of the 'north arm', which does not have any nodes associated to it, since it is represented by a single node, the one the animal was released from in the south arm (the rat senses each of these two arms in the same direction— north). The three nodes for each of the other arms represent a conjunction of head direction and wall information. Nodes in the extremities are coding for the end of an arm and head directionality. Since in this case no landmarks are available, the head direction information is used to distinguish the several arms.

22.4 Discussion

Our analysis of the role of hippocampus and parietal cortex in the rat has been informed both by our analysis of the monkey parietal cortex and by a broader systems view of the components of a cognitive map that go beyond signaling 'you are here'. In reviewing the distinction between the taxon and locale system we noted that affordances:

(1) generalize taxes and enable the rat to navigate in novel circumstances; and
(2) may refine plans inferred on the basis of a cognitive map by providing explicit information on actions possible in the current environment.

We note here a parallel with the way in which AIP may use current input to refine general grasp strategies that IT may outline on the basis of general object characteristics.

We rejected the McNaughton–Nadel model (Fig. 22.2a) by observing that MLC cells do not strongly encode place information. However, by analysing data from *monkey* parietal cortex, we were able to hypothesize *two* systems in *rat* parietal cortex: one detecting affordances (corresponding to cells that fire in preparation for a movement); and one based on optic flow and vestibular cues during the movement. This latter information corresponds in part to a new model by McNaughton *et al.* (1996), which pays attention to vestibular, but not optic flow, information, and posits a parietal system for 'path integration', updating the animal's estimate of head direction in a fashion remarkably similar to the dynamic remapping for saccades in monkey LIP. We note here that Touretzky and Redish (1996) have developed the CRAWL model of rodent navigation, which gives a functional non-biological analysis of the path integration mechanisms for spatial position (as distinct from head position), which underlie the ability of animals to find a direct path home after a complex outward trajectory. However, in more complex environments, a direct path is seldom adequate to reach home or some other goal. The WG theory offers key ideas for analysis of motivated behaviour in complex environments. In moving *beyond* path integration—selecting a complex path rather than constructing a straight path home—we may expect to encounter the problems of 'sequence management' (which, in our study of primate grasping, we suggested were the domain of interactions between pre-SMA and the basal ganglia.)

TAM–WG provides a model that can be used to answer how behavioural and spatial representations are compiled and how they are selected for use. Moreover, TAM–WG can be used to explain much spatial behaviour without requiring an *a priori* system for organizing sensations into an absolute spatial framework, as postulated by O'Keefe and Nadel (1978). For this reason, the model can be used as a modelling environment for the investigation of motivated spatial behaviour. It can also be viewed as a tool for development of biologically testable models of the cooperative computation of multiple brain regions as the animal explores its world in a goal-driven way.

With this, we have established the fruitfulness of a 'cooperative computation' model which:

(1) sees many parietal subregions as specialized for computing specific classes of affordances;

(2) stresses the interaction between these subregions, as well as the dynamic interaction of parietal cortex with other neural systems;

(3) learns from cross-species comparisons; and

(4) points up the importance of neural architectures which may implement related schemas (functional units such as dynamic remapping and path integration) in different species and, perhaps, within different brain regions in a given brain.

Acknowledgments

This work was supported in part by a Program Project (P20) grant from the Human Brain Project (P01MH52194), and in part by the National Science

Foundation (IRI-9221582). My thanks to Peter Dominey for his work on the saccade model; to Andrew Fagg for his work on the FARS model, and to Giacomo Rizzolatti and Hideo Sakata for their discussion of unpublished data; to Paul Rothemund for suggesting the role in navigation of parietal systems for detection of visual motion; and especially to Alex Guazzelli, Mihail Bota and Fernando Corbacho for valuable discussion which led to the results in Guazzelli *et al*. (1998).

References

Apicella, P., E. Scarnati, T. Ljungberg and W. Schultz (1992). Neuronal activity in monkey striatum related to the expectation of predictable environmental events. *Journal of Neurophysiology* **68**(3), 945–60.

Arbib, M. A. (1972). *The Metaphorical Brain: Cybernetics as Artificial Intelligence and Brain Theory*. New York, Wiley-Interscience.

Arbib, M. A. (1997). From visual affordances in monkey parietal cortex to hippocampo-parietal interactions underlying rat navigation. *Philosophical Transactions Royal Society of London B*, **352**, 1429–36.

Arbib, M. A., Erdi, P. and Szentágothai (1997) *Neural Organization: Structure, Function and Dynamics*. Cambridge, MA, MIT Press.

Arbib, M. A. and D. H. House (1987). Depth and detours: an essay on visually guided behavior. In (M. A. Arbib and A. R. Hanson, ed.), *Vision, Brain and Cooperative Computation*. pp. 129–63. Cambridge, MA, Bradford Book/MIT Press.

Arbib, M. A. and I. Lieblich (1977). Motivational learning of spatial behavior. In (J. Metzler, ed.), *Systems Neuroscience*, pp. 221–39. New York, Academic Press.

Baizer, J. S., L. G. Ungerleider and R. Desimone (1991). Organization of visual inputs to the inferior temporal and posterior parietal cortex in macaques. *Journal of Neurosciences* **11**, 168–90.

Barto, A. G. (1994). Adaptive critics and the basal ganglia. In (J. C. Houk *et al*., ed.), *Models of Information Processing in the Basal Ganglia*, pp. 215–32. Cambridge, MA, MIT Press.

Barto, A. G., S. Richard and C. W. Anderson (1983). Neuronlike adaptive elements that can solve difficult learning control problems. *IEEE Trans. on Systems, Man, and Cybernetics* **SMC-13**, 834–46.

Castiello, U., Y. Paulignan and M. Jeannerod (1991). Temporal dissociation of motor responses and subjective awareness: a study in normal subjects. *Brain* **114**, 2639–55.

Chen, L. L., L. H. Lin, E. J. Green, C. A. Barnes and B. L. McNaughton (1994*a*). Head-direction cells in the rat posterior cortex. 1. Anatomical distribution and behavioral modulation. *Experimental Brain Research* **101**(1), 8–23.

Chen, L. L., L. H. Lin, C. A. Barnes and B. L. McNaughton (1994*b*). Head-direction cells in the rat posterior cortex. 2. Contributions of visual and ideothetic information to the directional firing. *Experimental Brain Research* **101**(1), 24–34.

Colby, C. L., J. R. Duhamel and M. E. Goldberg (1993). Ventral intraparietal area of the macaque—anatomic location and visual response properties. *Journal of Neurophysiology* **69**, 902–14.

Dominey, P. F. and M. A. Arbib (1992). A cortico-subcortical model for generation of spatially accurate sequential saccades. *Cerebral Cortex* **2**, 135–75.

Droulez, J. and A. Berthoz (1991). A neural network model of sensoritopic maps with predictive short-term memory properties, *Proceedings of the National Academy of Sciences USA* **88**, 9653–7.

Eichenbaum, H., M. Kuperstein, A. Fagan and J. Nagode (1987). Cue-sampling and goal-approach correlates of hippocampal unit activity in rats performing an odor-discrimination task. *Journal of Neurosciences* **7**, 716–32.

Fagg, A. H. and M. A. Arbib (1998). Modeling parietal-premotor interactions in primate control of grasping. *Neural Networks*, in press.

Gibson, J. J. (1966). *The Senses Considered as Perceptual Systems*. London: Allen and Unwin.

Gnadt, J. W. and Andersen, R. A., (1988). Memory related motor planning activity in posterior parietal cortex of macaque. *Experimental Brain Research* **70**, 216–20.

Goldberg, M. E. and C. J. Bruce (1990). Primate frontal eye fields. III. Maintenance of a spatially accurate saccade signal. *Journal of Neurophysiol.* **64**, 489–508.

Graziao, M. S. A., R. A. Andersen and R. J. Snowden (1994). Selectivity of area MST neurons for expansion, contraction and rotation motions. *Investigative Ophthalmology and Visual Science* **32**, 823–82.

Guazzelli, A., F. J. Corbacho, M. Bota and M. A. Arbib (1998). Affordances, motivation, and the world graph theory. *Adaptive Behavior* **6**, 435–471.

Kase, C. S., J. F. Tronocoso, J. E. Court, J. F. Tapia and J. P. Mohr (1977). Global spatial disorientation: clinico-pathological correlations. *Journal of Neurological Sciences* **34**, 267–78.

Kolb, B., K. Buhrmann, R. McDonald and R. J. Sutherland (1994). Dissociation of the medial prefrontal, posterior parietal, and posterior temporal cortex for spatial navigation and recognition memory in the rat. *Cerebral Cortex* **4**(6), 664–80.

Lavoie, A. M. and S. J. Mizumori (1994). Spatial, movement- and reward-sensitive discharge by medial ventral striatum neurons of rats. *Brain Research* **638**(1–2), 157–68.

Lieblich, I. and M. A. Arbib (1982). Multiple representations of space underlying behavior. *The Behavioral and Brain Sciences* **5**, 627–59.

Lynch, J. C., Graybiel, A. M. and L. J. Lobeck (1985) The differential projection of two cytoarchitectonic subregions of the inferior parietal lobule of macaque upon the deep layers of the superior colliculus. *Journal of Comparative Neurology* **235**, 241–54.

Matelli, M., Luppino, G. and Rizzolatti, G. (1985) Patterns of cytochrome oxidase activity in the frontal agranular cortex of macaque monkey. *Behavioural Brain Research* **18**, 125–37.

Mays, L. E. and D. L. Sparks (1980). Dissociation of visual and saccade related responses in superior colliculus neurons. *Journal of Neurophysiol.* **43**, 207–32.

McNaughton, B. L. and L. Nadel (1990). Hebb–Marr networks and the neurobiological representation of action in space. In (Gluck, M. A. and Rumelhart, D. E., ed.), *Neuroscience and Connectionist Theory*, Chapter 1, p. 1–63. Norwood, NJ: Lawrence Erlbaum Associates.

McNaughton, B. L., B. Leonard and L. Chen (1989). Cortico-hippocampal interactions and cognitive mapping: a hypothesis based on reintegration of the parietal and inferotemporal pathways for visual processing. *Psychobiology* **17**, 230–5.

McNaughton, B. L., C. A. Barnes, J. L. Gerrard, K. Gothard, M. W. Jung, J. J. Knierim *et al.* (1996). Deciphering the hippocampal polyglot: the hippocampus as a path integration system. *Journal of Experimental Biology* **199**(Pt 1), 173–85.

Mirenowicz, J. and W. Schultz (1996). Preferential activation of midbrain dopamine neurons by appetitive rather than aversive stimuli. *Nature* **379**, 449–51.

Mishkin, M., L. G. Ungerleider and K. A. Mack (1983). Object vision and spatial vision: two cortical pathways. *Trends in Neuroscience* **6**, 414–7.

Muakkassa, K. F. and P. L. Strick (1979). Frontal lobe inputs to primate motor cortex: evidence for four somatotopically organized 'premotor' areas. *Brain Research* **177**, 176–82.

Muller, R. U., Kubie, J. L. and Ranck, J. B. (1987) Spatial firing patterns of hippocampal complex-spike cells in a fixed environment. *Journal of Neuroscience* **7**(7), 1935–50.

O'Keefe, J. (1983). Spatial memory within and without the hippocampal system. In (W. Seifert, ed.), *Neurobiology of the Hippocampus*, pp. 375–403. New York, Academic Press.

O'Keefe, J. and N. Burgess (1996). Geometric determinants of the place fields of hippocampal neurons. *Nature* **381**(6581), 425–8.

O'Keefe, J. and D. H. Conway (1978). Hippocampal place units in the freely moving rat: why they fire when they fire. *Experimental Brain Research* **31**, 573–90.

O'Keefe, J. and J. Dostrovsky (1971). The hippocampus as a spatial map. Preliminary evidence from unit activity in the freely moving rat. *Experimental Brain Research* **34**, 171–5.

O'Keefe, J. and L. Nadel (1978). *The Hippocampus as a Cognitive Map*. Oxford: Clarendon Press.

Ranck, J. B. (1973). Studies on single neurons in dorsal hippocampal formation and septum in unrestrained rats. I. Behavioral correlates and firing repertoires. *Experimental Neurology* **41**, 461–535.

Rizzolatti, G., R. Camarda, L. Fogassi, M. Gentilucci, G. Luppino and M. Matelli (1988). Functional organization of inferior area 6 in the macaque monkey II. Area F5 and the control of distal movements. *Experimental Brain Research* **71**, 491–507.

Sakata, H., M. Taira, A. Murata and S. Mine (1992). Neural mechanisms of visual guidance of hand action in the parietal cortex of the monkey. *Cerebral Cortex* **5**, 429–38.

Sakata, H., H. Shibutani, Y. Ito, K. Tsurugai, S. Mine and M. Kusunoki (1994). Functional properties of rotation-sensitive neurons in the posterior parietal association cortex of the monkey. *Experimental Brain Research* **101**(2), 183–202.

Schultz, W., R. Romo, T. Ljungberg, J. Mirenowicz, J. R. Hollerman and A. Dickinson (1995). Reward-related signals carried by dopamine neurons. In (J. R. Houk *et al.*, ed.), *Models of Information Processing in the Basal Ganglia*, pp. 233–48. Cambridge, MA, The MIT Press.

Sharp, P. E. and C. Green (1994). Spatial correlates of firing patterns of single cells in the subiculum of the freely moving rat. *Journal of Neurosciences* **14**, 2339–56.

Sutton, S. S. (1988). Learning to predict by the methods of temporal differences. *Machine Learning* **3**, 9–44.

Swanson, L. W. and G. J. Mogenson (1981). Neural mechanisms for the functional coupling of autonomic, endocrine and somatomotor responses in adaptive behavior. *Brain Research Reviews* **3**, 1–34.

Taira, M., S. Mine, A. P. Georgopoulos, A. Murata and H. Sakata (1990). Parietal cortex neurons of the monkey related to the visual guidance of hand movement. *Experimental Brain Research* **83**, 29–36.

Taube, J. S., R. U. Muller and J. B. J. Ranck (1990*a*). Head-direction cells recorded from the postsubiculum in freely moving rats. I. Description and quantitative analysis. *Journal of Neuroscience* **10**, 420–35.

Taube, J. S., R. U. Muller and J. B. Ranck, Jr (1990*b*). Head-direction cells recorded from the postsubiculum in freely moving rats. II. Effects of environmental manipulations. *Journal of Neuroscience* **10**(2), 436–47.

Tolman, E. C. (1948). Cognitive maps in rats and men. *Psychological Review* **55**, 189–208.

Touretzky, D. S. and A. D. Redish (1996). Theory of rodent navigation based on interacting representations of space. *Hippocampus* **6**, 247–70.

Wiener, S. I. (1993). Spatial and behavioral correlates of striatal neurons in rats performing a self-initiated navigation task. *Journal of Neuroscience* **13**(9), 3802–17.

23

Visuospatial processing in a pure case of visual-form agnosia

A. David Milner, H. Chris Dijkerman and David P. Carey

23.1 Introduction

Visual form agnosia refers to a variety of apperceptive agnosia in which the patient's ability to perceive, discriminate and recognize the shape of objects is grossly impaired (Benson & Greenberg 1969). Detailed case descriptions of such patients have been given by Goldstein & Gelb (1918), Adler (1944), Benson & Greenberg (1969), Landis *et al.* (1982) and Milner *et al.* (1991), and extensive experimental studies of their perceptual abilities have been presented by the same authors, as well as by Gelb & Goldstein (1938), Efron (1969), and Campion & Latto (1985). There is a remarkable similarity among these patients, both in their pathology and in their visual symptoms. In all cases the brain damage has been bilateral and in most cases caused by carbon monoxide poisoning, the principal exceptions being the patients of Goldstein & Gelb (missile injury) and Landis *et al.* (mercury poisoning). Also in all cases the profound deficit in form perception is seen without any appreciable deficit in auditory or tactile perception, and in most cases without any appreciable deficit in other domains of visual perception, including colour, motion, stereopsis and even visual acuity.

In addition to these preserved visual domains, the loss of visual form processing itself turns out not to be absolute. Visual discrimination performance is dependent on the behavioural response through which it is measured. This has been discovered through testing one exceptionally pure case of form agnosia, the young woman D.F. (Milner *et al.* 1991). In D.F., the processing of size and of orientation (whether manipulated in the picture plane, the horizontal plane, or the sagittal plane) appears to be severely compromised when tested using a range of conventional perceptual tasks. Yet these same dimensions are processed at a high level when tested using visuomotor tasks under normal conditions (Goodale *et al.* 1991; Milner *et al.* 1991; Carey *et al.* 1996; Dijkerman *et al.* 1996). These striking dissociations have led to the hypothesis that while visual form agnosia must involve severe damage to the occipito-temporal areas of the 'ventral' cortical processing stream as identified in the monkey (Ungerleider & Mishkin 1982; Morel & Bullier 1990; Felleman & Van Essen

1991; Tanaka 1997), it may leave the occipito-parietal regions that constitute the 'dorsal stream' largely intact (Goodale & Milner 1992; Milner & Goodale 1993, 1995). This interpretation is supported by findings of occipito-temporal damage in neuroimaging studies of other cases of apperceptive agnosia (Grossman *et al.* 1996).

This hypothesis is predicated on the premise that the dorsal stream in primates has the principal function of processing visual information for the purpose of controlling and guiding action (for related proposals, see also Glickstein & May 1982; Bridgeman 1992; Jeannerod & Rossetti 1993). In our view, then, the intact visuomotor abilities seen in D.F. are attributed to and identified with the human homologue of this dorsal system. Conversely, patients with optic ataxia, whose lesions invariably include damage to the superior region of the parietal lobe around the intraparietal sulcus, have visuomotor deficits that may be attributed to a disruption of this dorsal control system (Milner & Goodale 1995). While the damage to D.F.'s brain is not entirely restricted to the occipitotemporal region, her main visual symptoms can be seen as resulting from a selective disconnection which deprives visual form perception systems in the temporal lobe of their inputs from the primary visual cortex (Milner & Goodale 1995). The intact visual functions in D.F. may be mediated by a relative sparing of the 'parvocellular-blob' channel within the ventral stream (allowing her to perceive surface characteristics of objects like their colour and visual texture), along with the bulk of the dorsal stream pathway (allowing her a large measure of visuomotor control).

This hypothesis about D.F.'s functional lesion is consistent with our knowledge of the two streams of visual processing in the monkey as derived from both electrophysiological and neurobehavioural research (Milner & Goodale 1995; Milner & Dijkerman 1998). Our argument can therefore be turned on its head, in that one can regard D.F.'s lesion as an 'experiment of nature', which may shed light on the operating principles of the dorsal stream in the human brain. In other words, according to Milner & Goodale's hypothesis, investigating D.F.'s visual abilities could provide a rare opportunity to study the human dorsal stream in action, out of the shadow of the normally dominant ventral stream (Milner 1998).

The particular issue that we consider in this chapter is the nature and extent of D.F.'s visuospatial abilities, and what these may tell us about the visual function of the dorsal stream in the normal human brain. To put the question crudely: Does D.F. retain 'where' processing, and if so, what kinds of 'where' processing?

23.2 The dorsal stream and visual space

The majority of visually-driven neurones in the monkey's posterior parietal cortex (PPC) appear to contribute to the coding of egocentric spatial location for the purpose of directing motor acts. It has been known since the work of

Hyvärinen & Poranen (1974) and Mountcastle *et al*. (1975) that there are major classes of neurones in the PPC which are associated with:

(1) saccadic eye (and probably head) movements;
(2) pursuit eye (and probably head) movements;
(3) directed ocular fixations to particular parts of body-centred space; and
(4) reaching movements of the arm.

These classes of neurones have received detailed study since that time, and while all of them require some form of visuospatial analysis, the current view is that those analyses are not provided by a single all-purpose system in the PPC. Instead, it seems clear that there are multiple visuospatial coding systems in PPC, each associated with a different visuomotor modality (Rizzolatti *et al*. 1994; Colby & Duhamel 1997; Andersen 1997).

   For example, when a monkey is trained to respond to a given static stimulus in its visual field either by directing an eye movement or a hand movement to it, different subsets of neurones in the PPC are activated by the visual stimulus (Snyder *et al*. 1997). Similarly, moving stimuli are not processed in a uniform all-purpose way, even within the so-called 'motion area' (MT or V5). Already at this stage the signal is beginning to be analysed separately for different motor purposes. Thus Gruh *et al*. (1997) have found that although electrically microstimulating a given locus in area MT generally influences an ongoing saccadic or pursuit eye movement in mutually consistent ways, i.e. as if to allow for a particular movement of the target, occasionally it affects the two response modalities in quite different ways. Presumably this must reflect the activation of overlapping but distinct cell groups each passing different information regarding stimulus motion on to specialized saccadic and tracking systems in PPC areas such as 7a and LIP. Recent neuroimaging studies indicate that much the same is true in the human posterior parietal cortex: that is, there are quite separate visual representations for guiding eye movements and for guiding hand movements towards the same stimulus locations (Kawashima *et al*. 1996). When both eye and hand are allowed to move, both of these areas, located in different sectors of the human intraparietal sulcus, are activated.

   How is visual information coded in order to guide these different kinds of eye, head, and limb movements? We have reviewed elsewhere (Milner & Dijkerman 1998) the evidence from the laboratories of Andersen (see Andersen 1995) and of Galletti (see Battaglini *et al*. 1997) showing that several sub-areas of PPC contain visually-driven neurones that are modulated by gaze location. In other words, the neurones take some account of the eye's position in the orbit. By this means ensembles of cells could code visual location with respect to the head, and not only with respect to the retina. Furthermore, Brotchie *et al*. (1995) have shown that the monkey's head position can also influence the visual and saccade-related responses of some neurones in a comparable fashion, perhaps by virtue of proprioceptive or vestibular signals from the neck.

This modulation of neuronal responses by head position would therefore allow the representation of space in a body-centred coordinate system. Still other PPC areas contain neurones whose visual responsiveness is defined entirely in head-based coordinates, and not at all by the absolute location of the stimulus in the retina (Galletti *et al*. 1995; Duhamel *et al*. 1997).

These different ways of coding spatial location in PPC probably correspond to the different purposes to which the information is put (cf. Colby & Duhamel 1997). For example, neurones that explicitly code head-centred location may provide the necessary visual control for reaching, while assemblies of gaze-modulated retina-centred neurones may be used to provide the necessary visual control of saccadic eye movements. But all of these forms of spatial coding, of course, will only be of value over rather short time spans, since they relate the stimulus to the current location and body posture of the animal. Every time the animal moves its body as a whole, the usefulness of the coding will be lost. That is, all forms of egocentric spatial coding, while ideal for guiding action in the present and immediate future, will be counter-productive for storing spatial information for use very far in the future. Coding in egocentric coordinates on the other hand provides the necessary precise information about object location for calibrating the amplitude and direction of an immediate movement of the eye, head, or limb, and indeed for the on-line control and correction of such movements. Such egocentric coding therefore seems to be admirably suited to the visuomotor role that the dorsal visual pathway appears to play.

In contrast, movements that depend on visual information gathered during an earlier behavioural episode clearly have to depend on allocentric coding, since the animal is likely to have moved its own location and/or posture. In other words, the only reliable form of visual coding for spatial memory over timescales beyond a few seconds will be with respect to landmarks within the visual array. On this view, all movements that are delayed or postponed must depend on information about the relative location of the target object *vis-à-vis* other objects in the world. Presumably, whenever we encounter an important target object, therefore, it will make sense for the brain to encode the location of the object in *both* of these two different ways. The question is, does the spatial information for allocentric coding derive from the egocentric processing that we know occurs within the dorsal stream, or is it processed quite separately and in parallel with that dorsal-stream coding? Milner & Goodale (1993, 1995) have hypothesized that the latter is the case, and specifically suggested that allocentric coding may depend critically upon the ventral stream. In contrast, the 'where' characterization of the dorsal stream (Mishkin 1972; Ungerleider & Haxby 1994) argues for the former position, i.e. that the dorsal stream provides the necessary spatial information for both egocentric and allocentric coding.

We have examined D.F.'s visuospatial abilities with these two opposing views in mind, and have tried to compare both her immediate versus delayed use of location information and also her abilities to use allocentric versus egocentric forms of coding. Obviously her spatial abilities can only provide a lower bound on the capacities of the normal human dorsal stream for visuospatial coding, since there is likely to be some degree of damage to the dorsal system in her brain. Nonetheless our hope is that some general principles can be extracted from this programme of research which may provide pointers as to the operating characteristics of the intact system.

23.3 Manual reaching and saccadic eye movements

The first prediction that we must make about D.F.'s spatial abilities is that if she has a largely intact dorsal stream, then her immediate use of visual information for guiding her hand and eye towards target stimuli should be good, at least under normal testing conditions, despite her profound perceptual impairments. To this end, we have examined D.F.'s saccadic and reaching responses to targets located in different locations in her visual field. We have also varied the conditions under which she was asked to make her hand and eye movements, so as to explore the limits of the system she is using.

Movements made to peripheral visual targets

D.F.'s ability to make visuomotor responses to single visual targets was assessed using a series of different tasks. In the first task D.F. was required to make saccadic eye movements towards a target presented on a VDU screen at eight locations along the horizontal axis (Dijkerman *et al*. 1997). A fixation cross was situated in the centre, with four targets on either side. The inter-target distance was 2.5°. Two testing conditions were used. In the first condition, the subject was asked to make a saccade from the fixation cross towards the stimulus as soon as it appeared (immediate saccade task). D.F.'s performance on this task was very similar to that of two age- and sex-matched healthy control subjects (see Fig. 23.1 top). In the second block of trials, subjects were instructed to wait 5 s after stimulus disappearance before making the saccade (the delayed saccade task). Although the control subjects continued to direct their eye movements accurately towards the target location, D.F. performed this task considerably less accurately, sometimes making errors of several degrees in magnitude, and overall showing a greatly reduced gain (see Fig. 23.1 bottom).

The second task required D.F. to make manual pointing responses towards single targets presented at eight different locations. The targets consisted of LEDs mounted within a rectangular piece of black perspex which was placed in the frontal plane of the subject. The LEDs were only visible when lit. Again D.F. was asked to perform this task under two different conditions:

(1) to respond as soon as the target appeared; or

(2) to respond after a delay of 10 s.

A. D. Milner *et al.*

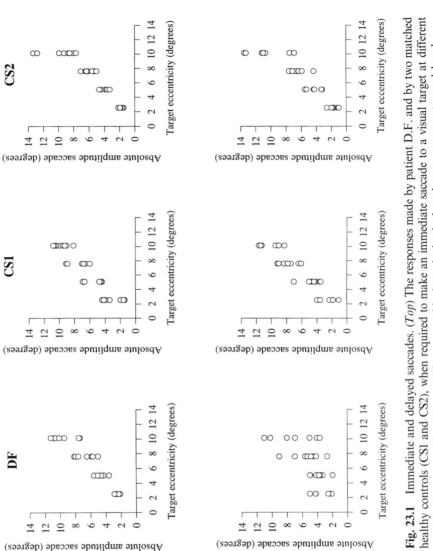

Fig. 23.1 Immediate and delayed saccades. (*Top*) The responses made by patient D.F. and by two matched healthy controls (CS1 and CS2), when required to make an immediate saccade to a visual target at different lateral eccentricities. (*Bottom*) The comparable data obtained when the eye movement was delayed.

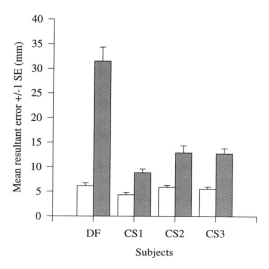

Fig. 23.2   Immediate and delayed pointing. The ordinate represents the mean error in mm of pointing responses to target LEDs presented at locations along the horizontal. The *open bars* of the histogram show the errors for immediate pointing, and the *filled bars* for delayed pointing. CS1, CS2, and CS3 are three matched healthy controls.

Her movements were recorded at 100 Hz using an Optotrak 3020 opto-electronic recording system (Northern Digital, Inc.). D.F.'s performance on these two tasks mirrored that seen in the saccadic eye movement tasks. Her immediate pointing responses were as accurate as those of three healthy control subjects, but her pointing became considerably less accurate when there was a delay between stimulus presentation and the pointing movement (see Fig. 23.2).

Movements made to visual targets lying in depth

Given recent findings that some dorsal stream mechanisms for sensorimotor control seem to depend critically on binocular vision (Sakata *et al.* 1997), we have examined D.F.'s processing of visual distance information in the depth dimension, to see to what extent it is preserved, and to what extent it may depend on the use of binocular vision (Carey *et al.*, in press).

In the first experiment, we used the same stimulus board as was used for pointing to lateral locations. This time it was placed flat on the table with its long axis lying sagittally, thus creating an array of stimuli lying horizontally in depth. D.F. was asked to make an immediate pointing response towards a single lit LED presented at 16 different positions. The task was performed under both binocular and monocular (dominant eye) viewing conditions. Again the Optotrak recording system was used to analyse the movements. D.F.'s performance under binocular viewing conditions was slightly less accurate than that of the three normal control subjects, but her errors were almost twice as large under monocular viewing conditions as under binocular viewing conditions (see Fig. 23.3). In contrast, the removal of binocular vision resulted only in a marginal decrease in pointing accuracy in the control subjects.

We also examined the velocity profiles of the pointing movements. Under binocular viewing conditions, the maximum resultant velocity of the hand during the movement was highly correlated with target distance in D.F. ($r = +0.81$, $P < 0.001$; as compared with $r = +0.87$, $+0.86$, and $+0.66$ for the three healthy control subjects; all correlations significant at $P < 0.001$). In contrast to the results for endpoint accuracy, the removal of binocular vision did not result in any major changes in these correlations between peak velocity and target distance ($r = +0.85$, $P < 0.001$ for D.F., and $r = +0.85$, $+0.69$, and $+0.67$, for the three controls, again all significant at $P < 0.001$). Although showing the normal high correlation with distance, however, D.F.'s peak velocities were lower than those of our control subjects (averaging 67.9 cm/s overall, as opposed to 92.8, 127.2, and 152.4 cm/s for the three controls).

Inspection revealed that most of her terminal errors were due to her falling short of the target. Thus it may be that her visuomotor system is subject to a consistent under-estimation of the distance of targets, especially under monocular conditions, rather than to an increase in random error. This would partly explain the lower velocities of her reaching movements, given the normal tendency for people to reach more slowly to closer targets.

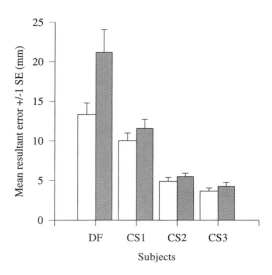

Fig. 23.3 Pointing in depth. The ordinate represents the mean error in mm of pointing responses to target LEDs presented at locations arrayed in the sagittal plane. The *open bars* of the histogram show the errors made under binocular viewing conditions, and the *filled bars* under monocular conditions. CS1, CS2, and CS3 are three healthy controls (not the same as in Fig. 23.2).

In a second experiment, we examined reaching and grasping for solid objects located in depth, so that we could examine D.F.'s processing of both distance and object size in parallel. We asked her to reach out and grasp cubes of three different sizes (3, 5 and 7 cm^3) placed one at a time at five different distances (16, 22, 28, and 34 cm) on the table in front of the subject. Head position was stabilized using a chin rest, and subjects were required to use their index finger and thumb (precision grip) for each grasp. They were tested in six blocks of trials, alternating between binocular and monocular viewing conditions. Movements were again recorded using the Optotrak 3020 system. Subjects also participated in a distance estimation task, modelled after the grasping task procedure, except that instead of reaching, they estimated in inches the distance of the object from the same start position as used in the grasping trials. Subjects were shown an inch on a ruler before testing began.

The results of this experiment were clear (Carey *et al.*, in press). In the grasping task, D.F. scaled her movements as accurately as the controls. Just as in the pointing experiment, her peak velocity was highly correlated with object distance under both binocular and monocular viewing conditions ($P < 0.001$ in both conditions in all subjects). Thus, the data from both of these experiments agree in showing that on this measure D.F.'s visuomotor system was processing 3-D distance rather efficiently for the purpose of programming and guiding her reaches. In sharp contrast, however, D.F.'s verbal estimates of distance correlated well with actual object distance only under binocular viewing conditions, and even here the correlation was lower than normal ($r = +0.73$, as opposed to $+0.93$ and $+0.95$ in the controls: all significant at $P < 0.001$). In fact, although her estimates tended to increase with increasing object distance, they typically fell short of the actual distances by 40–50 per cent. Under monocular conditions, the correlation fell to $+0.29$ in D.F., a value only just significant at $P < 0.05$, while the correlations in the controls remained very high ($+0.98$ and $+0.96$, both $P < 0.001$).

Thus the results of this experiment are consistent with those of the previous experiment, in that they show that D.F.'s ability to calibrate the velocity with which she reaches to visual targets in depth is not severely disrupted even under monocular viewing; but in contrast they show that her *perception* of depth can be severely disrupted, especially when binocular information is unavailable. These data suggest the possibility that 'pictorial' depth cues can be used by neurologically intact subjects to guide monocular grasping, and that such cues may depend on an intact ventral stream for their processing. This hypothesis suggests that illusions of pictorial depth should affect grasping in depth more under monocular than binocular conditions.

Summary: locating single visual targets

We may conclude from this series of experiments that under normal conditions D.F. is able to direct her saccadic eye movements and manual reaching movements quite accurately in space, as one would expect if her dorsal stream has remained largely intact. However it is also clear that there are severe limitations on these abilities. First, the imposition of a delay greatly reduces her response accuracy, both when she is reaching towards a target and when she is making a saccadic eye movement towards it. Second, when her use of binocular viewing is prevented, D.F.'s terminal accuracy at reaching in depth towards targets placed at different distances is quantitatively impaired, though she remains able to scale her reaching velocity well as a function of distance. Yet despite this partly preserved visuomotor guidance of reaching in depth, D.F. is clearly impaired when she has to estimate the same distances verbally, especially when reliant upon monocular vision.

These results are broadly consistent with previous studies carried out with D.F. Thus Goodale *et al.* (1994) reported that D.F.'s ability to calibrate her anticipatory finger-thumb grip size when reaching out to grasp blocks of different width fell to chance when a delay of as little as 2 s was imposed on her. This is a dramatic result, given the normality of D.F.'s grip calibration under normal circumstances (Goodale *et al.* 1991). Taking these results with three different response modalities (finger grip, arm reach, and saccadic eye movement) together, it can be argued that the visuomotor systems that D.F. is using must be highly time-limited. Of course a short time constant of this kind is exactly what would be expected if the dorsal stream is designed to control movements in the 'here and now' rather than providing a more generalized visual representation of space.

The second finding, of a loss of accuracy when monocular viewing is used, is also consistent with previous research. Thus both Dijkerman *et al.* (1996) and Marotta *et al.* (1997) have shown that D.F. becomes substantially less accurate in her grasping behaviour when viewing a target object monocularly. This finding holds good for both the control of grip aperture when reaching to grasp blocks placed at different distances in depth (Marotta *et al.* 1997), and for the control of grip orientation when reaching to grasp a square plaque tilted at different orientations in depth (Dijkerman *et al.* 1996). It may be assumed that in both tasks our ability to make an accurate grasp under monocular conditions will depend critically on the processing of pictorial depth cues, i.e. information such as visual perspective and context. These monocular cues will be available to normal observers, but perhaps not to D.F. The corollary of this interpretation is that the dorsal stream in isolation must be highly dependent on *binocular* cues to depth. Such a conclusion would fit well with the discoveries by Sakata and his colleagues (1997), who have shown that many visually-driven PPC neurones that are selectively sensitive to the orientation of surfaces in depth lose this selectivity under monocular viewing conditions.

Our data also show, however, that D.F.'s *subjective estimates* of distance are very severely disrupted under monocular viewing conditions. Dijkerman *et al.* (1996) similarly reported that D.F.'s accuracy when asked to make a manual match to a target oriented in depth suffered a severe deterioration under monocular viewing conditions. It is possible that even under these ostensibly 'perceptual' testing conditions D.F. is actually still using her visuomotor system to guide her responses, e.g. through the mediation of motor imagery. We have gathered some data supporting the idea that she sometimes spontaneously uses such a strategy when trying to make perceptual judgements of size and orientation (Dijkerman & Milner 1997; Dijkerman *et al.*, in preparation). Presumably when D.F. imagines reaching for an object viewed monocularly, these motor images will be less precise than images she can produce under binocular conditions, just as her real reaches are less precise. Thus if she is using an imagined reach when making distance estimates, then her accuracy would be expected to deteriorate under monocular conditions.

Multiple responses

In a recent abstract, Murphy & Goodale (1996) reported that D.F. was able to point to any designated one of a set of differently coloured circular tokens set out randomly on a square board in front of her (see also Murphy *et al.* 1998). We have confirmed and extended this observation (Carey *et al.*, in preparation). Not only could D.F. point correctly (and with spatial precision) to any single named token in such a display, she was also able to point to up to five such tokens in a nominated sequence, and also to point simultaneously to any two of them using the forefingers of her two hands together. Fingertip accuracy was confirmed using the Optotrak motion analysis system. D.F. was every bit as accurate as the two age- and sex-matched control subjects on all three of the pointing tasks (single-target pointing, serial pointing, and bimanual pointing).

While it is true that in pointing simultaneously to two locations in this task, D.F. might be said to be taking into account the separation between two stimuli in space and separating her effectors in accordance with that inter-stimulus separation, it would not follow that she was using allocentrically coded spatial information to perform the task. It is equally possible, and arguably more probable, that she is using the egocentrically coded location of each target stimulus in guiding her two responses. Parsimony therefore dictates that we cannot use these findings as evidence for intact allocentric coding. In order to seek more definitive evidence that D.F. may have the use of such coding, it is necessary to use more complex tasks.

23.4 Perception of spatial relationships

In the same study, Murphy & Goodale (1996) also reported that D.F. was unable to reproduce the sets of tokens set out in front of her, when asked to do so on a separate but identical board situated immediately to the right of the stimulus array. We have replicated and extended these observations by asking D.F. and two age- and sex-matched control subjects to respond to multi-target arrays in a number of different ways (Carey *et al.*, in preparation). In the first task, subjects were required first to enumerate the number of tokens present in the display, and then to judge which two tokens were closest to one another, and which two were farthest apart. Several of these judgements were quite difficult. Surprisingly, D.F. performed well on both of these tasks. She gained 91 per cent correct responses, in comparison with 100 per cent for each of the two controls on counting; and 75 per cent correct responses, in comparison with 87 per cent and 91 per cent for the two controls, on relative separation judgements. Nonetheless, it was notable on the videorecordings of her behaviour that she made large and frequent head movements during these tasks, behaviour that was not noticeable in the controls. Furthermore, she usually enumerated the tokens by first saying what colours she saw, and then apparently counting the number of colour words she had just uttered. It is possible therefore that her success in these apparently allocentric tasks may again have been based on a strategy in which she moved her gaze in a sequential manner which she could then use to link a colour (and thus an individual object) with a fixation (eye/head) location. Her relative separation judgements might then have been 'read off' as proprioceptive distances between her successive head positions.

Like Murphy & Goodale (1996), we have found that when asked to reproduce an entire target array as precisely as possible on the separate blank board using an identical set of coloured tokens, D.F. performed very slowly and inaccurately. Furthermore, we also found that she performed poorly in a task where she had to indicate the spatial locations of *individual* target stimuli on the response board. In this task, subjects were required to point to the equivalent position of a specified target or targets; for example, if a red target was specified, the subject was required to point to the absolute position that the target would occupy if the stimulus array was translated to the right by its own width. Yet despite the absolute inaccuracy of her responses, D.F.'s pointing positions tended to bear some resemblance to the relative spatial positions of the targets; for example, if a blue target was below and to the right of a red target, her response when asked for blue would be roughly below and to the right of where she pointed when asked to point to where the red token was on the blank array. Her reproductions of the arrays resulted in similar errors: relative positions of tokens (e.g. blue token is to the left and above the red token) were often reasonably preserved in her copy, while the absolute distances between the tokens were much less accurately copied. D.F.'s errors occurred in spite of the fact that the target array was always present and could be continuously referred to while reproducing the arrays on the blank surface.

These data suggest that if D.F. does have allocentric spatial information available to her, it is very crude. It might be said to be of a 'categorical' nature rather than of a 'coordinate' nature (Kosslyn 1987). But as before, the pattern of results as a whole could equally well be seen as reflecting an egocentric strategy in which she was able to register spatial relationships only by monitoring her own movements while successively fixating the individual stimuli. It is her consistent introspective report that she deals with one token at once in these tasks, and is unable to inter-relate the whole set as a visual pattern. It may be, however, that she can form a supramodal spatial representation using kinaesthetic monitoring of her actions—actions that are guided by egocentric visual information.

It appears from these experiments that D.F. has a particular difficulty in making judgements of the positions of targets within a square array, unless she is allowed to make an egocentrically-driven visuomotor response to that target. In contrast, normal subjects are quite capable of making such judgements regarding the target array and using the information to guide visuomotor responses with respect to a separated response array. They can also of course readily relate the tokens together as an overall *gestalt* within the stimulus array, which they can use to help them reproduce the absolute spatial positions of the targets.

It could be argued that it is unfair to expect D.F. to perform *perceptual* tasks involving allocentric coding of space, given that as a visual-form agnosic, she has—by definition—a profound impairment of visual perception. It might be fairer to offer D.F. the opportunity instead to make manual responses that could be *guided* by allocentric spatial coding. We therefore designed a new visuomotor task that was intended to maximize the opportunity for D.F. to use allocentric spatial processing, but which at the same time would minimize the usefulness of egocentric spatial information. The task requires her to make a range of direct manual responses on the basis of different spatial arrangements in the visual array.

23.5 Visual coding of spatial relationships for action

We devised a set of circular discs (13 cm diameter) made of transparent perspex, each of which had circular holes cut in it. We presented the discs singly to D.F. in the frontal plane, and asked her to reach out and grasp them by inserting her fingers through the holes, which were painted red for clarity. In this way we were able to look for evidence for accurate visual guidance of her fingers during the prehension movement with respect to both the separation of pairs of target holes and the angle formed by a line joining them. Given that D.F. is skilled at orienting her wrist and opening her finger-thumb grip in order to grasp objects of different shapes, sizes and orientations, this task seemed well suited to her visuomotor abilities. There were two levels of task difficulty, in which we used either discs with three holes (for the forefinger, thumb and middle finger), or with two holes (for the forefinger and thumb only). In both tasks the forefinger–thumb distance was varied (see Figs 23.4 and 23.5). In addition, the forefinger–thumb axis was either placed vertical, or tilted 45° to the left or right. Also, two different positions of the middle finger hole were used in the three-finger task (diagonally above or below the index-finger hole). In the two-finger task, the two holes were situated either in the centre, or 2 cm to the left or to the right of the centre of the disc. Since all of the holes were painted red, D.F. had no possibility of 'colour coding' each location. The prehension movements were videotaped and analysed frame by frame (Dijkerman *et al.* 1998).

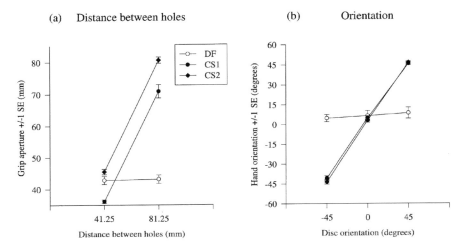

Fig. 23.4 Grasping three-hole discs. (a) The separation between forefinger and thumb as the hand approaches the disc (two frames—40 ms—before contact). The two healthy control subjects (*filled symbols*) open their grip to match the separation between the appropriate holes in advance of contact with the disc. D.F., however, shows no such ability to match her grip to the distance between the holes (*open circles*), tending to keep her finger and thumb at a default separation corresponding to the smaller inter-hole distance. (b) The orientation of the hand at the same point during the reach. The two controls match the hand orientation to the relative positions of the holes almost perfectly, while again D.F. shows almost no tendency to do this, tending to maintain her hand near a default vertical orientation.

The results were clear. D.F. was completely unable to adjust her grip or hand orientation on the basis of the positions of the holes in the three-finger task (Fig. 23.4). While the controls opened their forefinger–thumb grip, and oriented the hand, so as to closely match the appropriate holes, D.F. showed no such tendency. Instead, she had to correct her hand posture on contact with the disc, using tactile cues. In contrast, she did orient her hand correctly, and also aimed her hand to the left or right when required, in the two-finger task (Fig. 23.5b–d). Yet even in the two-finger task, she still remained quite unable to modulate her forefinger-thumb grip scaling as a function of the inter-hole distance (Fig. 23.5a). Although there was now a significant trend to match the distance, she still had to depend on tactile contact to insert her fingers into the holes. Particularly striking was the observation that on many trials (55.6 per cent in the three-hole task, 39.5 per cent in the two-hole task) D.F. inserted the *wrong* finger into one or more hole(s), e.g. inserting the forefinger into the hole lowest on the disc intended for the thumb. Control subjects never made this mistake.

It thus seems clear that D.F. was quite unable to extract any allocentric spatial information from the pattern of holes set in the stimulus discs. She was

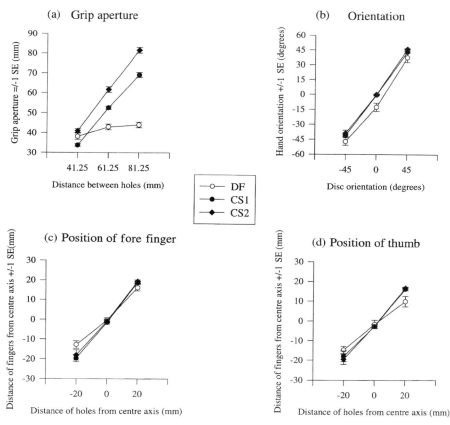

Fig. 23.5 Grasping two-hole discs. (a) Shows the separation between forefinger and thumb as the hand approaches the disc. The two healthy controls (*filled symbols*) again open their grip to match the separation between the two holes in advance of contact with the disc, while D.F. (*open circles*) shows only a minimal tendency to match her grip to the distance between the holes. (b) Shows the orientation of the hand as it approaches the disc. Here D.F. is as accurate as the two controls in matching her hand to the orientation formed by the two holes. (c) and (d) Depict the accuracy with which D.F. aims for the part of the disc (left, centre or right) where the holes are located. It is clear that she is almost as accurate as the controls in doing this, especially with her forefinger.

Thus she can locate the holes reasonably well in egocentric space.

only able to extract egocentric information sufficient to allow her:

(1) to direct her hand to the appropriate left/right part of the disc (see Fig. 23.5c and 23.5d); and

(2) to orient her hand with respect to a single pair of holes (see Fig. 23.5b).

When three holes were present in the display, this ability to orient the hand was lost (Fig. 23.4b).

But why should D.F. be able to respond well to the orientation of the dipole formed by two holes, yet not be able to respond to their separation? One possibility is that the two holes, of similar colour, provided some energy within a low spatial frequency bandwidth, and that this was sufficient to activate orientation selective neurones within the magnocellular channel and hence the dorsal stream. Such neurones would have allowed her to achieve what she did achieve in the two-hole condition, i.e. accurate reaching to the correct part of the disc and accurate turning of the hand to the correct orientation. But they would not have allowed her to deal with three-hole discs (in which presumably no clear axis was formed by the holes). Neither, probably, would they have enabled D.F. to adopt a suitable finger-thumb grip aperture in either of the two conditions.

We believe that the accurate performance of the complete act of disc-grasping requires an allocentric coding of the pattern of holes, and consequently the participation of the ventral as well as the dorsal stream. The dorsal stream can guide the forefinger (usually the leading digit) accurately into one of the holes, and can cause the wrist to rotate to the correct orientation. This can all be done egocentrically. But the opening of the forefinger-thumb grasp, let alone the choice of the correct hole for the forefinger to enter, requires allocentric information processed via the ventral stream. Not having the benefit of that form of coding, D.F. was quite unable to perform these aspects of the task. It is notable that even normal subjects do not find the task an easy or natural one to perform—it does not have the effortless feel of some of our other visuomotor tasks such as grasping solid objects. Thus we tentatively conclude that the task is not one that the dorsal stream has evolved to cope with alone: the task also needs guidance from perceptual processes within the ventral stream.

In other words, it may be that even a simple motor task, if it requires allocentric coding, forces the observer to use his or her ventral stream. Yet of course we found in the previous set of experiments that D.F. could successfully point to two separate tokens when using the forefingers of her two hands. Presumably, therefore, she could have pointed to the two holes in the disc-grasping experiment using her two forefingers. Each hand would then be performing a separate act of egocentric localization, and no allocentric coding would be required. But one cannot point to two places at once with one hand, except by coding the separation of those two places, i.e. using allocentric coding.

These findings suggest an interesting limitation on dorsal stream visual processing. While D.F. can use the size of a single object to calibrate her finger-thumb aperture with exquisite accuracy (Goodale *et al.* 1991; Carey *et al.* 1996), it appears that she cannot use the distance between two objects for the same purpose. In other words, D.F. can control her grip as a function of visual *size*, but she cannot do so as a function of visual *distance*. Indeed the 'unnaturalness' of forming a grip in order to match a spatial separation rather than a size that was experienced by our healthy controls in the disc-grasping task suggests that the two tasks present very different visuomotor problems to the observer. One can be solved without conscious perception; the other perhaps cannot. Accordingly, we find it difficult to accept the recent suggestion that the automatic grip calibration exhibited by normal people during reaching for an object is a response to the spatial separation between the contours of the object, rather than to its size *per se* (Brenner & Smeets 1996).

23.6 Discussion

One of the major questions over our attribution of D.F.'s pattern of visual abilities to her use of a relatively-intact dorsal stream (Milner & Goodale 1995), is the extent of her visuospatial ability. We have argued that the dorsal stream carries out computations on the visual array to furnish the necessary information for guiding actions with respect to individual objects, but that the actual perception of visual properties, including their spatial relationships, is governed by the ventral system. Accordingly there would be no expectation that D.F. should be able to achieve spatial percepts, despite being well able to guide her actions in space. Furthermore, we have argued that the dorsal stream has evolved for the guidance of action in *egocentric coordinates*, in order to expedite 'on-line' an animal's dealings with its visual world. We have conceptualized the ventral stream, on the other hand, as providing the visual information for longer-term spatial coding, which necessarily has to be largely allocentric, so that location is linked to landmarks rather than to the (more mobile) observer. In contrast, the currently prevalent view (Ungerleider & Mishkin 1982; Ungerleider & Haxby 1994) is that the visual processing of space, of all kinds and for all purposes, is mediated by the dorsal stream.

The data we have summarized here suggest that although D.F. is well able to code locations in her visual field for the guidance of immediate eye and hand movements, she begins to have difficulties when the movement has to be preceded either by a delay or by the mediation of a recoding operation in which the response is relocated elsewhere in movement space. She also performs poorly when the task requires the exact coding of the distance between two or more stimulus elements. Thus our data are consistent with the idea that allocentric spatial coding is not possible in D.F., perhaps as a consequence of the fact that such processing is parasitic upon the perceptual processing of the array. It is true that in our 'allocentric' tasks of token reproduction and disc grasping, D.F. seems to be able to match the orientation formed by pairs of stimuli with better than chance accuracy—but parsimony dictates that the egocentric strategy of kinaesthetically coding her direction of gaze shift between elements could handle this aspect of spatial relationships without the need for truly visual allocentric coding. When distances have to be matched (either with tokens or with the digits in the disc-grasping task) D.F. falls to something approaching a chance level of performance.

Of course there are other possible interpretations of our data. In particular, it is possible that frontal-lobe damage interferes with D.F.'s spatial working memory. We know from structural MRI evidence that she does have diffuse bilateral prefrontal damage, though relatively mild (Milner *et al*. 1991), and both lesion and electrophysiological evidence indicate that short-term working memory for spatial location depends on prefrontal mechanisms (e.g. Funahashi *et al*. 1989, 1993). Therefore it might be predicted that her frontal damage would cause D.F. to be impaired at making delayed reaches and saccades. On the other hand, it is difficult to see how D.F.'s problems with the wide range of spatial perceptual tasks (including tasks that have no memory component) that we have described could be attributed to prefrontal damage. Furthermore if D.F.'s frontal damage were severe enough to cause a profound disruption of spatial coding then one would expect it also to cause disinhibitory effects, such as incorrectly directed saccades in an anti-saccade task (Guitton *et al*. 1985). In other words, when instructed to move her eyes to the mirror-image location with respect to a visual stimulus, she should tend to make incorrect saccades *towards* the stimulus instead. But although we have found that D.F.'s eye movements are very inaccurate in *magnitude* in such an anti-saccade task (Dijkerman *et al*. 1997), we did not observe any occasions when she made saccades in the wrong *direction* (i.e. towards the stimulus). Instead she moved the eyes away from the stimulus (correctly), but generally to default locations around the middle of the range.

We conclude that our data are consistent with the idea that allocentric visuo-spatial information is not processed within the dorsal visual stream *per se*. In reaching this conclusion, we are not of course denying that allocentric spatial information can influence motor acts. What we are suggesting is that the motor system may only be able to use such information after it has first been processed by the perceptual system (which we assume is not available in D.F.).

There are a number of published reports on healthy observers indicating that visuomotor responses—when made immediately—depend preferentially upon egocentrically-coded spatial information, while perceptual judgements or delayed motor responses tend to be driven by allocentric information. Thus illusions of spatial location (e.g. the moving-frame illusion or the Roelofs effect), while spectacularly able to fool our perceptual system, do not deceive our saccadic eye movement system (Wong & Mack 1981), nor do they, in general, cause errors of immediate manual pointing (Bridgeman *et al*. 1981, 1997). These illusions do, however, come into play when our motor responses are delayed (Wong & Mack 1981; Bridgeman *et al*. 1997). Delays of a few seconds seem to cause a qualitative shift in the visual programming of spatially-directed action, rather than just a quantitative loss of accuracy. Indeed this qualitative change can become apparent even without the help of visual illusions. For example, Rossetti (1998) has reported that subjects distribute their errors when making immediate pointing responses in a quite different way from the errors they make when responding after a delay of more than 1 s. While the errors made in immediate pointing tended to be related to the starting position of the hand, those made following a delay showed a greater dependence on visual contextual factors, i.e. the spatial arrangement of the target array.

Yet while there is a meaningful qualitative distinction to be made in such experiments between egocentric and allocentric coding, there is no doubt that the two forms of coding can act together in guiding a given action. Indeed it will be rare under normal conditions for any given task to tap only one or the other component. A good example is provided by the work of Gentilucci and his colleagues (1997). They have shown that the presence of Muller-Lyer 'fins' causes illusory overshoot or undershoot errors when subjects point to the end of a line, and that while these errors increase with delay, they are still present even during immediate pointing. The authors argue that these illusory effects reflect allocentric coding of the location of the endpoint of the line. If so, then their results suggest that although the influence of this form of coding can be increased by certain manipulations, it can probably never be removed altogether, at least in a visual array where multiple stimulus elements are present. Only isolated single stimuli could ever be totally free of some degree of allocentric coding. In all other situations, allocentric coding may in fact be obligatory, though its influence may vary under the strategic control of the subject, e.g. through the operation of selective spatial attention (Gentilucci *et al*. 1997). The important point for the present discussion, however, is that while an act may be under the simultaneous control of both egocentric and allocentric representations of location, this does not imply that both of these representations are mediated by the same brain system.

Implicit in all of the studies that tease apart two separate visuospatial processing systems by means of visual illusions of location is that what is visually *experienced* by the observer is not (or not entirely) what controls his or her *response*. In these studies, the experimental manipulation shifts the subjective location of the target but not its true position. But dissociations between awareness and action have also been reported in complementary studies where an experimental manipulation alters the *true* location of the target but not its *perceived* location. For example, a lateral shift of an LED target during an eye movement may be unperceived due to saccadic suppression, but will still result in a seamless pointing response that is indistinguishable both to the observer and the experimenter from responses made to unperturbed targets (Goodale *et al*. 1986). It is as if the pointing response has its own 'unconscious' visual control independent of the visual processing that yields our awareness of spatial location.

In summary, the literature is consistent with the idea expressed above that egocentric localization is tied closely to immediate visuomotor control, while allocentric coding is associated with tasks that require perceptual judgements and/or a delayed response. The data from D.F. that are summarized in this chapter support the view that when the perceptual system is severely compromised by brain damage, then allocentric spatial coding will be disrupted along with the coding of other perceptual attributes. This suggests that the two forms of spatial coding are achieved in parallel rather than through a single visual pathway. While the dorsal stream may have rapid and automatic control over actions directed in egocentric space, the organism may depend on perceptual processing within the ventral stream for coding stimulus location with respect to the visual context. Our data do not of course speak to the question of how the ventral stream may achieve this allocentric coding, still less how this form of coding is able to influence action.

23.7 Conclusions

The evidence we have described here leads us to conclude that D.F. does not have any residual ability to code spatial locations in allocentric coordinates. She can cope remarkably well in her spatial world by using egocentric systems to code location, apparently with increasingly complex strategies for putting such information together. Of course, as we pointed out in the Introduction, this conclusion does not *force* us to reject the idea that the human dorsal stream might provide the visual information for spatial perception and cognition in healthy individuals. For example, it is quite possible that D.F. has damage to her dorsal stream that might impair its functioning. Nonetheless, the dissociations that we have described here are striking. Even a sequence of five pointing responses can be accomplished accurately providing that the targets are held in verbal short-term memory (e.g. blue, yellow, black, red, green). Yet the separation of finger and thumb to match two holes in a disc that has to be grasped is essentially random. The qualitative difference between D.F's performance on these two tasks seems more plausibly to be related to a difference in kind than a difference of degree. It seems unlikely that a degraded system would do well in one task and close to chance in the other, when the two tasks would appear to be of comparable complexity.

The data, then, are at least consistent with the hypothesis that the ventral stream is needed for the coding of spatial relationships between the elements of a visual scene (Milner & Goodale 1995). Nonetheless there is no doubt that parietal damage, especially in the right hemisphere, can result in a range of other disorders of visuospatial perception and visuospatial cognition. One possibility for understanding this is that there may be a representational system in the inferior parietal lobule (areas 39 and 40) of the human brain, which integrates at a high level information derived from a range of visual areas in *both* of the cortical streams (Milner 1997; Turnbull *et al.* 1997). This system may be able to put together and manipulate information about perceptually segregated elements of a visual display, in order to construct abstract spatial representations of the visible world for a variety of cognitive purposes.

A parietal location for this high-level spatial system would not of course imply that it is more closely associated with the dorsal than the ventral processing stream. There is strong evidence now that the human dorsal stream terminates not in such inferior parts of the parietal lobe, but instead in more superior parts in and around the intraparietal sulcus (Milner & Goodale 1995). Not only do lesions in this superior region impair visually-guided arm movements, hand movements, eye movements, and finger movements, but also the same regions become metabolically active during performance of these acts by healthy individuals (Thier & Karnath 1997). Lesions in the inferior parts of the right parietal lobe are frequently associated with neglect symptoms, rather than these kinds of visuomotor impairments (Milner 1997; Perenin 1997). This double dissociation indicates that the inferior parietal system is both anatomically and functionally distinct from the dorsal stream. We suggest that the human dorsal stream may nonetheless provide important inputs into this hypothesized system for spatial cognition, though the most crucial visual inputs may come from the ventral stream and associated medial temporal structures.

References

Adler, A. 1944 Disintegration and restoration of optic recognition in visual agnosia. *Arch. Neurol. Psychiatr.* **51**, 243–59.

Andersen, R. A. 1995 Encoding of intention and spatial location in the posterior parietal cortex. *Cerebral Cortex* **5**, 457–69.

Andersen, R. A. 1997 Multimodal integration for the representation of space in the posterior parietal cortex. *Philos. Trans. R. Soc. Lond.* **B352**, 1421–8.

Battaglini, P.-P., Galletti, C. & Fattori, P. 1997 Neuronal coding of visual space in the posterior parietal cortex. In *Parietal Lobe Contributions to Orientation in 3D Space* (ed., P. Thier & H.-O. Karnath), pp. 539–53. Heidelberg: Springer-Verlag.

Benson, D. F. & Greenberg, J. P. 1969 Visual form agnosia: a specific deficit in visual discrimination. *Arch. Neurol.* **20**, 82–9.

Brenner, E. & Smeets, J. B. J. 1996 Size illusion influences how we lift but not how we grasp an object. *Exp. Brain Res.* **111**, 473–6.

Bridgeman, B. 1992 Conscious and unconscious processes: the case of vision. *Theory Psychol.* **2**, 73–88.

Bridgeman, B., Kirch, M. & Sperling, A. 1981 Segregation of cognitive and motor aspects of visual function using induced motion. *Percept. Psychophys.* **29**, 336–42.

Bridgeman, B., Peery, S. & Anand, S. 1997 Interaction of cognitive and sensorimotor maps of visual space. *Percept. Psychophys.* **59**, 456–69.

Brotchie, P. R., Andersen, R. A., Snyder, L. H. & Goodman, S. J. 1995 Head position signals used by parietal neurons to encode locations of visual stimuli. *Nature* **375**, 232–5.

Campion, J. & Latto, R. 1985 Apperceptive agnosia due to carbon monoxide poisoning. An interpretation based on critical band masking from disseminated lesions. *Behav. Brain Res.* **15**, 227–40

Carey, D. P., Harvey, M. & Milner, A. D. 1996 Visuomotor sensitivity for shape and orientation in a patient with visual form agnosia. *Neuropsychologia* **34**, 329–38.

Colby, C. L. & Duhamel, J. R. 1997 Spatial representations for action in parietal cortex. *Cogn. Brain Res.* **5**, 105–15.

Dijkerman, H. C. & Milner, A. D. 1997 Copying without perceiving: motor imagery in visual form agnosia. *NeuroReport* **8**, 729–32.

Dijkerman, H. C., Milner, A. D. & Carey, D. P. 1996 The perception and prehension of objects oriented in the depth plane: I. Effects of visual form agnosia. *Exp. Brain Res.* **112**, 442–51.

Dijkerman, H. C., Milner, A. D. & Carey, D. P. 1997 Impaired delayed and anti-saccades in a visual form agnosic. *Exp. Brain Res. Supp.* **117**, S66 (abstract).

Dijkerman, H. C., Milner, A. D. & Carey, D. P. 1998 Grasping spatial relationships: loss of allocentric coding in a patient with visual form agnosia. *Consciousness & Cognition*, in press.

Duhamel, J.-R., Bremmer, F., BenHamed, S. & Graf, W. 1997 Spatial invariance of visual receptive fields in parietal cortex neurons. *Nature* **389**, 845–8.

Efron, R. 1969 What is perception? *Boston Studies in the Philosophy of Science* **4**, 137–73.

Felleman, D. J. & Van Essen, D. C. 1991 Distributed hierarchical processing in the primate cerebral cortex. *Cerebral Cortex* **1**, 1–47.

Funahashi, S., Bruce, C. J. & Goldman-Rakic, P. S. 1989 Mnemonic coding of visual space in the monkey's dorsolateral prefrontal cortex. *J. Neurophysiol.* **61**, 331–49.

Funahashi, S., Bruce, C. J. & Goldman-Rakic, P. S. 1993 Dorsolateral prefrontal lesions and oculomotor delayed-response performance: evidence for mnemonic 'scotomas'. *J. Neurosci.* **13**, 1479–97.

Galletti, C., Battaglini, P. P. & Fattori, P. 1995 Eye position influence on parieto-occipital area PO (V6) of the macaque monkey. *Eur. J. Neurosci.* **7**, 2486–501.

Gelb, A. & Goldstein, K. 1938 Analysis of a case of figural blindness. In *A Source Book of Gestalt Pychology* (ed., W. D. Ellis), pp. 315–325. London: Kegan Paul, Trench, Trubner.

Gentilucci, M., Daprati, E., Saetti, M. C. & Toni, I. 1997 On the role of the egocentric and the allocentric frame of reference in the control of arm movements. In *Parietal Lobe Contributions to Orientation in 3D Space* (ed., P. Thier & H.-O. Karnath), pp. 339–354. Heidelberg: Springer-Verlag.

Glickstein, M. & May, J. G. 1982 Visual control of movement: the circuits which link visual to motor areas of the brain with special reference to the visual input to the pons and cerebellum. In *Contributions to Sensory Physiology, Vol. 7* (ed., W. D. Neff), pp. 103–145. New York: Academic Press.

Goldstein, K. & Gelb, A. 1918 Psychologische Grundlagen hirnpathologischer Fälle auf Grund von Untersuchungen Hirnverletzter. *Z. Neurol. Psychiatr.* **41**, 1–142.

Goodale, M. A. & Milner, A. D. 1992 Separate visual pathways for perception and action. *Trends Neurosci.* **15**, 20–5.

Goodale, M. A., Pélisson, D. & Prablanc, C. 1986 Large adjustments in visually guided reaching do not depend on vision of the hand or perception of target displacement. *Nature* **320**, 748–50.

Goodale, M. A., Milner, A. D., Jakobson, L. S. & Carey, D. P. 1991 A neurological dissociation between perceiving objects and grasping them. *Nature* **349**, 154–6.

Goodale, M. A., Jakobson, L. S. & Keillor, J. M. 1994 Differences in the visual control of pantomimed and natural grasping movements. *Neuropsychologia* **32**, 1159–78.

Grossman, M., Galetta, S., Ding, X.-S. *et al.* 1996 Clinical and positron emission tomography studies of visual apperceptive agnosia. *Neuropsychiat. Neuropsychol. Behav. Neurol.* **9**, 70–7.

Gruh, J. M., Born, R. T. & Newsome, W.T. 1997 How is a sensory map read out? Effects of microstimulation in visual area MT on saccades and smooth pursuit eye movements. *J. Neurosci.* **17**, 4312–30.

Guitton, D., Buchtel, H.A. & Douglas, R.M. 1985 Frontal-lobe lesions in man cause difficulties in suppressing reflexive glances and in generating goal-directed saccades. *Exp. Brain Res.* **58**, 455–72.

Hyvärinen, J. & Poranen, A. 1974 Function of the parietal associative area 7 as revealed from cellular discharges in alert monkeys. *Brain* **97**, 673–92.

Jeannerod, M. & Rossetti, Y. 1993 Visuomotor coordination as a dissociable visual function: experimental and clinical evidence. In *Visual Perceptual Defects (Bailliere's Clinical Neurology, Vol. 2, No. 2)* (ed., C. Kennard), pp. 439–460. London: Bailliere Tindall.

Kawashima, R., Naitoh, E., Matsumura, M. *et al.* 1996 Topographic representation in human intraparietal sulcus of reaching and saccade. *NeuroReport* **7**, 1253–6.

Kosslyn, S. M. 1987 Seeing and imaging in the cerebral hemispheres: a computational approach. *Psychol. Rev.* **94**, 148–75.

Landis, T., Graves, R., Benson, D. F. & Hebben, N. 1982 Visual recognition through kinaesthetic mediation. *Psychol. Med.* **12**, 515–31.

Marotta, J. J., Behrmann, M. & Goodale, M. A. 1997 The removal of binocular cues disrupts the calibration of grasping in patients with visual form agnosia. *Exp. Brain Res.* **116**, 113–21.

Milner, A. D. 1997 Neglect, extinction, and the cortical streams of visual processing. In *Parietal Lobe Contributions to Orientation in 3D Space* (ed., P. Thier & H.-O. Karnath), pp. 3–22. Heidelberg: Springer-Verlag.

Milner, A. D. 1998 Neuropsychological studies of perception and visuomotor control. *Philos. Trans. R. Soc. Lond.* **B355**, in press

Milner, A. D. & Dijkerman, H. C. 1998 Visual processing in the primate parietal lobe. In *Comparative Neuropsychology* (ed., A. D. Milner), pp. 70–94. Oxford: Oxford University Press.

Milner, A. D. & Goodale, M. A. 1993 Visual pathways to perception and action. In *Progress in Brain Research, Vol. 95. The Visually Responsive Neuron: From Basic Neurophysiology to Behavior* (ed., T. P. Hicks, S. Molotchnikoff & T. Ono), pp. 317–337. Amsterdam: Elsevier.

Milner, A. D. & Goodale, M. A. 1995 *The Visual Brain in Action*. Oxford: Oxford University Press.

Milner, A. D., Perrett, D. I., Johnston, R. S. *et al.* 1991 Perception and action in 'visual form agnosia'. *Brain* **114**, 405–28.

Mishkin. M. 1972 Cortical visual areas and their interaction. In *The Brain and Human Behavior* (ed., A. G. Karczmar & J. C. Eccles), pp. 187–208. Berlin: Springer-Verlag.

Morel, A. & Bullier, J. 1990 Anatomical segregation of two cortical visual pathways in the macaque monkey. *Vis. Neurosci.* **4**, 555–78.

Mountcastle, V. B., Lynch, J. C., Georgopoulos, A. P., Sakata, H. & Acuña, C. 1975 Posterior parietal association cortex of the monkey: command function of operations within extrapersonal space. *J. Neurophysiol.* **38**, 871–908.

Murphy, K. J. & Goodale, M. A. 1996 Egocentric versus allocentric spatial analysis in visual form agnosia. *Invest Ophthalmol Vis Sci* **37**, 4985 (abstract).

Murphy, K. J., Carey, D. P. & Goodale, M.A. 1998 The perception of allocentric spatial relationships in a visual form agnosic. *Cogn. Neuropsychol.* **15**, in press.

Perenin, M.-T. 1997 Optic ataxia and unilateral neglect: clinical evidence for dissociable spatial functions in posterior parietal cortex. In *Parietal Lobe Contributions to Orientation in 3D Space* (ed., P. Thier & H.-O. Karnath), pp. 289–308. Heidelberg: Springer-Verlag.

Rizzolatti, G., Riggio, L. & Sheliga, B. M. 1994 Space and selective attention. In *Attention and Performance XV. Conscious and Nonconscious Information Processing* (ed., C. Umiltà & M. Moscovitch), pp. 231–265. Cambridge, MA: MIT Press.

Rossetti, Y. 1998 Implicit perception in action: short-lived motor representations of space. *Consciousness & Cognition*, in press.

Sakata, H., Taira, M., Kusunoki, M., Murata, A. & Tanaka, Y. 1997 The parietal association cortex in depth perception and visual control of hand action. *Trends Neurosci.* **20**, 350–7.

Snyder, L. H., Batista, A. P. & Andersen, R. A. 1997 Coding of intention in the posterior parietal cortex. *Nature* **386**, 167–70.

Tanaka, K. 1997 Mechanisms of visual object recognition: monkey and human studies. *Curr. Opin. Neurobiol.* **7**, 523–9.

Thier, P. & Karnath, H.-O. 1997 *Parietal Lobe Contributions to Orientation in 3D Space.* Heidelberg: Springer-Verlag.

Turnbull, O. H., Carey, D. P. & McCarthy, R. A. 1997 The neuropsychology of object constancy. *J. Int. Neuropsychol. Soc.* **3**, 288–98.

Ungerleider, L. G. & Haxby, J. V. 1994 'What' and 'where' in the human brain. *Curr. Opin. Neurobiol.* **4**, 157–65.

Ungerleider, L. G. & Mishkin, M. 1982 Two cortical visual systems. In *Analysis of Visual Behavior* (ed., D. J. Ingle, M. A. Goodale & R. J. W. Mansfield), pp. 549–586. Cambridge, MA: MIT Press.

Wong, E. & Mack, A. 1981 Saccadic programming and perceived location. *Acta Pychol.* **48**, 123–31.

Author Index

Reference pages are italicised.
Entries of contributors' chapters are in bold.

Abbott, L.F. 130, *143*, *146*
Abraham, L. 385, *401*
Abrahams, S. 255, *257*, **259–86**, *286*, *288*
Abzug, C. *319*
Acuna, C. 27, 91, 95, 97, *102*, 445, *465*
Adams, R.D. 33, 36, 40, *46*, 347, *358*
Adler, A. 443, *463*
Agid, Y. *126*
Aglioti, S. 44, *48*
Aguirre, G.K. 256, *257*, 397, *398*, 405, 408, 410, 412, *413*
Aimard, G. 37, 45, *47*
Aizawa, S. *245*
Akbarian, S. 386, *398*
Albright, T.D. 5, *28*
Alexander, M. 35, *47*, 186
Alkon, D.L. 222, *243*
Allen, G.L. *414*, *441*
Alleva, D.C. *244*
Alsop, D.C. 256, *257*, 397, *398*, 405, 408, 410, 412, *413*
Altman, G.A. 43, *46*
Alyan, S. 168, *184*
Amaral, D.G. 9, 11, 19, *25–6*, *28*, 222, *243*, 256, *257*, 290, 293–4, 296, 298, *299–302*, 305, *318*, 321, 323, 335, 337, 339, *340–1*, *343–4*, 345, *358*, 394, *403*
Amari, S.I. 209, *215–16*
Amit, D.J. 337, *340*
Amorim, M.A. 385, 394, *398–9*, *402*
Anand, S. 460, *463*
Andersen, P. 264, *288*
Andersen, R.A. 7, 15, *25–6*, 31, 44–5, *46*, 51, 64, 66, 68, *86*, **90–101**, *101–3*, 105, 109, 113–14, 116–17, *122–4*, *126*, 130–1, 133, 142, *143–6*, 326, *340*, 381–3, 390, *398*, 412, 418, 423, *440–1*, 445, *463*, *466*
Anderson, B. 24, *25*
Anderson, C.W. 429, 434, *440*
Anderson, D.J. 224–5
Anderson, E. 223, *244*
Andre-Deschays, C. 382, *400*
Angelelli, P. 35–6, 42, *46*
Angeli, S.J. 259, 269, *286*, 296, *299*
Angulo, J.C. 187, *201*
Anslow, P. 346, *357*
Antonucci, G. 37, 42–5, *47–8*, 51, *66*
Anwyl, R. 353, *357*
Apicella, P. 427, *440*

Argadona, E.D. 187, *201*
Arai, K. 209, *215*
Arbib, M.A. 22, 105, 107, *125*, *145*, 303, **416–40**, *440–1*
Arguin, M. 75, *86*, 128–9, 139–40, *143*, 377, *379*
Arolfo, M.P. 168, *184*
Asanuma, C. 91, *101*, 133, 142, *143*
Assad, J.A. 109, *124*
Attneave 69, 81, 83, *86*
August, D.A. 317, *318*
Austin, K.B. 211, *215*
Azzopardi, P. 378, *380*

Babb, T.L. 274, 284, *286*
Bach, L. 256, *258*
Bachevalier, J. 19, 27, 296, *300*, 345, 349, *356–7*
Baddeley, A.D. 24, *25–6*, 265, *286*, *288*, 294, *301*
Bailey, P. 292, *299*
Baizer, J.S. 416
Baker, S.C. 408–9, *414*
Balonov, L.J. 43, *46*
Banks, M.S. 91, 96–8, *101–2*
Bannerman, D.M. 223–5, 237, 242, *243*
Barash, S. 91, *101*, 114, *122*, 383, 390, *398*
Barbieri, C. 377, *379*
Barbieri, S. 36, 42, *49*
Barlow, J. *215*
Barnes, C.A. 18, *26–7*, 167–8, 171, 174, *184*, 199, *201*, 204, 206–8, 210–12, 214, *215–17*, 222, **305–17**, *318–19*, *341*, 424–5, 433, 439, *440–1*
Barozzi, S. *48*, 140
Barth, T. 131, *144*
Barto, A.G. 429, 434, *440*
Barton, J.J.S. 54, *65*
Bashir, Z. *340*
Basso, M.A. 117, *125*
Batchelor, A.M. 355, *356*
Batista, A.P. 93, *103*, 445, *466*
Battaglini, P.P. 37, *46–7*, 51, *64*, 133, *144*, 445–6, *463–4*
Baudonniere, P.M. 387, *398*
Baudry, M. *244*
Baumgartner, C. 73, *89*, 393, *403*
Baylis, G.C. 70, 72, 76, 78, 83, *86–7*, 105, *126*, 140–1, *144*, *379*

Bear, M.F. 222, *243*
Becker, J.T. 231, *245*, 273, *289*, *401–2*
Becker, W. 385, *401–2*
Behrmann, M. 45, *47*, *65*, 84, *86*, 105–6,
    122, *125–6*, 129, 142, *145*, 377, *379–80*
Bench, C. 408, *414*
Bender, M.B. *86*
BenHamed, S. *124*, 446, *464*
Benhamou, S. 158, *165*
Benson, D.F. 404, *414*, 443, *463*, *465*
Benson, P.J. 378, *380*
Beritoff, J.S. 385, *398*
Bernardini, B. 39–40, *48*
Berry, W. *341*, *343*
Berthoz, A. 16, 20, 22, 31, 209, *216*, 256,
    257, 303, 334–5, 339, *341*, **381–98**,
    398–402, 410, *414*, 418, *441*
Berti, A. 35, *46*, 52, *66*, *122*
Beschin, N. 24, *26*
Best, P.J. 17, *26*, 171, 174, *185*, 203, *218*,
    316, *319*
Bevan, R. 378, *380*
Bianchi, L. 105, 109, *125*
Biederman, I. 377, *379*
Biegler, R. 168, *184*, 227–8, *243*
Binkofsky, F. 42, *47*
Bioulac, B. 95, *103*
Bisiach, E. 12, 23, *26*, 34, 37, 41, 43–4, *46*,
    48, 58–9, *66*, 67, 70, *86–7*, 104–5, *122*,
    129, 139, 142, *143–4*, 350, *356*, *379*
Bito, H. 240–1, *243*
Black, A.H. 172–3
Black, J. 222, *243*, *245*
Black, S.E. 54, *65*
Blair, H.T. 151, *165–6*, 198, *202*, 206,
    215–16, 385, *402*
Blakenburg, M. *124*
Blatt, G. 91, *101*
Bliss, T.V.P. 221–2, 240, *243*, *245*
Bloomberg, J. 382, 388, 391, *398*, *402*
Blum, K.I. 224, *244*
Bolhuis, J.J. *340*
Boller, F. *46*, *87*, *122*
Bonda, E. 397, *399*
Bonin, G.V. 292, *299*
Book, A. 408, *414*, 440, *464*
Bordl, F. *340*
Born, R.T. 445, *464*
Bostock, E. 167, 171, *184*, 193, 200, *201*, 210,
    217, 333, *341*
Bota, M. *440–1*
Bottini, G. 33, 36, 39, 41–2, 44–5, *46*, *48–9*,
    105, *125*, 386, *399*, *402*, 404, *414*
Boussaoud, D. 5, *26*
Bower, G.H. *318*
Bower, J.M. *343*
Bowers, D. 23–4, *27*, *47*
Bowery, N. *245*
Bowes, D. 350, *357*

Bracewell, R.M. 91, *101*, 114, *122*, 383, 390,
    398
Bradley, D.C. 68, *86*, 91, 96–8, 100, *101*, *103*,
    105, 109, *122*
Branch, M. *185*
Brandt, T. 392, *399*
Bransford, G.D. 240, *243*
Bremmer, F. 113, *123–4*, 131, *144*, *464*
Brenner, E. 459, *463*
Brent, V.A. 240, *245*
Bridgeman, B. 444, 460, *463*
Brion, S. 345–6, 349, 351, *356*
Brodemann, R. 235, 241, *244*
Brooks, B.S. 42, *47*
Brotchie, P.R. 15, *26*, 92, *101*, 117, *123*, *126*,
    131, *144*, 445, *463*
Brown, I.S. 290, *302*
Brown, M. 238, *244*
Brown, M.A. 160, *165*
Brown, M.W. 19, *26*, 349, *356*
Brown, R. 242, *243*
Brown, T.H. 353, *356*
Brown, W.J. 274, 284, *286*
Bruce, C.J. 106, 117, *124*, *126*, *215*, 305, 418,
    441, 460, *464*
Brunn, J. 84, *87*, 104, *124*, 129, 139, 141–2, *144*
Brutton, C.J. *286*
Bub, D. 75, *86*, 128–9, 139–40, *143*, 377, *379*
Buchtel, H.A. 460, *464*
Buckley, M.J. 349–50, 354, *356–7*
Buckner, R.L. 408, *414*
Buhrmann, K. 432, *441*
Bullier, J. 117, *126*, 443, *465*
Bullock, P. 269–70, *288*
Bulthoff, H.H. 378, *379*
Bunsey, M. 256, *257*
Bures, J. 17, 147, **167–84**, *184–5*
Buresova, O. 174, *184*
Burgess, N. **3–25**, *28*, **31**, *86*, 134, *144*, **147–64**,
    165–6, 167, *185*, 227, 260, 273, *288*,
    303–4, 334, *340*, 407–8, 412, *413–4*, 432,
    442
Burke, T. *165*, 247, *257*, 404, 407, *414*
Burnod, Y. 107, *123*
Burnett-Stuart, G. 138, 142, *144*
Burton, H.L. 198, *202*
Burwell, R.D. 11, *26*
Bushnell, N.C. 114, *123*
Butcher, S.P. 221, 223–5, 237, *243–4*
Butters, N. 291, *301*
Buxbaum, L.L. 13, *26*, 85, *86–7*, 377, *379*
Byrne, J. *341*, *343*

Cahusac, P.M.B. 256, *258*, 324–6, 335–6, 339,
    340–2, 394, *401*
Cain, D.P. 222–3, 226, 233, *243*, *245*, 353,
    358
Calvanio, R. 129, 139, *144*, 266, *287*
Camarda, R. 113, *124*, 408, 419, *414*, *442*

Caminiti, R. 105, 107, 109, *123*, *125*
Cammalleri, M. 408, *414*
Campbell, B.A. *244*
Campbell, R. *288*
Campion, J. 443, *463*
Capitani, E. *26*, 142, *144*
Cappa, S. 37, 39, 44, *46*, *49*, 105, *125*, 386, *399*, *402*, 404, *414*
Carew, T.J. 222, *243*
Carey, D.P. **443–63**, *463–6*
Caritu, Y. 387, *402*
Carletti, M. 377, *379*
Carpenter, P. 84, *87*, 104, *124*, 129, 139, 141–2, *144*
Cartwright, B.A. 150, 164, *165*, 206, *216*
Castaigne, P. 34, *46*
Castelluci, V.F. 240, *244*
Castiello, U. 420, *440*
Castro, C. *340*, 377
Cave, C.B. 265, *286*
Celani, M.G. 33, 42, 45, *48*
Celebrini, S. 131, *146*
Cermak, L. *300*, *302*
Cesarani, A. 40, *48*
Chalmers, D.J. 35, *46*
Chamizo, V.D. 229, *245*
Chandler, H.C. 7, *28*
Chang Chui, H. 35, *46*
Changeux, J.P. *341*
Chapuis, N. 385, *400*
Charade, O. 382, 385, *400*
Charles, N. 37, 45, *47*
Chedru, F. 53
Chen, D.F. 224, *245*
Chen, L. *184*, 422, 425, 433, *440–1*
Cheng, K. 206, *215*
Chetkowitch, D.M. *243*
Christ, K. *27*, 37, *47*, 51, 58, *65*, 127, 139, 141–2, *145*
Church, R. *244*
Cipilotti, L. 381, 394, *400*
Ciurli, P. 105, *125*
Claiborne, B. 337, *340*
Clower, R.P. 296, *302*
Cocchini, G. 24, *26*
Cockburn, J. *301*, *357*
Cohen, B. *401*
Cohen, L. 105, *126*
Cohen, N.J. 203, *216*, 222, *243*, 264, 285, *287*, 290, *299*, 317, *318*
Colby, C. 16, 31, **104–22**, *123–4*, 127, 133, *144*, 381, 390, *399*, 419, *440*, 445–6, *463*
Coles, M. *88*
Collett, T.S. 151, 164, *165*, 206, *216*
Collingridge, G.L. 222, 240, *243–4*, *342*
Collins, G.H. 251, *257*, 347, *358*
Connelly, A. 291, 294–5, 298, *299–301*
Connor, C. *143–4*, 378, *379*
Connors, B.W. 312, *318*

Conquet, F. *340*
Conway, D.H. 167, 174, *185*, 422, *442*
Conway, M. *288*
Corbacho, F.J. *440–1*
Corell, R. *287*
Corkin, S. 42, *46*, 247, *257*, 260, *287*, 290, *299–300*
Cornacchia, L. 44, *46*
Cornu, P. 393, *401*
Corpinot, K. 394, *398*
Corsellis, J.A.N. 284, *287*
Corsi, P.M. 247, *257*, 260, *287*
Corwin, J.V. 7, *28*
Coslett, H.B. 13, 24, *26*, 377, *379*
Cotterill, R.M.J. *342*
Court, J. *88*, 416, *441*
Courtney, S.M. 383, 395, *399*
Cowan, J. 209, *216*
Cowan, J.D. *165*, *219*
Cowan, W.M. 11, *28*, 91, *101*, 293, *300*
Cowey, A. 105, *123*
Cox, T. 273, *286*
Craik, F.I.M. 238, *244*, *246*
Crane, J. **247–56**, *257*
Cressant, A. 151, 164, *165*
Crisp, J. 70, *88*
Critchley, M. 5, *26*, 34, *46*
Crivello, F. 256, *257*, 382, 384, 395, 397, *399*, *401*, 410, *414*
Cross, H.J. 295, *299*
Crowell, J.A. 96, 100, *102*
Cubelli, R. 35, *47*
Cummings, J.L. 404, *414*

D'Amelio, M. 408, *414*
D'Esposito, M. 256, *257*, 397, *398*, 405, 408, 410, 412, *413*
Damasio, A.R. 35, *46*
Damasio, H. 35, *46*
Danek, A. *399*
Daniel, H. *340*
Danysz, W. 223, *243*
Daprati, E. 460, *464*
Davidson, M. 348, *358*
Davies, C.H. 67, *340*
Davis, C. 71–3, *87*
Davis, G. 70, *87–8*
Davis, M. 222–3, *244*
Davis, S. 221–3, *243–4*
Dayan, P. *143*, *146*
De Jong, B. *414*
De Luca, M. 35, 42, *46*
De Renzi, E. 266, *287*, 377, *379*, *414*
de Waele, C. 387, *398*
Deadwyler, S.A. 203, *216*
Dean, P. 70, 152, *165*
Deecke, L. *401*, *403*
Deglin, V.L. 43, *46*
Degos, L.D. *46*

Deisseroth, K. 240–1, *243*
Delay, J. 345–6, 349, 351, *356*, 360, 362, 367, 373
Dell, G.S. 240, *245*, 298, *300*
Della-Sala, S. 24, *26*
Denis, M. 394–5, 397, *399*, *401*
Denzler, P. 53, *65*
Derosier, C. 387, *402*
Desimone, R. 5, *26*, 95, *101*, 256, *258*, 378, 416, *440*
Detre, J.A. 256, *257*, 397, *398*, 405, 408, 410, 412, *413*
Deutsch, D. *300*
Deutsch, J. *300*
di Pellegrino, G. 37, *46*, 113, *124*, 127, *144*
Diamond, A. 269, *287*
Dichgans, J. 55, *64–5*
Dick, H. 60, *64–5*
Dickinson, A. 227, *243*, *442*
Dienes, Z. *88*
Dieterich, M. *399*
Dijkerman, H. **443–63**, *464*
Diller, L. 53, *65*
Ding, X.S. 444, *464*
DiScenna, P. *245*
Dolan, R. 238, *245*, *399*, 408–9, *414–15*
Dominey, P.F. 417–18, *440–1*
Donnett, J. **149–64**, *165–6*, 407–8, 412, *413–14*
Dostrovsky, J. 17, *28*, 149, *166*, 167, *185*, 186, *202*, 405, *415*, 421, *442*
Doudet, D. 95, *103*
Douglas, R. *464*
Drain, M. 84, *87*
Driver, J. 13, *25*, 31, 60, *66*, **67–86**, *86–9*, 104, *123*, 128–9, 140–2, *144*, 377, *379*
Droulez, J. 209, 381, *399*, 418, *441*
Dubois, B. 105, *126*
Duchen, L.W. 345–6, *358*
Dudchenko, P.A. 206, *218*
Duffy, C.J. 91, 96–7, *101*
Duhamel, J.R. 105, 107–8, 111–15, 117–20, *123–4*, *126*, 127, 133, *144*, 381, 390, *399*, 419, *440*, 445–6, *463–4*
Duncan, J. 70–2, *87*, 95, *101*, 285, *300–1*
Durbin, R. *217*, *342*

Ebert, V. 290, 298, *302*
Eccles, J.C. *465*
Edelman, J.A. 209, *215*
Eekman, F.H. *343*
Efron, R. 443, *464*
Egeth, H. 377, *379*
Egly, R. 70, *87*
Ehrenstein, W.H. 60, *65*
Eichenbaum, H. 203, 211, *216*, *218*, 256, 264, 285, *287*, 422, *441*
Eifuku, S. 90, *103*
Elga, A.N. 211, *216–17*

Ellis, S. 105, *123*
Ellis, W.D. *464*
Elman, J. *218*
Emslie, H. 265, *286*
Engel, J. *286*
Ergenzen, N. 408, *414*
Erickson, R.G. 97, *103*
Ermentrout, B. 209, *216*
Erminio, F. 386, *399*
Errington, M.L. 240, *245*
Eskandar, E.N. *124*
Essick, G. 25, *101*, 133, 142, *143*
Etienne, A.S. 152, *165*
Etkin, D. *166*, 198, *202*, 385, *402*
Evans, A.C. 256, *257–8*, *399*, *415*

Fadiga, L. *46*, 107, 113, *124*, 127, *144*
Fadlallah, H. 391, *402*
Fagan, A. *216*, 422, *441*
Fagg, A.H. 419, *440–1*
Faglioni, P. 377, *379*, 404, *414*
Fahy, F.H. 19, *26*
Falconer, M.A. 261, *287*
Farah, M. *26*, 84–5, *86–7*, 104, *124*, 129, 139, 141–2, *144*, 266, *287*, 377, *379*
Farne, A. 377, *379*
Fattori, P. 37, 51, *46–7*, *64*, 445–6, *463–4*
Faugier-Grimaud, S. 386, *399*, *402*
Fazeli, M.S. 222, *243*, *342*
Feig, S. 235, *243*
Feigenbaum, J.D. 256, *258*, **259–86**, *287–8*, 325–6, 335–6, 339, *340–2*, 394, *401*
Felleman, D.J. 443, *464*
Felton, R. *300*, *302*
Fenton, A. **167–84**, *184–5*, 199, *201*
Ferraina, S. 105, 107, 109, *123*, *125*
Ferraguti, F. *340*
Fetter, M. 55, *64–5*, 388, *400*
Field, P. 131, *144*, 173, *185*, 359
Finch, D.M. 409, *415*
Findlay, J.M. 53, *66*
Fischer, B. 67, *88*, 104, *125*, 129, *145*
FitzGibbon, E. *123*
Flanders, M. 105, *126*
Flandrin, J.M. 43–4, *49*, 51, 58, *66*
Fletcher, F. 238, *245*, 383, *399*, 408–9, *414–15*
Fogassi, L. 37, *46*, *101*, 107, 113, *122*, *124–5*, 127, *144*, 383, 389, *398*, 419, *442*
Forrest, E. *340*
Fortin, W.F. 211, *215*
Foster, D. 337, *342*
Foster, T.C. 327, 337, 339, *340*
Fox, P.T. 249, *257*
Fox, S.E. 190, *201*
Frackowiak, R.S.J. 36, *46*, *165*, 238, *245*, 256, *257*, 383, 386, 397, *399*, *401*, 405–12, *414–15*
Francis Turner, L. 168, *184*
Frasca, R. 37, 45, *47*, 51, *66*

Freund, H.J. 42, *47*
Freund, J.R. *399*
Frey, S. 397, *399*
Frey, U. 19, 37, 39, 147, 164, **220–43**, *244*, 353
Friedrich, F.A. 70–1, *88*, 377, *380*
Frith, C.D. 36, *46*, 149, *165–6*, 238, *245*, 256, *257*, 383, 386, 397, *399*, *401*, 405–13, *413–15*
Fukada, M. *257*, *341–2*, 393, *402*
Fukuda, Y. 91, 96, *3*
Funahashi, S. 460, *464*
Furukawa, T. 63, *65*
Fuster, J.M. 95, *102*, 388, *401–2*

Gabriel, M. *218*
Gabrieli, J.D.E. 290, *299*
Gadian, D.G. **290–9**, *299–301*
Gaffan, D. 19, 23, *26–7*, 221, 230, 238, 242, *244*, 248, 256, *257–8*, 296, *300*, 303, 320–1, 325, *340*, *343*, **345–56**, *356–8*
Gaffan, E. 321, *340*, 355, *357*
Gage, H. 259, 267, *289*
Galetta, S. 444, *464*
Gallant, J.L. 44, *143*, 378, *379*
Gallese, V. 37, *46*, 107, *124–5*, 127, *143–4*
Galletti, C. 37, *46–7*, 51, *64*, 133, *144*, 445–6, *463–4*
Galli, C. 107, *123*
Gallistel, C.R. 167, *184*, 206, *215–16*, 259, *287*
Gallse, V. 113, *124–5*
Gangitano, M. 408, *414*
Garcia, R. 387, *402*
Garcin, R. 34, *47*
Garling, T. 408, *414*
Garrard, P. 149, *166*
Garrud, P. 256, *258*, 259, *288*
Garthwaite, J. 355, *356*
Gattass, R. 105, *123*
Gaulin, S.J.C. 206, *218*, 230, *245*, 409, *415*
Gavrilov, V.V. 387, 389–90, *399*
Gaymard, B. 392, *399–401*
Gazzaniga, M. *25*, *46*, *88*, 104, *124*, *301*, *343*
Geesaman, B.L. 91, *101*
Geiger, S.T. *440*
Gelade, G. 134, *146*
Gelb, A. 443, *464*
Gentilini, M. 377, *379*
Gentilucci, M. 37, *46*, 61, *66*, 106, 113, *124–5*, 127, *144*, 419, *442*, 461, *464*
George-Francois, P. 327, 330–3, 337, *340*, 381, 385, *398*
Georgopoulos, A. *27*, 91, 95, 97, *102*, *165*, 416, *442*, 445, *465*
Gerber, D. 224, *245*
Gerrard, J.L. 168, *184*, 206, 209, *217*, *318–19*, 424–5, 439, *441*
Gettner, S.N. 106, *125*, 141, *145*, **359–78**, *379–80*
Ghaem, O. 256, *257*, 395, 397, *399*, 410, *414*

Gibson, B.S. 96, *101*, 187, *202*, 377, *379*
Gibson, J.J. 416, *441*
Gilberto Gonzalez, R. 290, *299*
Gilchrist, I.D. 72, *88*
Giles, C. *165*
Girosi, F. 130, *145*
Gladden, V.L. 167, *184*, 199, *201*
Glasauer, S. 383, 385, 389, 394, *398–401*
Glickstein, M. 444, *464*
Glisky, E.L. 298, *300*
Gluck, M. *166*, 256, *257*, 285, *287*, *441*
Gnadt, J. 91, *101*, 114, 116, *122*, *124*, *398*
Goddard, N.H. 273, 285, *287*
Goelet, P. 240, *244*
Goldberg, M.E. 16, *26*, *101*, 105–6, 111–14, 117–18, 120, *123–4*, *126*, 127, *144*, 381, 390, *399*, 418–19, *440–1*
Goldman-Rakic, P.S. 6, 11, *26*, *28*, 388, *399*, 460, *464*
Goldstein, K. 443, *464*
Golob, E.J. 206, *218*
Gomez, C. 187, *201*
Good, M.A. 224–5, 237, *243*
Goodale, M. 5, 8, *26*, *29*, 50–1, *66*, 105, *125*, 130, *144*, *258*, *289*, 443–4, 446, 452–4, 458–9, 461–2, *463–6*
Goodman, S.J. 15, *26*, 92, *101*, *123*, 130–1, *144*, *340*, 445, *463*
Goodrich, S.J. 72, *87*, 89, 141, *144*, 377, *379*
Goodridge, J.P. 140, 206, *216*, *218*
Gothard, K.M. 167–8, *184*, 203, *216–17*, 307, 316, *318*, 424–5, 439, *441*
Gottlieb, J.P. 16, *26*
Goulet, S. 296, *300*
Gowling, E.A. 353, *357*
Grady, C.L. 383, *400*
Graf, W. *123–4*, *399*, 446, *464*
Grafman, J. *46*
Grant, S.G. 240, *245*
Grasby, P.M. 238, *245*, 383, *399*, 408–9, *414–15*
Grasso, R. 381, 385, *398*, *402*
Graves, R. 443, *465*
Gray, C.M. 308, *318*
Gray, J.A. 264, *288*
Graybiel, A. *102*
Graydon, R. 261, *287*
Graziano, M.S.A. 37, *47*, 91, 96, *101*, 106–7, *124*, 127, 133, *144*, 423, *441*
Green, C. 425, *442*
Green, D. 136, *144*
Green, E.J. 309, 312, 316, *318*, 425, 433, *440*
Greenberg, J.P. 443, *463*
Greengard, P. 240, *246*
Greenstein, Y.J. *166*
Gregory, R.L. 186, *201*
Gresty, M. 385, 393, *401*
Grice, G.R. 353–4, *357*
Gross, C.G. 5, *28*, 37, *47*, 95, *103*, 105–7, *123–4*, 127, *144*, 266, *287*

Grossenbacher, P.G. *465*
Grossman, M. 444, *464*
Grudman, M. *166*
Gruh, J.M. 445, *464*
Grunewald, A. 95, *102*
Grunewald, R.A. 295, *300*
Grusser, O.J. 386, *398–400*
Guariglia, C. 14, 24, *26*, 29, 37, 40–5, *47–8*,
    51, 58–9, *66*, 395, *400*
Guazelli, A. *441*
Guedry, F.E. *401*
Guigon, E. 105, *125*
Guiton, D. 209, *217*
Guitton, P. *217*, 460, *464*
Guldin, W.O. 386, *398–400*
Gulyas, B. 386, *400*
Gurd, J.W. 240, *245*
Gutnikov, S.A. 353–4, *357*

Habib, M. 20, *26*, 149, *165*, 394, *400*, 404, 407,
    414
Habib, R. 238, *246*
Hadji-Dimo 34, *47*
Halligan, P. 35, *47*, 51, *65*, 67–8, 77–81, *87–8*,
    104–5, *123–4*, 129, 138, 142, *144–5*, 370,
    380
Halliwell, R.F. *245*
Hamann, S.B. 298, *300*
Hammond, K.M. 266, *287*
Hampson, R.E. 203, *216*
Hampton, R.R. 409, *414*
Handelmann, G.E. 231, *245*, 273, *289*
Hanson, A.R. *440*
Hanson, S.J. *165*
Harries, M.H. 378, *380*
Harrington, T.L. 91, 96, *102*
Harris, K.D. *287, 289*
Harris, L. 386, *399*
Harrison, S. 248, *257*, 321, *340*, 347, *357*
Hartje, W. *27*, 37, *47*, 51, 58, *65*, 127, 139,
    141–2, *145*
Harvey, M. 443, 456, *463*
Hasboun, D. 387, *402*
Hasselmo, M.E. *146*, *217*, 378, *379*
Hawkins, R.D. 164, *166*, 208, *218*
Haxby, J.V. 383, 395, *399–400*, 446, 459, *466*
Hayman, C.A.G. 291, 298, *300–1*
Hebb, D.O. 186, 188, *201*, 345, 352–4, *356–7*
Hebben, N. 443, *465*
Hecaen, H. *400*
Heide, W. 117, *124*
Heilman, K.M. 23–4, *27*, 34–6, 42–4, *47*, 70,
    88, 104, *124*, 127, 136, 138, *145*, 350, *357*
Heimbrand, S. 385, *402*
Hellawell, D.J. 377, *380*
Helmholtz, H. 16, 114, *125*
Hendler, T. 187, *202*
Henn, V. 133, *146*
Hepp, K. 133, *146*

Herrero, M.T. 11, *27*
Herscovitch, P. 249, *258*
Heyser, C.J. 203, *216*
Hicks, T.P. *123*, *465*
Hietanen, J.K. 378, *380*
Hikosaka, K. 91, 96, *103*
Hikosaka, O. 376, *380*
Hill, A.J. 17, *26*, 200, *201*, 211, *216*, 316, *318*
Hillis, A.E. 84–5, *87*
Hodges, H. 264, *288*
Hoesing, J.M. 206, *218*
Hoffmann, K. 131, *144*
Hollerman, J.R. 427, *442*
Holliger, P. 382, *400*
Hommer, D.W. 376, *380*
Horel, J.A. 293, *300*, 349, *357*
Hornak, J. 19, 23, *27*, 54, *65*, 303, **345–56**, *357*
Horner, M.D. 298, *300*
Hotwitz, B. 383, *400*
Houk, J.C. *440, 442*
Houle, S. 238, *244, 246*, 254, *258*
Hu, X.T. *124*
Huang, Y.Y. 241, *244*
Huber, W. 54, *65*
Huerta, J. *246*, 363
Huerta, M.F. *379*
Hughes, A. *143*, 152, *165*
Humphrey, D.R. *399*
Humphreys, G.W. 72, *88*, 370, *379*
Hurtig, R. 53, *66*
Husain, M. 35, *47*, *88*, 129, 142, *145*
Huston, J.P. 174, *184*
Hyman, B.T. 290, *299*
Hyvarinen, J. 14, 105, 445, *465*

Imbert, M. 131, *146*
Incisa della Rochetta, A. *299*, 381, 394, *400*
Incoccia, C. 37, 45, *47*, 51, *66*
Ingle, D.J. *29*, *258*, *289*, *466*
Inoue, Y. 223, *245*
Insausti, R. 11, *27*, *257*, 293, *300*
Inui, T. *123*
Iriki, A. 109, *125*
Isaacs, E.B. 295, *299*
Isaacson, R.L. *287*, *301*
Ishiai, S. 53, *65*
Ishikuza, N. *340*
Ishiyama, K. 106, *125*
Israel, I. 381–2, 385, 388, 390–2, *398*, *400–1*
Ito, I. 23, *245*
Ito, Y. 423, *442*
Iversen, S.D. 23, *27*, *340*, 352, *357*
Ivy, G. 409, *414*
Iwai, E. 91, 96, *103*
Iwamura, Y. 109, *125*

Jackson, G.D. 295, *299–301*
Jacob, O. *398*
Jacobs, L.F. 230, *244–5*, 409, *415*

Jacobson, A. *88*
Jakobson, L.S. 443, *464*
Jalinke, M.T. 53, *65*
Jander, R. 168, *184*
Jarosz, J. 273, *286*
Jarrard, L.E. 11, *27*, 149, *165*, 273, 277, *287*
Jeannerod, M. *27*, 43–4, *49*, 51, 58, *65–6*, 105, 107, *124–5*, *145*, 420, *440*, 444, *465*
Jeffery, K. **3–25**, **31**, **147–64**, *165*, 222, *244*, **303–4**
Jetme, B. *26*
Johnson, K.A. 107, 109, *123*, *125*, 290, *299*
Johnson, P.B. 105, 107, 109
Johnsrude, I. **247–56**
Johnston, C.W. 53, *65*
Johnston, M.K. 240, *243*
Johnston, R.S. 443, 452, 458, 460, *465*
Jones, E.G. 291, *300*
Jones, G.V. 264, *287*
Jones-Gotman, M. 260–1, 265–6, *287*
Jordan, M.I. *146*
Josephs, O. 407, *415*
Jung, M.W. 168, *184*, 206, 209, *217*, *287*, 424–5, 439, *441*

Kaas, J.H. 363, *379*
Kairiss, E.W. 353, *356*
Kakei, S. 7, *27*
Kalina, M. 284, *286*
Kamin, L.J. 227, *244*
Kaminsky, Yu. **167–84**, *184–5*
Kandel, E.R. 164, *166*, 208, *218*, 224, 240–1, *244–5*
Kant, I. 83–4, *88*
Kapur, S. 238, *244*, 254, *258*
Karczmar, A.G. *465*
Karnath, H.O. 12–13, *27*, *29*, 31, 37, 43, *47–8*, **50–63**, *65–6*, 67, *87–9*, 104, *123–5*, 127–9, 139–42, *145*, 382, *401–2*, 412, *463–6*
Kase, C.S.J. 416, *441*
Kaseda, M. 107, *124–5*
Kawano, K. 91, 96–7, *102*, 390, *400*
Kawarasaki, A. 95, *102*
Kawashima, R. 445, *465*
Keenan, C.L. 353, *356*
Keil, K. 383, 395, *399*
Keillor, J.M. *464*
Keller, E.L. 209, *215*
Kennard, C. 35, *47*, *88*, *343*, *465*
Kertesz, A. *47*
Kesner, R.P. *215*, 256, *258*, 325–6, 334–5, 339, *341–2*, 387, *401*
Kettner, R.E. 158, *165*
Khurgel, M. 409, *414*
Kilduff, P. 35, *47*
Kimura, D. 247, *257*
King, D.J. 117, *126*
King, M.D. *299*, *301*
King, V. 7, *28*

Kinsbourne, M. 12, *27*, 44, *47*, 52, 61, *65*, 70, 75, *88*, 142, *145*, 290, 298, *300*, *302*
Kirch, M. 460, *463*
Kishimoto, K. 209, *216*
Kitu, T. 90, *102*
Kleinbaum, D.G. 310, *318*
Knierim, J.J. 151, *165*, 167–8, *184*, 206, 209, 211, *217–18*, 424–5, 439, *441*
Knowlton, B. *245*
Koch, C. 134, *145*
Koch, K.W. 95, *102*
Koenig, E. 388, *400*
Kohler, S. 254, *258*
Kohonen, T. 209, *216*
Kolb, B. 5–6, *27*, *165*, 409, *415*, 432, *441*
Komatsu, H. 91, 97, *102*
Kompf, D. 117, *124*
Konczak, J. 60, *64–5*
Konishi, M. *341*
Kooistra, C.A. 44, *47*
Korshunov, V.A. 387, *402*
Kosslyn, S.M. 24, *27*, 454, *465*
Kramer, A.F. 70, *88*
Krauzlis, R.J. 117, *125*
Krug, M. 235, 241, *244*
Kubie, J.L. 151–2, 160, 164, *166*, 167, 170–1, *184–5*, 186, 189–90, 193, 197, 199–200, *201–2*, 203, 210, *216–18*, 256, *258*, 316, *319*, 333, *341*, 432, *441*
Kubik, S. 173, *185*
Kudrimoti, H.S. 150, *165*, 167, *184*, 209, 211, *218*, 316, *318*
Kulik, S. 242, *243*
Kunesch, E. 42, *47*
Kuperstein, M. *216*, 422, *441*
Kupper, L.L. *318*
Kurylo, D.D. 91, *102*
Kurz, E.M. 305, *319*
Kushiya, E. 223, *245*
Kusunoki, M. 15–16, *26*, *28*, 106, *125*, 423, *442*, 449, 452, *466*
Kutsuwada, T. 223, *245*

Lacquaniti, F. 105, *125*
Ladavas, E. *47*, 67, 83, *88*, 104, *124*, 129, 139, 141–2, *145*, *379*
Lagae, L. 96, *102*
Lamassa, M. 33, 42, 45, *48*
Landis, T. 404, *414*, 443, *465*
Lang, W. 382, *400*
Laplane, D. *46*
Latto, R. 443, *463*
Lavie, N. 70, 72, *88*
Lavoie, A.M. 427, *441*
Le Bihan, D. 386–7, *400*
Le Peillet, E. 264, *288*
Leblanc, M. 53, *65*
Lee, G.P. 42, *47*
Leen, T. *144–5*, *218*

Lefebre, J.C. 386, *399*
Leiberman, K. 24, *26*
Leonard, B. 167, 171, *184*, 210, *216*, 309, 312, 316, *318*, 427, *441*
Leonard, G. 248, *257*
Leroy-Willig, A. 386–7, *400*
Levine, D.N. 129, 139, *144*, 266, *287*
Levy, W.B. 317, *318*
Lewald, J. 60, *65*
Lewis, J.W. 113, *125*
Lhermitte, F. 53, *65*
Li, C.S. *103*
Li, W. 94, 141, 45
Liebelt, B. 53, *65*
Lieblich, I. 417, *440–1*
Lin, L.H. 425, 433, *440*
Lincoln, N.B. 53, *66*
Linden, J.F. 95, *102*
Lipscomb, B.W. 206, *215*
Lipsitz, M. 382, *400*
Lipton, P. 235, *243*
Liu, Z. 168
Ljungberg, T. 427, *440*, *442*
Lobeck, L.J. *102*
Lobel, E. 386–7, *400*
Logie, R.H. 24, *26*
Logothetis, N.K. 200, *201*, 378, *379*
Lomo, T. 221
Long, G.M. 187, *201*, *243*, *245*
Longuet-Higgins, P. 240, *244*
Loring, D.W. 23–4, *27*, 42, *47*, 350, *357*
Lortie, C. 105, *126*
Lueschow, A. 378, *380*
Luppino, G. 37, *46*, 107, 113, *124–5*, 127, *144*, 419, *442*
Luzatti, C. 12, *26*, 129, 139, 350
Lynch, G.S. *244*, *342*, 418
Lynch, J.C. 91, 95, 97, *102*, 445, *465*

Ma, Y. 90, *102–3*, 130, *145*, 326–7, 334–5, *341–2*, 354, *357*, 387, *400–1*
MacAndrew, S.B.G. 264, *287*
MacDonald, C.A. 290, 298, *300–1*
Mack, A. 460, *466*
Mack, K.A. 432, *441*
Mackintosh, N.J. 227, 229, *244–5*
Macko, K. 129, *145*, 381, *401*
Madison, D.V. 240, *244*
Maes, H. 96, *102*
Magnotti, L. 37, 40–2, 44–5, *48*
Maguire, E.A. 20, 22, 149, *165–6*, *257*, 284, 303, 397, *401*, **404–13**, *414*
Mahut, H. 348, *358*
Maisog, J.M. 383, *400*
Maldonado, P.E. 383, *318*
Malenka, R.C. 222, *243*
Malinow, R. 240, *244*
Maljkovic, V. 377, *380*
Malkova, L. 296, *300*

Manabe, T. 223, *245*
Mansfield, R.J.W. 29, *258*, *289*, 466
Margerison, J.H. 284, *287*
Margules, J. 206, *216*
Marin, O.S.M. 66
Mark, V.W. 34, 43, *47*
Markham, J. 249, *258*
Markowitsch, H.J. 238–9, *246*
Markowska, A.L. 348, *357*
Marks, C. 71, *88*
Markus, E.J. 167, *184*, 199, *201*, 203, 210, *216*
Marotta, J.J. 452, *465*
Marquis, M. 309, 312, 316, *318*
Marr, D. 21, *27*, 69, 73, 78–9, 81, *88*, 208, *216*, 260, *287*, *289*, 303, 305, *318*, 377, *380*
Marrett, S. 251, *258*
Marshall, J.C. *27*, 35, *47–8*, 51, *65*, 67, 77–8, *88–9*, 105, *124*, 129, 138, 142, *144–5*, 370, *380*
Martin, W.R.W. 249, *258*
Martin-Elkins, C.L. 293, *300*
Martinez, J.L. *215*
Matelli, M. 37, *46*, 61, *66*, 113, *124–5*, 419, *442*
Matin, L. 141, *145*
Matsumura, M. 446, *465*
Matthies, H. 235, 241, *244*
Mattingley, J.B. 60, *66*, 67, 70–3, *87–8*
Matzel, L. 221–2, *245*
Maunsell, J.H.R. 95, *102*
Maurer, R. 152, *165*
Mauritz, K.H. 53, *65*
Maxwell, M. 91, 96–8, 100, *101*
May, J.G. 444, *464*
Mayes, A.R. 264, *289*, 407, *414*
Mayford, M. 164, *166*, 208, *218*, 224, *245*
Mays, L.E. 418, *441*
Mazoyer, B. 256, *257*, 382–4, 394–5, 397, *399–401*, 410, *414*
Mazzoni, P. 94, *103*, 130, *145*
McCarthy, R.A. 460, *466*
McClelland, J.L. 20–1, *27*, *123*, 208, *215*, *217*, 273, 285, 305, 317, *318*, 338, *341*, 378
McClosky, M. 317, *318*
McDonald, R. 432, *441*
McFarlane, S. 382, 388, *398*
McGaugh, J.L. *342*
McGlinchey, L. 353, *357*
McGlinchey-Berroth, R. *47*
McHugh, T.J. 224, *244*
McKoon, G. 298, *300*
McLaren, I.P.L. 229, *245*
McLeod, P. 70, *88*
Mc Mackin, D. *357*
McNaughton, B.L. 18, 20–1, *26–7*, 149–50, 164, *165–6*, 167–8, 171, 174, *184–5*, 199–200, *201–2*, 203–4, 206–11, *215–19*, 221, *244*, 259–60, *287*, *289*, **305–17**, *318–19*, 326–7, 338, *340–1*, 422, 424–5, 433, 439, *440–1*

Meador, K.J. 23–4, *27*, 42, *47*, 350, *357*
Meldrum, B.S. 264, *288*
Mellet, E. *257*, 394–5, 397, *399*, *401*, 410, *414*
Melville-Jones, G. 382, 388, 391, *398*, *402*
Meltzer, J. 167, 174, *184*, 308, *318*
Mercer, E. *245*
Mergner, T. 385, *401–2*
Metcalfe, T. 385, 393, *401*
Metzler, J. 271, *289*, *440*
Meunier, M. 19, *27*, 296, *300*, 349, *357*
Meyer, C.A. *257*
Miall, C. *217*, *342*
Miezin, F.M. 408, *414*
Milberg, C.R. 206, *218*
Milberg, W.P. 35, *47*
Miller, E.K. 256, *258*, 378, *380*
Miller, S. 385, *401*
Milner, A.D. 5, 23–4, *27*, 31, 50–1, *64*, *66*, 105, *125*, 130, *144*, **443–63**, *463–5*
Milner, B. 18, 20, *28*, 42, *46*, 147, 149, *166*, **247–56**, *257–8*, 260–1, 264–6, *288–9*, 290, *300–1*, 305, *319*, 320, *343*, 345, 349, *358*, 381, *402*, 407–8, *415*
Mine, S. 7, *28*, 106, *126*, 416, 423, *442*
Mintum, M.A. 249, *258*
Miotto, E.C. 269–70, *288*
Mirenowicz, J. 427, *441–2*
Mirring, S. 386, *400*
Mishina, M. *245*
Mishkin, M. 5–6, 19, 21, *27*, *29*, 130, *145*, 147, 248, 251, *258*, 259, 266, 269, 284–5, *286*, *288–9*, **290–9**, *299–301*, 320, *341*, 345–6, 349, 354, *356–8*, 381, *401*, 432, *441*, 443, 446, 459, *465–6*
Mitchison, G. *218*
Mittau, M. 376, *380*
Mittelstaedt, H. 168, *185*, *215*, *217*, 385, *401*
Mittelstaedt M.L. 168, *185*, *215*, *217*, 385, *401*
Miyachi, S. 376, *380*
Miyashita, K. 376, *380*
Miyashita, Y. 256, *258*, 324–6, 335–6, 339, *340–2*, 394, *401*
Mizumori, S.J.Y. 149, *166*, 309, 312, 316, *318*, 427, *441*
Mogenson, G.J. 427, *442*
Mohr, J.P. 416, *441*
Molotchnikoff, S. *123*, *465*
Mondin, G.W. 187, *201*
Montgomery, M.W. 13, *26*, 377, *379*
Moore, K.M. 167, 84, *216*, 316, *318*
Moray, N. 71, *88*
Morel, A. 117, *126*, 443, *465*
Morris, R.G. 17, 20, 147, **259–86**, *286–9*
Morris, R.G.M. 19, 147, 149, 164, *165–6*, 168, *184*, 206, 208, 214, *217*, **220–43**, *243–5*, 256, *258*, *288*, *341*, 353
Morton, N. 266, *288*

Moscovitch, M. 45, *47–8*, 84, *86*, 104–5, *122*, *125*, 129, 139, 141–2, *143*, 145, *145*, 238, *245*, 254, *258*, *379–80*, *465*
Moser, E. 264, *288*
Moser, M.B. 264, *288*
Moss, M. 348, *358*
Motter, B. 91, *102*
Mountcastle, V.B. 14, *27*, 48, 91–2, 95, 97, *102*, 105, *340*, *399*, *440*, 445, *465*
Mozer, M. 142, *145–6*, *217–18*
Muakkassa, K.F. 419, *441*
Muller, C. 393, *403*
Muller, K.E. 310, *318*
Muller, R.U. 17, *29*, 147, 149–52, 160, 164, *165–6*, 167, 170–1, *184–5*, **186–201**, *201–2*, 203, 206, 209–10, *217–18*, 316, *318–19*, 333, 385, *341*, *402–3*, 432–3, *441–2*
Munoz, B.P. 209, *217*
Murata, A. 7, 15, *28*, 106–7, *124–6*, *442*, 449, 452, *466*
Muri, R. *401*
Murphy, K.J. 453–4, *465*
Murray, E.A. 19, *26–7*, 248, 256, *258*, 259, 269, 284–5, *286*, *288–9*, 296, *299–300*, 320, *341*, 346, 348–50, 352, 354, *356–8*
Musen, G. *245*
Myers, C.E. 256, 285, *287*

Nadel, L. 17–19, 24, *28*, 90, *102*, 149, 164, *166*, 167, *185*, 186, *202*, 203–4, 210, *217*, 221, 226, 229, 238–9, 242, *245*, 248, *258*, 260, 271, 284–5, *286–8*, 305, *319*, 334, *341*, 347, 350, *358*, 381, *401*, 405, *415*, 417, 422, 424–5, 439, *441–2*
Nagode, J. *216*, 422, *441*
Naitoh, E. *465*
Nakamura, H. 106, *126*
Nakamura, K. 90, *103*, 327, *341*, 393, *402*
Nakayama, K. 377, *380*
Nalwa, V. 378, *379*
Nardi, G.L. 385, *401*
Neelin, P. 249, *257–8*
Neff, W.D. *464*
Nerad, L. 168, *184*
Netto, C.A. 264, *288*
Newsome, W.T. 91, 97, *102*, 445, *464*
Nickerson, R.S. *26*
Nico, D. 43, 45, *48*, 58–9, *66*
Niki, H. 107, 24, *258*, 324–6, 335, 339, *340–3*, 394, *401*
Nimmo-Smith, I. 265, *286*
Nishihara, H.K. 90, *380*
Nishijo, H. 90, *102–3*, 327, *341*, 393, *402*
Nolan, J.R.M. 247, *257*
Nunn, J. **259–86**, *287–8*

O'Dell, I.J. 240, *245*, *300*
O'Donnell, B.F. *202*

O'Keefe, J. **3–25**, *28*, **31**, 90, *102*, **149–64**, *165–6*, 167, 171, 174, *184–5*, 186, *202*, 203–4, 207, 210, *217*, 221, 226, 229, 238–9, 242, *245*, 248, 256, *258*, 259–60, 271, 273, 285, *288*, **303–4**, 305, 307–8, *318–19*, 326, 333–4, *340–1*, 347, 350, *358*, 381, *401*, 405, 407–8, 412, *413–15*, 417, 421–2, 425–6, 431–2, 436, 438–9, *442*
O'Regan, J.K. 376, *380*
O'Reilly, R.C. 20, 21, *27*, 208, *217*, 317, *318*, 338, *341*
Ohtsuka, H. 106, *125*
Olbrich, A. 393, *403*
Olson, A. 72, *88*
Olson, C.R. 105–6, *123*, *125*, 131, 141, *144–5*, **359–78**, *379–80*, 409, *415*
Olton, D.S. 174, *185*, 231, 239, *245*, 259, 269, 271, 273, *289*, *342*, 348, *357–8*
O'Mara, S.M. 90, *102*, 326–7, 334–5, *341–2*, 387, *401*
Ono, T. 90, *102*, *123*, *257*, 285, 327, *341–2*, 393, *402*, *465*
Oram, M.W. 378, *380*
Orban, J.A. 96, *102*
Orssaud, C. 382–4, *401*
Ostergaard, A. 298, *300*
Ostry, D. 71, *88*
Otto, T. 203, *216*
Ovadia, D. 40, *48*
Owen, A.M. 408, *415*
Owen, M.J. 251–2, 256, *257–8*, 321, *340*
Oxbury, S. 23, *27*, 352, *357*
Oxbury, L. 23, *27*, 352, *357*

Pach, J. *217*
Padovani, A. 24, *26*, 395, *400*
Paillard, J. *123*, *217*, *341*
Paladini, R. 35, *47*
Pallis, C.A. 394, *401*
Palmer, E.P. 404, *414*
Palmer, S.E. 83, *88*
Pandya, D.N. 6, 11, *28*, 291, *301*
Pantano, P. 24, *26*, 395, *400*
Panzeri, S. 337, 339, *343*
Papagno, C. 40, 43, *48*
Parasuraman, R. *87*
Parker, A. 349, 351, *357–8*
Parkinson, J.K. 248, *258*, 269, 285, *289*, 296, *300*, 320, *341*
Parsons, C.G. 223, *243*
Passerini, D. 42, *48*
Passingham, R.E. 386, *399*
Paterson, A. 394, *401*
Patterson, A. 404, *415*
Paulesu, E. 36, *46*, 386, *399*
Paulignan, Y. 420, *440*
Pauls, J. 378, *379*
Pause, M. 42, *47*, 386, *399–400*

Pavio, A. 265, *289*
Pavlides, S. 158, *166*, 306, *319*
Paxinos, G. 169, *185*, 189, *318*
Pedotti, A. 37, *46*
Peery, S. 460, *463*
Pelisson, D. 209, *217*, 461, *464*
Perani, D. 35, *48*, 51, *66*, *122*, 129, *144*, 350, *356*
Perenin, M.T. 37, 45, *47*, 50–1, *66*, *463*, *465*
Perett, D. *257*, 423, 460, *465*
Peretti, V. 142, *144*
Perez-Vicente, C. 337, *342*
Perin, C.T. 353, *358*
Perlmutter, J.S. 249, *257*
Pesce, M. 129, 139, *145*
Peterhans, E. 73, *89*
Peters, T.M. 249, *257*
Petersen, S.E. 408, *414*
Peterson, M.A. 187, *202*
Petit, L. 382–4, *400–1*
Petrides, M. 247, 251–2, 256, *257–8*, 260, 284, *286*, *289*, 320, *341*, 397, *399*, 408, *415*
Petrone, P. 129, 139, *144*
Petronio, A. 377, *379*
Petsche, T. *146*
Phillips, J. *165*, 404, 407, *414*
Pickering, A. 255, *257*, 273, *286*, *288*
Pierrot-Deselligny, C. 388–91, *399*
Pietrini, P. 383, *400*
Pietrzyck, U. 382, *400*
Pigarev, I.N. 105, *124*
Pigott, S. 247, *258*, 264, *289*
Pillon, B. *126*
Pizzamiglio, L. 24, *26*, 37, 40–5, *47–8*, 51, *66*, 105, *125*, 395, *400*
Plum, F. *399*, *440*
Poggio, T. 130, *145*, 255, *257*, 261, 265–6, 269–71, 285, 378, *379*
Polkey, C.E. *286*
Popov, K. 382, *400*
Poranen, A. 14, *27*, 445
Porta, E. *26*, 142, 44
Posner, M.I. *66*, 70–1, *88*
Potegal, M. 385, *401*
Poucet, B. 150, 164, *165*
Pouget, A. 15, 31, 67, 73–6, 78, 82–3, **127–43**, *145–6*, 365, 368, 377, *379–80*
Powell, T.P.S. 291, *300*
Prablanc, C. 461, *464*
Preddie, D. *143–4*, 378, *379*
Presson, C.C. 408, *415*
Pribram, K. *287*
Price, C. 407, *415*
Prince, D.A. *318*
Prokasy, W.F. *245*
Provinciali, L. 129, 139, *145*
Pytko-Joiner, D.E. 349, *357*

Qin, Y.L. 21, *184*, *216*, 303, **305–17**, *319*
Quintana, J. 388, *401–2*

Quirk, G.J. 152, 160, 164, *166*, 167, *185*, 199, *202*, 208, 210, *217*, 256, *258*, 316, *319*, 333, *341*

Radant, A.D. 376, *380*
Rafal, R.D. 67, 70–1, 76, 78, 81, *87–8*, 140–1, *144*, 377, *379–80*
Raichle, M.E. 249, *257–8*, *341–2*, 408, *414*
Raieli, V. 408, *414*
Raiguel, S. 96, *102*
Raimondo, D. 408, *414*
Rains, G.D. 247, *258*, 265, *289*
Ramsay, M. 224–5, 237, *243*
Ramus, S.J. 296, *302*, 321, *344*
Ranck, L.B. *29*, 149–50, 160, 164, *166*, 167, *185*, 190, 197, *201–2*, 203, 206, 208, *216–18*, 256, *258*, 312, 316, *319*, 386, *402*, 422, 432–3, *442*
Rand, M.K. 376, *380*
Rasmussen, T. 42, *46*
Ratcliff, R. 298, *300*
Rawlins, J.N.P. 149, *166*, 208, *217*, 256, *258*, 259, *288*
Recce, M. 153–4, 157–8, 163, *165–6*, 167, *185*, **259–86**, *287*, *289*, 307–8, *319*, 334, *340*
Redish, A.D. 18, 147, 163, *166*, **203–15**, *216–18*, 439, *442*
Reep, R.L. 7, *28*
Reese, H.W. *415*
Reichert, H. 53, *65*
Rempel-Clower, N.L. 290, 294, 296, 298, *301–2*
Requin, J. *400*
Rescorla, R.A. 227, *245*
Reuter-Lorenz, P.A. 84, *87*
Reymann, K. 235, *244*
Ricci, S. 33, 42, 45, *48*
Richard, S. 90, 147, 429, 434, *440*
Riches, I.P. 19, *26*, 349, *356*
Riddoch, M.J. 72, 85, *88*, 370, *379*
Riesenhuber, M. *146*
Riggio, L. *125*, *380*, 445, *465*
Righetti, E. 33, 42, 45, *48*
Rivaud, S. 388, 390–3, *399–401*
Rizzo, M. 53, *66*
Rizzolatti, G. 35, *46*, 52, 61, *66*, 105–7, 113, *124–5*, 377, *380*, 419, *440*, *442*, 445, *465*
Robbins, T.W. 3, *28*, 37
Roberts, A.C. 3, *28*
Robertson, I.H. *27*, *47–8*, *65*, 67, *88–9*
Robertson, L.C. 76, *88*
Robertson, R.G. 327, 330–3, 337, 339, *340–3*
Robinson, D.L. 105, 114, *123*, *126*
Rock, I. 83, *88*
Rode, G. 37, 45, *47*
Rodman, H.R. 5, *28*
Rodrigo, T. 229, *245*
Roland, P.E. 386, *400*

Rolls, E.T. 18, 21, 90, *102*, 208, *217–18*, 256, *258*, 259–60, 285, *289*, 303, **320–39**, *340–3*, 355, *358*, 378, *379–80*, 387, 393–4, *401–2*
Romani, C. 72, *88*
Romo, R. 427, *442*
Rondot, P. 394, *400*
Ropper, A.H. 33, 40, *46*
Rorden, C. 60, *66*
Rorden, R. 70–2, *87–8*
Rosinski, R.R. 408, *414*
Ross, R.G. 376, *380*
Rossetti, Y. 444, 460, *465*
Rossier, J. **167–84**, *185*
Rostas, J.A.P. 240, *245*
Rotenberg, A. 17, 147, 164, *166*, **186–201**, 208, *218*
Rowan, M.J. 353, *357*
Rowland, L.P. 33, 36, 40, *47*
Royden, C.S. 96, *102*
Rubens, A.B. 14, *28*, 37, 39, *48*, 51, *66*
Rumelhart, D.E. *166*, *287*, *441*
Rupniak, N.M.J. 320, *343*
Rusconi, M.L. 14, *29*, 34, 36–7, 39–45, *46*, 48–9, 142, *144*, 386, *402*

Sacchetti, B. **167–84**, *185*
Saetti, M.C. 460, *464*
Saito, H. 96, *103*
Sakata, H. 7, 15, *27–8*, 91, 95–7, *102–3*, 105–7, 113, *124–6*, 326, *343*, 419–20, 423, *440*, *442*, 445, 449, 452, *465–6*
Sakimura, K. 223, *245*
Saksida, L.M. 206, *218*
Salamon, G. 382, *401*
Salinas, E. 130, *143*, *146*
Salmon, D.P. *343*
Salsbury, K. 349, *357*
Samsonovich, A.V. 203–4, 206–9, 211, *218*
Sanders, H.I. *343*
Sandroni, R. 36, 42, *49*
Sasaki, M. 97, *102*, 390, *400*
Satoshi, E. 90, *102*
Saucier, D. 226, 233, *245*, 353, *358*
Saunders, R.C. 248, *257*, 320–1, 325, *340*
Saypoff, R. 186, *201*, *217*
Scandolara, C. 113, *124–5*
Scarnatti, T. 427, *440*
Schacher, S. 240, *244–5*
Schacter, D. 220–1, *246*, 290, 298, *300–1*
Schall, J.D. 117, *126*, 200, *201*, 361, *380*
Schenk, F. 180, *185*
Schenkel, P. 67, *88*, 104, *125*, 129, *145*
Schlag, J. 132–3, *146*, 361, *380*
Schlag-Rey, M. 132–3, *146*, 361, *380*
Schmahmann, J.D. 6, *28*
Schreiter, U. 386, *400*
Schroeder, H. 241, *244*
Schulman, H. 240, *245*

Schultz, W. 427, *440–2*
Schwartz, A.B. 158, *165*
Schwartz, M.L. 11, *26*
Schweigart, G. 385, *402*
Scoville, W.B. 18, *28*, 149, *166*, 269, *287*, 290, *301*, 305, *319*, 345, 349, *358*, 407, *415*
Seal, J. 95, *103*
Segal, B. 382, 387, *398*
Seguinot, V. 152–3, 158, *165*
Seifert, W. *216*, *341*, *442*
Sejnowski, T.J. 15, 31, 67, 73–6, 78, 82–3, **127–43**, *145–6*, 377, *380*
Selemon, L.D. 6, 11, *26*, *28*
Seltzer, B. 6, 11, *28*
Schacher, S. *244*
Shallice, T. 24, *28*, 238, *245*, 383, *399*, 408–9, *413–15*
Shapiro, M.L. 211, *215*, *218*
Sharp, P.E. 151, 160, *165–6*, 167, *185*, 189, 198–9, *202*, 206, 208, *215–16*, *218*, 386, *402*, 425, *442*
Sheliga, B. *125*, *380*, 445, *465*
Shen, J. 18, *26*, 204, 206, 208, 211–12, 214, *215*, 305–6, *319*
Shenoy, K.V. 91, 96–9, *101*, *103*
Shepard, R.N. 271, *289*
Sherry, D.F. 230, *245*, 409, *414–15*
Shettleworth, S.J. 409, *414*
Shibutani, H. 91, 96, *102–3*, 423, *442*
Shields, S. *340*
Shikata, E. 106, *126*
Shimamura, A. *301*, *343*
Shinoda, Y. 7, *27*
Shipp, S. 412, *414*
Shoqeirat, M. *289*
Shors, T.J. 221–2, *245*
Siegal, A.W. 408, *414–15*
Siegel, R.M. *101*, 133, 142, *143*
Simmen, M.W. 337–8, *343*
Sipila, P. 211, *218*
Sirigu, A. 20, *26*, 105, *123*, *126*, 149, *165*, 404, 407, *414*
Skaggs, W.E. *184*, *201*, 209, 211, *216*, *218*, **305–17**, *318–19*
Skavenski, A.A. 91, *102*
Skidmore, B. 412, *414*
Small, M. 80, 105, *123*
Smania, N. 44, *48*
Smeets, J.B.J. *463*
Smith, B.A. 150, 164, *165*, 206, *216*
Smith, M.L. 247–8, *258*, 260–1, 264–6, 283, *289*, 320, *343*, 381, *402*
Smolensky, P. *218*
Snowden, R.J. 91, 96, *101*, 423, *441*
Snyder, L.H. 15, *26*, 68, *86*, 92–3, *101*, 105, 109, 117, *122–3*, *126*, 131, *144*, 445, *463*, *466*
Soechting, J.F. 105, *126*
Solier, R. *185*, *201*
Soul, J. 382, 388, *398*

Soulie, D. 387, *402*
Spackova, N. 284, *286*
Sparks, D.L. 133, *146*, 418, *441*
Speakman, A. 151, 153, *166*, 174, *185*
Spear, N. *301*
Sperling, A. 460, *463*
Spiegler, B.J. 296, *301*
Spinelli, D. 35, 42, *46*
Squire, L.R. 19–20, 23, *28*, 221, 238–9, *245*, *257*, 259, 264–5, 269, 273, *286–7*, *289*, 290, 294, 296, 298, *300–2*, 305, *319*, 321, 335, *341–4*, 345, 349, *358*, 394, *403*
Squires, N.K. 187, *202*
Stackman, R. *218*
Stanton, G.B. 114, 117, *126*
Staunton, H. *165*, 404, 407, *414*
Stead, M. *217*
Steele, R.J. 231–2, *243*, *245*
Stein, J.F. 104–5, *126*, 127, *146*
Steinhof, N. 393, *403*
Stelmach, J. *400*
Stepankova, J. 284, *286*
Sterzi, R. 33, 36–7, 39, 41–2, 44–5, *46*, 48–9, 386, *399*, *402*, 404, *414*
Steward, O. *28*, 235, *245*
Stewart, C. *340*
Stoner, G. 91, *101*
Stricanne, B. 94, *103*, 131, *146*
Strick, P.L. 419, *441*
Sugiyama, H. *245*
Suomi, S.J. 348, *358*
Suster, M.S. 18, *26*, 204, 206, 208, 211–12, 214, *215*, *318*, 306, *319*
Sutherland, R.J. 167, 174, *184*, 206, *218*, 308, *318*, 409, *415*, 432, *441*
Sutton, S.S. 429, 434, *442*
Suzuki, W.A. 11, 19, *28*, **290–9**, *301–2*, 321, 323, *343–4*
Suzuki, W.E. 256, *258*
Suzuki, Y. 133, *146*
Swanson, L.W. 11, *28*, 427, *442*
Swash, M. *343*
Sweatt, J.D. 241, *243*
Swets, J. 136, *144*, *289*

Tabossi, P. *48*
Taira, M. 15, *28*, 106, *126*, 419, *442*, 449, 452, *466*
Takaoaka, Y. *102*
Takayama, C. *245*
Takei, Y. 385, *402*
Talairach, J. 251, 254–5, *257–8*
Talbot, W.H. 91, 97, *102*
Tamura, R. 259, 327, *341*, 393, *402*
Tanaka, K. 91, 96, *103*
Tanaka, M. 109, *125*
Tanaka, Y. *28*, 106, *125–6*, 444, 449, 452, *466*
Tanila, H. 211, *218*
Tapia, J.F. 416, *441*

Taube, J.S. 17, *29*, 149, 151, *166*, 198, *202*, 206, 210, *217–18*, 271, *289*, 333, *341*, 386, *402*, 433, *442*
Tees, R.C. *165*
Tesauro, G. *144–5, 218*
Teuber, H.L. 43, *48*, 290, *300*
Teyler, T.J. 221, *245*, 305, *319*
Thier, P. 27, *29*, *48*, 51, *64–6*, 67, *87*, *89*, 97, *103*, 113, *123–4*, *126*, 382, *401–2*, *463–6*
Thompson, E.E. 42, *47*
Thompson, L.T. 171, *185*, 203, *218*, 316, *319*
Thompson, W.O. 42, *47*
Thomson, J. 385, *402*
Thorpe, S. 131, *146*
Timsit, S. 393, *401*
Tipper, S.P. 105, *122*, *126*, 129, *146*, 377, *379–80*
Tlauka, M. 408, *415*
Tolman, E.C. 158, *166*, 352–4, *358*, 417, *442*
Tom, C. 224, *245*
Tomie, P.D.B.A. *319*
Tomko, D. *401*
Tonegawa, S. 223–4, *244–6*
Toni, I. 460, *464*
Toppino, T.C. 187, *201*
Torre, E.R. 235, *245*
Touretzky, D. 18, *144–6*, 147, 163, *166*, **203–15**, *216–18*, 439, *442*
Tournoux, P. 251, *258*
Tovee, M.J. 355, *358*, 378, *380*
Tran Ba Huy, P. 387, *398*
Treisman, A. 134, *146*
Tremblay, L. **359–78**, *380*
Treue, S. 91, *101*
Treves, A. 260, 285, *289*, 321–3, 325, 333, 336–9, *342–3, 358*
Trillet, M. 37, 45, *47*
Tronosco, J.F. *441*
Tropper, J. 391, *402*
Trotter, Y. 131, *146*
Tsien, J.Z. 224, *243–6*
Tsien, R.W. 240–1, *244–5*
Tsukagoshi, H. 53, *65*
Tsurugai, K. 423, *442*
Tsuzuku, T. 381, 385, *398*
Tulving, E. 220–1, 230, 238–9, *244, 246*, 290–1, 298, *300–1*, 409, *415*
Turnbull, O.H. 462, *466*
Tzanetos, D.B. *166*, 198, *202*, 385, *402*
Tzortzis, C. 394, *400*
Tzourio, N. 256, *257*, 382–4, 394–5, 397, *399–401*, 410, *414*

Ullman, S. *145*
Umeno, M.M. 117, *126*
Umilta, C. *122*, *125*, 377, *379*, *465*
Ungerleider, L.G. 5–6, *26*, *29*, 129, *145*, 251, *258*, 266, *289*, 381, 383, 395, *399–401*, 416, 432, *440–1*, 443, 446, 459, *466*
Uno, T. 90, *103*

Vaina, L.M. *216*
Valenstein, E. 35, 43, *47*, 70, *88*, 104, *124*, 127, 136, 138, *145*
Vallar, G. 13–14, *29*, 31, **33–46**, *46*, *48–9*, 51, 58–60, *66*, 67, *87*, *89*, 104–5, *122*, *125*, 142, *144*, 386, *399*, *402*
Van Essen, D.C. 113, *125*, *143–4*, 378, *379*, 443, *464*
Van Hoesen, G.W. *258*, 291, *301*, 323, *343*
Van Opstal, A. 133, *146*
Van Paesschen, W. 295, *299*, *301*
Vandenberghe, R. 407, *415*
Vanderwolf, C.H. 308, *319*
Varay, A. 34, *47*
Vargha-Khadem, F. **290–9**, *301*
Vazquez, M. 187, *201*
Ventre, J. 43–4, *49*, 51, 58, *66*, 386, *399*, *402*
Verfaellie, M. 35, *47*
Vermersch, A.I. *401*
Victor, M. 33, 40, *46*, 294, 298, *301*, 347, *358*
Vidal, P.P. 387, *398–9*
Vieville, T. *398*
Vighetto, A. 37, *47*
Villa, P. 404, *414*
Visser, R.S.H. 261, *289*
Vitte, E. 385, 387, *399*, *402*
Vitu, F. 376, *380*
Von der Heydt, R. *89*
Voss, K. 240, *245*
Voytko, M.L. 349, *357*

Wagner, A.R. 227, *245*
Walaas, S.I. 240, *246*
Walker, J.A. 70–1, *88*, 259, 267, *289*, 377, *380*
Walker, R. 53, *66*
Wallace, C.S. 235, *245*
Wallace, M.A. 84, *87*, 104, *124*, 129, 139, 141–2, *144*
Wan, H.S. 203, 206–7, *218*
Wannier, T. 7, *27*
Warburton, E. 36, *46*
Ward, R. 72, *89*
Warrington, E. *343*, 345–6, *358*, *402*
Warrington, K. 381, 394, *400*
Watanabe, T. 324, *343*
Watkins, J. *244*
Watkins, K.E. 291, 294, 298, *299*, *301*
Watson, M. *185*
Watson, R. 43, *47*, 70, *88*, 104, *124*, 127, 136, 138, *145*, 169, 189
Watt, S. 54, *65*
Weaver, K.L. 306, *319*
Weber, J. 337, *341*
Weigend, A. *218*
Weinberger, N.M. *342*
Weiskrantz, L. 3, *28*
Welch, J. 377, *380*
Whishaw, I.Q. 6, *27*, 409, *415*

White, S.H. 169, 374, 408, *415*
Whiteley, A.M. 394, *402*
Wiener, S. 203, *218*, 385, 387, *399*, *402*, 427, *442*
Wiest, G. 393, *403*
Williams, J. *47*, 149, *166*
Wilner, J. 305, *319*
Wilson, A. *244*
Wilson, B. 294, *301*
Wilson, F.A. 19, *26*, 349, *356*
Wilson, H.R. 209, *219*
Wilson, M.A. 149, *166*, 171, *185*, 200, *202*, 207, 209–11, *219*, 224, 259, *289*, 306–8, 316, *318–19*
Wilson, P.N. 408, *415*
Winson, J. *166*, 306, 308, *319*
Wise, R. *46*, *415*
Wise, S. 131, *144*
Witter, M.P. 9, 11, *25–7*, *257*, 305, *318*, 321, 337, *340*
Wolfe, J.B. 353, *358*
Wong, A.B. 84, *87*, 104, *124*, 129, 139, 141–2, *144*
Wong, E. 460, *466*
Wood, F. 290, 298, *300*, *302*
Worsley, K.J. 251, *258*
Wurtz, R.H. 91, 96–7, *101–2*, 117, *125*

Xiao, D.K. 96, *102*
Xing, J. 68, *86*, 94, *103*, 109, *122*

Yagi, T. 223, *245*
Yamashita, M. *102*, *400*
Yap, G. *47*, 97, 106–7, *124*, *144*
Yin, T.C.T. 91, 97, *102*
Young, A.W. 53, *66*
Young, D.A. 377, 376, *380*
Young, L. 385, *403*
Yukie, M. *103*

Zajaczkowski, W. 223, *243*
Zangwill, O.L. 404, *415*
Zee, D. *398*
Zeki, S. 412, *414*
Zeloni, G. 377, *379*
Zhang, K. 208, *219*
Zilles, K. 307–8, *319*
Zimmermann, E. 117, *124*
Zinyuk, L. **167–84**, *184–5*
Zipser, D. 92, *103*, 130, *146*
Zoccolotti, P. 105, *125*
Zola, S.M. 290, 294, 298, *301*
Zola-Morgan, S. 19, *28*, 221, 238, *245*, 259, 269, 287, 294, 296, 298, *301–2*, 321, 335, *343–4*, 345, 348–9, *358*, 394, *403*

Subject Index

Most entries for specific cortical areas will be found as subentries under the following main entries: *Brodmann areas, frontal region, hippocampal region, occipital region, parietal region, temporal region, visual cortex.*

acceleration signals 16, 386
acuity (visual) 376, 443
affordance 22, 416–40
agnosia 404, 443–63
algorithm 169, 433
allocentric, *see* frame of reference
allothetic signals 186, 198
amnesia 18–19, 149, 290–9, 305, 320, 345–6, 349, 394, 407
  hemiamnesia 352
  retrograde amnesia 305
amygdala 9–11, 19, 205, 260–1, 274, 284, 323, 345, 349, 352
angular position, of place fields 189, 192–201, 198
animals, subjects of study; *see also* species differences/similarites
  birds 385–6, 409
  humans 33–86, 127–146, 247–302, 345–56, 381–463
  primates 90–146, 290–302, 320–39, 359–78, 416–40
  rodents 149–206, 303–17, 345–56, 416–40
anosognosia 37
anoxia 284, 345–7
anterior thalamus 10, 17, 205–6, 215, 348, 351, 386, 424
arousal 11, 13, 14
ataxia 5, 12, 15, 23, 50–1, 63, 444, 465
attention 11–13, 51–4, 70–2, 114–22, 143, 220, 229, 237–9, 294, 359, 377–8, 390, 394, 439, 461
attractant field 427
attractor dynamics 164, 209–11, 305
audition 11, 33, 43, 59–60, 85, 90–1, 93–5, 100, 129, 153, 200, 321, 323, 443
autoassociation 164, 303, 322–39
axis
  horizontal 52–6, 62, 364, 447
  intrinsic 69, 79, 81
  object-based 80–3
  predominant 81–3
  principal 79, 80, 83
  vertical 43–4, 133, 334, 364
  see also coordinates; frame of reference

basal ganglia 36, 64
  in motivation 427

in motoric aspects of navigation 160, 412–13
in sequence management 421–4, 439
basis functions 129–31, 133, 135, 137, 139, 141, 143
bias
  egocentric, in neglect 52, 55, 60–3, 76–86, 133–4, 137
  orientation, in rats 426, 431–2
binding problem 157
binocular vision 18, 113, 187, 449–53
birds, *see* animals
bisection, line 64, 137–9, 142
blocking, in conditioning 226–7, 229, 237
blood-flow 249, 251–2, 254, 256, 382–3, 405–6, 412; *see also* imaging
body, *see* coordinates; frame of reference; position
body axis 12, 57–9, 61, 63, 326
brainstem 11, 393
Brodmann areas
  BA 1 5, 6, 35
  BA 2, 2v 5, 6, 35, 386
  BA 3–5 6, 35
  BA 6 6, 35, 386, 419
  BA 7 5, 6, 35
  BA 7a 5, 10, 15, 16, 22, 27, 91–3, 101, 133, 386, 398, 416, 445
  BA 7b 5–7, 416
  BA 8–20 6, 35
  BA 27, *see* hippocampal region, anatomy, pre- and postsubiculum
  BA 28 323; *see also* entorhinal cortex
  BA 35–36, 11
  BA 37 35, 254, 255
  BA 39 5, 35, 462
  BA 40 5, 35, 462; *see also* parietal region, anatomy, supramarginal gyrus
  BA 41–43 6
  BA 44 6, 35; *see also* premotor cortex
  BA 45 6
  BA 46 390, 421
  BA 47 6
  BA 48, *see* pre- and postsubiculum
  BA 49, *see* parasubiculum

CA1, CA3, *see* hippocampal region, anatomy
caloric stimulation 13, 14, 36, 142, 383
Cartesian space 79–80, 142–3; *see also* coordinate; frame of reference

cerebellum 7, 411
charts, model of hippocampal function 203,
    207, 211, 214–15, 422
cingulate cortex and gyrus 35, 291, 351, 363,
    382, 387, 397–8, 406–11
coarse coding 421, 430, 432–3, 435
cognitive map 17–19, 204–11, 226–7, 260, 352,
    417–26
    and allocentricity 260, 271, 417
    and event timing 18–19
    and Hebbian synapse 353–6
    in humans 285
    location of items within 17–18, 224–30
    long term memory in 305
    memory and understanding in 239
    mental visualisation 394
    neural elements of 17–18, 285
    new information assimilated into 200, 224–30,
        237–42
    and place cell activity 184, 186
    and primates 334
    and reversal learning 436–8
colour
    discrimination, and lesions/pathology 350,
        443–4, 454–8
    vs object/location coding in SEF 369–76
command, motor, see motor
compensation
    for eye and head movements 96–100, 418
    in memory systems in development 299
    by sensory stimulation in neglect 13–14, 51
competition
    hemispheric 76, 81, 377
    between map-based and orientation
        systems 426
    in network models 135–7, 157, 207, 433
computational modelling, see models
computer simulated environment 407, 410, 412
consciousness and space 16, 23, 35, 45, 50, 238,
    304, 459
consolidation, see memory
contrast enhancement 433
coordinate systems 14–16, 23–4, 43, 67–70,
    92–101, 106–22, 381
    and integration 92–101
    and memory 23–4, 116
    in neglect 37, 51, 67–86
    network modelling of 127–43, 209–14
    transformation/translation of 15–16, 43, 51,
        92, 96–8, 104, 116, 122, 132–43
    see also axis; frame of reference
coordinates (system type)
    allocentric 326, 394, 462
    arm-centred 14, 37, 107
    cartesian 79–80, 142–3
    craniotopic, see head-centred
    body-centred 51, 92, 131, 446
    egocentric 14, 23, 79, 326, 446, 459
    environment-centred (with respect to
        gravity) 142

eye-centred 94, 115, 127, 132, 446
head-centred 14–16, 37, 92, 94, 97–8, 112,
    113, 127, 131–2, 392, 442
motor 104, 121–2, 130
non-retinal 51, 75
object/shape-centred 79–81, 131, 142
oculocentric, see eye-centred
observer-independent 106
page-based 69
receptor surface 104
retinocentric 15, 67, 69, 74, 94, 97–8, 104,
    131, 142
truncocentric 67, 142
world-centred 51, 93, 131, 331
cornu ammonis, see CA1 and CA3
corollary discharge, see motor command
cortex (see cortical regions e.g. parietal region,
    temporal region)
corticocortical
    ensemble activity 305–17
    projections 5–11, 91, 242

darkness
    effect of ∼ on spatial behaviour 152, 168
    place cell firing in 150–2, 167–83
    pointing in 61–2
    saccades in 94, 382–4, 388–90, 392–4
    spatial view cell (monkey) firing in 332–4
    spontaneous visual search in 54, 58
declarative, see memory
delayed response, spatial 259, 269, 461
dendrites, role in memory 222, 233–6
dentate gyrus 9, 10, 205–15, 292–3, 322, 336,
    338
    role in orthogonalizing inputs 205–15
depth
    effect of ∼ on retinal-expansion focus shift 96
    cells encoding rotation in ∼ 423
    estimation in visual form agnosia 449–53
development
    phylogenetic ∼ of hippocampal/parietal
        function 18, 24
direction
    heading 17, 149–64, 204–6, 425–39
    in cognitive map 17, 260
    vs distance encoding 383–6
    to goal in rodent navigation 149–64, 170
    head ∼ vs spatial view in primate
        hippocampus 326–33
    of heading corresponding to retinal focus of
        expansion 96
    imagined in neglect 23–4, 350
    multimodal ∼ preferences in LIP cells 94
    neuronal level encoding
        of allocentric heading ∼ in rats, see
            head-direction cells
        of gaze ∼ in 7a/LIP, modulation 92, 93
        of heading computation in MSTd 96–100
        of ∼ preferences in LIP 94

of ~ preferences in VIP 109–14
of ~ selectivity in MIP 107–9
of ~ selectivity in SEF 359–78
of directionality in rat subiculum 425
object-centred ~ selectivity 361–78
oculocentric ~ selectivity 361–3, 365–9
displacement
  angular 168, 381–5, 425
  linear 152–3, 248, 381–98
  see also path integration system
distance
  angular ~, place field determinant 188, 199
  vs direction encoding 383–6
  between locations, hippocampal role in 21,
    227–30, 248
  and hippocampal navigation model 154–63,
    432–4
  vs motor sequence coding 381
  neglect dependent on 105
  perception in form agnosia 447–59
  reaching ~ affects MIP cells 107–9
  'ultranear' neurons in VIP 113
  to walls, place field determinant 17, 150–2,
    188, 432
distributed representation 91–4, 100–1, 133,
    188, 355, 376, 419
  and impression of unitary space 101, 104
dopamine in reinforcement 241–2, 427, 441
dorsal visual pathway/stream 5, 21–4, 50, 292,
    303, 383, 444–63
drive reduction, model 428–34

EEG 153, 158, 307–8, 312
efference copy, see motor command
egocentric, see coordinates; frame of
  reference
electrical stimulation 37, 39, 91, 113, 221, 387
electroencephalogram, see EEG
encoding, see memory
entorhinal
  cells in rat navigation model 154–64, 205–9
  cortex in memory 251–6, 261, 283, 290–9,
    322–3, 336, 349
exploration 36, 51–63, 155, 160–3, 168, 180,
    207–9, 226–9, 237–9, 332, 381, 405–9
external signals
  and hippocampus 147, 152, 167–84, 198–200,
    212, 214
  and neglect 36–9, 54
  and parietal cortex 114, 121
exteroceptive signals, see external signals
extrapersonal space 25, 33–4, 37, 42–6
eye
  centred, see coordinates; frame of reference
  movement
    in affordance-graph model 416–19
    corollary discharge of ~ command, and
      remapping 116–22
    exploratory, in neglect 52–5, 6–61

responsive neurons in MST 91
  supplementary eye field in 361–78
  see also saccades and pursuit
position, see position, eye
velocity 100, 418

feature detector 433–4
feedback
  sensory ~ from movement 16, 109, 122, 434
  projections 109, 122, 434
  visual 17
figure
  vs ground 78, 83
  visuospatial testing 69, 76–9, 261, 346, 378
fMRI 386–7, 406
forearm 40, 43–4
forgetting 248, 285; see also amnesia
form agnosia 443–63
fornix, see hippocampal region, anatomy;
  lesions
fovea 70, 111, 117, 360, 362
frame(s) of reference
  and alignment 12–16, 58–63, 82, 92–101,
    110–14, 121
  impaired in neglect 33–86, 127–46, 350–2
  rotation vs translation 13, 43–4, 56–64
  in intraparietal areas
    AIP, grasp-related 106–7
    LIP, eye-centred 114–17
    MIP, arm-centred 107–9
    VIP, head-centred 109–14
  mismatch/conflict between 17, 94, 121, 147,
    167–84, 198–201, 375, 385
  multiple
    integration of 44, 90–101, 147, 293, 316,
      390–3
    and hippocampal navigation model 203–15
    requirement for 20–4, 104–6
    simultaneous single representation of
      90–101, 127–46
  and remapping
    hippocampal 164, 171, 193, 206
    parietal 16, 116–21, 417–19, 421, 425, 439
  and transformation 13, 92–100, 116–21, 160,
    409
  translation between 14–17, 90–101, 127–46
  see also axis; coordinate
frame of reference, system type
  action-based 104–26, 359–78, 416–63
  allocentric 12–24, 79–85
    and local body-surface space 104–6
    and long-term memory 23–4, 303–4,
      443–63
    and memory in humans 259–86
    in hippocampus (monkey) 325–39, 394
    and navigation 151–64, 404–13
    in place cells (rat, model) 151–64
    spatial learning system 226–30
    in supplementary eye field 359–78
    in visual form agnosia 453–62

frame of reference, system type (*cont.*)
  arena 17, 168–84, 227, 432
  body-centred 15–16, 51, 92–9, 104, 131, 144,
    359, 412, 445–6
  craniocentric, *see* head-centred space
  egocentric 12–24, 417, 444–7
  in hippocampus (monkey) 326
    and long-term memory 23–4, 303–4, 443–63
    and motion perception 99
    in navigation 160
    and neglect 31–86
    orientation system (rat/model) 426
    and parietal cortex 33–146, 412–13, 444–6
    and posterior cingulate 409
    and short-term memory 23–4, 350–2
    and spatial memory strategies 270–2, 285–6
    in visual form agnosia 454–62
  eye-centred, *see* oculocentric; retinal
  global 24, 76, 207, 251, 416
  head-centred 14–16, 73, 92–4, 104, 109–16,
    127, 131–5, 446
  object-based/centred 13, 18, 22–3, 31, 67–86,
    128–9, 140–2, 361–78, 420
  oculocentric 127, 132, 141, 360–9, 372, 375
  retinal
    and heading computation in MSTd 96–9
    and LIP and 7a 15–16, 92, 114–17
    in parietal model 15, 127–46
    and object-centred representation 69–85
    and remapping 14, 109–17, 418
    and retrieval of visual memory 350–2
    retinotopy 36, 42, 44, 73–4, 428
    and supplementary eye field 359–65
    and VIP 14, 109–14
    see also eye-centred
  somatotopic 36
  trunk-centred 12–14, 25, 37, 43–4, 61–3, 67,
    104, 127–8, 385, 422
  world-centred 16, 23, 51, 93, 116–17, 131
frontal region 13, 22–3, 35, 106, 109, 117, 189,
  220–1, 238, 242, 323, 359–61, 387–98,
  409, 412, 419
  F1 7, 181, 282
  F2 421
  F4 113, 419
  F5 7, 419–23
  F6 421
  frontal eye field (FEF) 117, 351, 382–3, 390–1,
    418
  precentral gyrus 382, 387, 397, 419; *see also*
    FEF
  prefrontal area 3, 6, 10–11, 205, 291–3, 388–93,
    409, 423, 427
  premotor area 5–7, 35–7, 106–7, 113, 127,
    361, 383, 387, 397, 416, 421, 423–9
  supplementary eye field (SEF) 106, 303,
    360–78, 382, 390–3
  supplementary motor area (SMA) 6, 35, 361,
    387, 397
functional imaging, *see* imaging

gain fields and modulation 15, 92–8, 127–46,
  390
galvanic stimulation 386–7
gaze 50–5, 60, 92–100, 112, 131, 330–1, 351,
  360–3, 378, 445–6, 454, 459
glutamate 222, 242
goal cells in navigation model 154–64
goal-directed movement 51, 60–1, 174, 180–1,
  220, 226, 237, 240, 392, 427

hand, *see* coordinate; frame of reference
  movement 15, 106, 126, 127, 419, 442, 459,
    463
head centered space, *see* coordinate; frame of
  reference
head direction
  in humans 385–7
  and primate hippocampal units 326–7, 330–2
  system in rodent and models 149, 151–2, 158,
    198, 200, 204, 206, 425, 432–3, 438–9
head-direction cells 17, 149, 151, 158, 200
heading computations in MSTd 96–101
Hebbian learning 154, 158, 209–10, 227, 229,
  237, 352–6, 433
hemiamnesia 352, 356
hemianaesthesia 33–4, 36, 39, 44–5
hemianopia 33–6, 44–5, 64, 74, 351
hemineglect, *see* neglect
hemiplegia 33, 37, 45
hemispace 52–4, 60–1, 63, 127–8
hidden unit 130, 365, 368–9
hippocampal region, anatomy
  anatomical description 4–11, 291–3, 322–3,
    336–8
  CA1 and CA3 9–11, 163, 169, 190, 205–15,
    223, 243, 284, 292, 305, 308, 321–2,
    333–9, 345–6, 421, 424
    CA3 and chart model 205–15
    CA3 in autoassociation memory 332–9
  commissure 9
  dentate, *see* dentate gyrus
  fornix 9–10
  hippocampus proper 9–11, 205, 321, 336,
    407–8, 412, 422
  human pathology 247–9, 259–64, 290–5,
    345–7
  parahippocampal gyrus 11, 16, 20, 90, 93,
    247–9, 251–5, 261, 277–8, 283–4, 322–3,
    325, 333, 335, 404–11
  parasubiculum 10, 205, 208, 292
  perforant path 9–11, 221, 322, 333, 336, 338
  pes hippocampi 8, 260–1, 283
  postsubiculum 205–6, 387, 433
  presubiculum 10–11, 16–17, 90, 93, 149, 292,
    387, 425
  recurrent collaterals 163–4, 337
  subicular complex 9–10, 292
  subiculum 9–10, 163–4, 205, 208, 284, 292,
    322–3, 386–7, 394, 425
  uncus 274

hippocampal region, functional roles in
  cognitive mapping, *see* cognitive map
  directional orientation, subicular complex 7,
    149–215, 381–440; *see also* direction;
    head direction; head-direction cells
  distance coding 21, 154–63, 227–30, 248,
    432–4
  localisation, *see* entorhinal cells; hippocampal
    region, anatomy, subiculum place cells
  learning and memory 220–356, 381–423;
    see also memory
  navigation 17, 22, 149–64, 203–15, 256, 303,
    334–5, 393–8, 416–40
  place avoidance/preference tasks 174–84
  perception/representation
    in allocentric reference frame 22–5,
      151–64, 325–39
    of environmental shape 150–2, 157, 163–4,
      312, 436
    of large-scale space 20, 22, 393–8, 404–13
  separation of inputs 164, 204–15, 242, 338
  see also lesions
homing 168, 384–5
hypothalamus 11, 427–8, 435; *see also*
  mammillary nuclei

idiothetic signals 167–83, 186, 198–9, 215, 382,
  398, 440
imagery, memory, and perception 4, 24, 142, 408,
  453
imaging, functional, in human brain
  of cingulate region 397–8
  and episodic memory 240
  of frontal region 238, 382, 397–8
  of hippocampal region 20, 22, 147, 149,
    247–56, 303, 393–8, 404–13
  and insular region 397–8
  and macro-environment tasks 20, 22, 393–8,
    404–13
  and object location memory 247–56
  and methodological issues 284, 339
  of occipital region 397
  of parietal region 22, 147, 303, 382–93, 397
  and saccadic tasks 382–3
  of vestibular region 386–8
  and vestibular tasks 393–8
inhibition
  altered in neglect 52
  in network models 135, 137, 207, 208, 428
insula 36, 387, 397–8
integration
  multimodal 44, 90–101, 147, 293, 390–3
  path, *see* path integration
  sensorimotor 15, 316
  temporal 356
intention 12, 16, 31, 117–22, 369
internal representation 45, 149, 317, 405
  of direction 433
  of macro-environment 149, 412

  in neglect 34, 54, 351
  in parietal cortex 408
  shifted/remapped 16, 114, 116, 121
internal signals and place cell firing 17, 18, 147,
  152, 186, 198, 212; *see also* idiothetic
  signals; vestibular system;
  proprioception
interneurons 190, 312, 418
intralaminar thalamic nuclei 7, 132
intraparietal, *see* parietal region, anatomy
ischaemia 264, 345, 347

kinaesthesia 454, 459
kinematics 60, 61

labyrinths, vestibular 385, 387
landmarks
  array of 226–9, 237
  associative relationships between 226
  and direction 394, 432, 438
  and distance, 432, 433
  extra-maze, influence of 169, 171
  and topographical memory 394–7, 404–11
  location/layout and spatial map 18, 20,
    226–9, 436
  and long-term spatial memory 446, 459
  and object-location memory 252–5
  in navigation 168, 204, 226–9
  visual 93, 306, 393–398
language 24, 33–4, 230, 239, 247, 260–1, 265,
  277, 294–8, 397
lateralization 33, 43, 60, 254, 277, 284–6
learning, *see* memory
learning (types)
  autoassociative 338–9
  associative 220–42, 247, 335–6, 347–56
  configural 349
  and coordinate transformation 92–6
  landmark ∼ 227–30
  mechanisms in navigation model 154–60,
    208–14, 426–40
  place ∼ 167–84
  procedural 23, 293
  reinforcement, *see* reinforcement
  rapid 20, 237
  reversal ∼ 426, 429–31, 436–8
  semantic, in amnesic case 290–1
  spatial 154–63, 184, 215, 220–43, 247, 256,
    261, 318, 340, 347, 349, 415, 427
  and temporal contiguity 352–53
  topographical 256, 405–13
lesions
  of fornix impair spatial/scene memory 19, 22,
    248, 320–1, 345–55, 431
  of frontal cortex 117, 127, 460
  of hippocampus; *see also* fornix
    and item-location memory 247–56,
      259–86, 320–3

lesions (*cont.*)
    and episodic/scene memory 290–302,
      345–56
    impair navigation 17, 149
    and LTP experiments 222–3
    of labyrinths 385
    and lateralisation effects
      contralesional 13, 33–45, 50–63, 67, 70–2,
        76, 117, 142
      ipsilesional 37, 40, 43–4, 50–63, 70–6, 117
    of occipito-temporal region 443–63
    of parietal cortex 90
      effects on saccade tasks 389–91
      inferior parietal lobule (neglect) 11–14,
        33–46, 50–64, 67–76, 104–5
      modelled 127–46
      object-space impairment 420
      somatosensory areas (neglect) 33–46
      superior parietal lobe (visuomotor
        impairments) 11–12, 50, 463
    of parietotemporal cortex 392–3
    of perirhinal cortex and item recognition
      memory 296–99, 345–56
    of posterior cingulate cortex impair
      navigation 409
    and topographical orientation 394, 407, 413
    and vestibular memory contingent saccade
      task 389–93
lobectomy, *see* lesions
local view 204–15, 335, 424, 432
locale system 204, 226, 417, 425–27, 438
location-specific cells, *see* place cells; *see also*
    entorhinal cells; hippocampal region,
    anatomy, subiculum
long-term memory, *see* memory
long term potentiation, *see* synaptic changes
    and learning

magnetic resonance imaging (MRI) 45, 249–50,
    261–84, 290–302, 386–7, 406, 411
mammillary nuclei 10, 205, 323, 346–8, 355,
    386, 406
map
  cognitive, *see* cognitive map
  motor 132
  somatosensory 105
maze
  radial arm 267, 273, 437–8
  T-maze 22, 426–38
  watermaze 17, 164, 206, 214, 220–43
memory, processing
  autoassociation 322–39
  consolidation 21, 206, 220, 240–2, 316–17
  encoding, mnemonic
    and allo- vs egocentric systems 18, 22–3,
      271, 446
    context 220–42, 276–7
    dual encoding 265
    location in old vs young rats 206

  vs long-term storage 18, 22–3, 285
  macro-environment, and hippocampus 20
  mechanisms in mammals 220–42, 355
  rapid 237
  object location 250–3
  spatial response in monkey
    hippocampus 324
  stimulus location after offset in LIP 116
  topographical information 405–6, 408–11
recall
  and allo- vs egocentric systems, 22–5
  and autoassociation 323, 333–9
  delayed ∼ tasks 294
  in hippocampal model 208
  human spatial memory tasks 246, 261–7,
    394–8, 408–13
  orientation-modulated in neglect 24
  of saccade sequence 383
  in topokinetic and environmental
    memory 394–8
retention 229, 248, 265, 267, 298
retrieval
  vs encoding of object location 252–6
  hippocampal-neocortical interactions 21,
    238, 323. 338
  macro-environment, and hippocampus 20
  of place avoidance 175–80
  and primate hippocampus 333–7
  spatial, and temporal context in 19,
    237–8, 347–56
  in topographical memory 405–13
storage
  in allo- and egocentric systems 23–4
  capacity 321, 333
  in hippocampal model 208, 337–8
  hippocampal-neocortical interactions 21,
    305–17
  vs input and right hippocampus 285
  long-term and short-term 18, 22–4, 233,
    238–9, 297, 383
  in oculomotor and vestibular system 383
  rapid associational 220
  search pattern dependent on 160
  spatial context 322–3, 333–4
  synaptic mechanism of 233–6
memory, types
  associative 220–42, 290–302, 320–56
  declarative 20, 221, 239, 260, 264, 267, 273,
    290
  episodic 18–20, 220–43, 267, 273, 290–302,
    303, 321–3, 334–9, 346–55, 394, 407–11
  flashbulb 242
  long-term 20–4, 85, 220, 231–3, 237–8, 264,
    303–5, 317, 347, 351
  object location 21, 247–56, 259–86, 405–7, 446
  procedural 23, 282, 293
  recognition 19–20, 147, 247, 265, 273, 277,
    295–7, 335–6, 346–57
  reference 237, 275–7

scene 23–4, 320–1, 347–55
semantic 19–20, 35, 88, 147, 230, 242,
    290–301, 338, 394, 410–11
short-term 20, 24, 164, 200, 216, 220, 229,
    242, 303, 460, 462
snapshot 271, 321–3, 347
spatial 147, 230, 242, 247–56, 259–86, 297,
    347–55, 381–5, 390, 394–8, 446
topographic(al) 20, 381–98, 404–13
topokinetic 381–98
visual 19, 254, 265–7, 288, 350–1, 369, 381,
    391–3
working 26, 239, 259–86, 378, 388, 399, 421,
    460
mental rotation 13, 271–2, 277, 283
models, computational
    of hippocampus
        and autoassociative memory 18, 260,
            320–39
        and neocortical interaction 21, 160,
            305–17, 416–40
        and rodent navigation 17, 149–64, 203–15,
            260, 416–40
    of (posterior) parietal cortex 15, 76–8, 82–3,
        92, 127–46, 368–9, 416–40
    selection mechanism 132, 134, 136–7, 139
    winner-takes-all mechanism 135, 429, 431, 435
monkey, see animals
monocular vision 113, 449–53
motivation 417, 424–32
motor command 16, 92, 99, 114–21, 130, 385,
    398, 419–22, 425, 434
MRI, see magnetic resonance imaging; see also
    fMRI
multimodal integration, see integration

navigation
    episodic memory not linked to 230
    extero- and interoceptive influences on 167–84
    hippocampus in (accurate) 22, 256, 303,
        334–5, 404–13
    through large-scale environments 20, 393–8,
        404–13
    map-based 226, 417
    mental 393–8
    models of 149–64, 204–15, 416–40
    motion information used in 91–7, 383–6
    MST in 91, 96–7
    optical flow used in 96–7
    parahippocampal gyrus in 256
    parietal areas in 22, 91–7, 160, 303
    robot simulation of rat 149–64
    route-based 417
    short-range 334–5
    vestibular system in 383–6
neglect 12–13, 23–5, 31–86, 127–46, 303,
    345–56, 370, 377
    axis-based 78–86
    exploratory eye movements in 51–63

figure-based 77
framework rotation in 13, 43–4, 56–64
framework translation in 13, 33–46
gaze direction in 60, 351
gradient model of 12–13, 15, 44, 51–5, 61,
    73–7, 134–42
memory and 350–2
network model of 127–46
motor 34
object-centred 13, 67–86, 128, 140–1, 377
premotor theory 52
sensory stimulation, effects on 13, 36–46
somatosensation and 33–46
neural networks, see models
neuropsychology 19, 31, 33–89, 259–302,
    345–56, 381–98, 443–63
NMDA receptor 19, 220–41
novelty 19, 95, 149–51, 160, 207–9, 226–9, 237,
    240, 259, 317, 324–5, 335–6, 378, 405,
    438
nucleus accumbens 10, 205
nystagmus 37–9, 43

object-centred effects 76–8, 139–43,
    368–9
object location 21, 106, 122, 165, 247–56,
    296, 414–15, 446
object segmentation 71–4
occipital region 10, 31, 45, 73–8, 86, 397, 404–5
    see also visual
occipito-parietal region 266, 444; see also
    dorsal visual pathway
occipito-temporal region 266, 407, 410, 416,
    443–4; see also ventral visual pathway
oculomotor function 64, 93, 116–17, 351, 361,
    377, 388
olfaction 10, 153, 189, 321, 334, 426
optic ataxia 5, 12, 15, 23, 50–1, 63, 444
optic flow 16, 93, 97, 101, 416, 423, 439
optokinetics 13, 37, 40–6, 51
orbits, eye 92, 114, 363–71, 445
orientation
    in affordance and map-based motion-to-target
        model 416–40
    behavioural (taxon) system 425–40
    disorientation 206, 404, 407–9, 413, 416
    head; see also head-direction cells
        afferents to LIP 16
        in LIP and 7a 92–4
    and hippocampal view cells 259, 320–39
    of lines and neglect model 136–9
    in neglect, impaired 50–64
    and neuronal modulatory effects 15, 92–4,
        419
    of objects coded in
        intraparietal cortex 106
        supplementary eye field 359–78
    topographical 404–13
vector 426–37

orientation (*cont.*)
   vestibular system 16–141, 385–6
   in visual form agnosia, impaired 443–63
   see also angular position; direction
otoliths 398

parahippocampal gyrus, *see* hippocampal region
parasubiculum, *see* hippocampal region
parietal region, anatomy
   anatomical description 5–8, 11
   angular gyrus 5
   inferior parietal region 6–7, 11, 35, 37, 45, 51,
      61, 67, 387, 416, 462
   intraparietal
      AIP 5, 7, 14, 106–7, 122, 416, 419–23, 438
      LIP 5, 7, 8, 10, 15, 16, 91–6, 109, 114–22,
         127, 416–18, 421, 425, 439, 445
      MIP 5, 7, 14, 16, 106–9, 113, 116, 122
      PIP 106, 420
      VIP 5, 7, 8, 14, 106, 110–13, 122, 127, 133,
         416, 419, 421
      sulcus 5–6, 14, 106–7, 351, 383, 416, 444–5,
         463
   MST 7, 8, 91, 96–100, 423, 425
   parietal operculum 5–6
   parietoinsular cortex 386–7, 389, 392, 398
   parietotemporal region 51, 76
   postcentral area 5–6, 387
   posterior parietal cortex (PPC) 6, 14–15,
      90–101, 160, 293, 390–2, 416–40, 444–6
   precuneus 383, 397, 408, 410
   primary somatosensory area 5–7, 36, 42
   secondary somatosensory area 36, 416
   superior parietal region 5–7, 15, 23, 50–1, 63,
      102, 123, 383
   supramarginal gyrus 5, 35–6, 67
   see also Brodmann's areas
parietal region, functional roles in
   guidance and control of motor acts
      grasping 5, 14, 22–3, 106–7, 130, 416–23,
         438–9, 451–2, 458–9
      gripping 107, 419, 423, 451–2, 455–9
      pointing 14, 50, 60–3, 447–62
      pursuit, eyes 91, 96–101
      reaching 12–15, 23, 50, 60–1, 106–18, 195,
         416–17, 423, 435, 439, 445–63
      saccades 16, 94–5, 113–17, 127, 382–3,
         389–91, 416–18, 445, 460
      turning 422–5
   heading computations 96–101
   memory
      egocentric 350–2, 380–3
      short-term spatial 447–9, 459–63
   navigation 22, 91–7, 160, 303
   spatial perception/representation
      distance judgements 449–59
      in multiple frames of reference 33–146,
         350–2, 412–63; *see also* axis; coordinate;
         frame of reference

path integration system
   mechanisms 204–15, 381, 383–6, 439
   models 199, 204–15, 439
   in rodents 151–2, 167–8, 199, 204–15, 439
   role in sustaining place fields 151–2, 167–8,
      186, 199
pathology, *see* lesions
pattern
   completion 305
   recognition 199, 260
perceptual schema 432–3
peripersonal space 60–1, 105
peripheral space 36, 111, 119, 121, 175, 416, 447
perirhinal cortex
   anatomy 11, 19
   and recognition memory 256, 283–4, 292–3,
      321–2, 335–6, 345–56
phase coding 98, 138, 153–60
place cells
   description of 17–18, 149–50
   and environmental learning systems 227
   and maplike representation 184, 186, 421–3
   and memory 242, 303, 259–60, 305–17
   models of 154–64, 203–15, 421–3
   navigation driven by 150
   in rat vs monkey hippocampus 326–36, 393–4
place field
   influences, internal/external on 17–18,
      149–53, 167–84, 186–201, 432
   shape 150–64, 193
   stability 186–201, 205–14
plasticity and learning 158, 220–42, 299, 350–2
population coding
   parietal cortex 92, 97, 100, 133, 143, 368,
      419–20, 428
   in hippocampus 158–64, 333
position
   body 51, 55, 57–9
   eye
      and parietal activity 14, 60, 91–100,
         108–17, 130–43, 390–2, 418
      and primate hippocampus 327–32
   hand 61, 63
   head 92, 129, 139, 143, 279, 390, 439, 445–6,
      454
Positron emission tomography (PET) 20, 36,
      247–56, 382–97, 405–12; *see also* imaging
posterior cingulate area 397, 406–11
postrhinal cortex 11
postsubiculum 205–6, 387, 433; *see also*
      hippocampal region, anatomy
postural signals 105, 129–31, 142–3, 446, 456
potentiation, *see* synaptic changes and learning
prefrontal cortex, *see* frontal region
premotor cortex, *see* frontal region
prestriate cortex 251
primary visual cortex 5, 36, 444
primates, *see* animals
proactive interference 276–7

proprioception 14–17, 37, 42, 91–100, 131, 183, 385, 422, 445, 454
prosopagnosia 404
pursuit, eye movement 91, 96–101, 445

rat, *see* animals
reaction time 128–9, 135, 139, 361–2
receptor
  NMDA in learning 222–40
  surface, sensory 12–13, 104, 111, 114, 122
recognition memory, *see* memory
reinforcement and learning 154–8, 227, 237, 306, 353–4, 427–38
retina, *see* frame of reference
retrieval, *see* memory
retrosplenial cortex 10, 292, 293; *see also* posterior cingulate
reward 22, 95, 121, 151–61, 227–9, 348, 353–5, 393, 422–34
rhinal cortex 323, 349, 352; *see also* entorhinal; postrhinal cortex
robot 17, 147, 151–61, 326, 381
rodent, *see* animals
rotation
  body ∼, and vestibular-dependent memory 382–90
  of cues, effects on place cells 167–84, 186–201
  of frame of reference
    in neglect 13, 43–4, 56–64
    in rat spatial behaviour 167–84
    by sensory stimulation 13–14
  of head affects neglect 140–1, 150–2
  invariance in object-centred neglect 377
  mental, and item-location memory tasks 271–83
  of objects, perceptual effects 140–1
  responsive neurons
    in MSTd 96–100, 423
    in primate hippocampus 335
    in PPC 423
    as turn cells 423
    in VIP 110–11

saccades
  in visual form agnosia 446–61
  and area 6 and 8 in 383
  and attention 70, 117–22
  direction of 116, 141, 388–93, 460
  cingulate gyrus (median) in 382
  and egocentric coding 445–9
  eye fields in 382
  in hemianopia 351
  and intention 117–22
  LIP in 16, 94–5 113–17, 127, 416–18, 445
  and manual reaching 447–52
  memorised sequence of 22, 303, 382–3
  MT/V5 in 445
  in neglect 54, 351

object related 141–2, 359–78
  in parietal cortex 382–3, 445
  remapping of 16, 113–17, 416–21, 439
  and superior colliculus 418
  vestibular memory contingent ∼ task 388–93
  and visual constancy 16, 113–17, 416–18
  see also eye movement
scene
  memory 23–4, 320–1, 347–55
  visual analysis 16, 23–4, 53–4, 70–4, 83–5, 142, 376, 462
septum 9–11, 323
shape
  extraction in PPC 417
  object-∼ responsive neurons (AIP/PIP) 106–7, 122, 420–1
  and object-based neglect 69–85
  orientation by 436
  perception impaired in form agnosia 443
  place cells and 150–2, 157, 163–4, 312
  of place fields 150–64, 193
  of rooms and PET 407
simulation, *see* computer and models
single unit recording 90–126, 149–201, 305–39, 359–98
sleep and memory 21, 303–17
smooth pursuit 91, 97, 100
somatoparaphrenia 37
somatosensation and space 5–14, 33–45, 90, 93, 105–11, 153, 416, 425
space, *see* coordinate; frame of reference
spatial cells, *see* place cells; head-direction cells; spatial view cells
spatial view cells in primate hippocampus 323–39
species differences/similarities 220–1, 232–42, 384–5, 421–39
  hippocampal region 18, 24, 149–50, 220–42, 259, 295–7, 320–39, 345–9, 384–5,
  parietal cortex 24, 90, 104–6, 109, 116, 117, 127–30
speed
  eye velocity 100, 418
  of movement 155, 338, 386, 450–52
  of neural processing 200, 338
stimulation, *see* caloric stimulation; electrical stimulation; galvanic stimulation; vestibular system
stimulus control of place fields 167–201
striatum 10, 440
superior colliculus 5, 133, 135, 393, 418
symmetry and space 37, 54–5, 77–8, 151, 309, 351
synaptic changes and learning 147, 158–9, 164, 200, 207–14, 220–42, 316, 323, 336–8, 353–6

tactile sense 36–45, 111, 113, 334, 443, 456
taxon system 204, 417, 425–6, 438

taxon-affordance model 22, 416–40
temporal region, anatomy
  anatomical description 6–11, 291–3, 321–3
  areas
    MT 7, 256, 261, 445; see also visual, cortex; V5
    TE 292
    TEO 292
    TF 11
    TH 11, 248
  entorhinal, see entorhinal
  hippocampal region, see hippocampal region,
    anatomy
  inferotemporal
    cortex 7, 8, 78, 86, 107, 254–5
    neurons and object selectivity 378
  occipitotemporal, see occipital region
  perirhinal, see perirhinal cortex
  superior temporal region 5, 7, 26, 91, 103,
    379, 387, 391
  superior temporal sulcus (STS) 5, 200, 291–3
  temporoparietal junction 35, 387
temporal cortex/lobe, functional roles
  multiple specialisations in 290–302, 349–50
  in perception and memory 345–56
  in spatial memory 247–56, 259–86, 381–98,
    404–13
thalamus
  anatomical description 6–11
  nuclei, see anterior thalamus; intralaminar
    thalamic nuclei
theta rhythm in hippocampus 153–8, 190, 307–8,
    312
three-dimensional
  distance perception in form agnosia 451
  intepretation of 2-D image 72, 187
  perception in early-stage object
    recognition 377–8
  real ∼ environmental memory testing 271–7
  space, in neglect 59–60
touch 4, 107, 251–2, 268
trajectory 23, 63, 99, 111–13, 153, 204, 382,
    385–6, 396, 439
trunk axis 12
turns 4, 95, 157, 316, 352, 385, 394, 397, 422–6,
    443; see also rotation

unit recording, see single unit recording

velocity, see speed; direction
ventral visual pathway/stream 5, 21–3, 51, 78,
    107, 251, 304, 444–63
vestibular system
  cortex 386–7, 390–2
  signals 14–17, 22, 91–100, 131, 141–2, 303,
    334–5, 385–8, 422–5, 445
    and neglect 36–46, 51, 83
  stimulation 386–93
  contribution to direction 383–98
  see also head direction; head-direction cells

virtual reality 22, 25, 277, 286, 303, 408, 413
visual
  constancy 16, 92–101, 104–26
  cortex, general 5–8, 36, 86, 91–5, 107, 130,
    292, 350–1, 390, 416, 444, 462
  areas; see also occipital region; parietal
    region; temporal region
    V1 7, 8, 106, 140, 420
    V2 5, 7, 8, 106, 416
    V3 5, 7, 106, 416
    V4 7, 106, 143, 144, 378, 379
    V5 5, 7, 445; see also temporal region,
      MT
    V6 7, 464; see also parietal region
  crossmodal integration 44, 91–101
  dorsal stream/pathway, see dorsal visual
    pathway
  extinction 71–4
  features and object-centredness 369–71
  form agnosia 443–63
  guidance of grasping, AIP in 106–7
  influences on
    place cells (rat) 150–3, 167–75, 186–201
    primate hippocampal cells 320–39
  landmarks 93, 306, 393–8
  memory, see memory, types
  neglect 33–46, 50–64, 67–86, 127–46,
    345–56
  segmentation and neglect 71–8
  perceptual/mnemonic areas 23, 347–52
  receptive field 14–15, 91–4, 107–13, 131, 133–6,
    368
  search in neglect 51–6, 61, 134, 351
  signals and other modalities integrated 44,
    91–101
  space and dorsal stream 444–7
  targets, eye/hand movements to 107–9,
    382–93, 416–18, 447–53
  ventral stream/pathway, see ventral visual
    pathway stream
  see also coordinate; darkness; frame of
    reference; occipital region
visuomotor behaviour/visuospatial
    perception 36, 51, 61–3, 74–86, 104–22,
    139–41, 443–63
visuospatial neglect, see visual, cortex,
    neglect

walls
  influence on rat place fields 17–18, 150–64,
    167–73, 188–98, 432
  models, role in 150–64, 432–8
  and view cells in primate hippocampus
    326–33
  and watermaze strategy 225
way-finding, see navigation
Wechsler tests 294–5, 346
Wisconsin tests 348
world-graph model 416–40